An Integrated Approach to

Health Sciences

Second Edition

ANATOMY & PHYSIOLOGY

MATH

CHEMISTRY

MEDICAL MICROBIOLOGY

Supplements At-A-Glance

SUPPLEMENT	WHAT IT IS	WHAT'S IN IT
StudyWARE™ DVD	Software program (DVD in the back of the book)	• Quizzes with immediate feedback • Health-related videos • Animations • Interactive games • Crossword puzzles
Workbook	Print	• Review questions • Image labeling in selected chapters • Activities/labs • Extended concepts • "What Do You Think?" segments that pose ethical dilemmas for consideration
Mobile Downloads	Mobile downloads	• Mobile downloads for more than 300 medical terms
Instructor Resources	CD-ROM	• Electronic Instructor's Manual files • Electronic testbank • Slide presentations created in PowerPoint® with full-color art, animations, and video clips
WebTutor Advantage	Web access	• On Blackboard and WebCT platforms (other platforms available upon request) • Content and quizzes linked to each chapter • Comprehensive glossary • Video clips and animations • StudyWARE™ interactive games • Slide presentations created in PowerPoint® • Discussion questions • Midterm and final exams

An Integrated Approach to
Health Sciences

Second Edition

ANATOMY & PHYSIOLOGY

MATH

CHEMISTRY

MEDICAL MICROBIOLOGY

Bruce J. Colbert,
M.S., R.R.T.

and

Jeff Ankney, B.S., R.R.T.

Joe Wilson, B.S., M.S.

John Havrilla, B.S.,
M.Ed., M.A.

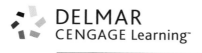

DELMAR
CENGAGE Learning™

Australia • Brazil • Japan • Korea • Mexico • Singapore • Spain • United Kingdom • United States

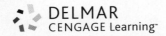

An Integrated Approach to Health Sciences, Second Edition

Bruce J. Colbert, Jeff Ankney, Joe Wilson, John Havrilla

Vice President, Career and Professional Editorial: Dave Garza

Director of Learning Solutions: Matthew Kane

Acquisitions Editor: Matthew Seeley

Managing Editor: Marah Bellegarde

Senior Product Manager: Debra Myette-Flis

Editorial Assistant: Samantha Zullo

Vice President, Career and Professional Marketing: Jennifer Baker

Executive Marketing Manager: Wendy Mapstone

Senior Marketing Manager: Kristin McNary

Associate Marketing Manager: Jonathan Sheehan

Production Director: Carolyn S. Miller

Content Project Manager: Thomas Heffernan

Senior Art Director: Jack Pendleton

Technology Project Manager: Patricia Allen

For product information and technology assistance, contact us at **Professional & Career Group Customer Support, 1-800-648-7450**

For permission to use material from this text or product, submit all requests online at **cengage.com/permissions**. Further permissions questions can be emailed to **permissionrequest@cengage.com**

Library of Congress Control Number: 2010942915

ISBN-13: 978-1-435-48764-2

ISBN-10: 1-4354-8764-8

Delmar
5 Maxwell Drive
Clifton Park, NY 12065-2919
USA

Cengage Learning products are represented in Canada by Nelson Education, Ltd.

For your lifelong learning solutions, visit **delmar.cengage.com**

Visit our corporate website at **cengagebrain.com**.

Printed in the United States of America
1 2 3 4 5 6 7 15 14 13 12 11

TABLE OF CONTENTS

SECTION ONE	FUNDAMENTALS OF ANATOMY AND PHYSIOLOGY

SECTION TWO   **FUNDAMENTALS OF MATHEMATICS**

SECTION THREE   **CHEMISTRY IN THE HEALTH SCIENCES**

I dedicate this book to my wife, Patty, for her love and support; my children, Joshua and Jeremy, for their inspiration; my deceased parents for their wisdom; and my brothers and sister for always being there.

—*Bruce J. Colbert*

I dedicate this book to my family, as well as to my former teachers, students, and friends, from whom I have learned much.

—*Jeff Ankney*

To my wife Theresa, for her 32 years of love and support; my children, Kim, Chris, Becca, and Kate, of whom I am so proud; and my students, from whom I have learned so much.

—*Joe Wilson*

I dedicate my portion of this textbook to my wife Barbara for her help and advice while I worked on the textbook.

—*John Havrilla*

PREFACE

Introduction

A book on the sciences and math should grab learners and show them why it is important to learn these sometimes confusing subjects. *An Integrated Approach to Health Sciences,* Second Edition is designed to do just that. By integrating subject matter and applying the theoretical to real-life clinical relevancy, learning becomes easier. When theories are grounded in the immediate skills learners will use in their chosen health fields, the relevance of these theories is made clear. With this connection made, learners become involved with the material, recognizing how important sciences and math are to their future successes in the health professions.

This project represents an innovative textbook, workbook, software, and instructor's resource. The writing style is easy-to-read and stimulating; humor is integrated to engage the learner. Numerous special features are also incorporated throughout the text to help you learn. See "About This Book" on page xvi for details.

Students in health-related programs and individuals interested in pursuing careers in the health professions are the primary audience for this text. While not intended to be used in an advanced course, this text does lay a solid foundation in health-related math and science on which to build in the future. This text is also an excellent review or preparatory book for adult learners who are beginning new careers in the health professions.

Designed and Organized for Learning and Success

This text and accompanying workbook were designed for a very important reason: to help you learn the subjects necessary for success in the health professions. Note the importance of the words *learn* and *success.* You do not need to be a genius in order to be successful in the health professions. It is more important that you possess determination and motivation. This implies a

"need to do more than just take this book home, read it, and return to class the next day." You will get much more from this course if you study and discuss the topics with other learners who share an interest in the health care field. Let's begin by discussing the process of learning.

True learning is not massive memorization with the goal of regurgitating material back to the instructor or simply passing an exam. Nor is true learning an oppressive chore to be dreaded. True learning comes from a desire to understand and a willingness to become an active part of the learning process. It takes place when you internalize what you are reading, discussing, and solving. Internalization means making the material a part of your life because you realize the importance of the material to your future success in your chosen health profession. In addition, becoming enthusiastic about learning makes learning a more natural and meaningful process.

We hope this book will help you in the process of true learning by presenting mathematics and the health sciences in a way that will make more sense to you. First, we have integrated the material to show how math and the health sciences relate to one another. You need to understand all of the health sciences, and if you are not good at math, it will affect your grades in the other sciences. Like a house foundation, if a few blocks are weak, the whole foundation can crumble.

Second, the text is broken down and organized in a logical fashion. The text consists of four sections pertaining to anatomy and physiology, mathematics, chemistry, and medical microbiology. Anatomy and physiology is an ideal leadoff not only because you will be dealing with the human body in your chosen health profession, but also because an understanding of anatomy and physiology will help you understand the examples used later in the chemistry, math, and medical microbiology sections. Likewise, math serves as a foundation for chemistry and applying some of the anatomy and physiology principles such as calculating mean arterial pressure. The medical microbiology section provides background in pathogens and infection control which relate to cellular structures in anatomy and physiology and chemical sterilization agents. The chemistry section examines topics such as molecules, enzymes, and acid-base relationships, and the gas laws which tie into and reinforce many of the concepts presented in the anatomy and physiology section.

Third, we use real-life analogies and health-related examples to reinforce the theoretical material presented. For example, understanding how the chemistry concept of acid and base applies to the analysis of blood to diagnose and treat disease helps to reinforce understanding of the underlying concept itself. Likewise, real-life analogies (to things such as a car or a house) help to illustrate potentially difficult mathematical and scientific concepts.

Finally, we have used a stimulating writing style, combining humor with presentation of theoretical and practical information so as to enhance motivational learning. We want you to not only learn but also to be able to define problems, analyze, generate ideas, and implement and evaluate solutions, as well as to develop your oral and written communication skills. In essence, we want you to become an effective thinker and communicator. Critical and creative thinking skills as well as communication skills are useful not only in your academic endeavors, but also in developing a meaningful and successful life.

Before closing, we want to stress that although the job market in health care is good, financial rewards are not the only criteria for success. If you do what you enjoy, monetary rewards can always follow. And remember: If you truly involve yourself in learning, not only will you be successful, but learning will actually become fun! Good luck in your explorations!

"I never knew anyone who was good at giving excuses, who was good at anything else."
—Ben Franklin

Major Changes to the Second Edition

■ Two new chapters on Medical Microbiology have been added to help learners understand the relationship between anatomy and physiology, chemistry, and living microorganisms, and how they relate to human health.

■ Physics Chapters 22 and 23 have been included in the Chemistry section as Chapters 21 and 24. Material related to physics and the special senses has been included in Chapter 9.

■ Numerous clinical-related math concepts have been added to show actual math application to health sciences and to enhance critical thinking.

■ A new feature called Quotes and Notes provides inspirational food for thought and unique health- and science-related "gee whiz" facts and stories.

■ An accompanying StudyWARE™ DVD has been created to offer additional practice through interactive quizzes and fun activities that correlate with each chapter in the book. Numerous anatomy, physiology and pathology animations, and health-related video clips reinforce related topics, provide clinical relevancy, and make difficult concepts come alive. Refer to pages xi–xii for a list of the animations and videos included on the StudyWARE™ DVD.

■ A StudyWARE™ Connection feature has been added to direct learners to related content on the DVD.

■ The workbook has been enhanced with additional questions, activities, ethical dilemmas, and labeling exercises.

■ A new Workbook Practice feature directs the learner to even more learning tools in the workbook including practice questions, additional activities/labs, and extended concepts.

Animations and Videos Included on the StudyWARE™ DVD

CHAPTER	ANIMATION TOPIC
1	Word Parts Work Together
1	Combining Word Roots
2	Body Planes
3	Typical Cell
3	Mitosis
4	The Skin
4	Tissue Repair

(continues)

CHAPTER	ANIMATION TOPIC
5	Types of Fractures
5	Synovial Joints
7	Neurotransmitters
7	Spinal Cord Injuries
7	Contra Coup Injury
8	Endocrine System
8	Pancreas
9	Vision
9	Hearing
10	Respiration
10	Asthma
10	Asthma in Child
11	The Heart
11	The Blood
11	Flow of Lymph
11	Congestive Heart Failure
12	Digestion
13	Urine Formation
13	Male Reproductive System
13	Female Reproductive System
13	Ovulation
21	Contrasting Solids, Liquids, and Gases
22	Separation of Alpha, Beta, Gamma Radiations by an Electric Field
23	Ions/Cations and Anions
23	Compounds and Molecules
25	Buffer Solutions
27	How Enzymes Work
29	Infection Control

CHAPTER	VIDEO TITLE
4	The Importance of Vital Signs
4	Digital/Electronic Thermometers
4	Bites, Burns, and Injuries
4	Lacerations and Puncture Wounds
6	Administering Intramuscular Injections
6	Body Mechanics

CHAPTER	VIDEO TITLE
8	Diabetic Emergencies
8	Blood Glucose Testing
9	Applying Eye Medications
9	Application of Ear Drops
9	Tympanic Thermometers
10	Respiration
10	Asthma Emergency
10	Oxygen Therapy
10	How to Use a Medicated Inhaler
11	Anatomy of the Heart
11	Pulse and Pulse Rates
11	Radial Pulse
11	Apical Pulse
11	Cardiac Cycle and ECG
11	Blood Pressure
11	Taking Blood Pressure
12	Requesting a Stool Sample
12	Occult Blood Test
13	Infant Examination
13	Urine Specimen
13	Urine Analysis
13	PAP Exam
14	Thermometers
14	Measuring Temperature
17	Pulse and Pulse Rates
28	Specimen Collection and Processing
28	Sputum Sampling
28	Throat Cultures
29	Sanitizing an Exam Room
29	Disinfecting Equipment and Cleanup
29	Infection Control Procedures
29	Pathogens
29	Controlling Disease
29	Cleaning Infectious Material
29	Removing Gloves and Gowns
29	Sterile Gloves and the Sterile Field

Additional Learning Resources

StudyWARE™ DVD

The DVD included in the back of each book provides numerous anatomy, physiology and pathology animations, video clips on many health-related topics, and interactive activities and quizzes for each chapter that provide additional practice, and fun, while learning. See "How to Use the StudyWARE™ DVD" on page xviii for details.

Also available: StudyWARE™ DVD Standalone to accompany *An Integrated Approach to Health Sciences,* Second Edition (**ISBN**: 1-1115-3736-4).

Workbook

The workbook has been enhanced with additional questions, activities, ethical dilemmas, and labeling exercises. Popular features such as extended concepts and "What Do You Think?" segments have been retained in this second edition.

Mobile Downloads

Downloadable audio has been created for more than 300 medical terms to help you learn even when you're on the go.

Premium Website

A Premium Website that is available to accompany the text includes the StudyWARE™, slide presentations in PowerPoint® with animations and video, and a link to mobile downloads.

Redeeming an Access Code:

1. Go to: http://www.CengageBrain.com
2. REGISTER as a new user or LOG IN as an existing user if you already have an account with Cengage Learning or CengageBrain.com
3. Select Go to MY Account
4. OPEN the product from the My Account page

ABOUT THE AUTHORS

Bruce Colbert is Associate Professor and Director of Allied Health at the University of Pittsburgh at Johnstown. He holds a Master of Science from the School of Health-Related Professions at the University of Pittsburgh. His emphasis was in Health Administration and Education and he received honors for his work on creative thinking.

Bruce has authored six textbooks, published several articles, and has given more than 200 invited lectures and workshops nationwide. Many of his workshops provide teacher training in making the health sciences engaging and relevant to today's students. He serves on several medical boards and has held numerous elected offices, most notably as President of the Pennsylvania Society for Respiratory Care.

Bruce enjoys spending time with his family, especially in outdoor activities such as fishing, hiking, and scuba diving.

Jeff Ankney is currently the Assistant Director of Allied Health Programs and Director of Clinical Education for the University of Pittsburgh at Johnstown Respiratory Care Program. Prior to holding this position, he was Program Coordinator of Pulmonary Rehabilitation and, later, Assistant Director of Cardiopulmonary Services at Somerset Community Hospital. He was also a public school teacher for many years.

Over the years, Jeff has lectured on lung anatomy and physiology, lung disease, the effects of smoking, and the respiratory care profession to public schools and various organizations. He also has served as a consultant on pulmonary rehabilitation and management concerns and currently serves as a member of the Patient Safety Committee at a local hospital. He was the recipient of the American Cancer Society Public Education Award.

An avid hunter and fisherman, Jeff can often be found wandering the Laurel Highlands of his native Somerset County with his son, Zack, and springer spaniel, Rusty.

Joe Wilson has been teaching mathematics at the University of Pittsburgh at Johnstown (Pitt-Johnstown) for the past 30 years. He holds a Master of Science in Mathematics, a Bachelor of Science in Education, and Pennsylvania teaching certificates in mathematics and physics. As the Natural Sciences scheduling coordinator for the past 20 years, he also assists students, faculty, and staff with a variety of schedule-related issues.

Joe is a member of the National Council of Teachers of Mathematics (NCTM), the Pennsylvania Council of Teachers of Mathematics (PCTM), and the Laurel Highlands Math Alliance (LHMA). He has presented at numerous venues over the years and chaired committees for both NCTM and PCTM.

Away from Pitt-Johnstown, Joe enjoys spending time in his woodshop, working on his pool game in the winter months, and walking the golf course in the summer.

John W. Havrilla has a Bachelor of Science degree in secondary education from Pennsylvania State University as well as a Master of Education in chemistry and a Master of Arts in physics from Indiana University of Pennsylvania. John spent two years in the Army Signal Corps prior to starting his teaching career. For one of the years he served in Vietnam.

John taught high school chemistry and physics the first ten years of his career. He then taught physics for seven years prior to transferring to the chemistry department where he worked for 19 years at the University of Pittsburgh at Johnstown. He retired from full-time teaching in 2007.

ACKNOWLEDGMENTS

The authors and Delmar Cengage Learning would like to thank those individuals who reviewed the second edition and offered suggestions, feedback, and assistance. Their work is greatly appreciated.

Reviewers

Ann Leslie Claesson, PhD, BSN, PSP, FACHE
Core Faculty
Capella University
Minneapolis, Minnesota

Jane W. Dumas, MSN, CCMA, CHI
Allied Health Department Chair
Remington College – Cleveland West Campus
North Olmsted, Ohio

Debbie Hartman, RN, MSN
Assistant Professor of Nursing
Blue Ridge Community College
Weyers Cave, VA

Karen Ruble Smith, RN, BSN
Health Science Consultant
Kentucky Department of Education
Division of Career & Technical Education
Frankfort, Kentucky

The authors would also like to thank Matt Seeley, Acquisitions Editor, for his belief in the concept of this project and his enthusiastic support. We especially want to thank Senior Product Manager Debra Myette-Flis for her invaluable guidance and assistance at every step of this process.

ABOUT THIS BOOK

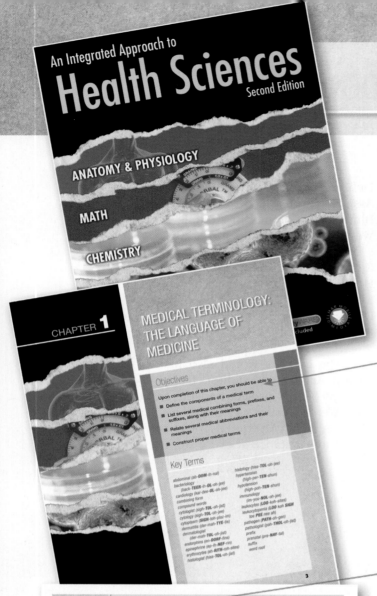

An Integrated Approach to Health Sciences, Second Edition integrates subject matter and applies the theoretical to real-life clinical relevancy to make learning easier. The writing style is easy-to-read and stimulating; humor is integrated to engage the learner; and several special features are incorporated throughout the text to enhance your learning experience.

Objectives and Key Terms

Objectives and key terms are presented at the beginning of each chapter to help you easily identify key topics *before* you read the chapter. Phonetic pronunciations follow selected key terms to assist you with pronouncing the terms correctly. It is also helpful to review the objectives and key terms *after* you have completed a chapter. Test yourself to see whether you can answer each objective and define each key term. If you cannot, you will know which areas to study again.

Special Focus

The Special Focus feature provides in-depth information on areas of particular interest that relate to concepts presented in the chapter. Two examples are "the fight-or-flight response" and "more than just the five senses."

Quotes and Notes

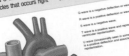

The Quotes and Notes feature gives health science related tidbits and facts along with learning hints and inspirational messages.

Clinical Relevancy

The Clinical Relevancy feature helps bridge the gap between theory and practice. Real-life analogies and examples illustrate how theoretical material applies to the health science field and encourages understanding of key concepts.

Professional Profile

The Professional Profile features describe a variety of health professions, and include information about where to visit online to obtain more information and learn more about the profession. Read these segments in the book and visit the suggested websites to discover health careers and opportunities that might interest you.

Stop and Review

The Stop and Review sections provide real-world application, feedback, and learning reinforcement through questions, reflections, and consideration of key material presented thus far before moving on in the chapter.

StudyWARE™ Connection

NEW! The **StudyWARE™ Connection** feature directs the learner to numerous anatomy, physiology and pathology animations, health-related video clips, interactive activities, and practice quizzes that reinforce material learned in the chapter.

Workbook Practice

NEW! The **Workbook Practice** feature directs the learner to even more learning tools in the workbook including practice questions, additional activities/labs, and extended concepts.

Full-Color Illustrations and Photos

Full-color illustrations and photos help clarify the text and visually reinforce concepts such as anatomy. Cartoons support learning through humor.

Chapter Review

The Chapter Review section includes review questions, a real-life issues and applications section, and suggested additional activities. This combined review approach helps learners assess their understanding of the chapter material and develop a health science mind-set and higher-order thinking skills, in addition to enhancing their creativity and critical-thinking skills.

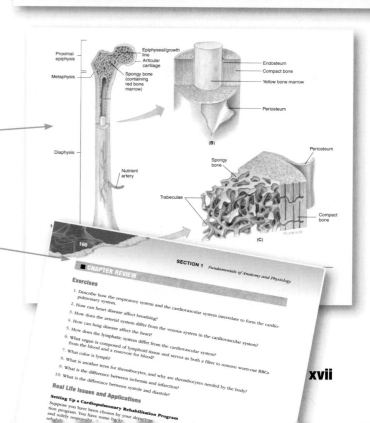

Professional Profile
Respiratory Care

The breath of life—that is what the respiratory therapist provides for those who either have difficulty breathing on their own or who have absolutely no ability to breathe.

Respiratory care practitioners work with patients of all ages. One minute they may be working with a baby that was born eight weeks too soon, and the next minute on a patient over 100 years of age!

This highly interesting profession requires vast knowledge of human anatomy and physiology, chemistry, physics, diseases and their effects on the respiratory and cardiovascular systems, as well as the types of respiratory medications and their effects on the human body. In addition, the respiratory care practitioner must be able to draw blood from arteries, perform CPR (cardiopulmonary resuscitation), and operate a myriad of advanced medical machinery such as breathing machines (also known as ventilators).

In bringing patients back from the precipice of death, the respiratory care practitioner experiences both excitement and a sense of accomplishment. This can provide these professionals with totally new ... that once seemed extremely impo ... more realistic perspectives.

Communication skills are ve ... respiratory care practitioner. The ... with physicians in developing gar ... ery of patients. A respiratory c ... responsible for educating pat ...

the proper use of respiratory medical equipment, equipment cleaning procedures, respiratory drugs, and tips on exercise and ways to improve activities of daily living.

Respiratory practitioners also are very much involved in community service. They often go to elementary and secondary schools to lecture on a variety of subjects including lung disease, asthma management, and the effects of smoking and air pollution. Furthermore, these professionals are active in developing employee wellness programs for business and industry.

Educational requirements vary for respiratory care practitioners. There are one-year certificate programs, associate degree programs, usually offered by community colleges or universities; and baccalaureate programs, offered by universities. There are two levels of respiratory care practitioners. *Technicians* are usually graduates of the certificate, or entry-level, programs while therapists are graduates of the advanced-level programs. Both, however, can be called *respiratory care practitioners.*

For more information regarding this fascinating and ... ssion, contact the American Association ... ol Row, Suite 122,

Stop and Review 10-4

a. What is the main breathing muscle called?
b. What is an accessory muscle?
c. Why is hemoglobin important?

StudyWARE CONNECTION

Go to your StudyWARE™ DVD and have fun learning as you play i... concepts you learned in this chapter.

| Workbook Practice | Go to your Workbook for more practice questions and activities. |

Labels on illustration: Proximal epiphysis, Metaphysis, Diaphysis, Nutrient artery, Epiphyseal/growth line, Articular cartilage, Spongy bone (containing red bone marrow), Endosteum, Compact bone, Yellow bone marrow, Periosteum, Spongy bone, Trabeculae, Periosteum, Compact bone

160

SECTION 1 *Fundamentals of Anatomy and Physiology*

■ CHAPTER REVIEW

Exercises

1. Describe how the respiratory system and the cardiovascular system interrelate to form the cardiopulmonary system.
2. How can heart disease affect breathing?
3. How does the arterial system differ from the venous system in the cardiovascular system?
4. How can lung disease affect the heart?
5. How does the lymphatic system differ from the cardiovascular system?
6. What organ is composed of lymphoid tissue and serves as both a filter to remove worn-out RBCs from the blood and a reservoir for blood?
7. What color is lymph?
8. What is another term for thrombocytes, and why are thrombocytes needed by the body?
9. What is the difference between ischemia and infarction?
10. What is the difference between systole and diastole?

Real Life Issues and Applications

Setting Up a Cardiopulmonary Rehabilitation Program
Suppose you have been chosen by your department... tion program. You have some back... and safely responsible... rehabili...

HOW TO USE THE STUDYWARE™ DVD

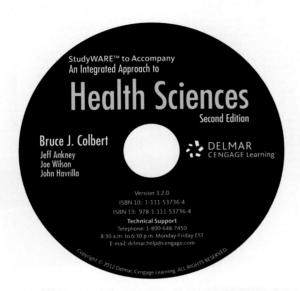

StudyWARE™ to Accompany
An Integrated Approach to

Health Sciences
Second Edition

Bruce J. Colbert

Jeff Ankney
Joe Wilson
John Havrilla

DELMAR
CENGAGE Learning™

Version 3.2.0
ISBN 10: 1-111-53736-4
ISBN 13: 978-1-111-53736-4
Technical Support
Telephone: 1-800-648-7450
8:30 a.m. to 6:30 p.m. Monday-Friday EST
E-mail: delmar.help@cengage.com

Copyright © 2012 Delmar, Cengage Learning. ALL RIGHTS RESERVED.

System Requirements

Minimum System Requirements

- Microsoft Windows XP w/SP 2, Windows Vista w/ SP 1, Windows 7
- Mac OS X 10.4, 10.5, or 10.6
- Processor: Minimum required by Operating System
- Memory: Minimum required by Operating System
- Hard Drive Space: 3.19GB
- Screen resolution: 1024 x 768 pixels
- DVD-ROM drive
- Sound card & listening device required for audio features
- Flash Player 10. The Adobe Flash Player is free, and can be downloaded from http://www.adobe.com/products/flashplayer/

Windows Setup Instructions

1. Insert disc into DVD-ROM drive. The software installation should start automatically. If it does not, go to step 2.
2. From My Computer, double-click the icon for the DVD drive.
3. Double-click the *setup.exe* file to start the program.

Mac Setup Instructions

1. Insert disc into DVD-ROM drive.
2. Once the disc icon appears on your desktop, double click on it to open it.
3. Double-click the *StudyWARE* to start the program.

Setup Instructions

1. Insert disc into DVD drive. The StudyWare™ installation program should start automatically. If it does not, go to step 2.
2. From My Computer, double-click the icon for the drive.
3. Double-click the *setup.exe* file to start the program.

Technical Support

Telephone: 1-800-648-7450
    Monday-Friday
    8:30 A.M.–6:30 P.M. EST
    E-mail: delmar.help@cengage.com

StudyWare™ is a trademark used herein under license.

Microsoft® and Windows® are registered trademarks of the Microsoft Corporation.

Pentium® is a registered trademark of the Intel Corporation.

Getting Started

The StudyWARE™ software helps you learn material in *An Integrated Approach to Health Sciences,* Second Edition. As you study each chapter in the text, be sure to explore the activities in the corresponding chapter in the software. Use StudyWARE™ as your own private tutor.

Getting started is easy. Install the software by inserting the DVD into your computer's DVD drive and following the on-screen instructions.

When you open the software, enter your first and last name so the software can store your quiz results. Then choose a chapter from the menu to take a quiz or explore one of the activities.

Menus

You can access the menus from wherever you are in the program. The menus include Quizzes and other Activities.

Quizzes. Quizzes include true/false, multiple-choice, and fill-in-the-blank questions. You can take the quizzes in both practice mode and quiz mode. Use practice mode to improve your mastery of the material. You have multiple tries to get the answers correct. Instant feedback tells you whether you're right or wrong and helps you learn quickly by explaining why an answer was correct or incorrect. Use quiz mode when you are ready to test yourself and keep a record of your scores. In quiz mode, you have one try to get the answers right, but you can take each quiz as many times as you want.

Scores. You can view your last scores for each quiz and print your results to hand in to your instructor.

Activities. Activities include image labeling, concentration, crossword puzzles, and Championship. Have fun while increasing your knowledge!

Animations and Video Clips. Numerous anatomy, physiology and pathology animations, and health-related video clips visually enhance the text material and reinforce learning.

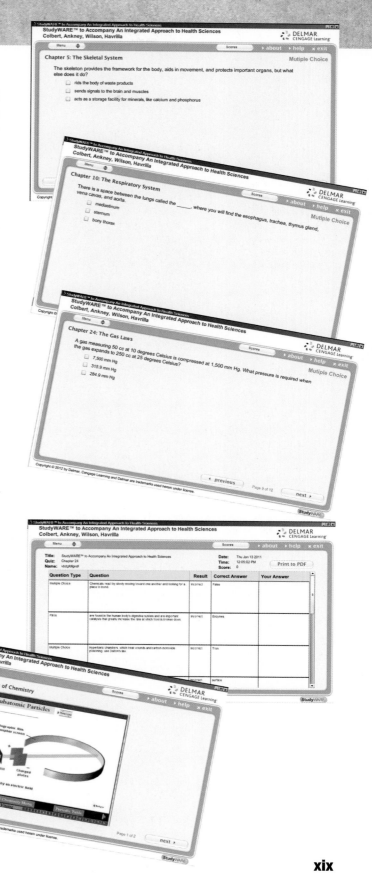

SECTION ONE

Fundamentals of Anatomy and Physiology

SECTION OVERVIEW

A basic understanding of human anatomy and physiology is crucial for anyone interested in the health sciences. This section presents an integrated and applied approach to anatomy and physiology. Rather than memorizing massive amounts of information, our approach emphasizes learning and understanding the material. Many analogies are used to aid in this process. We hope you enjoy this somewhat informal approach; after all, learning should be fun!

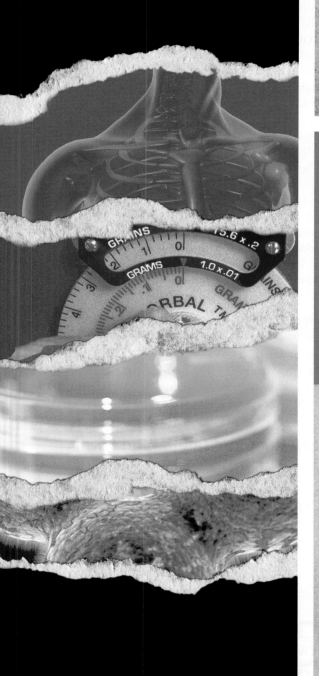

CHAPTER 1

MEDICAL TERMINOLOGY: THE LANGUAGE OF MEDICINE

Objectives

Upon completion of this chapter, you should be able to

- Define the components of a medical term
- List several medical combining forms, prefixes, and suffixes, along with their meanings
- Relate several medical abbreviations and their meanings
- Construct proper medical terms

Key Terms

abdominal (ab-**DOM**-ih-nal)

bacteriology
(back-**TEER**-ih-**OL**-oh-jee)

cardiology (kar-dee-**OL**-oh-jee)

combining form

compound words

cytologist (sigh-**TOL**-oh-jist)

cytology (sigh-**TOL**-oh-jee)

cytoplasm (**SIGH**-toh-plaz-im)

dermatitis (der-mah-**TYE**-tis)

dermatologist
(der-mah-**TOL**-oh-jist)

endorphins (en-**DORF**-fins)

epinephrine (ep-ih-**NEF**-rin)

erythrocytes (eh-**RITH**-roh-sites)

histologist (hiss-**TOL**-oh-jist)

histology (hiss-**TOL**-oh-jee)

hypertension
(high-per-**TEN**-shun)

hypotension
(high-poh-**TEN**-shun)

immunology
(im-you-**NOL**-oh-jee)

leukocytes (**LOO**-koh-sites)

leukocytopenia (**LOO** koh **SIGH**
toe **PEE** nee ah)

pathogen (**PATH**-oh-gen)

pathologist (pah-**THOL**-oh-jist)

prefix

prenatal (pre-**NAY**-tal)

suffix

word root

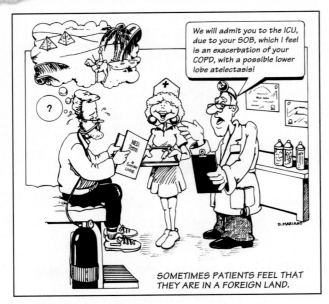

SOMETIMES PATIENTS FEEL THAT THEY ARE IN A FOREIGN LAND.

Source: Delmar/Cengage Learning

■ INTRODUCTION

Before beginning the discussion of anatomy and physiology in earnest, a short introduction to medical terminology is warranted. This chapter will help you to better understand those long medical terms that will soon become a part of your everyday conversations when you enter your given medical profession.

Imagine yourself in a foreign country where you do not speak the language. Even simple conversations would be difficult. For example, what if you need to explain how to drive a car to someone who does not know what certain words like *brake, tire,* and *steering wheel* mean? No matter how intelligent you are, you would look pretty silly making sounds and gestures to explain simple driving procedures.

Each profession has its own language and jargon that make it difficult for others to fully understand what is being said. Can you relate to Figure 1-1? It is important to realize, however, that this specialized language is needed in order to communicate accurately and concisely. You have chosen to pursue an interest in the medical profession, and it is important that you learn to "speak the lingo." On the StudyWARE™ CD-ROM you will find interactive games, a Spelling Bee activity with audio pronunciation for Chapters 1 to 13, and several other features.

The text, StudyWARE™ CD-ROM, and workbook together provide an extensive medical terminology review that will help you understand the fascinating language of medicine. In essence, you will learn medical terminology in a fairly painless and interesting manner.

What's in a Word?

What's in a word? The answer is "a lot" if it's a medical term. You will soon see how much information you can obtain from just understanding the medical origins of a single term.

The Word Root and Combining Form

If you understand medical terminology, one term can tell you quite a bit of information. Each medical term has a basic **word root** or stem that

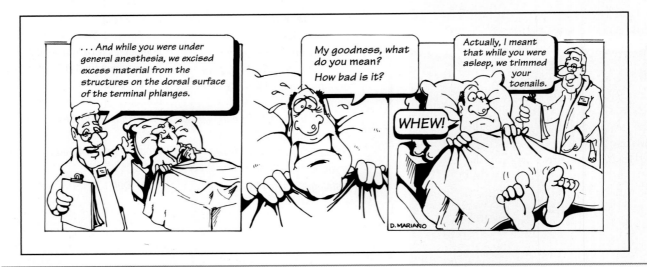

Figure 1-1

Source: Delmar/Cengage Learning

Special Focus

Humor in Medicine

It may seem strange to talk about humor in the medical professions. However, much scientific research is now being done to determine the benefits of humor in the healing process. Some research suggests laughter helps the immune system in warding off illness. This is not to say that humor therapy and positive emotions can replace medical treatment; they simply can enhance medical treatment and the body's positive response. Let's look at the process of laughter.

A good laugh has been shown to increase heart rate and improve blood circulation. Epinephrine levels in the blood also rise. Epinephrine is the body's arousal hormone, which stimulates the release of endorphins. Endorphins are the body's natural pain killers. Other immune system responses are also increased, and the entire respiratory system along with the facial muscles get a workout. These are some physiologic outcomes of laughter; but what about the psychological effects?

Humor has been shown to relieve tension and lessen anxiety. This is very important in a hospital environment, which can sometimes be frightening not only for the patient, but also for health science students. When appropriately used, humor can also help improve self-image and stimulate creativity. Some smoking cessation programs are now utilizing humor therapy to help cope with the nicotine withdrawal symptoms.

Don't forget to use humor to help you through this medical terminology chapter. The number of terms to memorize may seem overwhelming; but with practice and a positive attitude, you can easily master medical terminology. Use appropriate humor when you can, and remember that "what is learned with humor is not readily forgotten."

"Laughter is a vaccine for the ills of the world."

Joey Adams

usually comes from the Greek or Latin language. For example, the word root for heart is *cardi*. However, the term *cardi* is normally not used by itself. It is commonly combined with another word root, a **prefix** or **suffix**, to form a complete medical term.

The **combining form** consists of the word root and a connecting vowel to make it easier to pronounce and attach another root word or suffix. The combining form for heart is *cardi/o*; the combining form associated with cells is *cyt/o*; and the combining term associated with tissue is *hist/o*. Once again, the terms *cyt* and *hist* represent the word roots or foundations. The combining forms can now be put together with prefixes, suffixes, and other word roots to produce a multitude of medical terms. Table 1-1 shows some of the common word roots and their combining forms you may have already encountered.

Prefixes and Suffixes

A prefix is a part of a word that precedes the word root and changes its meaning. For example, the

prefix *ab* means "away from." If we combine this with the English word root *normal,* we have the term *abnormal.* This term now means "away from normal." Another common word root is *tension,* which in the medical professions can refer to blood pressure. If we insert the prefixes *hyper* ("increased") and *hypo* ("decreased"), we get the terms **hypertension** and **hypotension**, which mean respectively "high blood pressure" and "low blood pressure." Table 1-2 lists some common prefixes.

QUOTES & NOTES

Even the most current medical terms may have their roots in the ancient Latin language.

A suffix is a word ending that follows the word root and changes its meaning. A common suffix is *ology*, which means "the study of." **Cardiology**, therefore, is "the study of the heart." Remember, in order to combine the word root with another term, a vowel is needed in

TABLE 1-1
Common Word Roots and Their Combining Forms

COMBINING FORM	MEANING	COMBINING FORM	MEANING	COMBINING FORM	MEANING
aden/o	gland	hepat/o	liver	oste/o	bone
angi/o	vessel	hist/o	tissue	ovari/o	ovary
bacteri/o	bacteria	kinesi/o	movement	pancreat/o	pancreas
carcin/o	cancer	lapar/o	abdominal wall	phleb/o	vein
cardi/o	heart	leukocyt/o	white cell	proct/o	rectum
cholecyst/o	gallbladder	lymph/o	lymph vessels/fluid	pulmon/o	lung
cost/o	ribs	mamm/o	breast	py/o	pus
cyan/o	blue	mast/o	breast	rhin/o	nose
cyt/o	cell	melan/o	black	splen/o	spleen
dermat/o	skin	my/o	muscle	stern/o	sternum or breast-bone
encephal/o	brain	nephr/o	kidney	tendin/o	tendon
erythrocyt/o	red cell	neur/o	nerve or neuron	thorac/o	chest wall
gastr/o	stomach	onc/o	tumor or mass	thromb/o	clot
gynec/o	woman	ophthalm/o	eye	tox/o	poison
hem/o	blood	or/o	mouth	viscer/o	organ

TABLE 1-2
Common Prefixes

PREFIX	MEANING	PREFIX	MEANING
a	without or lack of	hemi	half
ab	away from	hyper	over or above
acro	extremity	hypo	under or below
ad	toward	inter	between
brady	slow	intra	within
contra	against	macro	large
di	two	micro	small
dia	through	mono	one
dys	difficult or painful	multi	many
ecto	outside	peri	around
endo	within	super	many or much
epi	upon or over	tachy	fast or rapid
eu	good or easy		

ology already has a vowel, the terms become **cytology** ("the study of cells") and **histology** ("the study of tissues"). The suffix term for a person who studies something is *ologist*. Therefore, a **cytologist** studies cells and a **histologist** studies tissues. Table 1-3 lists some common suffixes.

Also see Figure 1-2 which illustrates the parts of a medial term.

Compound Words

Compound words are made up of more than one word root. For example, referring to Table 1-1, we can take the combining forms for the colors white and red and combine these with the word root for cells. *Leuk/o* refers to white and *erythr/o* refers to red. So medical terminology for white blood cells and red blood cells is **leukocytes** and **erythrocytes**, respectively. Notice that these are compound words because they are made up of more than one word root.

In addition, you can add prefixes and suffixes to compound words. The term *penia* is a suffix that means "decrease in." A decrease in white blood cells is therefore termed **leukocytopenia**. Many more examples are given in the chapter review.

between the terms for readability purposes. The *wordroot/o* represents the combining form. In other words, if you wish to form the terms for "the study of cells" and "the study of tissues," you need to combine *cyt/o* and *hist/o* with the term *ology*, which means "the study of." Because

TABLE 1-3
Common Suffixes

SUFFIX	MEANING	SUFFIX	MEANING
al	pertaining to	oma	tumor
algesia	pain	opia	vision
centesis	surgical puncture	osis	abnormal condition of
crine	to secrete	pathy	disease
dipsia	thirst	penia	lack of
dynia	pain	phagia	eating or swallowing
ectomy	removal of	phasia	speech
emesis	vomit	phobia	fear
emia	blood condition	phonia	voice
esthesia	feeling or sensation	plast	surgical repair or formation
gram	a writing or record	plegia	paralysis
graph	instrument used for recording	scope	instrument to view or examine
graphy	process of recording	scopy	visual examination
ism	condition or state of being	spasm	involuntary contraction
ist	one who specializes	stasis	control or stop
itis	inflammation	stenosis	constriction or narrowing
lysis	breakdown or destroy	therapy	treatment
megaly	enlargement	tomy	incision or cut into
meter	instrument for measuring	toxic	poison
metry	act of measuring	trophy	development
oid	resemble	tension uria	pressure urine
ology	the study of		

Stop and Review 1-1

Define the following medical terms; notice how easy it is when you know a few basic word roots, prefixes, and suffixes.

a. cardiology

b. cardiomegaly

c. cardiogram

d. dermatologist

e. dermatitis

f. hypodermic

g. gastrology

h. gastroscopy

i. gastritis

j. acromegaly

k. acrocyanosis

l. dysphagia

m. thoracotomy

n. cholecystectomy

o. thoracentesis

p. melanoma

q. hypertension

r. hypotension

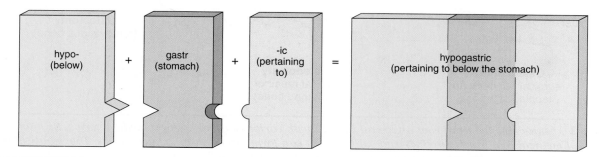

Figure 1-2 *A medical term may be taken apart to determine its meaning.* Hypogastric *means "pertaining to below the stomach."*

Source: Delmar/Cengage Learning

One advantage of learning medical terminology is that the terminology itself actually provides the definition of the term. Take the term **cytoplasm**, for example. Because *plasma* means "formative substance," the term *cytoplasm* literally means "the cell's formative substance." In Chapter 3 it will become evident that the substance responsible for forming a cell is the cytoplasm. By learning medical terminology, you will not have to memorize many definitions. If you know what the parts of the term mean, the medical term will actually give you the definition. While this book is not meant to be a dedicated medical terminology text, it does emphasize the majority of medical terms and concepts needed to facilitate your learning process. See Figure 1-3 for a graphic representation of medical terms related to the bone (*oste/o*).

General Hints on Forming Medical Terms

Even when you have learned the parts of medical terms and their meanings, it can sometimes be confusing trying to put the parts together to correctly form medical terms. It is important to note that most of the time, the definition indicates the last part of the term first, especially when a suffix is used. In other words, when using suffixes to construct medical terms, put the term parts together backward, or opposite to their occurrences in the definition. For example, an "inflammation of the skin" is **dermatitis**, not *itisdermato*. And "one who studies the skin" is a **dermatologist**, not an *ologistdermato*. "Pertaining to" (*al*) the abdomen is **abdominal**.

When using prefixes to form medical terms, you usually put the parts together in the order that you say the definition. For example, the medical term for "before" (*pre*) "birth" (*natal*) is **prenatal**. And, as shown previously, the term for "high blood pressure" is *hypertension,* which is put together as the definition is stated. As with any general rules, there are exceptions; but with practice you will become quite familiar and fluent in the proper construction of medical terms. See Figure 1-4 which shows various word roots for parts of the human body.

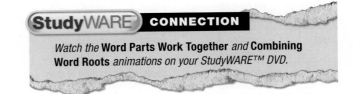

StudyWARE CONNECTION

Watch the **Word Parts Work Together** *and* **Combining Word Roots** *animations on your StudyWARE™ DVD.*

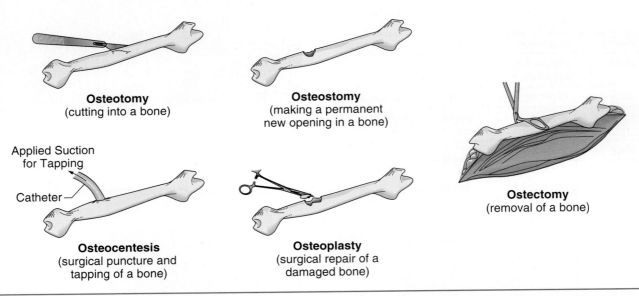

Osteotomy
(cutting into a bone)

Osteostomy
(making a permanent new opening in a bone)

Applied Suction for Tapping

Catheter

Osteocentesis
(surgical puncture and tapping of a bone)

Osteoplasty
(surgical repair of a damaged bone)

Ostectomy
(removal of a bone)

Figure 1-3 *Notice how the word root* osteo *can be used with various suffixes to form medical terms. By knowing a handful of medical root words, prefixes and suffixes, you can form hundreds of medical terms. The beauty of the system is that in forming the medical term, you automatically have the definition.*

Source: Adapted from Layman, Dale P., *Medical Language: A Programmed Body-Systems Approach.* Delmar/Cengage Learning, 1995.

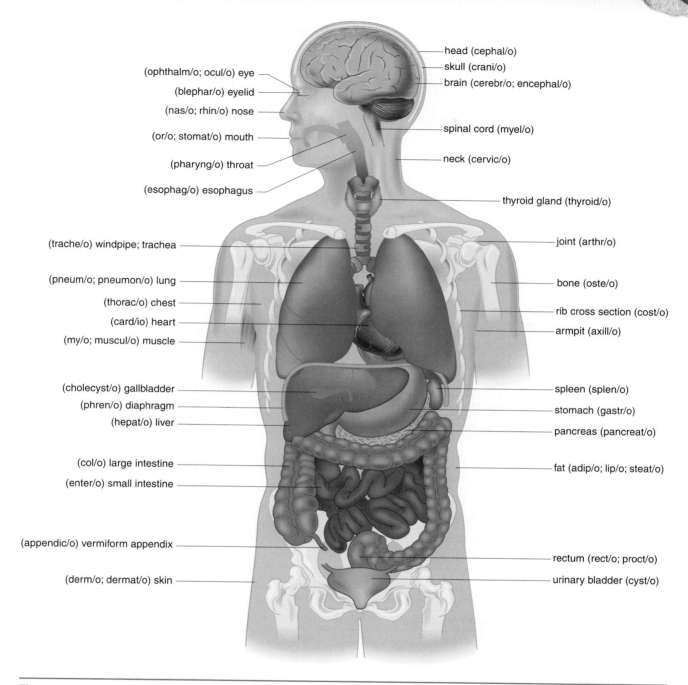

(ophthalm/o; ocul/o) eye

(blephar/o) eyelid

(nas/o; rhin/o) nose

(or/o; stomat/o) mouth

(pharyng/o) throat

(esophag/o) esophagus

(trache/o) windpipe; trachea

(pneum/o; pneumon/o) lung

(thorac/o) chest

(card/io) heart

(my/o; muscul/o) muscle

(cholecyst/o) gallbladder

(phren/o) diaphragm

(hepat/o) liver

(col/o) large intestine

(enter/o) small intestine

(appendic/o) vermiform appendix

(derm/o; dermat/o) skin

head (cephal/o)

skull (crani/o)

brain (cerebr/o; encephal/o)

spinal cord (myel/o)

neck (cervic/o)

thyroid gland (thyroid/o)

joint (arthr/o)

bone (oste/o)

rib cross section (cost/o)

armpit (axill/o)

spleen (splen/o)

stomach (gastr/o)

pancreas (pancreat/o)

fat (adip/o; lip/o; steat/o)

rectum (rect/o; proct/o)

urinary bladder (cyst/o)

Figure 1-4 *Word roots for parts of the human body.*
Source: Delmar/Cengage Learning

Medical Abbreviations

The medical profession, like all professions, uses its own set of abbreviations. These are helpful in shortening and simplifying long, complicated terms for diseases, procedures, or diagnostic tests.

Abbreviations are especially helpful with regard to charting. For example, a medical professional may take 50 blood pressures during the course of a busy day. It would simplify that professional's life to simply chart "BP 120/80" rather than "blood pressure is 120 millimeters of mercury over 80 millimeters of mercury." Table 1-4 lists some of the more common medical abbreviations.

Singular and Plural Endings

With everyday language, it is pretty simple to make a plural form of a word from a singular form. You simply add an "s" or "es" to the end of the word. However, making plural forms with medical terminology is a little more complicated. See Table 1-5 for examples of singular and plural forms of medical terms.

TABLE 1-4
Common Medical Abbreviations

ABBREVIATION	MEANING	ABBREVIATION	MEANING
AIDS	Acquired Immune Deficiency Syndrome	IV	intravenously
AMA	American Medical Association	lb.	pound
ASHD	arteriosclerotic heart disease	NPO	nothing by mouth
b.i.d.	twice a day	O_2	oxygen
BM	bowel movement	OR	operating room
BP	blood pressure	p.c.	after meals
CA	cancer	PE	physical examination/pulmonary emboli
CBC	complete blood count	p.o.	orally/by mouth
CCU	coronary care unit	p.r.n.	as required
CDC	Centers for Disease Control	pt.	patient
C&S	culture and sensitivity	q.	every
CNS	central nervous system	q.d.	every day
CO_2	carbon dioxide	q.h.	every hour
COPD	chronic obstructive pulmonary disease	q.2h.	every two hours
CPR	cardiopulmonary resuscitation	q.i.d.	four times a day
CVA	cerebrovascular accident	RBC	red blood cell
DOB	date of birth	ROM	range of motion
D_x	diagnosis	R_x	prescription
ECG/EKG	electrocardiogram	SOB	shortness of breath
EEG	electroencephalogram	t.i.d.	three times a day
EGG	white oval object produced by hens	UAO	upper airway obstruction
FUO	fever of undetermined origin	URI	upper respiratory infection
Fx	fracture	UTI	urinary tract infection
GI	gastrointestinal	VD	venereal disease
Gyn	gynecology	WBC	white blood cell
ICU	intensive care unit	Wt.	weight

TABLE 1-5
Singular and Plural Endings Along with Example Terms

SINGULAR ENDING	PLURAL ENDING	EXAMPLE
-a	-ae	*Vertebra* means a single spinal bone, whereas *vertebrae* means more than one spinal bone.
-ex or -ix	-ices	Each person has one *appendix*, and a surgeon removes several *appendices* annually.
-is	-es	The *prognosis* for the first patient seen looks favorable, while the *prognoses* for the next three patients seen are not positive.
-nx	nges	A health care students notes signs of irritation upon examination of the *pharynx* of a smoker, but he sees no such signs while examining several *phaynges* of nonsmokers.
-um	-a	The right *atrium* of the heart collects blood from the whole body, while both *atria* pump blood into the ventricles.
-us	-i	We each have a large airway called a main stem *bronchus* that branches into several smaller airways, or *bronchi*.

Stop and Review 1-2

Give the medical abbreviation for the following:

a. _____ a drug is to be given twice a day

b. _____ procedure performed on a pulseless person

c. _____ an electrical recording of the heart

d. _____ the unit patients are taken to when they have a heart attack

e. _____ as part of prep for surgery, patient is not allowed to eat or drink anything

Professional Profile
Medical Technology

Have you ever wished that you could be a detective? Do you enjoy reading mystery novels? If so, you may want to investigate the ever-growing field of medical technology. Medical technologists are highly skilled individuals who collect, prepare, and analyze biological specimens. Through the use of microscopes, computers, and other high-tech electronic equipment, they provide pieces to medical puzzles. In doing so they help solve mysteries such as what is ailing a patient or what caused a patient's death. Believe it or not, there is much uncharted territory in the human body, with many mysteries to be solved. With your investigative skills, you may be the one to unlock these secrets.

The term *medical technology* covers a broad range of procedures. These can include blood testing for things such as blood type; determining an individual's immune status (immunology); analyzing human tissue samples (histology); examining human cells for the signs or effects of disease (cytology); and studying how bacteria affects an individual (bacteriology). And this is just a small sampling of what these professionals do. You can see how important understanding anatomy and physiology at the cellular and tissue levels would be in this profession.

In addition to understanding anatomy and physiology, it is also important for medical technologists to be knowledgeable in the areas of microbiology physics and chemistry. Individuals working in a medical lab must ensure that the diagnostic equipment is functioning correctly. Some of these machines work on the principles of physics. Medical technologists also must work with chemicals in performing their duties.

Because mathematics is used when performing quality control and statistical analysis to check the accuracy of machines, an understanding of this area is also important to the medical technologist. Furthermore, math is needed anytime you deal with samples. How large is

(continues)

(continued)

the specimen? To what degree is a **pathogen** *(path/o* meaning "disease," *genic* meaning "producing") affected by various types and dosages of antibiotics? How are these values converted to metric values? Do the levels of arsenic in hair samples indicate death by foul play or natural causes? The need for math goes on and on.

Accuracy in obtaining, preparing, and analyzing specimens is of paramount importance in medical technology. Without accurate input from medical technologists, physicians who specialize in determining the natures of diseases and the effects of diseases on the human body (**pathologists**) cannot develop plans of action to treat patients. This information often must be rapidly provided. Inaccuracy or a delay may lead to the worsening of a patient's condition and even to death.

Educational requirements for medical technologists vary and include a certificate of completion from a technical school or hospital, a two-year associate degree from a college, or a four-year bachelor's degree. Some areas of specialization or research require more education, such as a graduate degree. You also may want to consider the field of education. Regardless of which path you choose, your first step is to get through school.

The American Medical Technologists (AMT) is a nonprofit certification agency and professional membership association that offers certifications in the following categories: Medical Technologists, Medical Laboratory Technicians, Medical Lab Assistants, Medical Assistants, Medical Administrative Specialists, Phlebotomy Technicians, Dental Assistants, Allied Health Instructors, and Clinical Laboratory Consultants. Visit their website for more information on this exciting field at www.amt1.com.

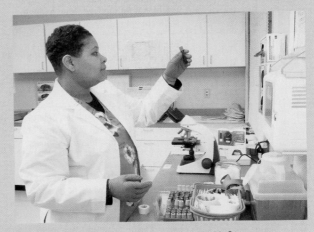

Source: McCutcheon, Maureen, *Exploring Health Careers.* Delmar/Cengage Learning, 1993.

■ CHAPTER REVIEW

Exercises

1. Using Tables 1-1 and 1-3, provide the correct medical terms for the following common (lay) descriptions. Remember, suffixes are placed at the end of the word, and the ending vowel is not used when the suffix begins with a vowel.

   a. the study of tissues

   b. white blood cells

   c. someone who studies the lung

   d. a decrease in red blood cells

   e. surgical repair of the nose

   f. pertaining to the nerves

   g. inflammation of the tendons

   h. a cancerous tumor

   i. an enlarged stomach

   j. pain in the nerves

   k. surgical puncture of the chest

   l. removal of the gall bladder

   m. an instrument used to record the brain

   n. stoppage of the blood flow

2. Using Tables 1-1, 1-2, and 1-3, provide the correct medical terms for the following lay descriptions.

   a. excessive (over or above) vomiting

   b. difficulty swallowing

   e. inflammation of many nerves

   f. condition of blue extremities

   c. less than (under or below) growth

   d. pertaining to between the ribs

   g. difficulty in speech

3. Provide the lay definition for the following medical terms.

a. bradycardia

b. gynecologist

c. lymphoma

d. kinesiology

e. laparoscopy

f. mammogram

g. myopathy

h. rhinitis

i. monocyte

j. toxicologist

k. microscope

l. phlebotomy

m. splenectomy

Real Life Issues and Applications

Explaining Medicalese in Plain English

You are working at a large urban medical center. The patient's doctor wants to explain the patient's condition to the patient's family. The problem is that the doctor speaks only "medicalese." Read the following excerpt from the patient's chart. Using common, nonmedical terms, how would you explain the patient's condition to the family?

"Pt. with COPD and ASHD admitted to hospital with lower rt. quadrant pain and FUO. EKG with normal parameters, slight hypertension noted. CBC normal with exception of elevated WBCs. Prepped for OR for laparoscopy. Procedure revealed appendicitis. Following excision, pt. returned to room. Will consult cardiologist and monitor for post-op complications."

Additional Activities

1. Make medical terminology flash cards. Put either a combining form, prefix, suffix, or medical abbreviation on one side of each card and the corresponding definition on the other side.

2. Make a list of 15 medical terms and 5 abbreviations that are not contained in this chapter. Provide definitions for each.

3. After reviewing a medical dictionary, discuss its various components and its usefulness.

4. Look up "physicians" in your phone directory and discuss what each specialist (ologist) does.

Downloadable audio is available for selected medical terms in this chapter to enhance your learning of medical language.

StudyWARE CONNECTION

Go to your StudyWARE™ DVD and have fun learning as you play interactive games, view animations and videos, and take practice tests to help reinforce key concepts you learned in this chapter.

Workbook Practice | *Go to your Workbook for more practice questions and activities.*

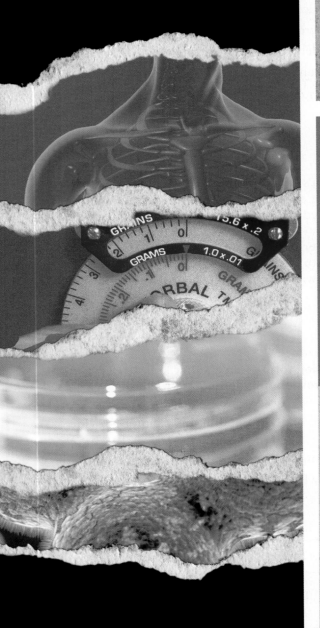

CHAPTER 2

OVERVIEW OF THE HUMAN BODY

Objectives

Upon completion of this chapter, you should be able to

- Define and differentiate the terms *anatomy* and *physiology*

- Define and state the relationship between cells, tissues, organs, and systems

- Describe the various directional terms in relationship to the human organism

- Discuss the concept of cyanosis

Key Terms

abdominal

acrocyanosis
(**AK** roh **SIGH** ah **NO** sis)

anatomy (ah-**NAT**-oh-me)

anterior (an-**TEER**-ee-or)

arterial (ar-**TEER**-ree-al)

body planes

caudal (**KAWD**-al)

cavity

cells

central cyanosis

cranial (**KRAY**-nee-al)

cyanosis (sigh-ah-**NO**-sis)

deoxygenated
(dee-**OK**-see-jen-**AY**-ted)

distal (**DIS**-tal)

dorsal (**DOOR**-sal)

erythrocyte (eh-**RITH**-roh-site)

frontal plane

hemoglobin
(**HE**-moh-**GLOW**-bin)

horizontal

inferior

lateral

medial (**MEE**-dee-all)

median plane (**MEE**-dee-an)

midsagittal plane
(mid-**SADJ**-ih-tal)

organ

pathophysiology

pelvic (**PEL**-vick)

peripheral (per-**IF**-er-al)

physiology (fiz-ee-**OL**-oh-gee)

posterior (pos-**TEER**-ee-or)

proximal (**PROCK**-sih-mal)

spinal

(continues)

superior

system

thoracic (tho-**RASS**-ick)

tissue

transverse plane (trans-**VERSE**)

venous system (**VEE**-nus)

ventral (**VEN**-tral)

vertebral (**VER**-teh-brall)

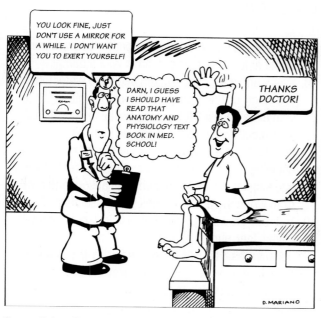

Source: Delmar/Cengage Learning

■ INTRODUCTION

The study of human anatomy and physiology is vitally important in all health science professions. In any health-related profession, you will be involved in some aspect of preventing, diagnosing, or treating disease processes. Because diseases disrupt normal operations of the body, it is necessary to first understand how a healthy body functions.

The human body is a wonderfully efficient and amazing organism. It is also a very complex organism. As a result, students may feel overwhelmed by the amount and complexity of information given to them when they begin studying human anatomy and physiology.

To make the study of human anatomy and physiology a little bit easier, we will be comparing the human body to everyday structures or machines that are familiar to you. This may seem a little odd, but you will begin to see some very interesting similarities. For example, you may better understand the hypothalamus and how it regulates body temperature within a narrow range when it is compared and contrasted to a home thermostat. The computer demonstrates some similarities to the human brain, and insulated electrical wiring corresponds well to the nerves

that carry the signals throughout the body. Many more analogies are utilized throughout this book. You may want to develop your own analogies to share with your classmates. This will greatly aid in learning the material.

QUOTES & NOTES

Although the amazing kidney is only about 4 inches long, 2 inches wide, and 1 inch thick, it filters approximately 180 quarts of fluid every day!

What Are Anatomy and Physiology?

What do the terms *anatomy* and *physiology* mean?

Definitions

Anatomy is the study of the form and structure of an organism. The study of the names and locations of the various bones in the human body is considered anatomy. Your body's skeleton can be compared to a house in which a wooden frame provides form and support. Just as the roof, walls, and doors are the anatomical features of the house, the skeleton, muscles, and skin are the comparable anatomical features of your body.

Physiology is the study of the processes of an organism, or in other words, "how and why something works." The transmission of nerve impulses from your brain to your eyelids so that you can blink is an example of a physiologic process. This could be compared to the way the wiring in a house conducts electricity from one area to another. You cannot see the conduction of the electricity, but you know the "process" is occurring. An area of study that is of great concern to health professionals is *pathophysiology*. **Pathophysiology** (*path/o* meaning "disease") is the study of why diseases occur and how the body reacts to them.

QUOTES & NOTES

Your stomach normally can hold 1-1/2 quarts when full. It uses hydrochloric acid to help digest food. How does the stomach keep from dissolving itself? It is lined with a mucous membrane that acts as a barrier between the acid and stomach tissue.

Special Focus

Amazing Facts of the Human Body

The study of human anatomy and physiology can be fascinating. To begin this journey, we have gathered some amazing facts for your consideration. The most amazing fact of all is life. As you learn about the human body throughout these first few chapters, we hope you marvel at the wonder of life.

1. Each day your lungs take in approximately 12,000 quarts of air!

2. Your lungs produce about a quart of mucus every 24 hours!

3. There are microscopic hairs (cilia) in your airways; these hairs beat back and forth like little oars at a rate of 1,500 beats per minute! This action moves that mucus up toward your pharynx (throat) at a rate of approximately 2 centimeters per minute!

4. When it gets to your pharynx, what happens to that mucus if you don't cough it out? YOU SWALLOW IT! You do this every day!

5. If you could take your lungs out, open up each little air sac, and lay those air sacs side by side on the ground, they would cover an area the size of a tennis court—approximately 70 square meters! Warning, do not attempt this at home; this should be done only by trained professionals!

6. If you don't think your heart is a hard worker, just take your pulse for a full minute. (Do this by feeling the beats at the radial artery located in your wrist.) Now let your hand imitate the squeezing action of your heart by fully opening and fully closing your hand at the same rate that your heart beats. Do this for 5 minutes. Do not stop and take a rest; your heart doesn't. How do the muscles in your hand and forearm feel after 5 minutes? Just a little reminder, if your heart rate is 80 beats per minute, your heart beats more than 115,000 times each day! If your hand gets tired during this little exercise, you can always switch to your other hand. But you only have one heart—so take good care of it.

7. If you possess an average appetite, you will consume at least 35 tons of food in your lifetime!

8. Ever wonder why your mouth begins to water when you think of thick juicy steaks or pepperoni pizza with extra cheese? It happens because the saliva in your mouth is actually a digestive juice. The minute hot, delicious pizza hits your mouth, with the help of chewing and saliva, the pizza starts to break down into substances that your body can absorb nutrients from when the pizza reaches your intestines.

9. Your hair grows approximately 1/4 inch each month! If you feel particularly hairy in the summer, it is because hair usually grows faster in the summer than in the winter. Hair also grows faster during the day than during the night. One word of caution: Putting fertilizer on your hair will not make it grow any faster, and will probably cause you to lose some friends!

10. Almost half the number of bones in your skeleton are found in your hands and feet!

11. Your fingerprints will grow in size during your lifetime, but unless your fingers are injured, the patterns of your fingerprints will remain the same. Those patterns are unique to you. No one else in the whole world has the same fingerprints as you do! Interestingly enough, no one else in the whole world has the exact same voice as you do, either. That makes you pretty special!

12. The three smallest bones in your body exist in each of your ears and take up an area about the size of a child's thumbnail. The names of these bones describe their shapes: the stirrup, the hammer, and the anvil.

13. Nerve impulses in your body can travel at speeds of up to 426 feet per second!

14. When you are resting, your body consumes about 250 ml of oxygen each minute. That is equivalent to a little over 1/2 pint of oxygen consumed every minute.

Makeup of the Human Body

What makes up the human body? The individual building blocks of the body are called **cells**. These are similar to the bricks required to build a house. It's hard to imagine what a house looks like by looking at one brick, yet thousands of them put together in a certain organized manner will shape a house. Cells, like bricks, come in all shapes and sizes and perform various functions. Figure 2-1 shows the different cell types found within the human body.

Cells can be joined together to form **tissues**. Just as bricks can be placed together in different patterns for different purposes, cells can be combined into structures, or tissues, that can perform special tasks or functions such as support, ventilation, and transportation of fluids.

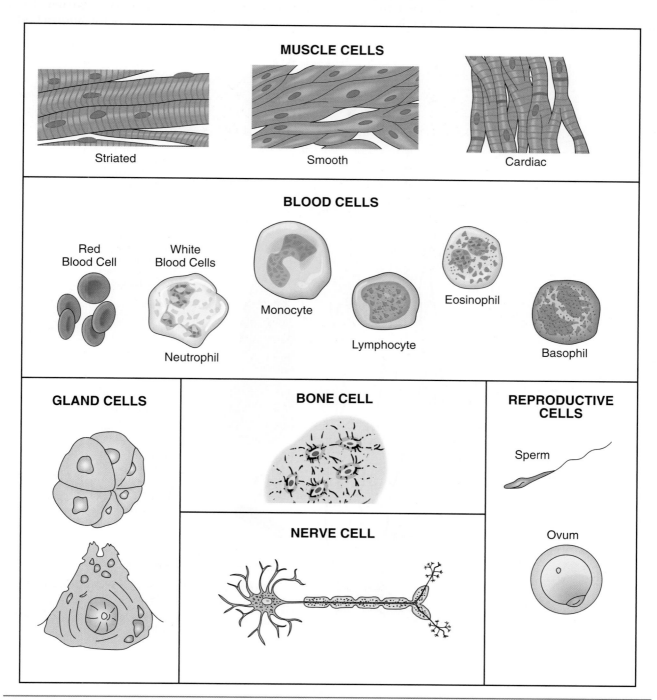

Figure 2-1 *Notice the diversity of cells found within the human body.*
Source: Delmar/Cengage Learning

The type of tissue structure depends on the function to be performed. This concept will be reinforced throughout this text: Structure, or "how something is put together," often relates to function. Two or more types of tissues can be joined together to form **organs**, which also have specific functions. The kidneys, heart, lungs, and stomach are all examples of organs within the human body.

The furnace in a home can be considered an organ that functions to generate heat for the home. However, more than just a furnace is needed to adequately and evenly heat a home. Additional materials such as fuel, electricity, duct work, and insulation are needed for a complete heating system. This is analogous to the way body organs work together in humans. Organs and other parts that join together to perform a specific body function are referred to as a **system**. These systems all function together to form the wondrous human organism (see Figure 2-2). We will explore the concepts of cells, tissues, organs, and systems in greater detail when we complete the overview of the human body.

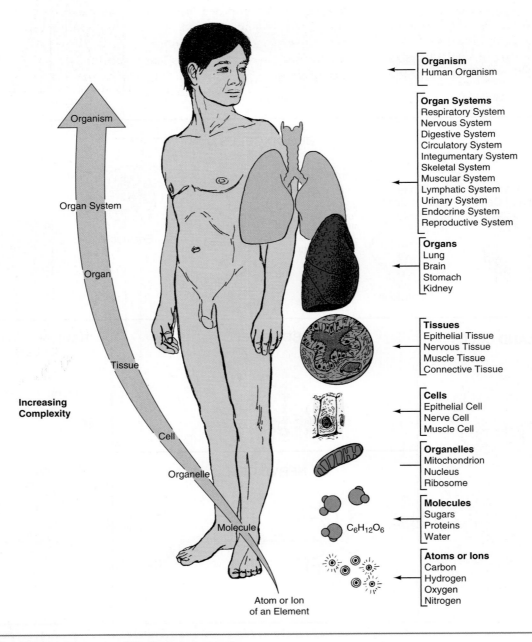

Figure 2-2   *The components of the human organism.*

Source: Delmar/Cengage Learning

Anatomical Landmarks

The design of any machine or structure requires a blueprint or plan. You must understand the terminology and directional terms contained in the blueprint in order to properly read and understand the design.

Body Planes and Directional Terms

The human body can be divided into **body planes**. Body planes are formed by imaginary lines dissecting the body into different regions for anatomical purposes. The three main body planes, as depicted in Figure 2-3, are the **transverse plane**, the **midsagittal (median) plane**, and the **frontal plane**. Directional terms can be used within these specific planes to identify where a structure is located or a surgical incision is to be made.

The transverse plane is a **horizontal** reference that divides the body into a top section and a bottom section. *Horizontal* means "lying flat and going from right to left or left to right," as does the horizon. The main directional terms defined by these regions are **superior (cranial)** and **inferior (caudal)**. *Superior* means "above" and *inferior* means "below." *Cranial* means "toward the head" and *caudal* means "toward the tail." The transverse plane, therefore, separates the body into a superior portion and an inferior portion. In addition, the terms can be applied when comparing structures that are above and below one another. For example, one can say that the nose is superior to the mouth, or that the mouth is inferior to the nose. This, of course, does not mean the mouth is less important than the nose.

The midsagittal, or median, plane is a vertical sheet that divides the body into a right side

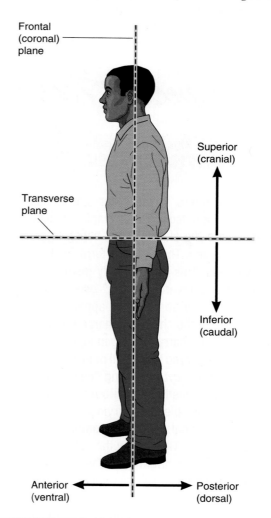

Figure 2-3 *The median (midsagittal) plane, the transverse plane, and the frontal plane with their corresponding directional terms.*

Source: Delmar/Cengage Learning

and a left side. The main directional terms in these regions are **medial** and **lateral**. *Medial* means "toward the middle" and therefore refers to structures and areas that are close to the midline. *Lateral* means "toward the side" and refers to structures and areas that are away from or to the side of the midline of the median plane. For example, the nose is medial in reference to the ear, and the ear is lateral to the nose.

The frontal plane is a vertical reference that divides the body into a front half and a back half. The directional terms defined by this region are **anterior, posterior, ventral,** and **dorsal**. *Anterior* and *ventral* refer to areas or structures on the front of the body. The chest and stomach are anterior, or ventral, regions. *Posterior* and *dorsal* refer to areas or structures on the back of the body. The spine is an example of a posterior, or dorsal, structure.

Other common directional terms are **proximal, distal,** and **peripheral**. These are reference terms that describe the relationship of structures to one another. *Proximal* means "near" or "in close proximity to" the reference point or point of attachment, whereas *distal* means "away from" the reference point or point of attachment. For example, if we choose the hip as our reference point, we can say the knee is proximal and the ankle is distal to the hip. Please refer back to Figure 2-3 to review all these planes and directional terms.

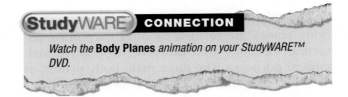

Watch the **Body Planes** animation on your StudyWARE™ DVD.

Body Cavities

The body can also be divided into regions according to certain spaces or **cavities** that house the organs. Just as the body is divided into the dorsal

Special Focus

Directional Terms, One Use of *Peripheral* Versus *Central*

Peripheral refers to the outer extremities such as the arms and legs. For example, a condition can exist where the skin appears bluish in color due to lack of oxygen. The medical term for this condition is **cyanosis**. This term literally means "condition of blue" (*cyan/o* meaning "blue," *osis* meaning "condition of"). The reason the skin appears bluish in color is because of the chemical characteristics of the cell responsible for carrying oxygen in the blood. This cell is known as the red blood cell or **erythrocyte** (*eryth/o* meaning "red," *cyte* meaning "cell"). The red blood cell contains mostly **hemoglobin**, which is the substance responsible for carrying oxygen throughout the body. Hemoglobin when combined with oxygen turns bright red. This is why the **arterial** blood (blood in the arteries) is bright red. When the red blood cell is not fully combined with oxygen, the cell has more of a darker red or, as we perceive it, a bluish tint. This is why veins in the **venous system**, which carry **deoxygenated** (decreased level of oxygen) blood back to the lungs to become reoxygenated, appear blue. When we cut ourselves, the oxygen in the air combines with hemoglobin and causes the blood to appear bright red—even if the blood is venous blood.

Venous blood is normally a dark red to bluish hue and, therefore that color is nothing to be concerned about. However, if there are abnormally low levels of oxygen in the body, arterial blood oxygen levels may become low and there will be more "bluish" blood (deoxygenated) in circulation. This can lead to a condition of blueness of the skin called *cyanosis,* which is of concern.

An important clinical assessment tool is being able to determine the difference between peripheral and central cyanosis. Someone can have just peripheral cyanosis, which causes only the extremities (arms and legs) to appear blue. This is also termed **acrocyanosis** (*acro* meaning "extremities"). If cyanosis is more severe, the whole body appears blue. This is termed **central cyanosis** and is a much more serious and a potentially fatal condition that requires immediate attention. More information on this important clinical subject will be provided in future chapters.

and ventral planes, body cavities can be classified as dorsal or ventral cavities. Remember, *dorsal* is a synonym for *posterior* and *ventral* is a synonym for *anterior*. The dorsal, or posterior, cavities can be further divided into the **cranial** cavity, which contains the brain, and the **spinal** or **vertebral** cavity, which houses the spinal cord (see Figure 2-4).

The ventral or anterior cavities can be further divided into the **thoracic** cavity, the **abdominal** cavity, and the **pelvic** cavity. The thoracic cavity contains the heart, lungs, and large blood vessels. The abdominal cavity houses the stomach, small intestine, a majority of the large intestine, liver, gallbladder, pancreas, and spleen. The pelvic cavity contains the urinary bladder, reproductive organs, and the final portion of the large intestine (see Figure 2-5).

Stop and Review 2-1

a. List five anatomical structures found on the anterior, or ventral, surface of the body.

b. List five anatomical structures found on the posterior, or dorsal, surface of the body.

QUOTES & NOTES

An additional important directional concept is left versus right. In assessing and treating patients, you ALWAYS refer to the patient's left and right. You can see the importance of this in the "Real Life Issues and Applications" section at the end of this chapter.

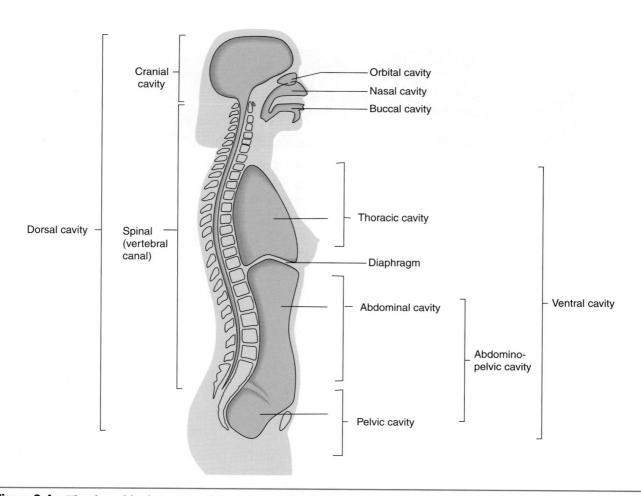

Figure 2-4 *The dorsal body cavities (cranial cavity and vertebral cavity) and the ventral body cavities (thoracic cavity, abdominal cavity, and pelvic cavity).*

Source: Delmar/Cengage Learning

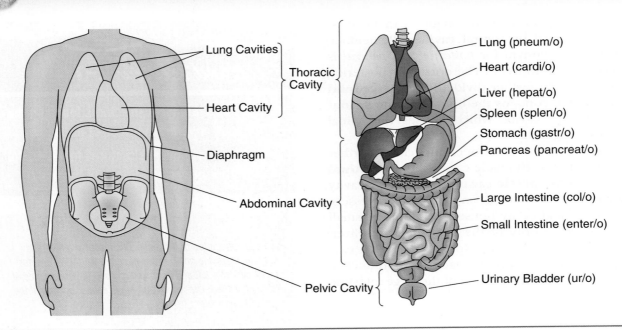

Figure 2-5   *Anterior view of organs within the body cavities.* Note: *If you removed the small intestine from the cavity and then stretched it out on the floor and measured it, it would be approximately 23 feet long!*

Source: Delmar/Cengage Learning

Clinical Relevancy

The Abdominal Quadrants

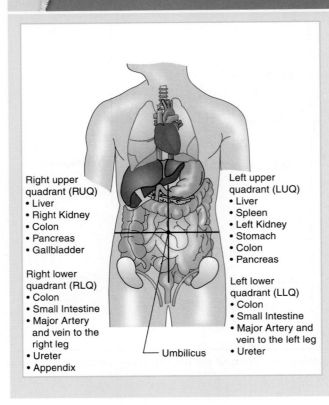

The abdominal cavity is such a large region and houses so many organs that it is even further subdivided into smaller units called *quadrants* (see Figure 2-6) for clinical assessment. These quadrants help identify the underlying problem. For example, a patient complaining of pain the right lower quadrant (RLQ) would need to be tested for appendicitis. Pain in the left upper quadrant (LUQ) would be suspicious for stomach problems.

Right upper quadrant (RUQ)
• Liver
• Right Kidney
• Colon
• Pancreas
• Gallbladder

Right lower quadrant (RLQ)
• Colon
• Small Intestine
• Major Artery and vein to the right leg
• Ureter
• Appendix

Left upper quadrant (LUQ)
• Liver
• Spleen
• Left Kidney
• Stomach
• Colon
• Pancreas

Left lower quadrant (LLQ)
• Colon
• Small Intestine
• Major Artery and vein to the left leg
• Ureter

— Umbilicus

Figure 2-6   *Abdominal quadrants and corresponding organs.*

Source: Delmar/Cengage Learning

QUOTES & NOTES

You can't hit a home run unless you step up to the plate. You can't catch a fish unless you put your line in the water. You can't reach your goals if you don't try.

—Kathy Seligman

Stop and Review 2-2

Give the opposite of the following terms:

a. central _____

b. distal _____

c. caudal _____

d. anterior _____

e. dorsal _____

f. medial _____

List the cavity where the following organs are found:

g. spleen _____

h. urinary bladder _____

i. lungs _____

j. large intestine _____

■ CHAPTER REVIEW

Exercises

1. A group of cells similar in structure and function can form (a/an):
   a. organ
   b. system
   c. tissue
   d. organism

2. Tissues can join together to form:
   a. cells
   b. systems
   c. an organism
   d. organs

3. Which of the following levels are needed to form a human organism: cells, tissues, organs, systems?
   a. cells and tissues
   b. tissues only
   c. cells, tissues, and organs
   d. cells, tissues, organs, and systems

4. What plane is divided by a horizontal sheet into superior and inferior regions?
   a. transverse
   b. median
   c. frontal
   d. midsagittal

5. Which of the following is not an organ?

   a. stomach

   b. bone

   c. skin

   d. heart

6. What cell carries oxygen in your body?

   a. leukocyte

   b. osteocyte

   c. erythrocyte

   d. cyanocyte

7. Differentiate between the terms *anatomy* and *physiology*.

8. List three anterior structures, three posterior structures, and three medial structures.

9. What two structures are found in the dorsal cavity?

10. What three cavities compose the ventral cavity? List a representative organ for each of these cavities.

Real Life Issues and Applications

The Importance of Medical Directional Terms

A patient with the diagnosis of peripheral vascular disease and diabetes presents to a physician's office. The diabetes has been poorly managed by the patient. An untreated wound to the patient's left foot has allowed gangrene to set in. Given the severity of the infection, the physician decides to amputate the lower left leg.

While prepping the patient for the operation the following day, a technician erroneously tags the patient's right leg because the technician was facing the patient, and instead of using the patient's left as a reference point, the technician used his own left as a reference point.

The right leg was then removed. When the patient was in recovery, the surgeon realized he had removed the wrong leg (which was the right leg!). The patient was immediately returned to the operating room and the correct (left), diseased leg was removed.

Do you see the importance of understanding medical directional terms? What are the legal and ethical issues involved here?

Additional Activities

1. Write three sentences using the terms *proximal* and *distal* within each sentence. *Hint*: Pick something as a reference point.

2. Write two sentences using the term *peripheral*.

3. Use anatomical landmark terminology (directional terms, body planes, or cavities) to describe an organ or body structure to another student or group of students. See if the other students can properly identify the organ or structure. Use concise descriptions.

4. Discuss the importance in the medical professions of being able to locate a specific region or area. Discuss what problems could arise if this is not done accurately.

Downloadable audio is available for selected medical terms in this chapter to enhance your learning of medical language.

StudyWARE CONNECTION

Go to your StudyWARE™ DVD and have fun learning as you play interactive games, view animations and videos, and take practice tests to help reinforce key concepts you learned in this chapter.

Workbook Practice   *Go to your Workbook for more practice questions and activities.*

CHAPTER 3

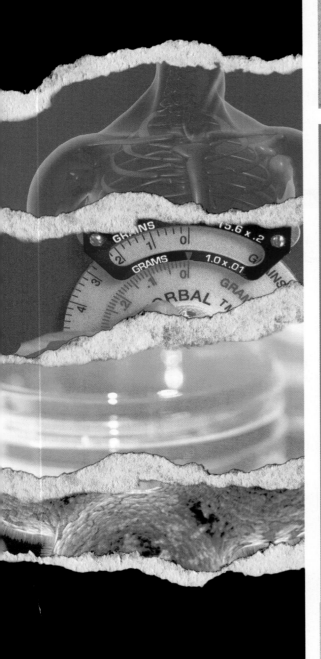

THE RAW MATERIALS: CELLS, TISSUES, ORGANS, AND SYSTEMS

Objectives

Upon completion of this chapter, you should be able to

- Discuss the various functions that cells need to perform

- Define and identify common cellular structures and their functions

- List and describe two methods of cellular transport across the cell membrane

- Describe the process of mitosis

- Define and discuss concepts pertaining to body tissues

- Differentiate epithelial, connective, muscle, and nerve tissues

- Differentiate organs and systems

- List and describe the organs contained within the body systems

- Relate medical terminology to body organs and systems

Key Terms

axon (**ACK**-son)
cardiovascular system
cartilage (**KAR**-tih-lidj)
cell
centriole (**SEN**-tree-ol)
centrosome (**SEN**-tro-sohm)

chromatin (**KRO**-mah-tin)
chromosomes
   (**KROH**-moh-sohmz)
connective tissue
deoxyribonucleic acid (dee **AWK**
   see **RYE** boh new **KLEE** ick)

(continues)

diffusion
endoplasmic reticulum
    (en-doe-**PLAZ**-mik ree-**TICK**-
    you-lim)
endothelium (en-doh-**THEE**-lee-um)
epithelium (ep-ih-**THEE**-lee-al)
genes
Golgi apparatus (**GOAL**-je)

lysosomes (**LIE**-so-sohmz)
microorganism
mitochondria (my-toe-**KON**-dree-ah)
mitosis (my-**TOH**-sis)
neurons (**NEW**-rons)
nucleolus (**NEW**-klee-OL-us)
nucleus (**NEW**-klee-us)
organelle (or-gah-**NEL**)

osmosis
protoplasm (**PRO**-toe-plaz-im)
respiration
ribonucleic acid (**RNA**)
ribosomes (**RYE**-boh-sohmz)
semipermeability
tissue

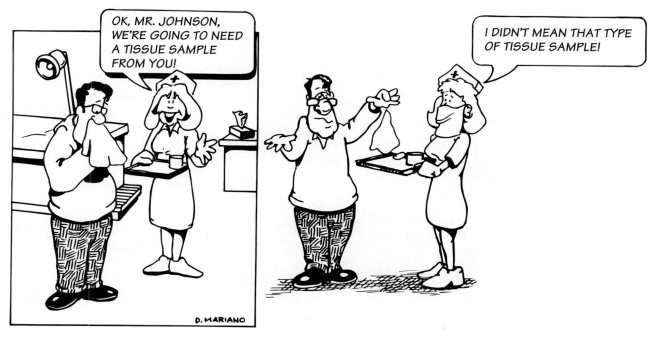

Source: Delmar/Cengage Learning

■ INTRODUCTION

The **cell** is the fundamental microscopic structure of life. The approximately 75 trillion cells found in the human body must carry on the processes associated with life. In addition, many cells perform specialized functions such as movement (muscle cells), communication (nerve cells), and oxygen transport (red blood cells). The common processes associated with most cells, regardless of type, are reproduction, taking in (ingestion) of food and oxygen, production of heat and energy, excretion, movement, and adaption to the environment.

QUOTES & NOTES

You may think that cell shapes are simple, but some plant cells have 13 sides, roughly forming a ball shape! Nerve and muscles cells can be several feet long!

Human Cell Variability

Just like the human organism itself, cells in the human body vary in shape, size, and function. For example, nerve cells are specialized to transmit electrical messages, red blood cells to transport oxygen, and white blood cells to help fight disease. Almost all cells are microscopic in size and range from 1/3 to 1/13 the size of the period at the end of this sentence. Nerve cells, however, may have projections, called **axons**, which can be as long as one yard. All cells, regardless of their size, shape, or specialization, generally contain an outer membrane, a fluid center (cytoplasm), and small structures called organelles inside the cytoplasm, which have specific functions. In addition, most cells contain a **nucleus**, which controls many cellular functions. Because cells die, the remaining cells of that particular type continually divide and replace the dead cells. For now, however, let's concentrate on the general components found in most cells. Figure 3-1 shows the major components of the cell.

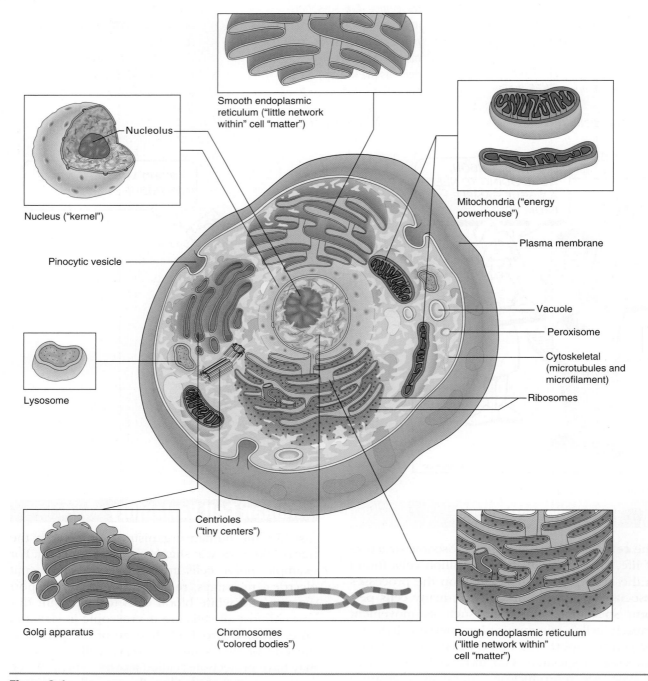

Figure 3-1   *Major components of the cell.*
Source: Delmar/Cengage Learning

Cellular Structures

There are many components to the human cell. We will discuss each component or structure and relate their importance to overall cellular function.

Cell Membrane

The parts of a cell are encased in a protective covering called the *cell membrane*, or *plasma membrane*, which also serves to give form to the cell. The cell membrane must allow certain materials

Special Focus

Microorganisms

Microorganisms (*micro* meaning "small") are living organisms so small that they can be seen individually only with the aid of a microscope. The microorganisms with which we are most familiar are human cells and bacteria. However, other microorganisms such as algae, bacteria, fungi, protozoa, viruses, and rickettsiae do exist. Table 3-1 provides a basic overview and descriptions of these other simple life forms. The Microbiology section of this textbook will go into much greater depth and clinical application.

One characteristic substance shared by all living things is **protoplasm**, which literally means "the original formative substance" (*proto* meaning "original," *plasm* meaning "formative substance"). The chemical ingredient list for protoplasm is quite simple, with oxygen, carbon, hydrogen, sulfur, nitrogen, and phosphorous being the main components. Amazingly, no one has yet been able to put these ingredients together to artificially produce protoplasm in the lab.

Cells also contain a special kind of plasm called *cytoplasm,* which means simply the cell's (*cyt/o*) formative substance. In addition to the chemicals found in the protoplasm, the cytoplasm contains water, food particles, and other specialized materials.

to enter and exit, while prohibiting other substances from passing through. This unique feature of selective passage is called **semipermeability**.

Organelles

Inside the cell is the cytoplasm, a slightly granular fluid environment containing water, proteins, carbohydrates, lipids (fats), and salts. Also within the cell are many smaller structures. These structures perform defined tasks for the cell similar to what organs do in the human body. In fact, these small structures are called **organelles**, meaning "small organs." Refer back to Figure 3-1 as we discuss the individual organelles.

Nucleus

The organelle that functions as the brain of the cell is called the *nucleus.* The nucleus controls most of the cellular activities and is especially important in the process of reproduction of the cell. Cells must be able to reproduce in order to carry on their existence and our existence. (Think what it would mean if the human population could not reproduce. In a hundred years or so, there would be no such organism as the human

TABLE 3-1		
Simplified Classification of Microorganisms		
CLASSIFICATION	**MICROORGANISM**	**DEFINITIONS**
Plant	Algae	Simple plants with few known disease-causing forms
	Bacteria	Microscopic, one-celled organisms that have both beneficial and harmful forms
	Fungi	Large group of simple plants that have some disease-producing forms. The fungi group includes mushrooms, bread molds, and yeast
Animal	Protozoa	One-celled animals much larger than bacteria; found in bodies of water; an amoeba is an example
Unclassified	Viruses	Smallest living things known; so small they can be viewed only through a special electron microscope; examples include measles, HIV, and the common cold
	Rickettsiae	Similar to bacteria but smaller; cannot exist outside of living host and are therefore parasitic; can cause typhus and Rocky Mountain spotted fever

being!) In addition, if cells could not repair and reproduce, every injury would be permanent and, in many cases, fatal.

In order to reproduce, an organism must have two main ingredients. First, the organism needs a blueprint or code to follow in order to reproduce the correct cells capable of the proper functions. Second, the organism must possess the ability to generate the material used to build the new cells. Within the nucleus of each cell is a material called **chromatin**. Chromatin contains **deoxyribonucleic acid (DNA)**. The DNA is the blueprint; it contains the information that defines the new cell and its characteristics. Chromatin eventually forms **chromosomes**. Chromosomes contain **genes**, which determine our inherited characteristics.

Another structure found inside the nucleus provides the raw material to build new cells and repair existing cells. This structure, called the **nucleolus**, contains **ribosomes**. Ribosomes are composed of **ribonucleic acid (RNA)** and protein. Ribosomes assist in the synthesis (production) of protein needed for cellular reproduction and repair.

Centrosome

A specific region within the cell that functions in cellular reproduction is the **centrosome**. Located near the nucleus, the centrosome contains **centrioles**, which play a major role in the division of the cell, and will be discussed shortly.

Mitochondria

Just as the human body needs to produce energy in order to survive and, hopefully, thrive, so does the cell. The energy powerhouse of the cell, called the **mitochondria**, is found throughout the cytoplasm. The mitochondria actually provides approximately 95% of the energy needed for cellular reproduction, repair, and movement. The concentration of mitochondria within a cell differs according to the cell's need. Liver cells, which require large amounts of energy, may have as many as 2,000 mitochondria each, whereas sperm cells, which need only minimal energy to swim to their destination, each have only one mitochondria coiled around the tail (flagellum).

From Figure 3-1, you can see that the mitochondria has a pleated or convoluted membrane, which significantly increases the surface area of the mitochondria. This is to allow for a barrier area for gas exchange, one of the most important

processes of your body. This is where special enzymes found nowhere else in the cell help to ingest oxygen and use it to generate energy for the cell and for you to survive. This process is known as cellular **respiration** and will be covered in detail in the Chemistry section. For now, think of cellular respiration as the combining of glucose (from foods) and oxygen to form energy for all essential cellular functions, which is referred to as cellular metabolism.

Golgi Apparatus

This energy generation and usage does, however, produce waste by-products. If we did not have a method to get rid of the waste products within our houses, we would soon be forced to move out, or possibly, become very sick due to the unsanitary conditions. As is the case with a house, each cell needs to be able to keep its microenvironment clean. The structure responsible for storing and packaging secretions for discharge from the cell is called the **Golgi apparatus**. The vacuole, or cellular storage spaces, can assist in this process. The Golgi apparatus can also concentrate and package needed secretory products for the body. Cells of glands having high levels of storage and secretion, as occurs in the digestive process, naturally have a larger number of these structures. The cells of the salivary, gastric, and pancreatic glands are therefore richer in this organelle.

Lysosomes

Lysosomes also assist in the removal of old debris and foreign material. Lysosomes contain a digestive enzyme that breaks apart and digests old cells and foreign material found within the cells. (Remember, *lysis* means "to break down or destroy.") This process is very important to the body's immune system.

Endoplasmic Reticulum

Finally, there is the **endoplasmic reticulum**, which deals with communication. The endoplasmic reticulum is actually a network of tubular structures within the cytoplasm. This network facilitates transport of materials in and out of the nucleus. It also helps in the synthesis and storage of proteins. There are two types of endoplasmic reticulum. The presence of ribosomes on the endoplasmic recticulum gives it a rough appearance and is aptly named rough endoplasmic recticulum. Smooth endoplasmic recticulum, of course, has no ribosomes. See Table 3-2 for an overview of cellular structure and function.

Clinical Relevancy

Examples of Cellular Transport Mechanisms

Because cell membranes are semipermeable, certain substances can move into and out of the cell. Two forms of transport are diffusion and osmosis. Diffusion results as an attempt to evenly disperse molecules of a substance throughout a given volume or environment. For example, a dead skunk in the middle of the road will be smelled throughout the whole neighborhood. A physiologic example is the movement of oxygen molecules from a high concentration in the lung to the blood which has a lesser concentration. See Figure 3-2 to illustrate the process of diffusion.

Osmosis is a little bit different because it is the movement of water in and out of the cell to reach equilibrium in the concentration of dissolved substances. If a highly concentrated solution (lots of dissolved material with little water) is on one side of a semipermeable membrane and a dilute or lower concentrated solution is on the other side, water from the lower concentrated side will move through the semipermeable membrane to make both sides equally concentrated. In other words, water moves from low concentration to high concentration to make both sides equal in concentration. See Figure 3-3, which illustrates the osmotic movement of water and how it can affect cells. Note that isotonic solutions have the same concentration both inside and outside the cell, while a hypertonic solution has a lower concentration of water surrounding the cell and so water leaves the inside of the cell to reach equilibrium (shrinks the cell). Whereas, if a hypotonic solution surrounds the cell, water will rush into the cell to attempt to reach equilibrium, which could result in swelling and bursting of the cell.

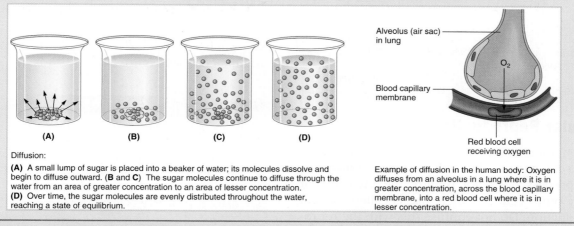

Diffusion:
(A) A small lump of sugar is placed into a beaker of water; its molecules dissolve and begin to diffuse outward. **(B and C)** The sugar molecules continue to diffuse through the water from an area of greater concentration to an area of lesser concentration.
(D) Over time, the sugar molecules are evenly distributed throughout the water, reaching a state of equilibrium.

Example of diffusion in the human body: Oxygen diffuses from an alveolus in a lung where it is in greater concentration, across the blood capillary membrane, into a red blood cell where it is in lesser concentration.

Figure 3-2 *The process of diffusion.*
Source: Delmar/Cengage Learning

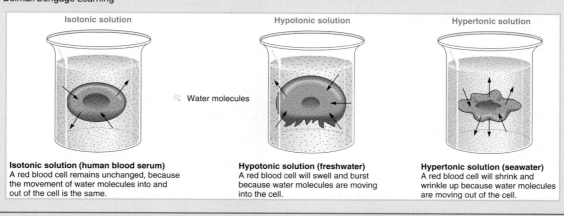

Isotonic solution (human blood serum)
A red blood cell remains unchanged, because the movement of water molecules into and out of the cell is the same.

Hypotonic solution (freshwater)
A red blood cell will swell and burst because water molecules are moving into the cell.

Hypertonic solution (seawater)
A red blood cell will shrink and wrinkle up because water molecules are moving out of the cell.

Figure 3-3 *The process of osmosis.*
Source: Delmar/Cengage Learning

TABLE 3-2
Cellular Structure and Function

CELLULAR STRUCTURE	CELLULAR FUNCTION	ORGANELLE TASKS
Plasma or cell membrane	Structure	Protective covering; allows for semipermeability
Nucleus	Control	Controls most cellular activity and reproduction
Chromatin	Reproduction	Found in nucleus and contains DNA; condenses to form chromosomes, which contain genes
Centrosomes	Reproduction	Contain centrioles, which play a major role in cell division
Nucleolus	Build and repair	Contains ribosomes made of RNA; synthesizes and produces protein
Mitochondria	Energy	Energy powerhouse found throughout cytoplasm
Golgi apparatus	Environmental control	Stores and packages secretions for removal
Lysosomes	Environmental control	Digest old cells and foreign material
Endoplasmic reticulum	Intracellular communication	Network of tubes that facilitates transport of materials in and out of nucleus; synthesizes and stores protein

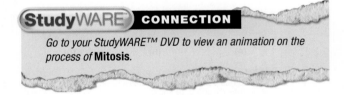

StudyWARE CONNECTION

Watch the **Typical Cell** *animation on your StudyWARE™ DVD.*

QUOTES & NOTES

One never finds life worth living. One always has to make it worth living.

—Harry Emerson

Cellular Reproduction

The ongoing process of replacing identical cells due to damage or cellular death is called **mitosis**. This process does not require the involvement of any other cell, and therefore is called asexual reproduction. Do not confuse this with the reproduction of a human being from sexual reproduction, also known as *meiosis*, which requires two different cells (sperm and egg) and will be covered in the Reproductive chapter.

Mitosis requires the replication of the genetic material (DNA) which is bundled in packages known as *chromosomes.* Chromosomes carry all the instruction for a cell and each new cell must have a copy of those instructions. When a cell is ready to divide, it first duplicates its chromosomes, and then enters into mitosis, which consists of four phases:

1. *Prophase* (*pro* = before). Here the nucleus disappears in the original cell and the chromosomes become visible. Centrioles separate and spindle fibers form to function as anchor lines.

2. *Metaphase* (*meta* = between). The chromosomes line up in the center of the cell.

3. *Anaphase* (*an* = without). The chromosomes split with the spindle fibers pulling them apart.

4. *Telophase* (*tele* = the end). Here the divided chromosomes go to the far end of the cell. The spindle fibers then begin to disappear, and the two nuclei reappear.

Now we have two identical cells formed from one original cell. See Figure 3-4.

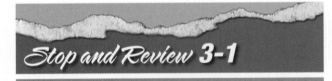

StudyWARE CONNECTION

Go to your StudyWARE™ DVD to view an animation on the process of **Mitosis.**

Stop and Review 3-1

The cell is often called the building block of life. It, therefore, should have several similarities to the finished product, or, in our case, the human body. See how many of the cellular structures can be related to the human organism. For example, the nucleus can be related to the brain and the cell membrane to the skin. Think of some more examples and describe the relationships. This will help you to truly understand cellular components and their functions.

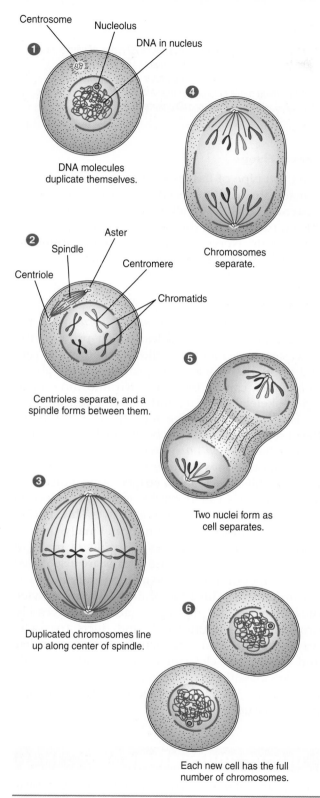

Figure 3-4   *The stages of mitosis. (1) Chromosome duplication. (2) Prophase. (3) Metaphase. (4) Anaphase. (5) Telophase. (6) Two new identical cells.*
Source: Delmar/Cengage Learning

Tissues

As stated earlier, a grouping of similar cells can form tissues that will have specialized functions in the human body. This section will discuss the various tissues that comprise the human body and the purposes they serve.

The Building Layers

If you wanted to construct a wall to cover a house, you would naturally need more than one brick to form the layers of the wall. The same is true of the human body. In order to form different types of layers, the body must combine similar cells together. Cells that are alike will join together to form **tissues**.

Before going further into the discussion of tissues, it is important to note that not all cells form tissues. Some cells, instead, remain "free floating." Examples of this type of cell include the red and white blood cells in our bloodstreams. However, many cells of a common type do combine to form tissues. The four main groups of tissues formed are epithelial, connective, nerve, and muscle.

Specific Tissue Types

Specific types of tissue include epithelial, connective, nerve, and muscle tissue.

Epithelial Tissue

Epithelial tissue is the type of tissue found in the skin that envelops the body. It also lines body cavities and organs such as the lungs and intestines and forms the glands in our bodies.

There are two types of epithelial tissue: **epithelium** and **endothelium**. Epithelium (*epi* meaning "outer") is the specialized type of epithelial tissue that covers the outside of the body. The skin is an example of epithelium tissue. Endothelium (*endo* meaning "within") is the specialized type of epithelial tissue that forms the lining of internal organs and blood vessels.

Connective Tissue

The primary purposes of **connective tissue** are support and protection. There are two types of connective tissue: *soft connective tissue*, which is also called adipose or fatty tissue, and *hard connective tissue*, which forms cartilage and bone.

Soft connective, or fatty, tissue serves several functions. This tissue stores fat, which can be used as an energy reserve if needed. In addition, soft tissue acts to pad our bodies, thus absorbing shocks and helping to maintain body heat by way of insulation properties. Finally, soft connective tissue holds together and connects various body parts and, thus, can be considered fibrous connective tissue. Ligaments and tendons are also examples of this type of tissue.

Hard tissue is bone and **cartilage**. Cartilage is the tough, semirigid yet elastic material found in the nose, ears, and voice box. The "Adam's apple" is a laryngeal cartilage that helps protect the "windpipe" from injury, such as a crushing blow, that could cut off air to the lungs. The flexibility of this cartilage also facilitates the process of swallowing. Although similar to cartilage, bone does have distinct differences. Whereas cartilage has some "give," bone is rigid; and bone has calcium salts, nerves, and blood vessels as part of its makeup, whereas cartilage does not.

Figure 3-5 shows types of epithelial tissue and connective tissue.

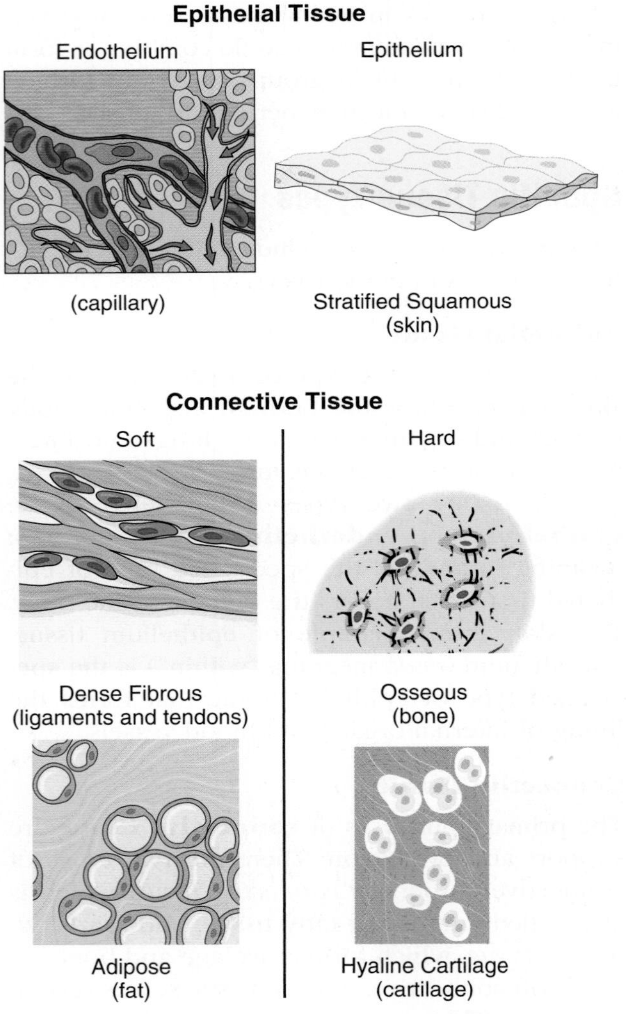

Epithelial Tissue

Endothelium   Epithelium

(capillary)   Stratified Squamous (skin)

Connective Tissue

Soft   Hard

Dense Fibrous (ligaments and tendons)   Osseous (bone)

Adipose (fat)   Hyaline Cartilage (cartilage)

Figure 3-5   *Types of epithelial and connective tissue.*
Source: Delmar/Cengage Learning

Nerve Tissue

The third type of tissue is *nerve tissue*. This tissue is made up of the specialized nerve cells called **neurons**. This tissue allows messages to be conducted to and from the brain and throughout the entire body. Nerve tissue is, of course, found in the nervous system, which comprises the brain, spinal cord, and various nerves.

Muscle Tissue

The final type of tissue is *muscle tissue*. This tissue composes your muscles, which produce the necessary movement that allows you to walk, run, and do work. Muscle tissue, which has the ability to contract, can be broken down into three main types: skeletal, cardiac, and smooth. *Skeletal muscle* is responsible for the movement of the body. Because this muscle can be controlled at will, it is classified as *voluntary muscle*. Skeletal muscles attach to our bones in order to accomplish motion. Because this muscle has a striped appearance, it is also sometimes called *striated muscle*. The second type of muscle tissue is *cardiac muscle*. This specialized tissue causes the heart to beat. Finally, there is smooth muscle, which lines the walls of many of our internal organs. Because organs are also called *viscera*, smooth muscle is sometimes referred to as *visceral muscle*. This type of muscle helps provide movement in the digestive tract, blood vessels, bronchial vessels (airways), and ducts (passageways) leading from the glands. Because cardiac and smooth muscles cannot be controlled at will, they are classified as *involuntary muscles*.

Figure 3-6 shows types of nerve tissue and muscle tissue.

Organs and Systems

Groupings of specialized tissues can now form organs that have specific functions within the human body. This section will discuss the various organs and describe their relationship to the system where they are contained. Additional or accessory structures needed for systems to fully function will also be covered.

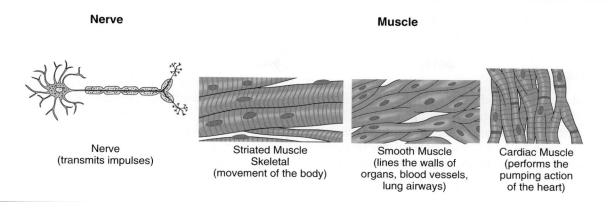

Figure 3-6 *Types of nerve tissue and muscle tissue.*
Source: Delmar/Cengage Learning

Organs

Just as cells combine to form tissues, tissues combine to form organs. The body has several organs, such as the heart, liver, kidneys, and lungs, each of which is made up of specialized tissues that help the organ to perform its given task or tasks.

Each body organ has a specific function or functions. For example, the heart is the main organ of the **cardiovascular** (*cardio* meaning "heart," *vascular* meaning "blood vessels") **system**; the heart performs the function of pumping blood throughout the blood vessels in the body. Figure 3-7 shows the major organs of the digestive system.

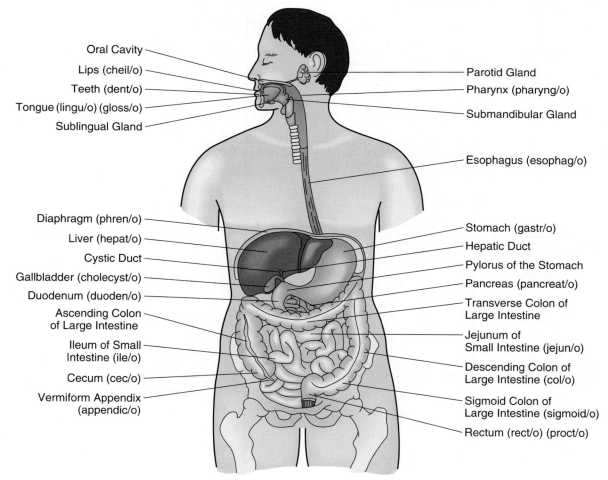

Figure 3-7 *The major organs of the GI system.*
Source: Delmar/Cengage Learning

(Organs and their specific functions are explored in greater detail in later chapters.)

Systems

The heart pumps blood, but without blood vessels, the blood would have nowhere to go. The master control organ, or brain, would be useless without nerves to send and receive messages. Just as a furnace in a house does not constitute a heating "system" until you add the necessary accessories (such as electricity, a thermostat, and heat circulation materials), organs need additional parts to form a complete system. Specific organs and the needed accessories form systems that have definite functions. Table 3-3 lists the body systems and their major functions, along with the major organs and accessory structures contained within each system. Medical terminology associated with the major components is also provided. Figure 3-8 shows the systems of the human body.

TABLE 3-3
Body Systems

BODY SYSTEM	MAJOR FUNCTIONS	MAJOR COMPONENTS
Integumentary	Protection, temperature regulation	Skin (*cutane/o* or *dermat/o*)
		Sebaceous glands (*seb/o*)
		Sweat glands (*hidr/o*)
		Hair (*pil/o*)
		Nails (*ungu/o*)
		Breasts (*mamm/o* or *mast/o*)
Skeletal	Support and protection, produces RBCs for oxygenation	Bones (*oste/o*)
		Joints (*arthr/o*)
		Cartilage (*chondr/o*)
Muscular	Movement of the body and its internal fluids	Muscles (*my/o*)
		Tendons (*tendin/o*)
Nervous	Control and coordination; receives input (sensory) and transmits output for appropriate responses	Nerves (*neur/o*)
		Brain (*encephal/o*)
		Spinal cord (*myel/o*)
		Eyes (*ophthalm/o*)
		Ears (*ot/o*)
Endocrine	Growth; sexual development; maintaining internal body metabolism	Adrenals (*adren/o*)
		Pancreas (*pancreat/o*)
		Pineal
		Pituitary
		Thyroid and parathyroids (*thyroid/o* or *thyr/o*)
		Thymus (*thym/o*)
		Gonads (*gonad/o*)
Respiratory	Oxygenation and excretion of carbon dioxide	Nose (*nas/o* or *rhin/o*)
		Pharynx (*pharyng/o*)
		Larynx (*laryng/o*)
		Trachea (*trache/o*)
		Lungs (*pneum/o*)
		Bronchi
		Alveoli

(continues)

TABLE 3-3 (*continued*)

Cardiovascular	Supplies oxygen and other nutrients to the body	Heart (*cardi/o*)
		Arteries (*arteri/o*)
		Veins (*ven/o* or *phleb/o*)
		Blood (*hem/o* or *hemat/o*)
		Red blood cells (RBCs) (*erythr/o*)
Lymphatic	Defense; breaks down RBCs	White blood cells (WBCs) (*leuk/o*)
		Lymph vessels and nodes (*lymph/o*)
		Spleen (*splen/o*)
		Tonsils (*tonsil/o*)
Gastrointestinal	Digestion; absorption of food nutrients; elimination of solid waste	Mouth (*or/o*)
		Esophagus (*esophag/o*)
		Stomach (*gastr/o*)
		Small intestine (*enter/o*)
		Large intestine (*col/o*)
		Liver (*hepat/o*)
		Bile (*chol/o*)
		Gallbladder (*cholecyst/o*)
Urinary	Formation and elimination of urine; water balance	Kidneys (*nephr/o* or *ren/o*)
		Ureters (*ureter/o*)
		Urinary bladder (*cyst/o*)
		Urethra (*urethr/o*)
Reproductive	Production of life	Testes (*orchid/o*)
		Ovaries (*ovari/o*)
		Uterus (*hyster/o*)
		Fallopian tubes (*salping/o*)

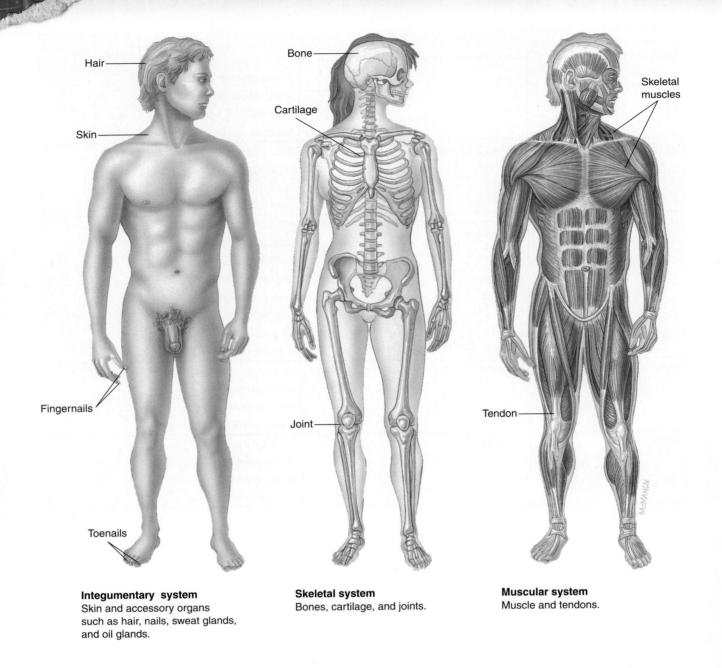

Integumentary system
Skin and accessory organs
such as hair, nails, sweat glands,
and oil glands.

Skeletal system
Bones, cartilage, and joints.

Muscular system
Muscle and tendons.

Figure 3-8   *(A) The integumentary, skeletal, and muscular systems of the body.*

Source: Delmar/Cengage Learning

(continued)

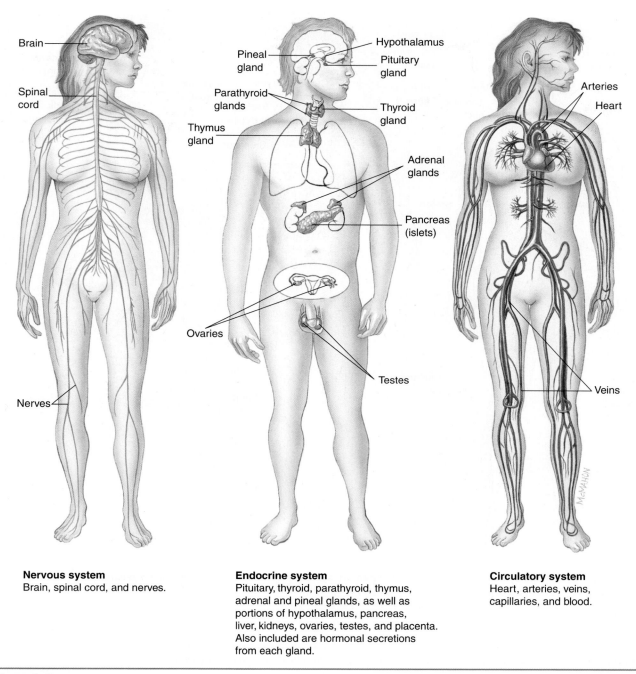

Nervous system
Brain, spinal cord, and nerves.

Endocrine system
Pituitary, thyroid, parathyroid, thymus,
adrenal and pineal glands, as well as
portions of hypothalamus, pancreas,
liver, kidneys, ovaries, testes, and placenta.
Also included are hormonal secretions
from each gland.

Circulatory system
Heart, arteries, veins,
capillaries, and blood.

Figure 3-8   *(B) The nervous, endocrine, and cardiovascular systems of the body.*
Source: Delmar/Cengage Learning

(*continued*)

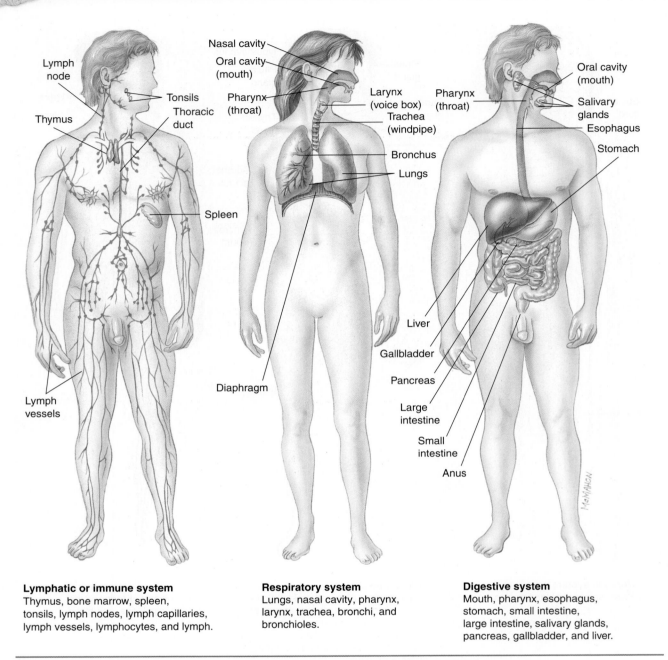

Lymphatic or immune system
Thymus, bone marrow, spleen,
tonsils, lymph nodes, lymph capillaries,
lymph vessels, lymphocytes, and lymph.

Respiratory system
Lungs, nasal cavity, pharynx,
larynx, trachea, bronchi, and
bronchioles.

Digestive system
Mouth, pharynx, esophagus,
stomach, small intestine,
large intestine, salivary glands,
pancreas, gallbladder, and liver.

Figure 3-8   *(C) The lymphatic, respiratory, and gastrointestinal systems of the body.*
Source: Delmar/Cengage Learning

(continued)

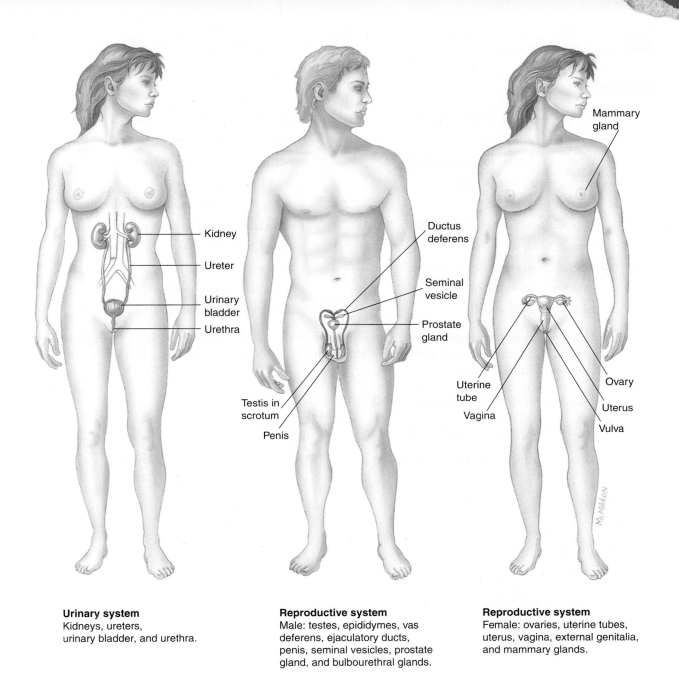

Urinary system
Kidneys, ureters,
urinary bladder, and urethra.

Reproductive system
Male: testes, epididymes, vas
deferens, ejaculatory ducts,
penis, seminal vesicles, prostate
gland, and bulbourethral glands.

Reproductive system
Female: ovaries, uterine tubes,
uterus, vagina, external genitalia,
and mammary glands.

Figure 3-8   *(D) The urinary and reproductive systems of the body.*

Source: Delmar/Cengage Learning

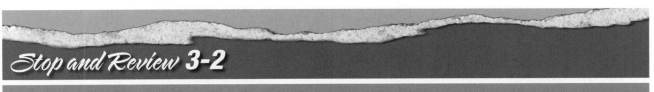

Stop and Review 3-2

What type of cells, tissues, and organs would you expect to find in the digestive system?

■ CHAPTER REVIEW

Exercises

1. Provide the term that best fits each of the following descriptions concerning the cell.

   a. "small organs"

   b. network of tubular structures that facilitates transport of materials in and out of the cell

   c. contain a digestive enzyme to help remove debris

   d. the energy powerhouse of the cell

   e. the cell brain or control center

   f. the blueprint of the cell

   g. the outermost layer of the cell

   h. helps in cellular absorption of larger protein and lipid molecules

   i. what the chromatin eventually forms

   j. structure found within the nucleus; provides raw material for cellular growth and reproduction

   k. structure responsible for storing and packaging cellular material

2. Write three separate paragraphs comparing cellular structure or function to that of your home environment. For example, one paragraph can compare your home's garbage disposal system to that of the cell. Think of two more.

3. List the four main groups of tissues found in the body.

4. What are the two types of epithelial tissue?

5. Of the answers to question 4, list which type will be found in each of the following:

   a. stomach

   b. glands

   c. blood vessels

   d. skin

6. Adipose tissue is:

   a. fat storage tissue

   b. muscle tissue

   c. transport tissue

   d. voluntary tissue

7. Hard connective tissue comprises:

   a. bone and cartilage

   b. ligaments and joints

   c. adipose or fatty tissue

   d. lymph and cardiac

8. Specialized nerve cells:

   a. are called neurons

   b. help to conduct messages

   c. are found in the brain and spinal cord

   d. all of the above

9. The type of muscle tissue responsible for movement of the body is:

   a. cardiac

   b. skeletal

   c. smooth

   d. nervous

10. The type of muscle that provides movement within the digestive system is:

    a. cardiac

    b. skeletal

    c. smooth

    d. endocrine

11. Using Table 3-3, list each system, develop 10 new medical terms per system, and provide a corresponding definition for each term. *Hint:* A medical dictionary will facilitate this project.

12. Contrast the various phases of mitosis.

Real Life Issues and Applications

An Ethical Question Concerning Organ Donation

A 52-year-old chronic alcoholic who was recently jailed for drunken driving has just been involved in an automobile accident where a father and his three young daughters were killed. Their mother has a severe head injury and most likely will be in a vegetative state forever. The alcoholic sustained severe liver damage and requires a transplant to save his life. Should the chronic alcoholic be a candidate for receiving an organ donation? What are the ethical arguments for and against this decision?

Additional Activities

1. A bill in your state legislature would automatically designate each licensed driver as an organ donor if killed in a car accident. Discuss your opinion regarding this type of legislation.

2. Write a paragraph about each body system, comparing the system to something outside of the body. For example, the skin can be compared to the earth's protective atmosphere in several ways. Your home or car can also be used. Be creative; it will help you to truly understand the body systems.

Downloadable audio is available for selected medical terms in this chapter to enhance your learning of medical language.

StudyWARE® CONNECTION

Go to your StudyWARE™ DVD and have fun learning as you play interactive games, view animations and videos, and take practice tests to help reinforce key concepts you learned in this chapter.

Workbook Practice   *Go to your Workbook for more practice questions and activities.*

CHAPTER 4

THE INTEGUMENTARY SYSTEM

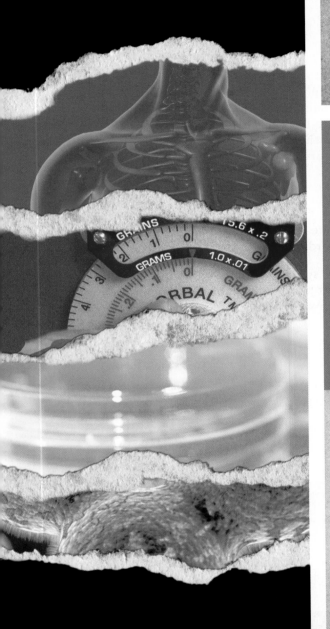

Objectives

Upon completion of this chapter, you should be able to

- Name the various components of the integumentary system

- List the functions of the integumentary system

- Discuss the terms associated with the disease process

- Relate medical terms and diseases of the integumentary system

Key Terms

acute disease
chronic disease
cicatrix (sih-**KAY**-tricks)
comedo (**KOM** ah doh)
contusion (kon-**TOO**-zhun)
core temperature
dermatitis
dermis (**DER**-mis)
diagnosis (dye-ag-**NO**-sis)
ecchymosis (eck-eh-**MOH**-sis)
endotoxins
epidermis (ep-ih-**DER**-mis)
etiology (ee-tee-**ALL**-oh-jee)
follicles (**FALL**-ih-kolz)
homeostasis
   (**HOH** me oh **STAY** sis)
hypermetabolism

hypothalamus
   (**HIGH** poh **THAL** ah mus)
idiopathic disease
   (ID-ee-oh-**PATH**-ic)
integumentary system
   (in-**TEG**-you-MEN-tair-ee)
keloid (**KEE**-loid)
keratin (**KER**-ah-tin)
laceration
   (**LASS** eh **RAY** shun)
latent disease
local infection
lunula (**LOO**-new-lah)
lymph vessels
nevus (**NEE** nus)
pathogen (**PATH**-o-jen)
pathology

(continues)

perfused
petechiae (pee-tee-**KEE**-ee)
prognosis (prog-**NO**-sis)
pruritus (proo-**RYE**-tus)
pyrogens (**PYE**-roh-genz)
rectal
remission
sebaceous gland (seh-**BAY**-shus)
squamous cells (**SKWAY**-mus)

subacute disease
subcutaneous fascia
    (sub-kyou-**TAY**-nee-us **FASH**-
    ee-ah)
sudoriferous glands
    (su-dor-**IF**-er-us)
systemic infection
tachycardia (tack-ee-**KAR**-dee-ah)
tachypnea (tah-**KIP**-nee-ah)

transdermal
urticaria (er-tih-**KAY**-ree-uh)
vascularization
    (vas-ku-lair-I-**ZAY**-shun)
vascularize
vasoconstrict
vasoconstriction
vasodilation
vital signs

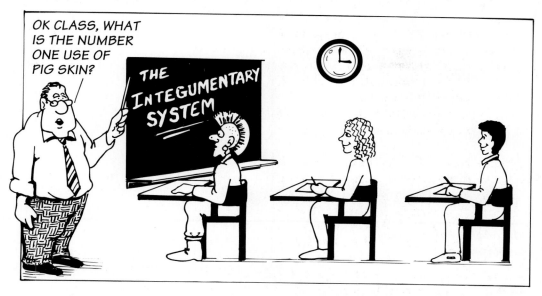

Source: Delmar/Cengage Learning

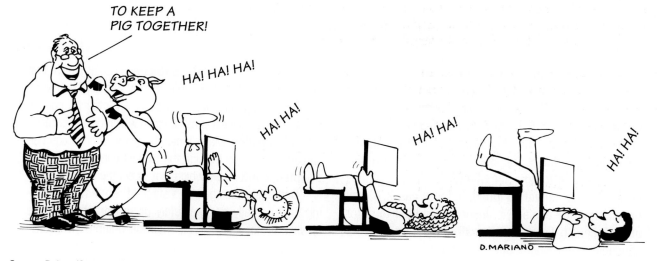

Source: Delmar/Cengage Learning

■ SYSTEM OVERVIEW

The outer surface of your body is normally covered by a layer of specialized cells known as skin. Your skin can be compared to the siding, stone, or bricks that cover your home. Just as the main purpose of siding, stone, or bricks is to provide protection for the insides of a building, skin helps maintain a safe internal environment for the rest of your body. Skin is a part of the **integumentary system** (from the Latin word meaning "a covering"), which also includes your fingernails, toenails, hair, **sebaceous** (oil) **glands**, **sudoriferous** (sweat) **glands**, and breasts (see Figure 4-1).

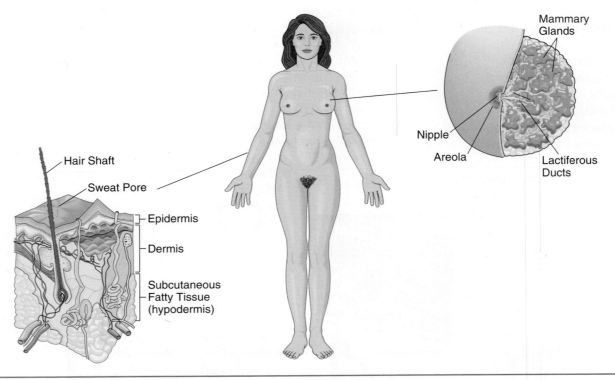

Figure 4-1   *The integumentary system.*
Source: Delmar/Cengage Learning

Special Focus

Disease Terminology

Because each chapter on the body systems includes a discussion of some of the major diseases that affect the system, a basic understanding of the terms relating to disease is warranted. **Pathology** is the study of diseases, including the structural and functional changes they cause. The study of the origin of a disease is called **etiology**. Sometimes the origin or cause of the disease cannot be found; in these cases, it may be said that the etiology is unknown. Another term for an untraceable disease is **idiopathic disease**. Until the causative agent was found, Legionaires' disease was considered an idiopathic disease.

A disease can be generally classified according to its severity and duration. An **acute disease** is usually severe but short in duration. A **chronic disease** will continue or progress over long periods of time. **Subacute diseases** fall somewhere between chronic diseases and acute diseases in terms of severity and duration.

As already discussed, a **pathogen** is an organism that can cause a disease. An infection is said to exist when harmful pathogens invade the body. An infection can be confined to a relatively small area, in which case it is called a **local infection**. Many times, however, an infection can spread, particularly through the bloodstream, and result in a **systemic infection**, which may affect the whole body.

Some diseases go into a stage of **remission**, meaning they partially or completely disappear. Although the disease is not active, it still has the potential to "come back"; thus it is referred to as a **latent disease**.

Finally, determining treatment for an illness or disease requires a **diagnosis**. The health care provider arrives at this conclusion by way of assessing the patient's signs and symptoms, history, chief complaints, and so on. When a diagnosis is made, treatment or therapy is instituted. How well the patient is expected to do is termed the **prognosis**. Hopefully, your prognosis for learning anatomy and physiology is excellent.

Functions of the Integumentary System

Your skin and the integumentary system in general serve important functions. The integumentary system protects your body from the introduction of germs, or pathogens, that can cause disease. It also protects your body from drying out by maintaining water to keep tissue deeper down in your body hydrated. Your skin and many of its parts also allow for sensory perception. The nerve endings in the skin let you feel pain, pleasurable sensations, pressure, and varying degrees of temperature. See Figure 4-2.

The integumentary system is a storage area for fatty tissue that is used for energy. Your skin (with a little help from sunshine) creates vitamin D. Vitamin D is important because it helps your body to utilize phosphorus and calcium. Both of these substances are necessary for proper growth and maintenance of the bones in your body.

In addition, the integumentary system regulates your body temperature. The maintenance of a fairly constant body temperature is one example of the very important physiologic concept of **homeostasis**. Homeostasis is the body's ability to maintain a normal state despite internal and external forces attempting to alter this state. Temperature, pulse, respiration, blood pressure, and various body chemical components are all maintained within narrow homeostatic ranges by your nervous and endocrine systems in order for the body to survive.

Temperature regulation is accomplished by changes in the size of the blood vessels in your skin. If you need to lose heat in order to cool off, the blood vessels get larger in diameter. This is known as **vasodilation** (*vaso* meaning "vessel," *dilation* meaning "enlargement"). In this way, more of your blood is exposed to the surrounding environment, which is usually cooler than the temperature of your body, and thus, more blood can lose heat through the skin. In addition to vasodilation, sweat glands in your skin excrete water and waste products, such as nitrogenous wastes and sodium chloride, onto the skin's surface in the form of sweat. It is not unusual to find 3,000 sweat glands per square inch of skin! Once on the surface, sweat evaporates, causing cooling.

If you are cold and need to warm up, the blood vessels in your skin get smaller in diameter (**vasoconstriction**) so that more body heat is retained. Muscles in the skin (*arrector pili*) that are attached to hair **follicles** constrict, and thus make the hair stand up straight, resulting in goose bumps. This erect hair traps a layer of noncirculating (stagnant) air right above the skin, which acts as dead air space. Dead air is nonmoving air, and, as a result, does not transfer or remove heat. Thus, this dead air space insulates your skin from the colder surrounding air. This works much the same way as goose down (feathers) provides warmth in winter jackets by creating dead air space between you and the cold winter winds.

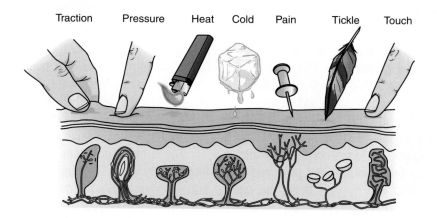

Traction   Pressure   Heat   Cold   Pain   Tickle   Touch

Figure 4-2 *Examples of different skin sensations.*
Source: Delmar/Cengage Learning

One important feature of the skin recently capitalized on by medicine is the skin's ability to absorb substances. Certain medications can be administered via patches placed on the skin. The skin slowly absorbs chemicals from the patch. (This method of administering medication through skin patches is called **transdermal** [*trans* meaning "across," *dermal* meaning "pertaining to the skin"] drug administration.) Slow absorption is advantageous when you want to spread out the release of medication to the body over a long period of time. You may have heard of the patch worn behind the ear for motion sickness, or of the chest or arm patch worn by patients with certain heart conditions. Chest pain due to cardiac problems is termed *angina pectoris* and results from lack of oxygen to the heart muscle. Nitrogylcerine vasodilates the coronary arteries that supply the heart with needed oxygen. Nitrogylcerine patches can help treat this condition by providing a constant level of this drug throughout the day (see Figure 4-3).

One of the most popular patches today is the nicotine patch worn by people who are trying to quit smoking. The medication released by this patch helps satisfy the addiction to the nicotine found in cigarettes without having to smoke and inhale thousands of other toxic chemicals. A secondary benefit of this patch is that it is making the air cleaner for others to breathe. Of course, any person using this patch must eventually be weaned from the need for the medication provided by the patch.

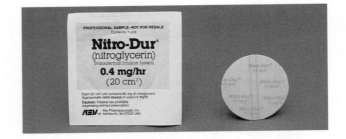

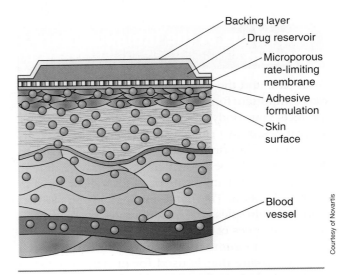

Backing layer
Drug reservoir
Microporous rate-limiting membrane
Adhesive formulation
Skin surface
Blood vessel

Courtesy of Novartis

Figure 4-3   *Nitro-Dur is an example of a transdermal patch containing a reservoir of nitroglycerine, a rate-controlling membrane to control absorption by the skin, and an adhesive layer.*
Source: Delmar/Cengage Learning

Clinical Relevancy

The Vital Sign of Temperature

Much can be learned from words. For example, **vital signs** are just that—signs that are vital to life. They show the overall status of the body. The major vital signs that are monitored include body temperature, heart rate (or pulse), respiration, and blood pressure.

Let's take a more in-depth look at the vital sign of temperature. As previously stated, the skin plays a major role in regulating body temperature. Body temperature is a balance between the heat produced by your body and the heat lost by your body. You can view your body as a house, or the proverbial temple if you wish. House temperature is dependent on several

factors such as insulation and construction materials, the heating system, and the outside weather conditions. The temperature of a house is controlled at a narrow range by a thermostat. If the inside temperature drops below the desired thermostatic setting, the furnace turns on and supplies more heat until the desired temperature is again established.

The human body does the same thing using different equipment. The **hypothalamus**, located in the brain, is your body's thermostatic control. It maintains the body at a narrow temperature range, normally 97.7–99.5°F. This range may fluctuate according to

(continues)

(continued)

hormonal variations, or what is called your *diurnal rhythm*. Typically your temperature is highest between 8:00 P.M. and 11:00 P.M. and lowest between 4:00 A.M. and 6:00 A.M. Have you ever noticed that many times your temperature will rise right before bedtime?

Fever is a disease-induced elevation of body temperature to greater than 100.5°F orally or 101.5°F rectally. **Rectal** temperature is 1°F higher because it more closely reflects body **core temperature**. Fever is most frequently caused by bacterial **pyrogens** (*pyro* meaning "fire" or "heat," *gen* meaning "producing"), which produce **endotoxins**. Endotoxins cause the hypothalamus to increase its body temperature setting. This condition, called *hyperthermia*, leads to faster breathing (**tachypnea**) and increased heart rate (**tachycardia**). Faster breathing is needed in order to ingest more oxygen from the atmosphere, which helps the body in this stressful period of increased work (**hypermetabolism**). The faster heart rate delivers much-needed oxygen to the tissues to maintain the metabolism and functioning of the body.

When a patient complains of a chill, it usually indicates a rapid rise in temperature. The reason for this is simple. The hypothalamus is sending signals to increase the temperature or turn up the thermostat. In order to increase heat within the body, the hypothalamus does two things. First, it causes the blood vessels in the peripheral areas of the arms and legs to constrict. Because much heat is lost in these areas, the body **vasoconstricts** (makes the tubes smaller) to minimize heat loss through the skin. This redirects more of the warmer blood to the central areas of the body. As a result, we feel cold in the peripheral areas and begin to shiver.

Second, the hypothalamus helps to increase body metabolism. This also produces extra heat to maintain the higher temperature setting. The reason the body shivers is that this process causes the muscles to become hyperactive and, therefore, produces heat for the body to increase its temperature. The vital signs are discussed in greater detail within their corresponding system chapters.

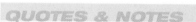

QUOTES & NOTES

Your skin weighs twice as much as your brain!

StudyWARE CONNECTION

Go to your StudyWARE™ DVD to view videos on **The Importance of Vital Signs** *and* **Digital and Electronic Thermometers***.*

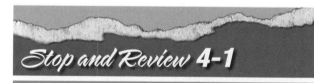

Stop and Review **4-1**

Describe how the integumentary system is vital in regulation of body temperature.

The Skin

The skin has several structures that support its vast array of functions. These structures along with their physiologic functions and purposes will now be discussed.

Structures of the Skin

Skin is composed of three main layers of tissue: (1) the epidermis, (2) the dermis, and (3) the subcutaneous fascia (Figure 4-4). The **epidermis** (*epi* meaning "upon," *dermis* meaning "true skin") is the outermost layer. This layer of skin is composed of even smaller layers of tissue. There are no blood vessels or nerve cells in the epidermis. Skin cells from the outer epidermis constantly shed; new cells grow from the innermost regions of the epidermis to take their place. This process is extremely important; in this way the skin can rapidly reproduce cells to repair itself from the damaging effects of climatic exposure, cuts, and abrasions.

The enlarged portion of Figure 4-4 illustrates the constant renewal process of this protective outer barrier. The **squamous cells** (flat, scaly epithelial cells) that make up the skin surface are actually dead cells because they are exposed to damaging environmental factors such as dry wind, heat, cold, and ultraviolet sun rays (the ideal environment for a cell is a wet and lukewarm area, such as the internal body). In fact, the ordinary acts of bathing, drying, dressing, and moving rub off about 500 million squamous cells a day. Just look at the fine white dust that collects in beds. These are collections of

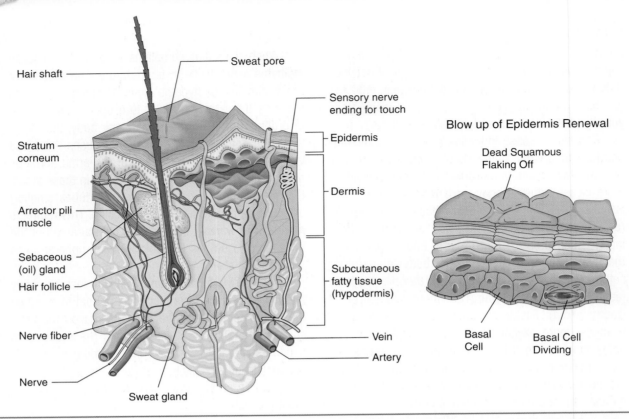

Figure 4-4   *The epidermal layer of the skin. Notice the continual sloughing off and renewal of the epidermal layer. The dead squamous cells make an excellent lunch for dust mites.*
Source: Delmar/Cengage Learning

sloughed off squamous cells. So how and why do we continue to renew this dead layer?

The "why" is simple. From Figure 4-4 it is apparent that these overlapping stacks of squamous cells would eventually form a nearly waterproof seal that would prevent internal fluids from leaking out. The "how" is just a little more complicated. The cells at the base of the layer (basal cells) continually reproduce to make new skin cells. These new cells are pushed away from the basal layer and become flattened as they are "sandwiched" between the basal layer and the skin surface. As they flatten, they slowly die, but they continue to be forced toward the surface, where they eventually replace the squamous cells that are continually flaking off the skin. Thus, your skin is constantly renewing itself by pumping up new cells from the basal layer, which will eventually replace the squamous cells that are worn off the surface.

The second layer from the outer surface of the skin is the **dermis**, which is also known as the corium, or "true" skin. This skin layer is directly beneath the epidermis and contains living tissue, involuntary muscles, tiny blood vessels known as

capillaries, nerve endings, and **lymph vessels**. Lymph vessels are needed to transport fluids from the various tissues of the body back to the blood circulatory system. Hair follicles, sudoriferous (sweat) glands, and sebaceous (oil) glands are also found in this skin layer. Sebaceous glands provide oil, called *sebum,* which normally keeps your skin from drying out. In addition, because sebum is somewhat acidic in nature, it also helps to destroy pathogens on the skin's surface.

The **subcutaneous fascia** (*sub* meaning "below," *cutaneous* meaning "skin," *fascia* meaning "band" or "layer") is the innermost layer of the skin. This layer is composed of elastic as well as fibrous connective tissue. Fatty tissue is also located here. This is the layer that is attached to the muscles underneath the skin.

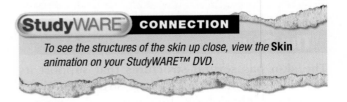

StudyWARE   **CONNECTION**

To see the structures of the skin up close, view the **Skin** *animation on your StudyWARE™ DVD.*

Skin Color

Skin color results from octopus-like cells called *melanocytes*. Melanocytes produce a brown-black pigment called *melanin* and inject this pigment into the basal layer, where skin cells divide. Everyone has approximately the same number of melanocytes; but, obviously, everyone does not have the same skin color. That is because skin shade depends on the level of melanin produced by the melanocytes. A mole is an example of a spot where melanocytes are concentrated in a small area. (A mole can also be a small, furry creature that burrows in the ground; but that's not important for this discussion!)

Sunburn results from the exposure of skin to high-energy ultraviolet rays. The high energy of the rays destroys exposed skin cells at a greater rate and can lead to loss of elasticity of the skin. This is why long-time sun worshipers often have sagging, leathery skin. Melanin helps absorb or trap this energy, thereby minimizing destruction to the skin. Therefore, the less melanin (lighter skin) you have, the greater your risk of damage from sunlight. A suntan, on the other hand, results from the increased production of melanin in an attempt to combat the excessive exposure to sunlight.

Hair and Nails

Hair is a fiber made up mainly of fibrous protein called **keratin.** Special cells in your skin form hair. These shafts of hair are held by sac-like structures known as hair follicles. Interestingly, the cells that make up your hair are dead cells. Imagine what it would be like if your hair was composed of living cells. Each haircut would prove extremely painful!

QUOTES & NOTES

If you counted the hairs on your head, they would probably add up to more than 100,000. Your fingernails are made of the same kind of material as a bull's horn.

Fingernails and toenails are plate-like structures also made up of keratin. Nails can be divided into three main sections: the nail root is located in a groove of the skin on the dermal surface; the nail body is the main part of the nail (the part that you see); and the free edge is the part that you trim. See Figure 4-5.

Fingernails grow about 1 millimeter a week. Growth occurs at the **lunula**. The lunula is the white, half-moon-shaped area on each fingernail. The purpose of fingernails and toenails is to serve as shields for the tips of your fingers and toes; however, they are also great for scratching itches.

Your nails are naturally pink because the tissue underneath is **vascularized** (that is, it contains many blood vessels through which blood flows). Because the nail beds represent the outermost regions of the body (the extremities), it is important to assess how well they are being **perfused** (that is, supplied with nutrients and oxygen as a result of a good blood supply). Blood turns darker, perceived as a bluish tint, when low in oxygen. Blue fingernails, therefore, can be a result of low oxygen levels in the blood and may indicate poor perfusion to the extremities. Perhaps now you understand why we observe the nail beds when looking for cyanosis. (Just make sure your patient doesn't have blue fingernail polish on!)

A quick clinical way of determining how well the extremities are being perfused is by pinching the patient's fingertip and letting go. Watch to see how long it takes for the nail bed to become pink again. The nail beds of poorly perfused individuals will take longer to "pink up" (reperfuse) than those of well-perfused individuals.

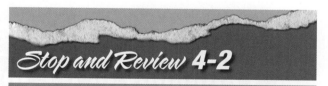

Stop and Review 4-2

Given a cubic centimeter of skin, list the various structures and their functions. Attempt to illustrate the three layers of the skin and their components.

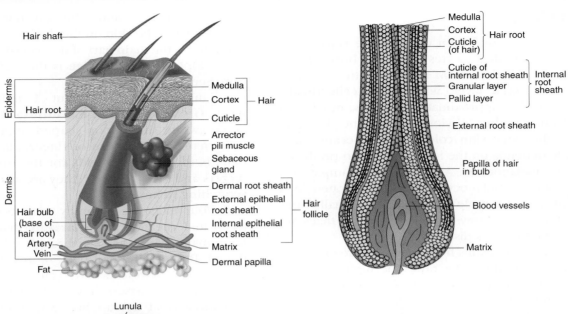

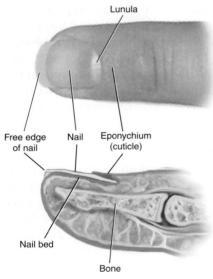

Figure 4-5   *Anatomy of the hair and nail and related structures.*
Source: Delmar/Cengage Learning

Clinical Relevancy

Pathology of the Integumentary System

It is very probable that during your career you will be exposed to terms relating to skin or diseases of the skin. Although this discussion touches on a fraction of the terms commonly used, it is a good starting point.

We have all heard news reports of fire victims suffering various degrees of burns. But what does *first-degree burn* really mean? The severity of a burn is determined by how much of the victim's body is burned, that is, the percentage of body surface area burned. A burn is considered serious if over 15% of the body surface area is affected, and many layers of skin are affected.

A first-degree burn is the least severe burn. No blisters form, but there is a reddening of the outermost

(continues)

(*continued*)

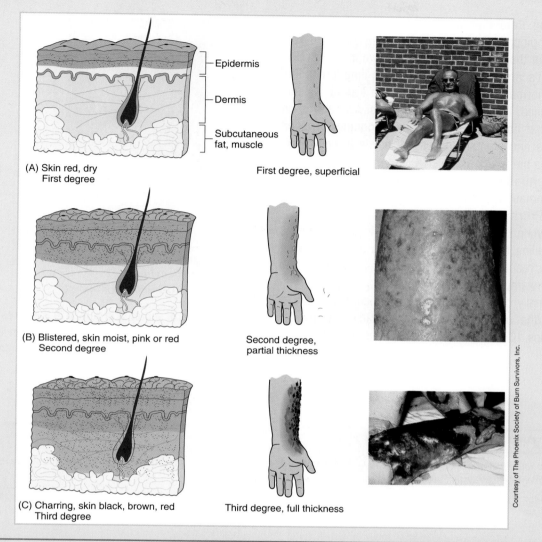

Courtesy of The Phoenix Society of Burn Survivors, Inc.

(A) Skin red, dry
First degree

Epidermis

Dermis

Subcutaneous fat, muscle

First degree, superficial

(B) Blistered, skin moist, pink or red
Second degree

Second degree, partial thickness

(C) Charring, skin black, brown, red
Third degree

Third degree, full thickness

Figure 4-6 *Examples of varying degrees of burns.*

Source: Delmar/Cengage Learning

epidermal layer. The victim may feel discomfort or pain, and there may be some mild swelling. A typical example of a first-degree burn is a sunburn. A second-degree burn is more severe. Blistering and swelling occur and there is damage to the epidermis and the dermis. The damage is not severe enough, however, to prevent regeneration of the skin. A third-degree burn is the most severe burn. It involves damage to every layer of skin as well as injury to the tissue below the skin. In some cases, growth cells may be destroyed. Fourth-degree burns penetrate to the bone and other underlying structures. See Figure 4-6. A newer classification includes first- and second-degree burns as "partial-thickness burns,"

while third- and fourth-degree burns are classified as "full-thickness" burns.

There are other important terms related to skin injuries. A laceration is a jagged opening or wound of the skin. It is not as smooth a wound as a cut or incision. Contusions are injuries that don't break the skin open. A contusion results in swelling and discoloration as well as pain or discomfort. (Think of the "goose egg" you may have gotten when you were younger and bumped heads with someone on the playground; that bump was actually a contusion.) An ecchymosis is the black-and-blue mark you get when you bump into a hard object. There is discoloration with no

(*continues*)

(*continued*)

swelling. **Petechiae** are tiny purple bruise marks the size of pinpoints. A scar that is normally formed as a result of the healing process is known as a **cicatrix**. Normal scars are red or purple and in time turn white. An abnormal scar growth is called a **keloid**. Keloids are raised, thick, and firm structures. A **nevus** is an area that has more than the usual number of blood vessels and pigmented cells. A nevus is commonly called a birthmark or mole.

Dermatitis (*derma* meaning "skin," *itis* meaning "inflammation") is a general term for skin inflammations. **Pruritus** is the term used for the itching sensation, while **urticaria**, or hives, are localized regions of swelling that itch. Hives are often associated with allergic reactions to bee stings or drugs. See Figure 4-7 for an example of a child with urticaria.

Finally, **comedo**, also known as the dreaded blackhead (the unfortunate teenage malady that usually develops 10 minutes before your date arrives), results

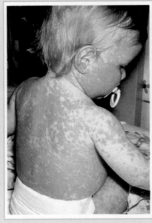

Courtesy of Robert A. Silverman, M.D., Pediatric Dermatology, Georgetown University.

Figure 4-7 *An example of urticaria.*
Source: Delmar/Cengage Learning

from a buildup of sebum and keratin in the pores of your skin. See Figure 4-8 which shows various skin lesions.

(*continues*)

StudyWARE CONNECTION

*Go to your StudyWARE™ DVD and view videos on **Bites, Burns, and Injuries**, and **Lacerations and Puncture Wounds** as related to the integumentary system. Also, view the animation on **Tissue Repair**.*

(continued)

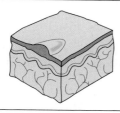 A **papule** is a small solid raised lesion that is less than 0.5 cm in diameter.

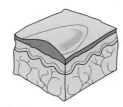 A **plaque** is a solid raised lesion that is greater than 0.5 cm in diameter.

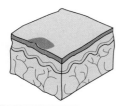 A **macule** is a flat discolored lesion that is less than 1 cm in diameter.

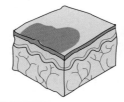 A **patch** is a flat discolored lesion that is greater than 1 cm in diameter.

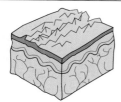 A **scale** is a flaking or dry patch made up of excess dead epidermal cells.

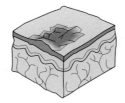 A **crust** is a collection of dried serum and cellular debris.

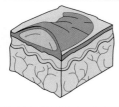 A **wheal** is a smooth, slightly elevated swollen area that is redder or paler than the surrounding skin. It is usually accompanied by itching.

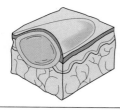 A **cyst** is a closed sack or pouch containing fluid or semisolid material.

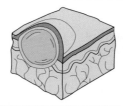 A **pustule** is a small circumscribed elevation of the skin containing pus.

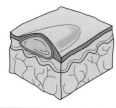 A **vesicle** is a circumscribed elevation of skin containing fluid that is less than 0.5 cm in diameter.

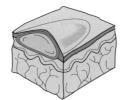 A **bulla** is a large vesicle that is more than 0.5 cm in diameter.

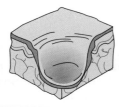 An **ulcer** is an open sore or erosion of the skin or mucous membrane resulting in tissue loss.

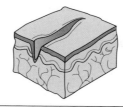 A **fissure** of the skin is a groove or crack-like sore.

Figure 4-8 *Examples of various skin lesions.*
Source: Delmar/Cengage Learning

■ CHAPTER REVIEW

Exercises

1. Provide the correct term for each of the following descriptions:

   a. germs, or what can cause disease

   b. blood vessels increasing in diameter

   c. what your blood vessels do when your body needs to conserve heat

   d. the outermost layer of skin

   e. another name for sudoriferous glands

   f. secretes sebum to keep the skin from dehydrating

   g. where fingernail growth occurs

   h. well supplied with blood

   i. inflammation of the skin

   j. hives

2. What is the most severe type of burn?

   a. first-degree

   b. second-degree

   c. third-degree

   d. fourth-degree

3. What is another term for a birthmark?

   a. laceration

   b. nevus

   c. keloid

   d. petechiae

4. A tiny, pinpoint, purple bruise mark on the skin is called a:

   a. laceration

   b. nevus

   c. keloid

   d. petechiae

5. A raised, thick growth resulting from a scar is called a:

   a. laceration

   b. nevus

   c. keloid

   d. petechiae

6. A jagged skin wound or opening is called a:

   a. contusion

   b. ecchymosis

   c. cicatrix

   d. laceration

7. What is the main purpose of sudoriferous glands?

8. List and give examples of the responsibilities of the integumentary system.

9. What is the fibrous protein that forms your hair?

10. Why do your fingernails normally appear pink?

Real Life Issues and Applications

Beauty Is More than Skin Deep

In a small but up-to-date community hospital, you care for a 17-year-old patient. This patient is very attractive, musically talented, and an excellent student. She has won many local and state competitions by way of her beauty and talent and has just received a full music scholarship to a prestigious university. An entertainment career was almost certain. However, she was severely burned in an accident; as a result, she is horribly scarred and her hands are severely injured. Years of extensive therapy may be necessary if there is to be even any hope of normal function returning to her hands.

Over the past several months, you and this patient have become very close. She has confided in you on numerous occasions and has responded to you better than to anyone else in the hospital. Recently, she has seemed quieter and more introverted than usual. When you ask her how she is doing, she looks you straight in the eyes and calmly states, "I can't stand it any longer. You are the only friend I can trust. Look at me; my future is ruined. As soon as I get out of here, I'm going to kill myself. Please don't say a word to anyone."

What would you do next? Would you tell anyone else? Would you break the trust she has placed in you?

Additional Activities

1. Contact a dermatologist and request information on diseases of the skin. Pick one disease and write a short report concerning the disease.

2. List several methods of protecting and caring for your "birthday suit."

3. Research the breakdown of the atmosphere's ozone layer, and pollution in general, and the possible impact of these things on the integumentary system. Discuss your findings with the class.

4. Discuss the social implications of skin disease. How much of an impact has advertising made?

 Downloadable audio is available for selected medical terms in this chapter to enhance your learning of medical language.

StudyWARE CONNECTION

Go to your StudyWARE™ DVD and have fun learning as you play interactive games, view animations and videos, and take practice tests to help reinforce key concepts you learned in this chapter.

Workbook Practice *Go to your Workbook for more practice questions and activities.*

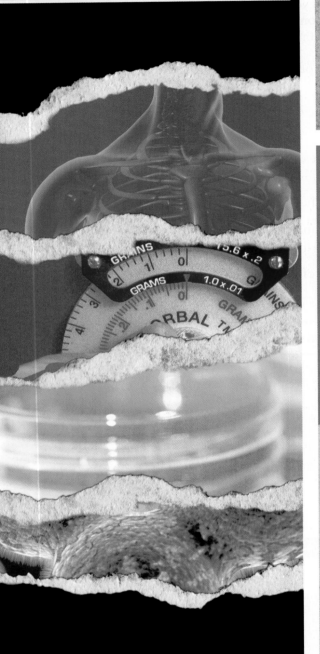

CHAPTER 5

THE SKELETAL SYSTEM

Objectives

Upon completion of this chapter, you should be able to

- List the purposes of the skeletal system
- Define the parts of a bone
- Describe the kinds of bones and their locations in the skeleton
- List and describe the kinds of joints
- Relate medical terms and diseases of the skeletal system

Key Terms

articular cartilage
(ar-**TICK**-you-ler)
articulation
(ar-**TICK**-you-**LAY**-shun)
bursa (**BER**-sah)
cartilage (**KAR**-tih-lidj)
compact bone
computerized tomography (**CT**)
congenital (kon-**JEN**-ih-tal)
cortical bone (**KOR**-tee-call)
diaphysis (dye-**AF**-ih-sis)
dislocation
endosteum (en-**DOS**-tee-um)
epiphyses (eh-**PIF**-ih-sees)
joint
ligament

magnetic resonance imaging
(**MRI**)
noninvasive
nuclear medicine
osteoblasts
osteoclasts
osteoporosis (**OSS**-tee-oh-por-
OH-sis)
periosteum
(per-ee-**OSS**-tee-um)
radiation therapy
radiology
radiopharmaceuticals
rickets (**RICK**-ets)
sonography
synovial fluid (sih-**NO**-vee-al)
X-ray

LIFE'S MOST EMBRRASSING MOMENTS (NO. 13 of 5,000)

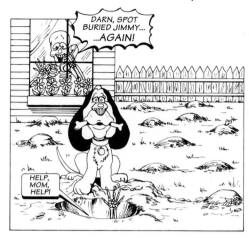

The trials and tribulations of the Osteo Family.

Source: Delmar/Cengage Learning

■ SYSTEM OVERVIEW

While the integumentary system is extremely important, without the skeletal system, our bodies would be nothing more than bags of water lying on the floor. Our skeletons provide the framework to support our muscles and skin, as well as allow for movement through the use of muscles, ligaments, tendons, and joints. This framework also protects vital organs. Your skull protects your brain, while your rib cage protects your lungs and heart. Certain bones in your skeleton contain bone marrow, which is responsible for producing red blood cells and white blood cells. The bones in your body also act as a warehouse for the storage of minerals, especially calcium and phosphorous. Do you remember which vitamin is necessary in order to utilize these two substances for bone growth? The answer of course is vitamin D.

Calcium is an extremely important mineral. It is needed for the heart to beat, the muscles to contract, and the blood to clot. The bones act as a "calcium bank" and supply the body with this mineral whenever needed. Of course, like borrowing from a bank, the body must pay back the bones by replacing the calcium borrowed with calcium from the bloodstream. If this does not happen, serious consequences can result, such as easily breakable brittle bones.

The skeletal structure can be divided into two major parts known as the *axial skeleton* and the *appendicular skeleton*. The axial skeleton provides form for the head and trunk and protects the organs of the body. These 80 bones include bones of the skull, thorax, and spinal column. The appendicular

skeleton is comprised of the 126 bones of the arms and legs (your appendages), as well as the bones of the shoulder and hips. Figure 5-1 shows the major components of the skeletal system.

Types and Composition of Bones

The organs of the skeletal system are the bones. Bones can be classified as organs because they utilize food and oxygen and perform specific functions. Bone is composed mainly of water, minerals, and organic matter. The main minerals are calcium, phosphorus, and magnesium. The organic material is a specific protein called *collagen*, which forms the intracellular "weave" or matrix, of the bone.

Not all of the 206 bones found in an adult's body are the same. The shape, size, and composition of a bone are dependent on its location in the body. The main types of bone found in your skeleton are *long bones, flat bones, short bones, and irregular bones.*

Flat bones are the *scapula* (shoulder blades), *sternum*, and bones of the skull. The bones provide flat surfaces to which muscles are attached. Flat bones also provide protection for organs of the body.

Short bones are irregularly shaped bones that compose your toes, ankles, and wrists. Irregular bones are oddly shaped and include the bones found inside the ear and the bones of the vertebrae. Figure 5-2 shows the bone types and shapes.

QUOTES & NOTES

Nearly half the bones in your body are in your hands and feet.

Long Bones

Long bones are found in the extremities (that is, the arms and legs). The *femur*, or thigh bone, is the longest bone in the human body and extends from the hip to the knee. The remaining long bones within the legs are the *tibia*, or shin bone, and the fibula. The long bones of the arm are the *humerus* (the upper arm) and the *radius* and *ulna* (both of the forearm).

Long bones are not solid bone but, rather, are composed of a variety of different cells. These bones are hollow. This hollow space is called the *medullary canal*. This canal is filled with yellow

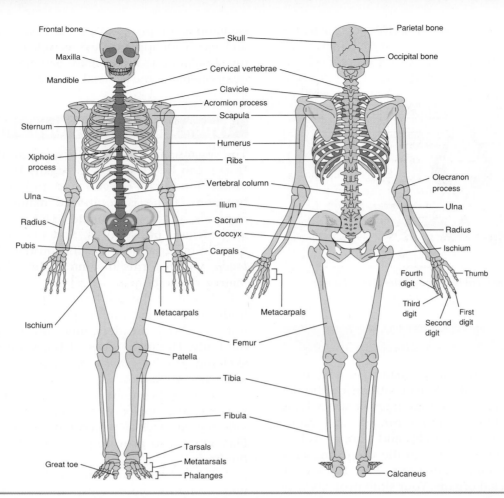

Figure 5-1 *The axial skeleton (blue) and the appendicular skeleton.*

Source: Delmar/Cengage Learning

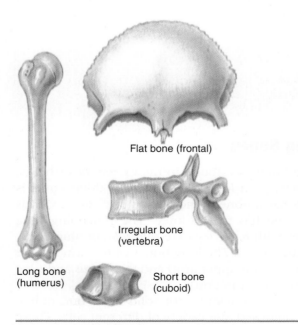

Figure 5-2 *Various bone shapes.*

Source: Delmar/Cengage Learning

marrow, which is mostly composed of fat cells. Yellow marrow is surrounded by a membrane called the **endosteum**.

The proximal ends (or **epiphyses**) of the long bones, such as the humerus and femur, contain red marrow. In addition, other non-long bones in the body (such as the ribs; the sternum, or breast bone; the shoulder blades, or scapula; and the bones of the spinal column, or vertebrae) also contain red marrow. Red marrow is very important because it produces red blood cells (RBCs), which carry oxygen, and a large number of white blood cells (WBCs), which fight infections. Millions of these blood cells are produced daily to replace dying blood cells. To give you an idea of the number of RBCs you have, there are about 25,000,000,000,000 (25 trillion) RBCs circulating in your blood! The average life of an RBC is 120 days, and your body must produce 3 million new RBCs every second! In cases of blood loss, your body can step up production to 10 times that rate. If the body's need for RBCs is greater than what the red marrow can supply, some of the fatty yellow marrow can be converted to red marrow. This is similar to having an army reserve or backup in times of crisis. See Figure 5-3 which details the parts of a long bone.

Compact bone forms part of the structure of long bones. It is very hard and dense. It is also very strong. **Cortical bone** (another name for compact bone) is the main component of the shaft (or **diaphysis**) of a long bone.

The outside of the bone is encased in a tough, white, fibrous membrane called the **periosteum** (*peri* meaning "around," *osteum* meaning "bone"). The periosteum contains blood vessels, lymph vessels, and nerves. The periosteum is responsible

for bone growth as well as for bone repair and nutrition. This covering is also where muscles, tendons, and ligaments attach to the bone.

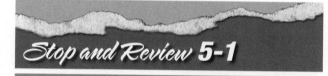

Stop and Review 5-1

a. List and describe the two main functions of the skeletal system.

b. What are the four main types of bone found in the skeleton? Give an example of each.

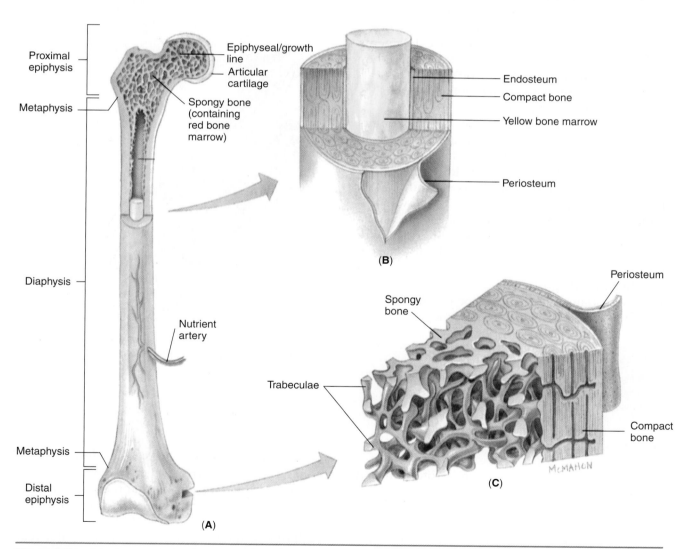

Figure 5-3 *(A) Components of a long bone. (B) Enlarged view of medullary cavity. (C) Spongy and compact bone.*

Source: Delmar/Cengage Learning

Articulations (Structures That Join Bones Together)

Movement is accomplished through the integration of bones and muscles. Bone joints must be structured in a specific manner to allow for the required movement. This section will discuss the makeup and various types of joints found in the human body.

Joints

Now that we have all 206 bones, they must be arranged in a way to allow for movement. This is where joints come into play. The area where two or more bones join together is known as a **joint**, or an **articulation**. Bones must be held together at the joint so they don't separate from each other every time there is movement. Bones are held together by **ligaments**, which are tough, whitish bands of connective tissue. Because ligaments hold the long bones together at the joints, they can come under a great deal of stress. This can cause the ligaments to stretch, which diminishes their function, or even to tear.

There are several different types of joints (see Figure 5-4). *Pivot joints* are found in the neck. *Ball-and-socket joints* are found in the shoulder and hip. *Hinge joints* are found in the knee and elbow. *Gliding joints*, which consist of flat or slightly curved bones that glide over each other to allow movement, are found in the wrist and ankle. Some joints do not move. Examples of nonmoving joints are *fibrous joints*, which hold the various bone plates of the skull together. Although these joints are fused together, they do possess minimal flexibility. In this way, these joints can absorb major stresses in much the same way as does an airplane wing.

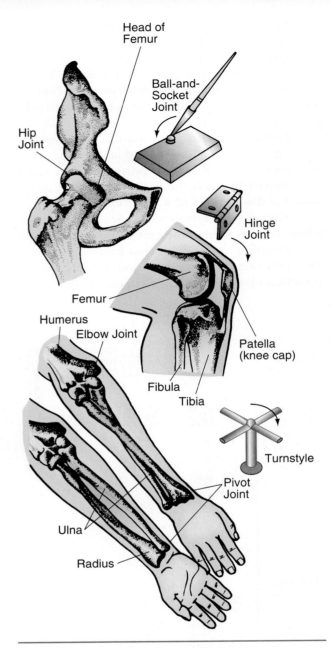

Figure 5-4   *Examples of types of joints.*
Source: Delmar/Cengage Learning

Cartilage

Another substance that provides protection and shape to the body is called **cartilage**. Cartilage is more flexible than bone and can be found in the flexible portions of your nose and ears. Cartilage acts as a connection between the ribs and the sternum. Because cartilage "gives" when pushed, it helps to prevent broken ribs when we collide with something.

Cartilage also provides a cushion between bones. In fact, **articular cartilage**, which is located on the ends of bones at the joints, acts as a shock absorber between bones. Without articular cartilage, your bones would grind together each time you moved, and eventually would wear away. The **bursa**, which is a sac found between bones at articulations, provides extra cushioning and secretes a lubricating substance known as

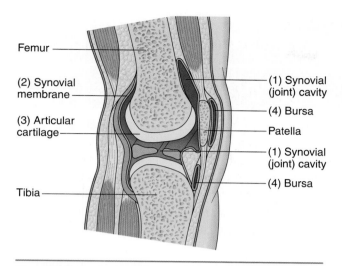

Femur

(2) Synovial membrane

(3) Articular cartilage

Tibia

(1) Synovial (joint) cavity

(4) Bursa

Patella

(1) Synovial (joint) cavity

(4) Bursa

Figure 5-5 *An example of a synovial joint. Note that the cartilage is utilized to cushion and protect the bones.*

Source: Delmar/Cengage Learning

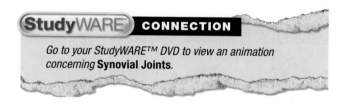 **CONNECTION**

Go to your StudyWARE™ DVD to view an animation concerning **Synovial Joints**.

synovial fluid. Without this fluid, we would all be like the Tin Man in the Wizard of Oz—we'd have to periodically oil our joints!

Through wear and tear, cartilage can progressively deteriorate and lead to joint pain, stiffness, aching, and strange sounds when the joint is moved. The medical term for this inflammation of the joint is *arthritis* or *osteoarthritis*. People with this condition commonly complain of pain when the weather changes. *Rheumatoid arthritis* is a chronic, intermittent inflammatory disease affecting mostly females between ages of 35 and 45. The etiology is not fully understood, but scar tissue and bone atrophy resulting from this disease can lead to severe pain and immovable joints. See Figure 5-6, which contrasts the two types of arthritis.

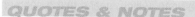 **QUOTES & NOTES**

Better to fail at something than to succeed in doing nothing.

—*Soundings*

Bone Growth and Repair

Our bones are constantly renewingg themselves. **Osteoblasts** are bone cells responsible for building new bone. Acting in opposition to these cells are **osteoclasts**. Osteoclasts are cells that continually tear down bone by excavating channels within the

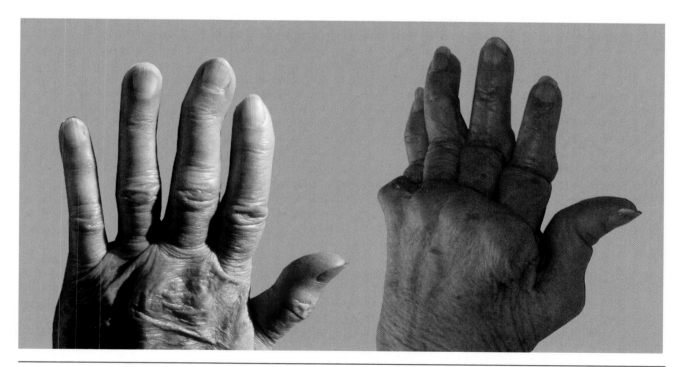

Figure 5-6 *Comparison of osteoarthritis (left) to rheumatoid arthritis (right).*

Source: Delmar/Cengage Learning

Clinical Relevancy

Bone Injuries

Not all bone fractures are the same. Broken bones result from trauma (either in the form of a direct blow or, indirectly, from the force of a blow that travels along the bone and fractures it at weak point), muscular contraction (if it is sudden and violent), or a disease process (in which case a spontaneous fracture can occur with no trauma).

Fractures can occur in varying degrees of severity. Bones can fracture completely (the whole way through the bone) or incompletely. Complete fractures may cause displacement of the bone, which means that a segment of the bone moves out of its normal position. Fractures do occur, however, in which the bone does not move out of its normal position.

Although there are many types of fractures, following are some of the more common breaks you may encounter (but, hopefully, not personally!). *Simple,* or *closed, fractures* occur without an open wound in the skin. A *hairline fracture* is a fine break that does not travel the whole way through the bone and does not result in displacement of the bone. As its name implies, this type of fracture shows up as a thin, hair-like line on an X-ray. *Spiral fractures* result from severe twisting of a bone. A *comminuted fracture*, in which the bone is splintered to pieces, can occur as a result of a crushing blow. A *compound fracture* (also known as an open fracture) is a break wherein the bone is forced through the skin, thus creating an open wound. A *greenstick fracture* means that the bone is only partially broken. This type of fracture often occurs in children due to their bones being more flexible, just like green sticks of wood. Now the next time people tell you to "break a leg" prior to a performance, you can ask them to be more specific!

Figure 5-7 shows the types of fractures.

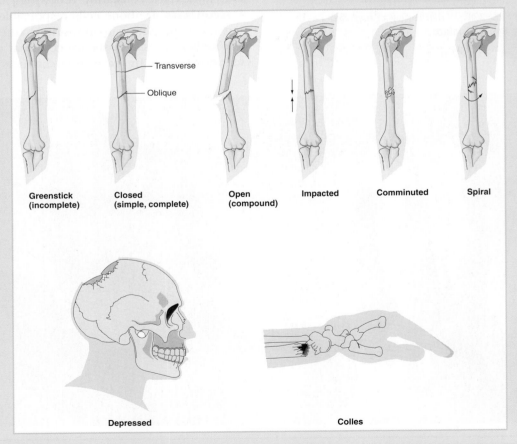

| Greenstick (incomplete) | Closed (simple, complete) | Open (compound) | Impacted | Comminuted | Spiral |

Transverse

Oblique

Depressed   Colles

Figure 5-7   *Examples of types of bone fractures.*

Source: Delmar/Cengage Learning

bone. Osteoblasts follow close behind, replacing the areas consumed by the osteoclasts. Up to 10% of your bone is eaten away and replaced per year. It is not that these bones are "bad"; it is just that your body has the ability to continuously build, repair, and even adapt itself to the stresses it faces. For example, a runner's leg bones thicken over time, and a horseback rider's bones may thicken at the points where they bang against the saddle. This can be compared to the development of skin callouses in areas of greater use or irritation. Similarly, immobilization can dramatically impact bone. We can see this when a cast is removed from an injured limb. With immobilization of only weeks, the bone, as well as the muscle, begins to slim and weaken.

QUOTES & NOTES

An easy way to not confuse osteoblasts and osteoclasts is to remember "B" for building, which is what osteo**B**lasts do.

Clinical Relevancy
Skeletal System Disorders

A **dislocation** is an injury that involves bones but is not a fracture. A dislocation results from movement of a bone out of its normal position in a joint. As is the case with fractures, dislocations can vary in type and severity. A compound dislocation can result when the joint is forced through the skin and is exposed to air. Dislocations that occur before or at birth are referred to as **congenital** (*con* meaning "with," *genital* meaning "birth") dislocations.

There are other bone conditions of which you may already be aware. **Osteoporosis** (*osteo* meaning "bone," *poro* meaning "passage full of pores," *osis* meaning "condition") is one such condition. This disease causes bones to lose density and increases bone porosity. The medical term literally means "a condition of bones with holes in them." These bones are brittle and are more prone to fracture than healthy bones. This disease is often associated with the aging population. Growing evidence exists that exercise and diet may help slow osteoporosis. See Figure 5-8.

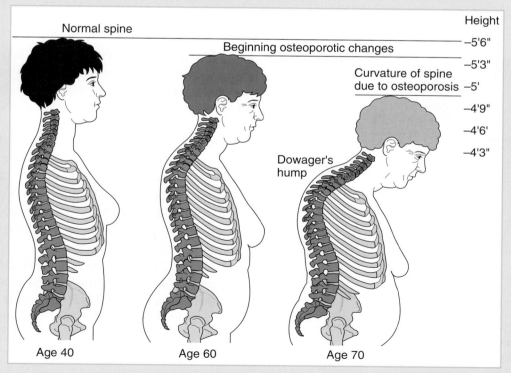

Figure 5-8 *Structural changes due to osteoporosis.*
Source: Delmar/Cengage Learning

(continues)

(continued)

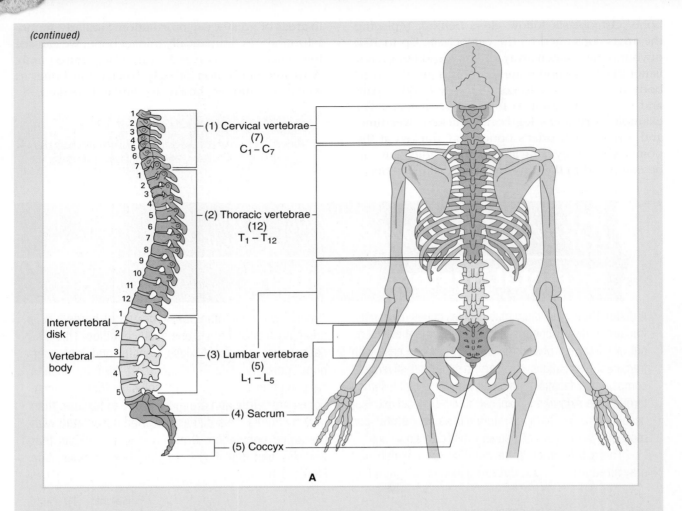

(1) Cervical vertebrae
(7)
$C_1 - C_7$

(2) Thoracic vertebrae
(12)
$T_1 - T_{12}$

Intervertebral disk

Vertebral body

(3) Lumbar vertebrae
(5)
$L_1 - L_5$

(4) Sacrum

(5) Coccyx

A

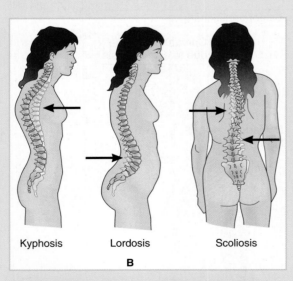

Kyphosis   Lordosis   Scoliosis

B

Figure 5-9   *(A) Normal vertebral column. (B) Spinal deformities.*

Source: Delmar/Cengage Learning

The spinal or vertebral column serves many important physiologic functions, but also serves as a central landmark and reference point of the body. Figure 5-9A shows a typical vertebral column with the corresponding types of vertebrae. For example, the branching of the lung takes place at T-5 and this fact is useful in interpreting an X-ray. The vertebral column can also be deformed as a result of birth defects, trauma, or disease processes. Figure 5-9B gives examples of *kyphosis* or humpback, *lordosis* or swayback, and *scoliosis* (an S curved or lateral displacement).

Another condition relating to the skeletal system is **rickets**. Rickets results from childhood deficiencies of calcium and vitamin D, and may cause softening of the bones that can lead to bow legs, among other pathologies.

Occupational or environmental sculpturing of this type helps us to discover how ancient people lived. For example, we know that constant squatting leaves a pattern of bumps and dents in hips, shinbones, and knees. This information led us to ascertain that our ancestors, the Neanderthals, did not sit but, instead, squatted.

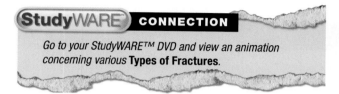

StudyWARE **CONNECTION**

Go to your StudyWARE™ DVD and view an animation concerning various **Types of Fractures***.*

Stop and Review 5-2

a. Differentiate the role of osteoblasts and osteoclasts.

b. _____ fluid serves as a joint lubricant.

c. A movement of a bone out of its normal position in a joint is called a _____.

d. The type of fracture where bone pierces through the skin is called a _____ fracture.

e. The major minerals and vitamins needed for strong healthy bones are _____, _____, and _____.

Professional Profile
Radiologic Technology

You may have heard the old cliché, "Beauty is only skin deep; ugly goes to the bone." In the health care setting, disease isn't always skin deep; it can also go to the bone. Oftentimes, in order for a physician to correctly decide what is occurring in a patient's body, it is necessary to obtain the clearest picture possible of bones, tumors, and tissue. To ensure this, the radiologic technologist must place the patient a precise distance from an **X-ray** machine and must time the exposure of radiation just right.

Taking X-rays (technically known as *radiographs*) of patients in an effort to identify illness is but one small part of the profession of **radiology**. **Magnetic resonance imaging** (or **MRI**) and **computerized tomography** (or **CT**) can provide amazingly detailed images of the human body. These two forms of imaging allow us to see parts of the body in three dimensions, rather like a sculpture as opposed to a photograph. The use of high-frequency sound waves (known as **sonography**) can produce images showing variations in tissue composition and shape.

Sonography is often used as a **noninvasive** way of determining the growth and condition of a baby before it is born or how well a heart is functioning. More involved forms of radiology include **radiation therapy** and **nuclear medicine**. Radiation therapy technologists deliver doses of radiation to help patients

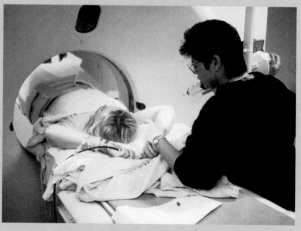

Source: Delmar/Cengage Learning

(continues)

(continued)

combat cancer. Nuclear medicine technologists are responsible for delivering specialized drugs (known as **radiopharmaceuticals**) for the diagnosis and treatment of various diseases.

Educational requirements for the profession of radiologic technology may include a certificate from a vocational school or hospital, an associate degree from a college, or a bachelor's degree. It is important to note that you must have a high school diploma (that is, your own—not somebody else's!) or equivalent regardless of which path you choose.

For more information on this dynamic field, visit the American Society of Radiologic Technologists at www.asrt.org.

■ CHAPTER REVIEW

Exercises

1. List the four main types of bone found in the body and give an example of each.

2. What material found in bones is responsible for the production of red blood cells?
   a. yellow matter
   b. gray marrow
   c. red marrow
   d. whatsamatter

3. What is another name for the shaft of a bone?
   a. epiphysis
   b. diaphysis
   c. periosteum
   d. medullary canal

4. The hollow space in long bones is called the:
   a. epiphysis
   b. diaphysis
   c. periosteum
   d. medullary canal

5. The tough white fibrous membrane that encases a bone is called the:
   a. epiphysis
   b. diaphysis
   c. periosteum
   d. medullary canal

6. List the five types of joints and give an example of each.

7. Differentiate between cartilage, ligaments, and bones.

8. What is an articulation?

9. What structures and substance are responsible for cushioning and lubricating the areas where bones are joined together?

10. Provide the best term for each of the following descriptions:
    a. movement of a bone out of its normal position
    b. a fracture resulting from twisting of the bone
    c. a fine fracture that does not travel through the bone
    d. a fracture where the bone is crushed and splintered
    e. a partial fracture that commonly occurs in children
    f. a common disease of the elderly that leads to brittle bones
    g. the vitamin responsible for bone growth and development
    h. the main mineral responsible for bone growth and development

Real Life Issues and Applications

Crushing Chest Injuries

The Emergency Department (ED) receives a motor vehicle accident (MVA) patient with crushing chest injuries and compound fractures of both femurs. The patient is tachypneic and has tachycardia with peripheral cyanosis and hypotension. The patient is initially stabilized and then rushed to the operating room (OR) to repair the internal injuries. What organs and systems are most likely to be affected by the crushing chest injuries? What precautions and treatments are needed to prevent the spread of infection before and after the repair of the compound fractures?

Additional Activities

1. Ask the radiology department of a local hospital to provide you with copies of X-rays showing several types of bone fractures.

2. Discuss how age affects bone structure.

3. Research the relationship between nutrition and bone development. Discuss your findings with the class.

Downloadable audio is available for selected medical terms in this chapter to enhance your learning of medical language.

StudyWARE **CONNECTION**

Go to your StudyWARE™ DVD and have fun learning as you play interactive games, view animations and videos, and take practice tests to help reinforce key concepts you learned in this chapter.

Workbook Practice *Go to your Workbook for more practice questions and activities.*

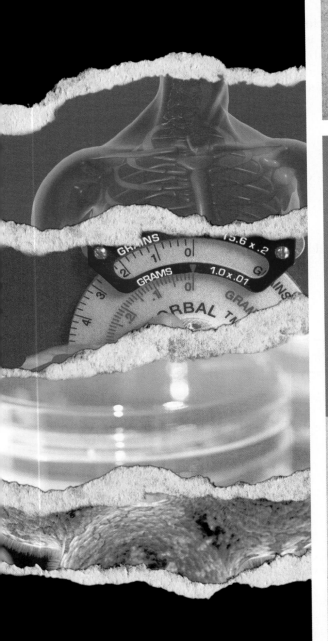

Objectives

Upon completion of this chapter, you should be able to

- List and describe the different types of muscle tissue
- Describe how muscles function
- Differentiate between voluntary muscles and involuntary muscles
- Describe various muscular movements
- Relate medical terms and diseases of the muscular system

Key Terms

abduction (ab-**DUCK**-shun)
adduction (add-**DUCK**-shun)
ataxia (ah-**TACK**-see-ah)
atrophy (**AH**-troh-fee)
cardiac muscle
cramp
electromyography (ee-**LECK**-tro-my-**OG**-rah-fee)
extension
flaccid (**FLAS**-sid)
flexion (**FLECK**-shun)
hernia (**HER**-nee-ah)
hypertrophy (hi-**PER**-tro-fee)
intercalated discs (in-ter-kah-**LAY**-ted)
muscles

myasthenia gravis (my-as-**THEE**-nee-ah **GRAH**-vis)
neuromuscular (new-roh-**MUS**-ku-lar)
paralysis (pah-**RAL**-ih-sis)
rotation
skeletal muscle
smooth muscle
spasm
tendinitis (ten-dih-**NIGH**-tis)
tendon (**TEN**-don)
tonus (**TOH**-nus)
vasoconstrict
vasodilate
visceral muscle (**VIS**-er-al)

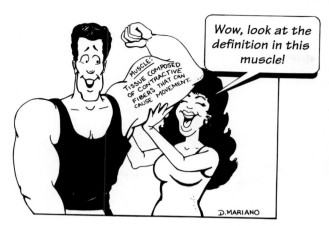

Source: Delmar/Cengage Learning

direction of the nervous system, provide form and motion of some type for your body. More than 600 muscles compose the muscular system (see Figure 6-1).

StudyWARE CONNECTION

Sometimes medicine can be injected directly into a muscle to be absorbed into the body for the desired effect. Go to your StudyWARE™ DVD to view a video on **Administering Intramuscular Injections**.

■ SYSTEM OVERVIEW

If your body possessed only an integumentary system and a skeletal system, you would then be simply a water-filled bag of bones with a couple of joints. You would still need some way of moving around. This is where **muscles** come into play. *Muscle* is a general term for all contractile tissue found in your body. The contractile property of muscle simply means it is capable of becoming short and thick as a result of a nerve impulse. Muscular tissue is constructed with bundles of muscular fibers. Each fiber is approximately the size of a human hair. These muscles, under the

QUOTES & NOTES

Muscles make up about half the weight of your entire body!.

Types of Muscles and Their Functions

Muscle can be divided into three groups: skeletal muscle, cardiac muscle, and smooth, or visceral, muscle. Skeletal muscle, as the name implies, attaches to the skeleton, cardiac muscle is of

---

Special Focus

Rigor Mortis

Have you ever heard of a dead body rising from a table or suddenly beginning to show signs of movement? This may sound like the opening for a movie about zombies or the "undead." Actually, it is a normal physiologic process that can be explained by science—not by science fiction. This process is called *rigor mortis*.

When the nervous system tells a muscle to contract, the signal causes the muscle fiber to open what are called *calcium ion channels*. This allows calcium ions to flow through these channels and into the muscle fibers. Because calcium causes the muscles to

contract, the muscle must get rid of calcium in order to return to its relaxed state. It does this by storing some calcium in the mitochondria and pumping the rest back through the channel.

When a body dies, however, the stored calcium cannot be pumped back out of the muscle via the channel. Therefore, excess calcium remains in the muscles throughout the body and causes the muscle fibers to shorten (contract) and stiffen the whole body. This stiffening process of the entire body is termed *rigor mortis*.

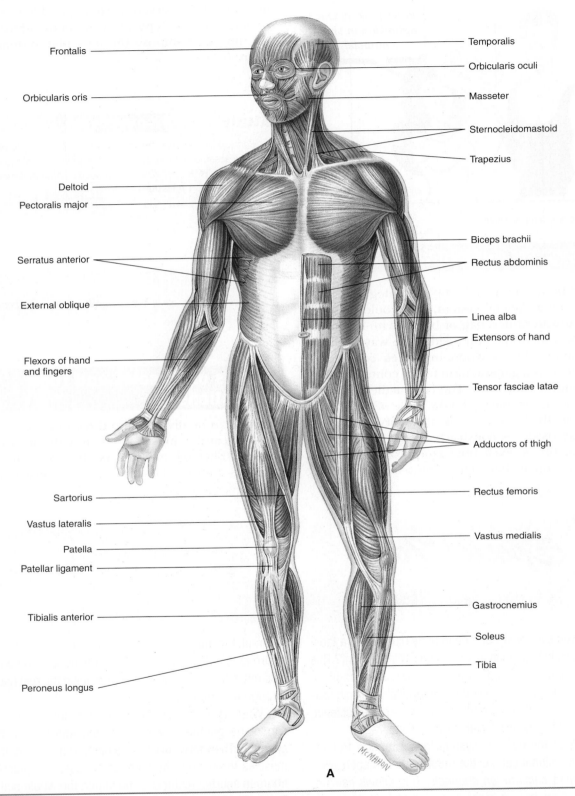

Frontalis

Temporalis

Orbicularis oculi

Orbicularis oris

Masseter

Sternocleidomastoid

Trapezius

Deltoid

Pectoralis major

Biceps brachii

Serratus anterior

Rectus abdominis

External oblique

Linea alba

Extensors of hand

Flexors of hand
and fingers

Tensor fasciae latae

Adductors of thigh

Sartorius

Rectus femoris

Vastus lateralis

Patella

Vastus medialis

Patellar ligament

Tibialis anterior

Gastrocnemius

Soleus

Tibia

Peroneus longus

A

Figure 6-1 *The major skeletal muscles of the body. (A) Anterior view.*

Source: Delmar/Cengage Learning

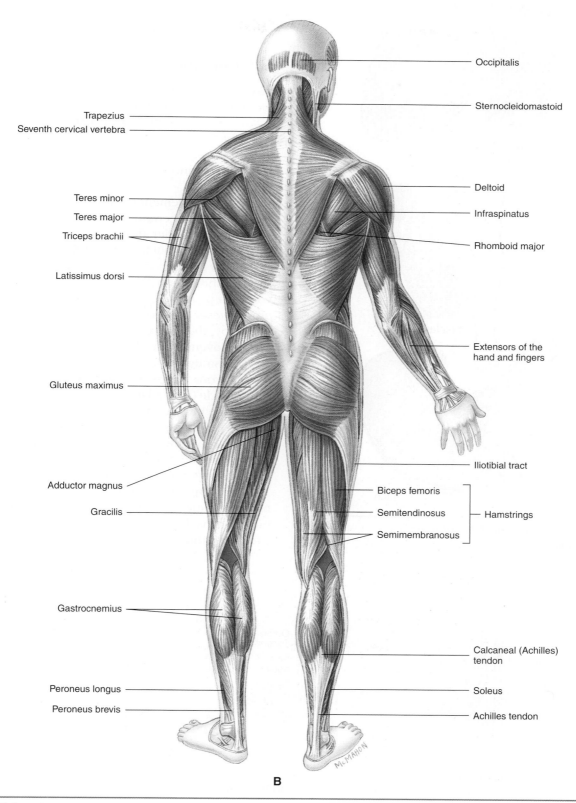

Figure 6-1 *The major skeletal muscles of the body. (B) Posterior view.*
Source: Delmar/Cengage Learning

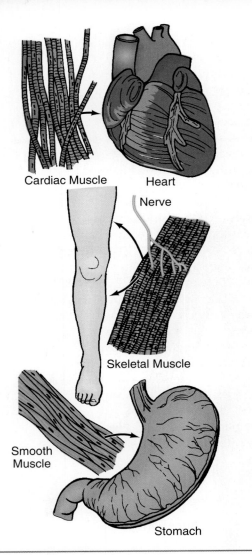

Figure 6-2   *The three types of muscle.*

Source: Delmar/Cengage Learning

course found in the heart, and smooth muscle lines the airways, vessels, glands, and organs in our bodies. See Figure 6-2.

Skeletal Muscles

Skeletal muscles are attached to bones and provide movement for your body. These are *voluntary muscles*, which means that you have control over their action. **Tendons** are fibrous tissues that attach skeletal muscle to bones. Tendons are very strong and do not stretch like cartilage or ligaments.

Body movement results from the contraction (shortening) of certain muscles and the relaxation of others. Consider the act of bending your arm so your fingers touch your shoulder. This is called *flexion*. In order to do this, your forearm is drawn to your shoulder as a result of the contraction of your biceps muscle, which is the *flexor* muscle or *prime mover* as shown in Figure 6-3A. Muscles, either by themselves or in muscle groups, that cause movement are known as *agonists*.

To straighten out that same arm requires you to relax your biceps muscle and to contract the triceps muscle (located underneath the humerus). The end of the muscle that is attached to the stationary bone is called the *point of origin* and can be seen in Figure 6-3B in the shoulder. The muscle end that is attached to the moving end is the *point of insertion* and is shown near the elbow in Figure 6-3B.

In straightening the arm, the triceps muscle now becomes the prime mover. Because the biceps muscle causes movement in the opposite direction when it contracts, it is called an

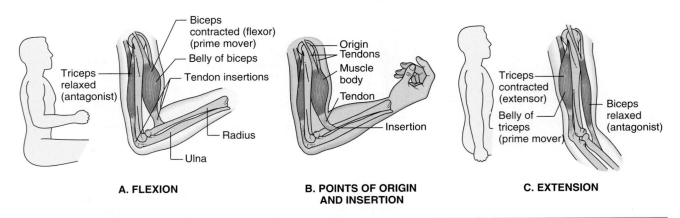

A. FLEXION

B. POINTS OF ORIGIN AND INSERTION

C. EXTENSION

Figure 6-3   *Coordination of antagonistic muscles to perform movement. (A) Flexion. (B) Points of insertion and origin. (C) Extension.*

Source: Delmar/Cengage Learning

antagonistic muscle. This brings us to an important concept. All movement is a result of contraction or relaxation of opposing muscles. In the previous example, for instance, you cannot forcefully contract the biceps muscle in order to straighten out your arm. If you doubt this, contract your biceps and actually try to straighten out your arm. Figure 6-3C illustrates this concept.

One very important and special skeletal muscle, which controls breathing, is the *diaphragm.* The diaphragm is both a voluntary and involuntary muscle. For example, most of the time you do not consciously think or control your breathing, but you can do so if you choose. This dome-shaped muscle separates the abdominal cavity and thoracic cavity and is responsible for performing the major work of bringing atmospheric air into the lungs. (Exactly how this process occurs is discussed in the respiratory system chapter.)

If skeletal muscle is damaged, it can regenerate itself. If the damage is extensive, however, scarring will occur.

Skeletal Muscular Movement

Certain terms are utilized to describe the direction of body movement.

Rotation describes circular movement that occurs around an axis. Rotation occurs when you turn your head from left to right or right to left.

Abduction (*ab* meaning "away") means to move away from the midline of the body. When you raise your arm to point out directions, abduction occurs.

Adduction (*ad* meaning "toward") means to move toward the midline of the body. When you bring your arm back down from pointing, adduction occurs.

Extension means to increase the angle between two bones connected at a joint. Extension is needed when you kick a football. Extension occurs when your leg straightens out during the kick. The muscle that straightens the joint is called the *extensor muscle.*

Flexion is the opposite of extension; it means to decrease the angle between two bones connected at a joint. Flexion occurs when you bend your legs to sit down. Flexion (and rotation) occurs when you move your arm into position to arm wrestle. The muscle that bends the joint is called the flexor muscle. Figure 6-4 illustrates the types of skeletal muscular movement previously discussed along with some additional movements.

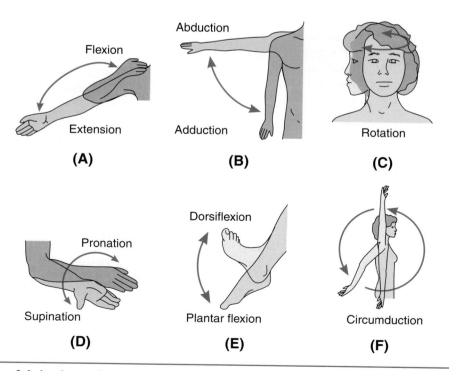

Figure 6-4   *Types of skeletal muscle movement.*

Source: Delmar/Cengage Learning

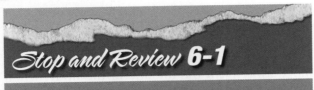

Stop and Review 6-1

Using skeletal muscular movement terms, write a paragraph describing the muscular movement required in a sport.

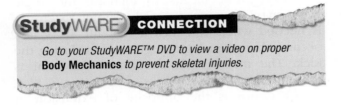

StudyWARE CONNECTION

*Go to your StudyWARE™ DVD to view a video on proper **Body Mechanics** to prevent skeletal injuries.*

Cardiac Muscle

Cardiac muscles create the walls of the heart. When these muscles contract, blood is squeezed out of the chambers of the heart, causing the blood to circulate throughout your body. Cardiac muscle is *involuntary* muscle, meaning that you do not have to consciously think about making your heart contract every time you need a heartbeat.

Cardiac muscle fibers are somewhat shorter than are the fibers of other muscle types. Because the heart must work constantly, cardiac muscles must receive a generous blood supply to get enough oxygen and nutrition, as well as to get rid of waste. In fact, cardiac muscle receives a richer supply of blood than does any other muscle in the body.

Cardiac muscle fibers are connected to each other by **intercalated discs**. As one fiber contracts, the adjacent one contracts, and so on. This is very similar to the "domino effect," or to the "human wave" often done at football games. The resulting wave of contraction squeezes out blood to the body.

Cardiac muscle does not regenerate after it has been seriously injured. If the blood supply going to the heart from the coronary arteries is blocked, damage to cardiac muscle can occur. This leads to scarring of the heart. Scar tissue cannot help when the healthy muscles of the heart contract. If the scarred area is big enough, there may not be enough healthy cardiac muscle remaining to efficiently pump

blood. An individual with this condition may experience severely diminished cardiac output, which could lead to death.

Visceral (Smooth) Muscle

Visceral, or **smooth**, **muscle** is found in the organs of the body, such as the stomach and other digestive organs. (It is not, however, found in the heart.) Visceral muscle is also found in the blood vessels and bronchial airways. Blood pressure can be affected by whether the smooth muscle within the blood vessels relax making the vessel become larger in diameter (**vasodilate**) or constrict to make it smaller in diameter (**vasoconstrict**). Vasodilation can lead to decreased blood pressure, while vasoconstriction can lead to increased blood pressure.

Smooth muscle is also found in the airways of your lungs. During an asthma attack, these muscles constrict, making it difficult to get air in and out of the lungs. This is what causes the wheezing sound heard during an attack. These muscles will be further discussed in the respiratory chapter.

A special form of smooth muscles called a *sphincter* is found throughout your digestive system. These donut-shaped muscles alternately contract, thus helping to move food and liquid through the digestive system. These muscles are discussed in greater detail in the gastrointestinal system chapter.

Smooth muscles are involuntary muscles; they do not contract as rapidly as do skeletal muscles. In fact, skeletal muscles can contract 50 times faster, once stimulated, than can smooth muscle. Because of their slower activity and lower metabolic rate, smooth muscles receive only moderate amounts of blood. When injured, smooth muscle rarely repairs itself and, instead, forms a scar.

Muscular Fuel

Muscle, like all tissue, needs fuel in the form of foodstuff and oxygen in order to survive and function. The body stores a carbohydrate called *glycogen* in the muscle. Glycogen is always on reserve waiting to be converted into a usable energy source. When needed, the muscle can convert glycogen to glucose, which releases energy for the muscle to function. Muscles with very high

Clinical Relevancy

Muscle Tone

Normally, all muscles exhibit muscle tone, or **tonus**. Tonus is the partial contraction of a muscle possessing resistance to stretching. Athletes who exercise regularly have increased muscle tone, which makes their muscles more pronounced. The muscle fibers in an athlete's muscles increase in diameter and become stronger. This is referred to as **hypertrophy** (*hyper* meaning "more than normal," *trophy* meaning "growth" or "development"). As muscles are used less and less,

they begin to lose their tone and become soft and flabby. This can occur in the clinical setting if a patient is required to remain in bed (i.e., bedfast) for an extended period of time or has a cast on for a prolonged period. Often muscles waste away from lack of use. This is referred to as **atrophy** (*a* meaning "without," *trophy* meaning "growth" or "development"). One of the reasons patients are made to get out of bed as soon as possible is to prevent atrophy.

demands (such as the leg muscles) also store fat and use it as energy. When energy is released, so is heat; this is why strenuous or prolonged exercise can overheat our bodies.

High-demand muscles are needed for endurance, such as is required for long-distance running. Therefore, in addition to using fat as an energy source, these muscles receive a very rich blood supply to provide much-needed oxygen. This rich blood supply gives the leg muscles a darker color relative to some other muscles in the body. For instance, muscles such as the hand, which are not in as great demand, receive a small supply of blood. These muscles utilize just the local blood supply for glucose and whatever glycogen is stored within. They therefore are lighter in color. Although these muscles are better at speed, they do not have endurance capabilities. To illustrate this point, the next time you take a long walk, keep pumping your hand. While the hand can move faster than the leg muscles, it will also tire more quickly. If you would like another illustration, consider the color of meat of the chicken versus the woodcock. The chicken, which does not fly, has white breast and wing meat and darker leg meat. This is not surprising because endurance is needed for the legs. Conversely, a woodcock, which is a migratory bird that transverses long distances, has dark breast meat for endurance. Now you know why a chicken's breast meat is white—when was the last time you saw a chicken flying overhead?

QUOTES & NOTES

The muscular system must work hand-in-hand with the nervous system for proper functioning. The junction of the nervous system and skeletal muscle is called the neuromuscular junction. You will learn more about this as it is explored in more depth in the next chapter.

Stop and Review 6-2

a. List two major types of involuntary muscles and describe their ability to regenerate.

b. Muscle wasting due to disuse is termed _____.

c. Muscle growth as a result of excessive usage is called _____.

d. Muscles store _____ to be converted to _____ for energy.

e. Vasodilation would cause _____ blood pressure, while vasoconstriction would cause _____ blood pressure.

Clinical Relevancy

Disorders of the Muscular System

Although you have already learned a few basics about muscles, following are some additional terms that may be useful to you in the future. Patients or victims of illness may be unable or unwilling to use their muscles over an extended period of time. As discussed earlier, their muscles become weak and begin to waste away, and this process is known as *atrophy.* You may have experienced a similar sensation if you ever had the flu and were bedridden for several days.

Ataxia (*a* meaning "without," *tax/o* meaning "coordination") is a condition wherein the muscles are irregular in their actions or there is a lack of coordination. Paralysis is the partial or total loss of the ability of voluntary muscles to move. Paralysis can be temporary or permanent. A muscle that suddenly and violently contracts is said to have a spasm or cramp. A spasm can occur in a single muscle or in a muscle group.

A hernia is a tear in a muscle wall through which an organ of the body protrudes. Tendinitis (*itis* meaning "inflammation of") is a condition wherein tendons become inflamed.

Electromyography (*electro* meaning "electric," *myo* meaning "muscle," *graphy* meaning "graph") is a diagnostic test wherein a group of muscles is stimulated with an electrical impulse. This impulse causes muscle contraction. The strength of the muscle contraction is then recorded. Certain diseases can alter the strength of muscles.

Several diseases involve the nervous system and the muscular system; these are termed neuromuscular diseases. Myasthenia gravis is a neuromuscular disease wherein the patient exhibits gradually increasing, profound muscle weakness. The first symptom of this disease often is drooping of one or both upper eyelids (called *ptosis*, meaning "downward"). There is also progressive paralysis. Interestingly, tendon reflexes almost always remain. *Muscular dystrophy* (*dys* meaning "disordered," *trophy* meaning "growth" or "nourishment") is an inherited muscular disease wherein muscle fibers degenerate and there is progressive muscular weakness. *Guillain-Barré syndrome* is a disorder of the peripheral nervous system that causes flaccid paralysis (limp muscles) and loss of reflexes. Interestingly, the paralysis is usually *ascending*, meaning that it starts in the feet or lower extremities and progresses toward the head. Paralysis usually peaks within 10 to 14 days. Although it may take several weeks or months, eventually most patients return to normal.

■ CHAPTER REVIEW

Exercises

1. List the three major muscle groups and give an example of each.

2. Contrast the terms *hypertrophy* and *atrophy* and give an example of how each situation could occur.

3. Explain how vasoconstriction and vasodilation affect blood pressure.

4. Cardiac muscle:

   I. is a voluntary muscle

   II. has intercalated discs to assist in contraction

   III. regenerates after injury

   IV. lines the blood vessels

      a. I only   c. II only

      b. I and II   d. I, II, III, and IV

5. A sudden or violent muscle contraction is called:

   a. a hernia

   b. paralysis

   c. a spasm

   d. atrophy

6. Partial or total loss of voluntary muscle use is called:

   a. a hernia

   b. paralysis

   c. a spasm

   d. atrophy

7. A tear in a muscle wall through which an organ protrudes is called:

   a. a hernia

   b. paralysis

   c. a spasm

   d. atrophy

8. Describe the difference(s) between abduction and adduction.

9. Define the term *neuromuscular disease.* List and describe one such disease.

10. What is the condition wherein muscle action is irregular or there is a lack of coordination?

Real Life Issues and Applications

Muscle Paralysis

One of your patients presents with ascending flaccid paralysis that began with tingling in the toes and muscle weakness. Loss of reflexes was also noted. What disease do you think this is? Knowing that this patient is losing the ability to use skeletal muscles, what life-threatening condition could occur? What vital signs will you need to monitor? What areas of patient care need to be addressed? What is the likely prognosis?

Additional Activities

1. Research the importance of nutrition and exercise with regard to proper muscle development. Discuss your findings with the class.

2. Pick a major muscle group and discuss how your life would be different if that group could not function properly because of a disease or accident.

3. Body building requires an extensive knowledge of muscles and muscle groups. Demonstrate five different exercises and explain the muscles they would develop.

4. Pair off with a partner and perform various muscle movements showing rotation, abduction, adduction, extension, and flexion. See if your partner can accurately classify each motion.

5. Invite a physical therapist to come in and demonstrate appropriate exercises and therapies to prevent or relieve back strain and promote good posture.

Downloadable audio is available for selected medical terms in this chapter to enhance your learning of medical language.

StudyWARE CONNECTION

Go to your StudyWARE™ DVD and have fun learning as you play interactive games, view animations and videos, and take practice tests to help reinforce key concepts you learned in this chapter.

CHAPTER 7

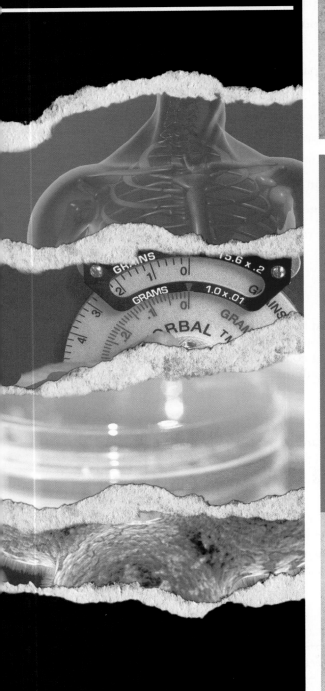

THE NERVOUS SYSTEM

Objectives

Upon completion of this chapter, you should be able to

- Differentiate between the central nervous system (CNS) and the peripheral nervous system (PNS)

- Describe the basic components of the nervous system at the cellular, tissue, and organ levels

- Contrast the types of neurons and their modes of conduction

- Define and describe the various components of the CNS

- Relate diseases of the CNS

- Describe the components and responses of the autonomic branch of the PNS

Key Terms

acetylcholine (**ACh**)
   (**AS**-eh-till-**KOH**-leen)
acetylcholinesterase (**AChE**)
   (**AS**-eh-till-**KOH**-lin-ESS-
   ter-ase)
action potential
aphasia (ah-**FAY**-zee-ah)
arachnoid membrane
   (ah-**RACK**-noid)
associative neurons
autonomic nerves
axon

brachial plexus
   (**BRAY**-kee-all **PLECK**-sus)
brain
cell body
central nervous system (**CNS**)
central processing unit (**CPU**)
cerebellum (ser-eh-**BELL**-um)
cerebral cortex
   (seh-**REE**-brawl)
cerebrospinal fluid (**CSF**)
cerebrovascular accident (**CVA**)
   (**SER**-eh-bro-**VAS**-kyou-lar)

(continues)

cervical plexus (**SER**-vih-kal)
choroid plexus (**KOH**-roid)
conductivity
corpus callosum
   (**KOR**-pus; kah-**LOW**-sum)
cranial nerves
dendrite
diencephalon (die-in-**SEF**-ah-lawn)
dorsal root
dorsal root ganglia
dura mater (**DOO**-rah **MAY**-ter)
emboli (**EM**-boh-lie)
encephalitis (en-**SEF**-ah-**LYE**-tis)
epinephrine (**E**-ih-**NEF**-rin)
fight-or-flight response
frontal lobe
ganglia (**GANG**-glee-ah)
glia cells (**GLEE**-uh)
gyri (**JIGH**-rye)
Heimlich maneuver (**HIME**-lick)
hemiplegia (hem-ee-**PLEE**-jee-ah)
homeostasis
   (**HOH**-me-oh-**STAY**-sis)

hypothalamus
   (high-poh-**THAL**-ah-mus)
irritability
lumbar plexus
meninges (meh-**NIN**-jeez)
meningitis (men-in-**JIGH**-tis)
midbrain
motor cortex
motor neurons
myelin sheath (**MY**-eh-lin)
nerve plexuses (**PLECK**-us-sus)
nerves
neuroglia (new-**ROG**-lee-ah)
neuron (**NEW**-ron)
neurotransmitter substance
norepinephrine (**NE**)
occipital lobe
olfactory (ol-**FAK**-toh-ree)
paraplegia (par-ah-**PLEE**-jee-ah)
parasympathetic nervous system
parietal lobe (pah-**RYE**-eh-tal)
peripheral nervous system (**PNS**)
peristalsis (per-ih-**STAL**-sis)
phagocytosis (fag-oh-sye-**TOH**-sis)

phrenic nerve (**FREN**-ick)
pia mater (**PEE**-ah **MAY**-ter)
piloerection
   (**PIE**-low-ee-**RECK**-shun)
quadriplegia
   (**KWAD**-rih-**PLEE**-jee-ah)
sacral plexus (**SACK**-ral **PLEX**-us)
sensory neurons
somatic muscles (so-**MAT**-ick)
somatic nerves
spinal cord (**SPY**-nal)
spinal nerves
stimulus
stroke
subarachnoid space
   (sub-ah-**RACK**-noyd)
sulci (**SUL**-kye)
sympathetic nervous system
synapse (**SIN**-apps)
temporal lobe
thalamus (**THAL**-ah-mus)
ventral root
white matter

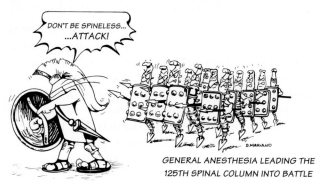

DON'T BE SPINELESS...
...ATTACK!

GENERAL ANESTHESIA LEADING THE
125TH SPINAL COLUMN INTO BATTLE

Source: Delmar/Cengage Learning

■ SYSTEM OVERVIEW

The nervous system and endocrine (glands) system together are responsible for control of the body. They coordinate all activities and help to maintain the internal environment in a state of equilibrium known as **homeostasis**. The cells in our bodies need a fairly constant set of conditions in order to properly function. For example, central body temperature must be maintained within a narrow range or cellular death will occur. Given that the cell is the basic unit of life, this would quickly cause organ and system failure, with resulting death of the individual. In addition to temperature,

there are many other body conditions that need to be maintained within a narrow range.

The nervous system, like all body systems, is composed of cells, tissues, and organs that act in a highly integrated manner. The cells of the nervous system are called **neurons**. The **nerves** can be considered the tissue; the main organs are the **brain** and **spinal cord**.

We live in an electronic age where computers are commonplace. Many people compare the computer to a human brain. While there are similarities, a comparison of the computer to the entire nervous system may be more appropriate (see Figure 7-1). Within a computer is a **central processing unit (CPU)**, which handles information from a variety of sources. The CPU, therefore, is comparable to the brain, which processes information from both the external (outside world) and internal (body) environments and then makes proper responses. The CPU receives its information from disks, keyboards, and other peripheral equipment; similarly, the brain receives information from the nerves and senses. The CPU responds to input through a maze of electronic circuitry and puts its output onto the computer screen; the nervous system responds via the massive network of nerves, which acts as a conduit of information within the nervous system.

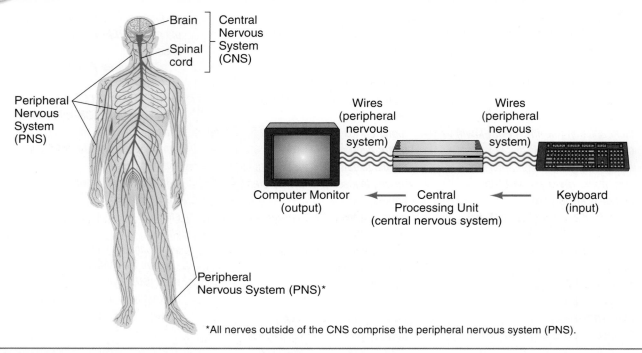

Figure 7-1　*The components of the nervous system with computer analogy.*
Source: Delmar/Cengage Learning

The nervous system is responsible for maintaining day-to-day functioning, that is, voluntary and involuntary activities. For example, you would not be able to attend class if not for the functioning of all components of the nervous system. All the voluntary activities that were required for you to get up, shower, prepare and eat breakfast, and drive or walk to school demanded extensive coordination of several muscle groups by the nervous system. At the same time, many functions were occurring that you did not consciously think about. For example, you did not need to keep telling your heart to beat or your lungs to breathe. These involuntary processes were also coordinated by the nervous system.

Stop and Review 7-1

a. Explain the fight-or-flight response.

b. Define the term *homeostasis*.

c. What is the responsibility of the nervous system?

Divisions of the Nervous System

The nervous system is divided into the **central nervous system (CNS)** and the **peripheral nervous system (PNS)**. The CNS is made up of the brain and spinal cord. As the term *central* implies, the CNS is the main processing unit of the body. The brain is the control organ, and the spinal cord is the main branch that transmits messages to and from the brain. These messages must come from or be sent to specific areas of the body; this is where the PNS is needed. Refer again to Figure 7-1, which illustrates the main components of the CNS and PNS.

The PNS is composed of the nerves that lie outside of (i.e., peripheral to) the CNS. In other words, the PNS connects your body to your brain and spinal cord. The PNS has both a voluntary component (the **somatic nerves**) and an involuntary component (the **autonomic nerves**). The somatic nerves control skeletal, or voluntary, muscles. The autonomic nerves control the involuntary processes such as heart beat, breathing, and digestion. The involuntary, or autonomic, component is further divided into the **sympathetic nervous system** and the **parasympathetic nervous system**. The sympathetic portion of the PNS is responsible for the fight-or-flight response, and as such, this system can be called on in emergency situations. The

Special Focus

The Fight-or-Flight Response

You have probably heard of the term **fight-or-flight response**; but even if you haven't, you have probably experienced it at least once in your lifetime. This survival response enables the body to prepare to face or flee from a perceived danger. For example, while walking down a dark alley, someone jumps out in front of you with a menacing scream. For a split second, you don't know whether this is someone playing a prank or someone who means you harm. Your brain senses this situation as a potential threat and instantaneously prepares to face or flee the threat. The *autonomic nerves* "kick" into high gear. These nerves operate without conscious control; in other words, you do not have to voluntarily tell them to turn on. If this process weren't instantaneous and the autonomic nerves had to wait for you to tell them to begin, precious seconds would be lost, possibly meaning the difference between life and death.

How does this process work? First, it is important to note that the fight-or-flight response results from an integration (working together) of the two main control systems of the body: the nervous system and the endocrine system (discussed in Chapter 8). Consider what would be needed to prepare yourself for a possible life-threatening situation. Your vision would need to be keen; the supply of oxygen to your muscles would need to be at its maximum; your heart, lungs, and brain would need to receive top priority; and nonessential systems such as the digestive tract would need to be temporarily ignored.

Now let's examine how your nervous and endocrine systems accomplish these ends. Following are some of the physiologic processes that occur during the fight-or-flight response. The pupils of the eyes dilate (become larger), thus allowing more light to be brought in for enhanced vision. The heart rate and force of contraction increase; not only does your heart speed up (tachycardia) to get more oxygen delivered to the body, but the force of each contraction increases, thus enhancing muscle perfusion. The airways of your lungs (bronchi) dilate to take in more oxygen from the atmosphere. The maximum amount of oxygen is being brought in by the lungs and delivered by the heart to areas that need to respond. Body metabolism is now at its peak.

At the same time, some nonessential areas are shut down; in this way all the energy can be concentrated where it is needed most. For example, your digestive, or gastrointestinal, tract is basically shut down. Blood flow to this region decreases because this area is not important in a life-threatening situation.

Finally, sweat gland production increases and the muscles attached to your hair contract, causing the hair to stand erect (a process known as **piloerection**); you have sweaty palms and you can feel the hair on the back of your neck stand up. With all essential systems at their peaks and nonessential systems minimized, your body is now ready to either confront or flee from the perceived danger. Your nervous system and endocrine system have successfully brought about the fight-or-flight response.

---

parasympathetic branch is primarily concerned with daily body maintenance and metabolic functioning. Some refer to this system as the "resting and digesting" system.

The nervous system also allows us to perform many higher functions such as reasoning, memory, and contemplation. Furthermore, it controls our special senses of taste, touch, smell, sight, and hearing. These senses allow us to detect changes in the environment. The brain can then react to these changes appropriately. The special senses are discussed in detail in Chapter 9. Figure 7-2 illustrates the divisions of the nervous system.

Functional Units of the Nervous System

The Neuron (Nerve Cells)

The basic functional unit of the nervous system is the neuron, or nerve cell. Neurons are primarily concerned with receiving and transmitting messages throughout the body. Aside from the common cellular components, the neuron has several specialized structures to facilitate its ability to communicate throughout the body. Each neuron has a central mass called the cell body.

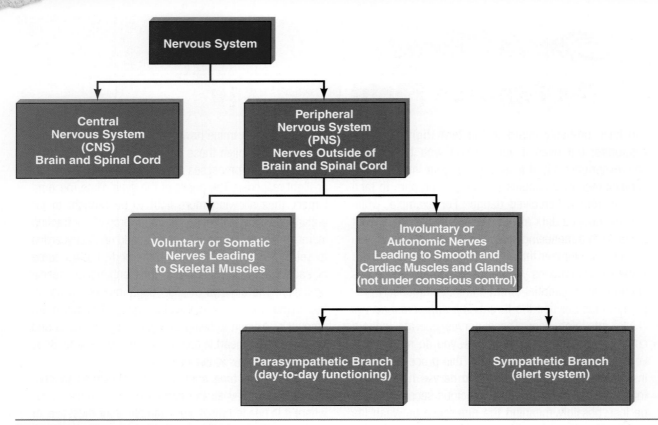

Figure 7-2 *The divisions of the nervous system.*
Source: Delmar/Cengage Learning

The **cell body**, which contains the nucleus, is the control center of the neuron. Extending from the cell body are numerous fibers called **axons** and **dendrites**. Dendrites carry signals toward the cell body, and axons transmit signals away from the cell body. While each neuron may contain several dendrites, there is only one axon.

A specialized covering protects the axon and allows signals to be conducted faster. This covering is called the **myelin sheath**. Myelin, a lipid (fatty) substance, is also called **white matter** because it gives the nerves a white appearance. Myelin stops signals from jumping to other nerves. This is very similar to the insulation that surrounds electrical wires; the insulation helps contain the signal and prevents the circuit from "shorting out" (see Figure 7-3).

Neurons possess several special properties that allow them to receive and transmit messages. Neurons demonstrate high levels of **irritability**. This does not mean they are easily angered, but, rather, that they can respond readily to a **stimulus**. A stimulus is anything that activates (excites) a nerve, thereby causing an impulse or signal to be sent. Neurons also have the ability

to pass on their signals; this is referred to as **conductivity**. The dendrites are the receivers in the system, and they pass the signal onto the cell body, where it can travel to the axon and be sent to either another neuron, a muscle, or a gland.

QUOTES & NOTES

*T*he amount of time needed for the brain to receive information and then act on it varies from person to person. To illustrate this point, hold a dollar bill downward by using your thumb and index finger. Have a friend position their index finger and thumb on opposite sides of the bill; the fingers should be halfway up but not touching the bill. Let go of the bill. Did your friend catch it? Now have your friend hold the dollar bill and you try to catch it. Were you able to?

Types of Neurons

There are three types of neurons, each with a different pathway and function. **Sensory neurons** (also known as *afferent neurons*) carry messages from all parts of the body toward the spinal cord and brain. These are found in the skin and sensory organs (eyes, ears, nose, and tongue) and give

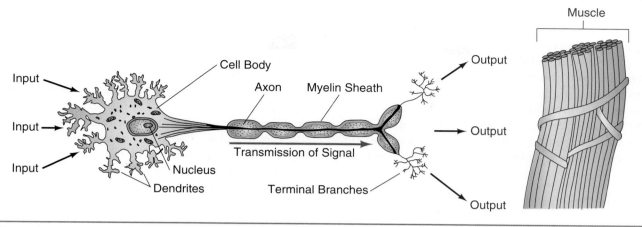

Figure 7-3 *The neuron and its signal transmission.*
Source: Delmar/Cengage Learning

input to the central processing areas (i.e., brain and spinal cord) of the body. Receptors located in sensory neurons help to initiate a response when stimulated by a change in the environment.

Motor neurons (also known as *efferent neurons*) carry messages from the brain and spinal cord to the muscles and glands. These are the output, or effector, nerves because they cause a response (provide the desired *effect*). They tell the muscle and gland what needs to be done. This is usually based on input from the sensory neurons.

Finally, **associative neurons** (also known as *connecting neurons*) simply carry signals from one neuron to another. Figure 7-4 illustrates the three types of neurons.

Most nerves contain both sensory and motor components. For example, your facial nerves are motor nerves when you smile or frown, because

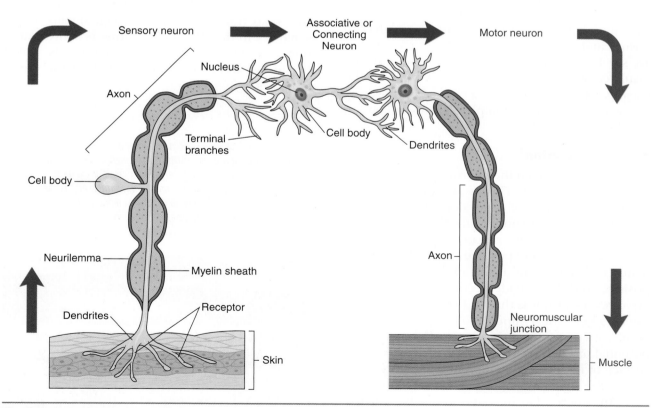

Figure 7-4 *Types of neurons.*
Source: Delmar/Cengage Learning

they tell the muscles in your face what to do. But when your tongue transmits taste to the brain via the facial nerves, these nerves act in a sensory capacity. And, while they are primarily motor nerves, even the nerves that supply the muscles must send signals back to the brain (sensory) to let it know the degree of muscular tone or contraction. Some nerves, however, are strictly sensory or motor in nature. For instance, the optic nerve in the eye contains purely sensory nerves.

Nerve Tissue

The functional units of the nervous system (i.e., the neurons) are grouped together to form nervous tissue known as nerves. Another type of cell found in the nervous system is called the **glia cell**. Glia cells are nonconducting and supportive cells. This means that they do not transmit signals but do support the neurons and, in essence, hold them together. In fact, when combined together to form tissue, these cells are called **neuroglia**, which literally means "nerve glue." During infections, neuroglia help combat infections by performing phagocytic functions. **Phagocytosis** (*phag/o* meaning "to eat") is the process of ingesting microorganisms.

Neurons are grouped together in bundles surrounded by connective tissue (neuroglia) to form actual nerves. These bundles, or nerve tracts, are similar to an electrical system wherein several insulated wires (individual neurons with myelin sheaths) are surrounded by a connective covering (neuroglia) to form a complete two-way conduit for electrical signals.

Nerve Conduction

The process by which the neurons pass on signals is called *conduction*. This is accomplished by a change in electrical charge along the length of the neuron. At rest (no signal), the inside of the neuron has an overall negative charge, and the outside has an overall positive charge. When stimulated or irritated, the inside of the cell becomes positive, and the outside becomes negative. This rapid reversal (in less than 1/1,000th of a second) causes an electrical impulse to be sent along. This is referred to as an **action potential**. An action potential is an electrochemical change on the surface of the plasma membrane of a neuron that causes the signal or impulse to be sent along.

Anywhere the message must be carried, whether from one neuron to another or from neurons to a muscle or gland, a small gap, or

synapse, occurs. This space is sometimes referred to as the *synaptic cleft*. The message needs some way of bridging this gap. This is accomplished via **neurotransmitter substances**, which are chemicals that can carry messages on to the next communication pathway. These chemicals are manufactured and stored at the terminal ends, or knobs, of the nerves, and their release is activated by the impulse. The three main neurochemical substances in our bodies that help transmit electrical impulses are **epinephrine**, **norepinephrine (NE)**, and **acetylcholine (ACh)**.

The actual neurochemical transmission is illustrated in Figure 7-5. Notice that when stimulated, the terminal branch of the axon releases ACh across the synapse to the other side. In Figure 7-5, the "other side" is a dendrite that will pass the signal on. There must also be some way to turn the signal off, or the stimulus would always be transmitting and, in essence, burn itself out. This is similar to an on/off light switch, which allows light to remain on only when needed. The "switch" in this case is *cholinesterase*, which breaks down ACh into an inactive form that cannot stimulate the membrane of the next nerve, muscle, or gland.

Acetylcholine is the neurotransmitter substance of the CNS. Acetylcholine and norepinephrine both transmit, or pass along, signals at the synapses in the PNS. Epinephrine is a circulating hormone produced by the adrenal glands; it will be further discussed in Chapter 8 on the endocrine system.

> **QUOTES & NOTES**
>
> **D**o not confuse acetylcholine (ACh) and **acetylcholinesterase (AChE)**. The ending "ase" is found on enzymes that break down substances. For example "lipo" means fat and lipase breaks down fats. ACh is the neurotransmitter that sends the signal along and AChE breaks it down or neutralizes its function.

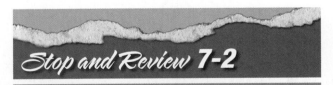

Stop and Review 7-2

a. What is a neuron?

b. What is the difference between afferent neurons and efferent neurons?

c. How are signals sent by nerves?

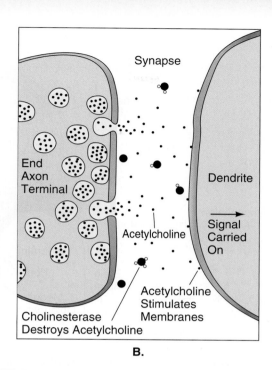

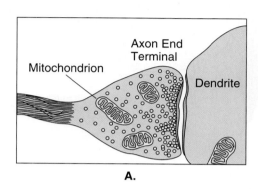

Figure 7-5 *The neurochemical transmission of a nerve signal or impulse.*
Source: Delmar/Cengage Learning

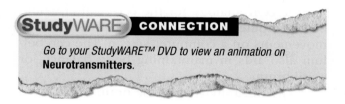

Go to your StudyWARE™ DVD to view an animation on **Neurotransmitters**.

The Central Nervous System

As previously stated, the CNS is composed of the brain and spinal cord. The brain is the most complex organ of the body and is responsible for every mental activity and almost every physical activity. The brain allows us to think, reason, remember, and feel emotion, among other things.

The spinal cord is responsible for bringing messages to the brain (input) via the sensory nerves and carrying messages from the brain (output) to either muscles (skeletal system) or glands (exocrine and endocrine systems) via the motor nerves. The spinal cord is also responsible for body reflexes.

The Brain

The brain is a very large organ, weighing approximately 3 pounds in an adult. It is composed of billions of neurons, which constantly send signals to each other via potentially trillions of connections. These signals can travel at an amazing 250 miles per hour!

The brain has four major divisions: the cerebrum, the **cerebellum**, the **diencephalon**, or interbrain, and the brain stem. Figure 7-6 shows the major divisions of the brain.

The cerebrum is the largest division of the brain. It consists of two hemispheres (*hemi* meaning "half") divided longitudinally (i.e., lengthwise) by a groove or fissure. A structure called the **corpus callosum** joins the right and left hemispheres and helps the right and left brain to communicate. The cerebrum has many folds, or convolutions, which greatly increase the surface area of the brain. By increasing the surface area, these folds, called **gyri**, allow for storage of more information. The furrows or fissures created by the folds are called **sulci**. Covering the entire cerebrum (including all the folds) is a thin layer of gray matter called the **cerebral cortex**. Gray matter is gray because it is composed of nerve cell bodies without myelinated sheaths, which would give a white appearance.

The cerebral cortex performs most of the higher brain functions and is divided into four specific lobes with specific functions. These are the **frontal lobe**, the **parietal lobe**, the **temporal**

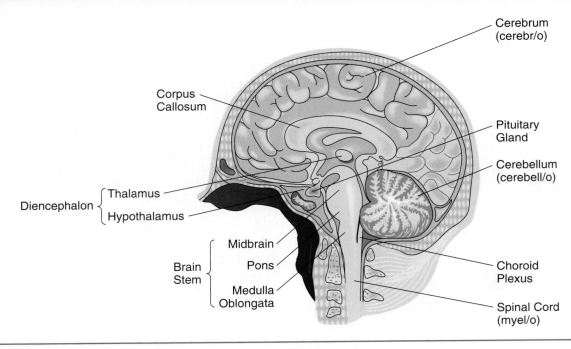

Figure 7-6   *Cutaway view showing the major divisions of the brain.*

Source: Delmar/Cengage Learning

lobe, and the **occipital lobe**. (Figure 7-7 shows the cerebral lobes as well as the major fissures, or grooves, that help to partition the cerebrum.) The frontal lobe, which contains the **motor cortex**, controls voluntary (i.e., skeletal) muscle movements. This lobe also contains speech areas. The parietal lobe is the sensory center for senses such as pain, pressure, and temperature. The temporal lobe is the auditory center, which interprets the sounds we hear from our ears. Finally, the occipital lobe is the visual center, which interprets input from our eyes. In summation, the cerebrum has several major higher functions including sensory perception and interpretation, muscular movement, emotional behavior, and memory.

Referring to Figure 7-7, the cerebellum is located in the back of the brain and is attached to the brain stem. The cerebellum works in conjunction with the cerebrum. The cerebrum begins muscular movement, and the cerebellum fine-tunes and coordinates this movement. The cerebellum is similar to the old tracking control on a VCR. The VCR heads (cerebrum) read and play the tape, but many times the picture needs to be adjusted by way of tracking (cerebellum) so that the tape plays better. Another more recent analogy for the cerebellum would be a computer mouse, which provides for finer movements on a computer screen. The cerebellum also aids in maintaining body balance, or equilibrium.

The third division of the brain is the diencephalon (also referred to as the *inner brain*). This area contains the **thalamus** and **hypothalamus** which help to interpret and transmit sensory input and regulate the endocrine system. All sensory input except **olfactory** (smell) is routed to the thalamus for processing and then transmitted to the cerebral cortex for interpretation. The hypothalamus (*hypo* meaning "beneath") is located beneath the thalamus and helps to regulate hormonal release. The hypothalamus also regulates the vital sign of temperature.

The final division of the brain is the brain stem, which is composed of the medulla oblongata, pons, and **midbrain**. The brain stem serves as a pathway, or junction box, that allows impulses to be conducted between the brain and spinal cord. This area regulates the remaining three vital signs of respiration, blood pressure, and heart rate.

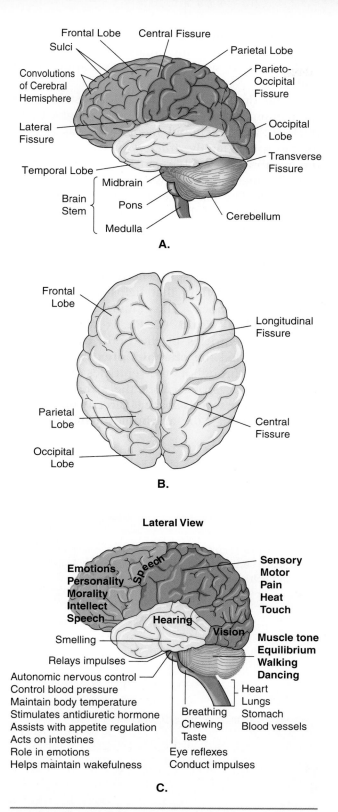

Figure 7-7 *Structural areas of the brain and their functions. (A) Lateral view of brain. (B) Superior view of brain. (C) Functional areas of cerebrum.*

Source: Delmar/Cengage Learning

The Spinal Cord

The spinal cord is the neural highway and message switching center of the body. Strategically located in the central area of the body, it receives sensory input from all parts of the body and passes this input up to (ascending) the brain. For this reason, *sensory nerve tracts* are also referred to as *ascending tracts.* Conversely, *motor tracts,* or *descending tracts,* carry directions or output from the brain down through (descending) the spinal cord and out to the target muscle or gland.

The spinal cord is located in the spinal cavity and contains specific vertebrae named for their particular locations. Figure 7-8 shows the specific regions of the spinal column. The three main

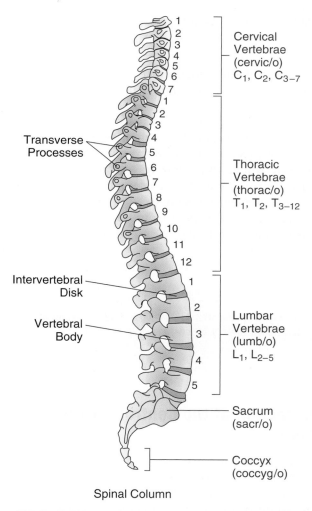

Spinal Column

Figure 7-8 *The spinal column.*

Source: Delmar/Cengage Learning

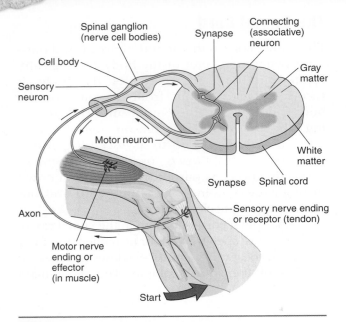

Figure 7-9   *The knee jerk reflex.*
Source: Delmar/Cengage Learning

functions of the spinal cord are reflex activities, sensory input to the brain, and motor output to the muscles or glands.

A reflex activity is an activity that basically bypasses the brain. For example, your patellar (knee) reflex gets its sensory input from the hit to your knee; this then travels to your spinal cord. Because this is a reflex pathway, however, the message is not sent to your brain. A direct message (motor) is sent from your spinal cord to cause your knee to jerk. See Figure 7-9.

QUOTES & NOTES

Courage is what it takes to stand up and speak; courage is also what it takes to sit down and listen.

—*Soundings*

Protection of the Central Nervous System

The CNS is vital to your existence; therefore, it must be carefully protected. We know that the bones of the skull and the vertebrae of the spine offer much protection against injury. There are, however, other structures that protect the CNS. The brain and spinal cord are surrounded by three layers of connective tissue called the **meninges**. The layers are called the **dura mater**, the **arachnoid membrane**, and the **pia mater**. The meninges act as a complete enclosure that seals the brain and spinal cord within.

The dura mater is the outermost layer of the meninges and is, therefore, the toughest and thickest. The arachnoid membrane was named for the spider family *Arachnida*. This is because the membrane resembles small spider webs. This web-like membrane allows fluid to easily travel through it. The pia mater is attached directly to the nerve tissue of the brain and spinal cord and has many tiny blood vessels. The pia mater supplies a large amount of the blood (perfusion) to the brain.

The brain and spinal cord are also bathed in a specialized fluid that helps act as a cushion against shock. This fluid, aptly named **cerebrospinal fluid (CSF)**, is manufactured inside the ventricles of the brain by a special structure called the **choroid plexus**. The fluid flows freely throughout the ventricles of the brain via a common space called the **subarachnoid space**. Of course, this space is directly under (*sub* meaning "under") the arachnoid membrane. See Figure 7-10.

StudyWARE CONNECTION

Go to your StudyWARE™ DVD to view animations on **Spinal Cord Injuries** *and a type of head injury known as* **Contra Coup Injury**.

Stop and Review 7-3

a. List the four major divisions of the brain.

b. Except for your olfactory sense, to which part of the brain is all sensory input routed for processing?

c. What are the three main functions of the spinal cord?

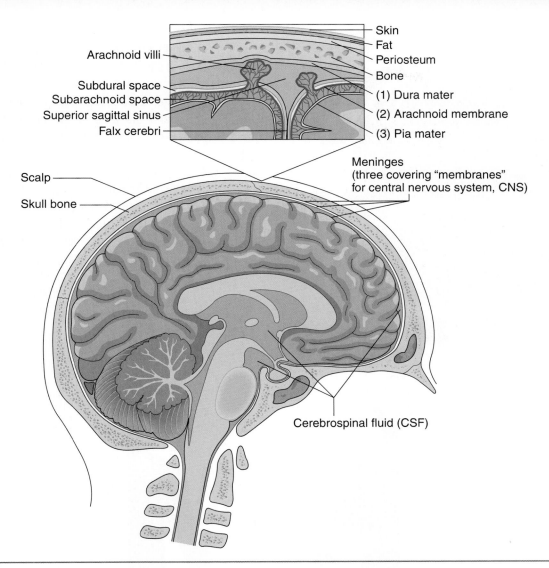

Arachnoid villi —
Subdural space —
Subarachnoid space —
Superior sagittal sinus —
Falx cerebri —
— Skin
— Fat
— Periosteum
— Bone
— (1) Dura mater
— (2) Arachnoid membrane
— (3) Pia mater

Meninges
(three covering "membranes"
for central nervous system, CNS)

Scalp —
Skull bone —

Cerebrospinal fluid (CSF)

Figure 7-10   *The meninges.*
Source: Delmar/Cengage Learning

Clinical Relevancy

Disorders of the Central Nervous System

Diseases of the CNS can affect the brain and/or spinal cord. An infection of the brain is called **encephalitis** (*encephalo* meaning "brain," *itis* meaning "inflammation"). These infections can be caused by viruses, bacteria, protozoa, and even fungi. Infection of the protective covering of the brain and spinal cord is called **meningitis**.

One of the most common brain disorders is called a cerebrovascular accident (CVA) or **stroke**. This is caused by a rupture of the blood vessels within the brain or some sort of blockage of blood flow. Blood clots, or **emboli** (blood clots that travel), can become lodged within the brain and disrupt blood flow to tissue, thereby resulting in tissue damage or death. A rupture or clot also builds up pressure within the brain, which can seriously affect the entire body. The pressure builds up rapidly because the brain, unlike other parts of the body, has very little "give";

(continues)

(continued)

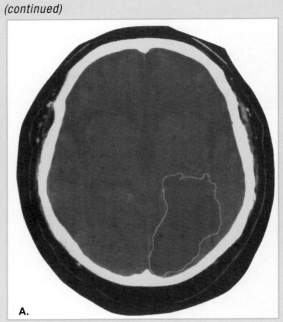

A.

it is encased within a rigid skull. Because it involves the brain and its blood supply, a stroke is also referred to as a **cerebrovascular accident**, or **CVA**.

The severity of a stroke depends on the extent of the damage and the area of the brain affected. Sometimes a stroke causes paralysis to the half of the body (hemi) opposite to where the brain was damaged. This is because, generally speaking, the right side of the brain controls the left side of the body, and vice versa. A right brain stroke, therefore, may cause **hemiplegia** (*plegia* meaning "paralysis") to the left half of the body. The stroke sufferer may also experience **aphasia** (*a* meaning "without," *phasia* meaning "speech") and, thus, lose the ability to speak, write, or effectively communicate. There are many forms of aphasia depending on the area of the brain affected. See Figure 7-11.

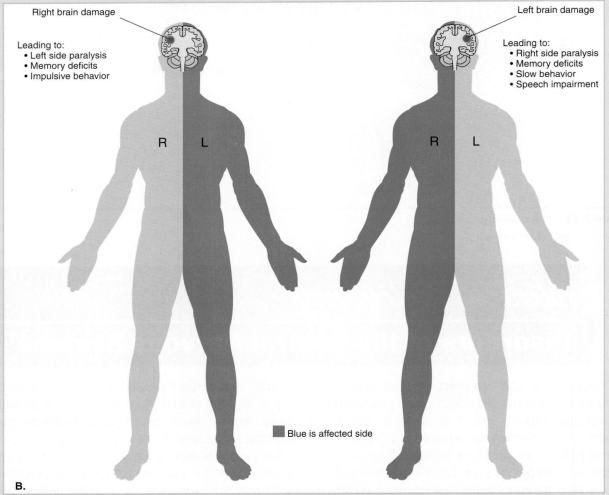

Right brain damage

Leading to:
• Left side paralysis
• Memory deficits
• Impulsive behavior

Left brain damage

Leading to:
• Right side paralysis
• Memory deficits
• Slow behavior
• Speech impairment

R   L

R   L

■ Blue is affected side

B.

Figure 7-11   *(A) An MRI of a visible bleed of the brain. (B) Symptoms of left and right CVA.*

Source: Delmar/Cengage Learning

(continues)

(continued)

Accidents, violence, and sports activities can lead to injury of the spinal cord. When an injury to the spinal cord occurs, the result can be loss of sensation and movement of body. If only the lower body is affected, this is called **paraplegia**; if all four limbs are affected, it is called **quadriplegia** (*quadri* meaning "four"). See Figure 7-12 for examples of spinal cord injuries.

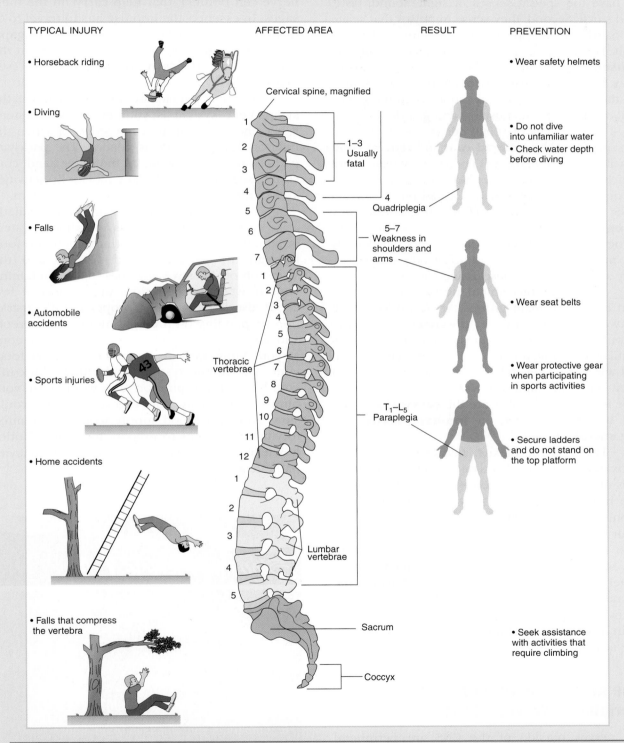

Figure 7-12 *Spinal cord injuries.*

Source: Delmar/Cengage Learning

The d Peripheral Nervous System

The PNS is made up of 12 pairs of **cranial nerves** found within the brain and 31 pairs of **spinal nerves** found along the spinal column. The cranial nerves perform four functions. First, they allow us to have the special senses of sight, sound, taste, and smell. Second, they sense impulses that relate to pain, temperature, touch, pressure, and vibration. Third, they control the voluntary or **somatic muscles**, which allow for body movement. Finally, they function in many involuntary activities such as those involving our involuntary muscles (i.e., smooth and cardiac muscles) and glands.

The 31 pairs of spinal nerves are attached to the spinal cord by a **dorsal root** and **ventral root**. Small masses of nerve cell bodies (gray matter) are attached to each dorsal root. **Ganglia** are collections of nerve cell bodies usually located outside of the CNS; these masses are therefore called **dorsal root ganglia**. They function in a sensory capacity to help bring input to the CNS. The ventral root functions as the motor nerve fiber that supplies output to voluntary and involuntary muscles and glands.

The numerous spinal nerves are interwoven into three main groups, or networks. These networks, called **nerve plexuses**, carry the impulses to various sections of the body. This is similar to an electrical junction box, which gathers wires from several sources into one area and then sends the signal onward to a specific area. The four main plexuses are the **cervical plexus**, the **brachial plexus**, the **lumbar plexus**, and the **sacral plexus**.

The cervical plexus, because of its close proximity to the head and neck, controls the muscles of the neck and receives sensory input from the head and neck. This plexus also innervates (connects) to the **phrenic nerve**, which controls your diaphragm, thus allowing you to breathe. The brachial plexus has numerous branches to the shoulder, arm, and hand. The lumbar plexus innervates the lower extremities. Finally, the sacral plexus contains the sciatic nerve, which gives some people with back problems shooting pain down the legs. Can you see why from looking at Figure 7-13?

The Autonomic Branch of the Peripheral Nervous System

All nerves outside of the CNS are peripheral nerves. Some of these nerves do not function under conscious control, but, instead, continually send and receive signals, thankfully with no voluntary effort on our parts. If you needed to think each time your heart beat or you took a breath, you would have little time to do anything else.

The autonomic nervous system (ANS) has special relay centers, or ganglia (masses of nerve cell bodies), that help carry on the messages. In essence, the impulse has to travel to or from the spinal cord over two synapses or gaps, whereas the sensory and motor input from the CNS has only one synapse to transverse (see Figure 7-14).

As noted previously in this chapter, the sympathetic system is your emergency system; it becomes active in times of stress or when the fight-or-flight response is needed. The parasympathetic nervous system, on the other hand, concerns itself mainly with daily metabolic activities and counterbalancing the sympathetic system.

For example, while you are eating quietly at a restaurant, your parasympathetic system is stimulating **peristalsis** (movement of food through the gastrointestinal system) and the secretion of digestive enzymes. It is maintaining your heart and respiration rate at normal levels. It also is maintaining proper pupil constriction (depending on the lighting or lack thereof) and airway and blood vessel tone. If someone at your table were to begin to choke on food, your sympathetic system would likely "kick in"; your heart and respiration rates would soar, your pupils would dilate, your digestive system would slow, and your blood supply would be shunted to vital areas so as to prepare for action. Notice how each of these actions opposes the parasympathetic actions.

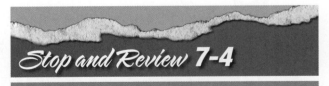

Stop and Review 7-4

Which nervous system:

a. speeds up peristalsis?

b. constricts the airways?

c. raises blood pressure?

d. moves your skeletal system?

e. constricts your pupils in bright light?

f. "kicks in" before a surprise test?

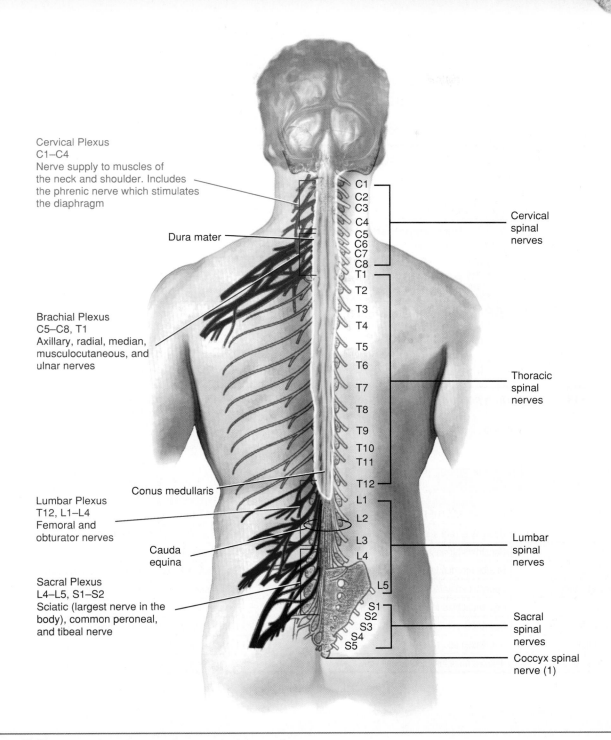

Cervical Plexus
C1–C4
Nerve supply to muscles of
the neck and shoulder. Includes
the phrenic nerve which stimulates
the diaphragm

Dura mater

Brachial Plexus
C5–C8, T1
Axillary, radial, median,
musculocutaneous, and
ulnar nerves

Conus medullaris

Lumbar Plexus
T12, L1–L4
Femoral and
obturator nerves

Cauda
equina

Sacral Plexus
L4–L5, S1–S2
Sciatic (largest nerve in the
body), common peroneal,
and tibeal nerve

C1
C2
C3
C4
C5
C6
C7
C8
T1
T2
T3
T4
T5
T6
T7
T8
T9
T10
T11
T12
L1
L2
L3
L4
L5
S1
S2
S3
S4
S5

Cervical
spinal
nerves

Thoracic
spinal
nerves

Lumbar
spinal
nerves

Sacral
spinal
nerves

Coccyx spinal
nerve (1)

Figure 7-13 *Spinal cord nerve plexuses and areas they serve.*
Source: Delmar/Cengage Learning

Hopefully, you know the **Heimlich maneuver** and can save the individual. After everything calms down, your body must be brought back to a normal state, or homeostasis. Your heart rate cannot remain at 150 for a prolonged time, and you must digest the large meal you have just consumed. Now the parasympathetic system must turn on and bring you back down from the state of heightened alert—that is, at least until you receive the bill!

See Table 7-1 for an overview of the actions of the sympathetic and parasympathetic branches of the autonomic system.

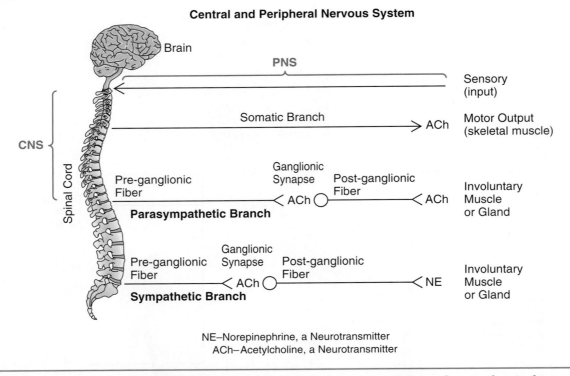

Figure 7-14   *Schematic representation of the CNS and the PNS showing synapses and neurochemical transmitter substances.*

Source: Delmar/Cengage Learning

TABLE 7-1
The Actions of the Parasympathetic and Sympathetic Nervous Systems

SYSTEM OR ORGAN	PARASYMPATHETIC ACTION	SYMPATHETIC ACTION
Heart	Decreases rate and force of contraction	Increases rate and force of contraction
Lungs	Constricts air passages	Dilates airways
Arteries	Dilates arteries to lower blood pressure	Constricts arteries, thus raising blood pressure
Gastrointestinal	Speeds peristalsis, increases digestion	Slows peristalsis and digestive activity
Urinary	Constricts bladder, thus encouraging urination	Relaxes bladder
Eye muscles	Constricts pupils, thus allowing less light to enter eyes	Dilates pupils, thus allowing more light to enter eyes
Sweat glands	Decreases secretion	Increases secretion
Hair muscles	Relaxes muscles, causes hair to lie flat	Contracts muscles and causes piloerection

■ CHAPTER REVIEW

Exercises

1. Describe how your brain is similar to a CPU.

2. What are the two main organs of the central nervous system?

3. Explain the difference between the PNS and the CNS.

4. The neuron is composed of what five main structures?

5. Describe the purpose of each of the structures listed in the answer to question 4.

6. What is the difference between the sympathetic nervous system and the parasympathetic nervous system?

7. What is the function of the cerebellum?

8. List the three layers of the meninges.

9. Which of the following body activities are controlled by the sympathetic nervous system and which by the parasympathetic nervous system?

   a. constriction of the bladder to encourage urination

   b. constriction of the pupils

   c. dilation of the airways

   d. decrease in force and rate of heart contraction

   e. piloerection

10. List the major chemical transmitter substances in the nervous system and tell where they are found.

Real Life Issues and Applications

Possible Spinal Cord Injury

While driving on a dark desert highway, you come across an unconscious accident victim who was apparently thrown from his vehicle. If the patient is not in immediate danger, why would you consider not moving him? If you need to perform CPR, what changes in technique may be necessary? If the patient sustained a spinal cord or neck injury and you moved him, what could be the outcome?

Additional Activities

1. Go to the library and research reflexes. Share your findings with the class. Demonstrate examples of reflexes.

2. Research how smoking, narcotics, and alcohol affect the nervous system. Share your findings with the class.

| Downloadable audio is available for selected medical terms in this chapter to enhance your learning of medical language. |

StudyWARE™ CONNECTION

Go to your StudyWARE™ DVD and have fun learning as you play interactive games, view animations and videos, and take practice tests to help reinforce key concepts you learned in this chapter.

Workbook Practice   *Go to your Workbook for more practice questions and activities.*

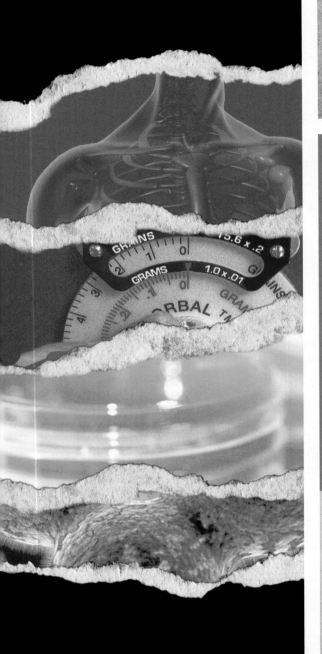

CHAPTER **8**

THE ENDOCRINE SYSTEM

Objectives

Upon completion of this chapter, you should be able to

- Differentiate between endocrine glands and exocrine glands

- List and describe the hormones and functions of the endocrine glands

- Relate the hazards of steroid abuse in athletic training

- Describe the process of hormonal secretion and regulation

- Differentiate between the types of diabetes and describe the corresponding clinical presentations

- Describe disorders of the endocrine system

Key Terms

acromegaly (ack-roh-**MEG**-ah-lee)
Addison's disease
adrenal cortex (ah-**DREE**-nal)
adrenal glands
adrenocorticotropic hormone (**ACTH**) (ad-**REE**-no-**KOR**-the-koh-trawp-ick)
aldosterone (al-**DOS**-ter-own)
alpha cells
anabolic steroids
anterior lobe
antidiuretic hormone (**ADH**)

beta cells
calcitonin
cortisol (**KOR**-tih-sol)
cretinism (**CREE**-tin-izm)
diabetes insipidus
diabetes mellitus
diuretic (die-you-**RET**-ick)
dwarfism
endocrine (**EN**-doh-krin)
epinephrine (**EP**-ih-**NEFF**-rin)
estrogen (**ES**-troh-jin)
exocrine (**ECKS**-oh-krin)

(continues)

exophthalmos (**ECKS**-of-THAL-mohs)

giantism

glucagon

glucocorticoids

glucose

glycosuria (**GLYE**-koh-**SOO**-ree-ah)

goiter (**GOI**-ter)

gonadocorticoids, or sex hormones (gon-ah-do-**KORT**-ih-**KOYDZ**)

gonads (ovaries and testes)

Graves' disease

growth hormone (**GH**)

hormones

hypercalcemia

hyperglycemia

hyperthyroidism

hypocalcemia

hypothyroidism

insulin

islets (islands) of Langerhans

isthmus (**IS**-mus)

ketones (**KEY**-tonz)

medulla (meh-**DULL**-ah)

melanocyte-stimulating hormone (**MSH**)

melatonin hormone (mel-ah-**TOE**-nin)

mineralcorticoids

myxedema (mick-seh-**DEE**-mah)

negative feedback loop

norepinephrine (nor-**EP**-ih-**NEFF**-rin)

osteoporosis (**OSS**-tee-oh-poh-**ROH**-sis)

oxytocin (auk-see-**TOE**-sin)

pancreas

parathyroid glands

parathyroid hormone (**PTH**)

pineal body (**PIN**-ee-al)

pineal gland

pituitary gland (pih-**TOO**-ih-tair-ee)

placenta

polydipsia

polyphagia

polyuria

posterior lobe

prolactin (**PRL**)

somatotropic hormone (so-**MAT**-to-troe-pick)

tetany

thymus

thyroid gland (**THIGH**-roid)

thyroid-stimulating hormone (**TSH**)

thyroxine

type I, or insulin-dependent, diabetes (juvenile diabetes)

type II, or noninsulin-dependent, diabetes (maturity-onset diabetes)

vasopressin (**VAY**-zoh-press-in)

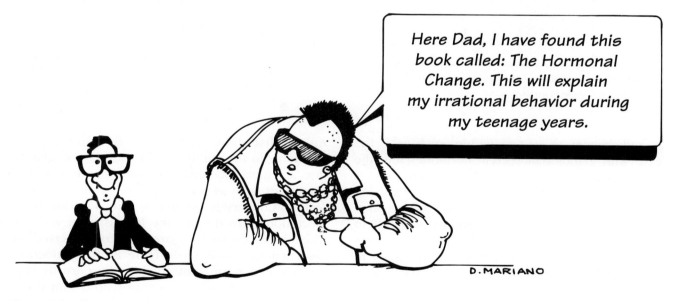

Here Dad, I have found this book called: The Hormonal Change. This will explain my irrational behavior during my teenage years.

D. MARIANO

Source: Delmar/Cengage Learning

■ SYSTEM OVERVIEW

The endocrine system is composed of eight important endocrine glands or groups of glands within the body. These are the **pituitary gland**, the **thyroid gland**, the **parathyroid glands**, the **thymus**, the **pancreas**, the **adrenal glands**, the **pineal gland**, and the **gonads (ovaries and testes)**, or sex glands (see Figure 8-1).

A *gland* is any organ that produces a secretion. Our bodies contain both **exocrine** and **endocrine** glands. The primary difference between the two can be found in the medical terms themselves. *Exocrine* (*exo* meaning "outside") literally means to secrete to the outside. We have already discussed exocrine glands such as the salivary and sweat glands, which secrete to the outside of the body in the forms of saliva and perspiration (see Figure 8-2A). *Endocrine* (*endo* meaning "within")

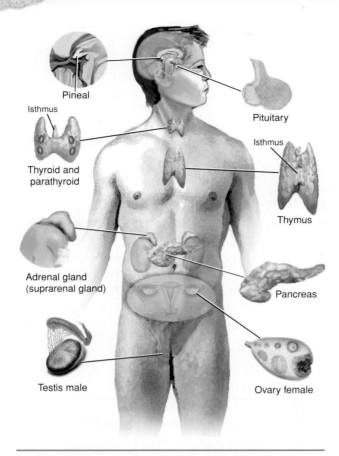

Figure 8-1   *Locations of the endocrine glands.*
Source: Delmar/Cengage Learning

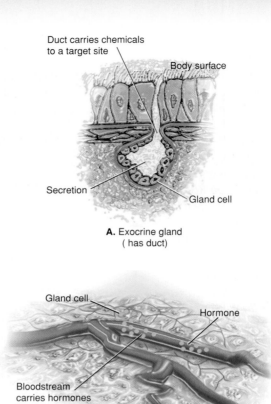

Figure 8-2   *Comparison of (A) an exocrine gland to (B) an endocrine gland.*
Source: Delmar/Cengage Learning

literally means to secrete within, such as is the case with glands that secrete hormones into the bloodstream and remain within the body.

Endocrine glands differ from exocrine glands in several other important ways. First, endocrine glands secrete **hormones**, which help to regulate and control body activities. A hormone is a chemical substance secreted by a gland in one part of the body that travels via the bloodstream to transmit its message to another area. This process can be compared to transmission within the nervous system; however, these chemical messengers travel via the bloodstream, while the electrochemical and neurochemical signals of the nervous system travel via nerve tracts. One example of hormone secretion can be traced to the adrenal glands, which secrete the hormone **epinephrine**. This hormone helps prepare the entire body for the fight-or-flight response. Each hormone has its own specific action or function.

Another major difference between endocrine and exocrine glands is the ways whereby the glands secrete. Exocrine glands have ducts (small

tubes) that allow secretions to flow into a body cavity or to the surface of the skin. Sweat glands are a typical example. Exocrine glands perform functions such as skin protection and body lubrication. Conversely, endocrine glands release their secretions directly into the bloodstream without the use of ducts; they are therefore referred to as ductless glands (see Figure 8-2B). Endocrine glands, which are controlled by the nervous system, work primarily to control body functions and maintain homeostasis. The endocrine system also stimulates long bone growth, develops sexual characteristics, regulates cellular activity, and maintains body water balance. In addition, this system regulates blood levels of sugar and minerals important to proper body functioning.

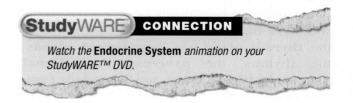

Watch the **Endocrine System** *animation on your StudyWARE™ DVD.*

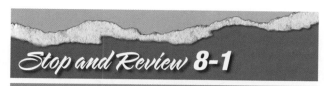

Stop and Review 8-1

a. What is a hormone?

b. What is a gland?

c. What are endocrine glands?

The Glands of the Endocrine System

The Pituitary, or Master, Gland

The pituitary gland, also known as the *hypophysis,* can be compared to the brain in the CNS. Although this gland is only the size of a pea, it controls the release of many of the hormones within the endocrine system. The pituitary gland has two parts, or lobes: the **anterior** (front) **lobe** and the **posterior** (rear) **lobe**. Each of these lobes produces several hormones. See Figure 8-3.

The anterior lobe is the controller lobe; it produces hormones that tell other glands what to produce. For example, the anterior lobe produces: **thyroid-stimulating hormone (TSH)**, which stimulates the thyroid gland to produce its specific hormone; **adrenocorticotropic hormone (ACTH)**, which stimulates the adrenal cortex to "turn on"; **growth hormone (GH)**, or **somatotropic hormone**, needed for bone and body growth; **prolactin (PRL)**, which stimulates the production of milk in the breast tissue of pregnant women; and **melanocyte-stimulating hormone (MSH)**. Melanin, as we learned in the chapter on the integumentary system, is responsible for skin color.

The posterior lobe produces **antidiuretic hormone (ADH)**, or **vasopressin**. A **diuretic** is a substance that promotes the excretion of fluid from the body. An antidiuretic, therefore, promotes retention of water. Antidiuretic hormone, when circulating in the bloodstream, thus causes the kidneys to retain (reabsorb) fluid within the body. Note: Alcohol inhibits ADH, thereby increasing the amount of fluid lost from the body. If you are for any reason instructed to drink plenty of fluids, alcohol is therefore not an appropriate choice because it will actually leave you with more of a fluid deficit. The posterior lobe also produces **oxytocin**, which causes contraction of the uterus to help deliver

Special Focus

Steroid Abuse

Some athletes turn to steroids to give them the competitive edge. More and more studies have shown, however, that the corresponding health risks and side effects far outweigh the temporary and questionable improvement an athlete may gain from the use of steroids.

Anabolic steroids are synthetic derivatives of the strongest male hormone called testosterone. In conjunction with athletic training, this hormone can stimulate muscle growth by reducing the amount of protein eliminated from the body. Because muscle is made of protein, the increased amount of protein in the body can be converted to muscle mass. The price for this increase in muscle mass, however, is very steep.

The hazard of taking a hormone not produced and regulated within the body is that it throws off the normal hormonal balance and confuses the body. Side effects of steroid misuse can include liver damage, physiological and psychological addiction, acne, cardiovascular disease, clogged arteries, liver and prostate cancers, headaches, dizziness, hypertension, and mood swings—certainly not characteristics of the ideal athlete! Males can also experience increased breast development, atrophied sexual organs, and sterility. Females can experience menstrual irregularities, increased facial hair growth, decrease in breast size, and deepening of voice.

So, for the slight gain in muscle, the question arises, "Is it worth it in the long run?" Why not train a little harder and longer and do it the right way—without the harmful side effects?

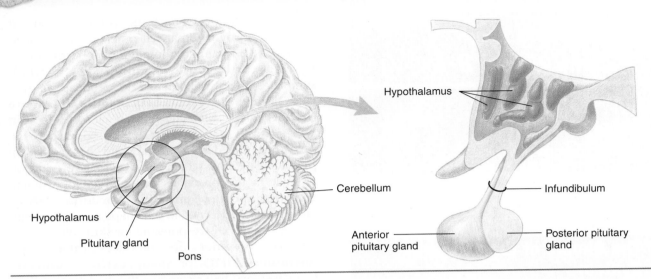

Figure 8-3   *The pituitary gland and its location.*

Source: Delmar/Cengage Learning

the neonate (*neo* meaning "new," *natal* meaning "pertaining to birth"). There are other hormones produced that will be discussed in the reproductive chapter. See Figure 8-4 which shows the various hormones secreted by the pituitary gland.

The Thyroid Gland

The thyroid gland is an H-shaped organ with two large lobes connected by a strip of tissue called an **isthmus**. This gland, the largest of the endocrine glands, surrounds the voice box. See Figure 8-5. Its major function is to regulate the production of heat and energy within our bodies. It accomplishes this by producing a hormone called **thyroxine**. In order to be produced, this hormone requires iodine. In the United States and some other countries, however, iodine is not abundant in the soil; our foodstuffs, therefore, do not contain adequate levels of iodine for proper thyroxine production. This is the main reason why we add iodine to salt (iodized salt)—because salt is so commonly used in cooking. The thyroid gland also produces **calcitonin**, which works with the parathyroid glands to regulate calcium levels in the body.

A deficiency of thyroxine causes the thyroid to work harder in an effort to produce more. This makes the gland hypertrophy and causes a **goiter**. A goiter is a swelling of the neck resulting from an enlarged thyroid. For a number of reasons, the thyroid may become overactive (**hyperthyroidism**) or underactive (**hypothyroidism**). With hyperthyroidism, the thyroid overproduces thyroxine, thus sending the individual into a "burnout" state. A common form of hyperthyroidism is **Graves' disease**, which is characterized by extreme nervousness, weight loss, excessive perspiration, and rapid pulse. All of these symptoms correspond to a hypermetabolic condition. The clinical appearance of an individual with Graves' disease is quite pronounced and includes a large goiter and bulging eyes (**exophthalmos**). See Figure 8-6 which shows exophthalmos and a goiter.

Cretinism results if the thyroid does not function in early life; the individual may become a dwarf, with or without mental deficiency. This disorder can be prevented via thyroid hormone replacement. If the thyroid atrophies during the adult years and thus secretes less hormone than normal, **myxedema** can occur. With myxedema, the individual becomes physically and mentally sluggish because the energy-producing hormone is not available in sufficient amounts. Myxedema can be cured via hormone replacement therapy.

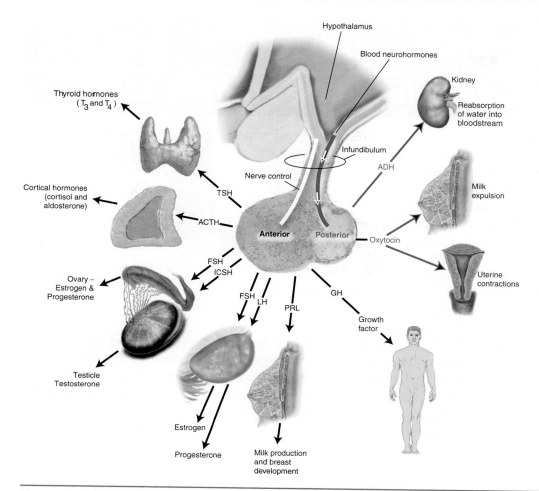

Hypothalamus

Blood neurohormones

Kidney

Thyroid hormones
(T_3 and T_4)

Reabsorption
of water into
bloodstream

Infundibulum

Nerve control

ADH

Cortical hormones
(cortisol and
aldosterone)

TSH

Anterior

Posterior

Milk
expulsion

ACTH

Oxytocin

Ovary –
Estrogen &
Progesterone

FSH
ICSH

FSH   LH

PRL

GH

Growth
factor

Uterine
contractions

Testicle
Testosterone

Estrogen

Progesterone

Milk production
and breast
development

Figure 8-4 *The pituitary gland and the hormones it secretes.*
Source: Delmar/Cengage Learning

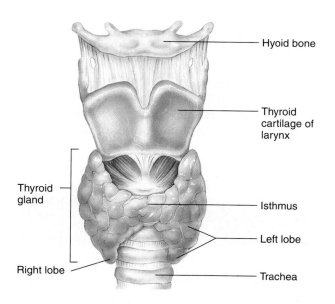

Hyoid bone

Thyroid
cartilage of
larynx

Thyroid
gland

Isthmus

Left lobe

Right lobe

Trachea

Figure 8-5 *The thyroid gland.*
Source: Delmar/Cengage Learning

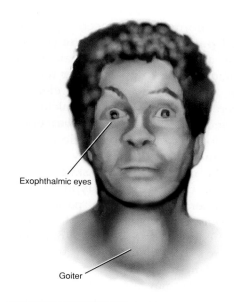

Exophthalmic eyes

Goiter

Figure 8-6 *An example of hyperthyroidism.*
Source: Delmar/Cengage Learning

Clinical Relevancy

Disorders Related to the Pituitary Gland

Several diseases are associated with a malfunctioning pituitary gland. If the gland does not produce enough growth hormone early in life, **dwarfism** can result. Dwarfism is characterized by a small body and underdeveloped sexual organs. See Figure 8-7. If the gland produces too much growth hormone, **giantism** can result. Giantism is characterized by extreme tallness and, again, underdeveloped sexual organs. Sometimes the pituitary gland becomes hyperactive and oversecretes in an adult after the majority of the growth process is compete. This leads to **acromegaly** (*acro* meaning "extremities," *megaly* meaning "enlarged"), which causes facial features and the bones of the hands and feet to enlarge. The pituitary gland can also reduce production of ADH. This would prevent the kidneys from reabsorbing water, thus resulting in **polyuria** (*poly* meaning "many or much," *uria* meaning "urine") and excessive body

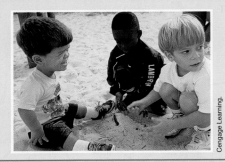

Figure 8-7   *An example of dwarfism.*

Source: Delmar/Cengage Learning

fluid loss. An individual suffering from this malady would experience **polydipsia** (*poly* meaning "many or much," *dipsia* meaning "thirst") and try desperately to correct the fluid imbalance. This often occurs in **diabetes insipidus.** Proper fluid balance can be restored via the use of ADH supplements.

The Parathyroid

Actually embedded in the thyroid gland are four parathyroid glands (*para* meaning "near"). See Figure 8-8. The hormone produced by these glands is called **parathyroid hormone (PTH).** It regulates the amount of dissolved calcium in the blood. Calcium is very important for muscular contraction, and an imbalance of this element can cause several problems. Too little calcium in the blood, a condition known as **hypocalcemia** (*hypo* meaning "low"), can lead to muscle spasms. These spasms can become increasingly longer in duration until the muscles reach a state of sustained contraction called **tetany.** Hypocalcemia results from underactivity of the parathyroid glands. Symptoms are dependent, of course, on the severity of the hypocalcemia. Treatment includes calcium replacement therapy to lessen the calcium imbalance.

Hypercalcemia may also exist, as in the case of a parathyroid tumor, causing overstimulation of these glands and excess calcium production. This will lead to elevated levels of calcium

in the bloodstream. While the kidney may be able to rid the body of this excess calcium, the calcium produced must come from some source. This source is the calcium-rich bones that will become weak and brittle as large amounts of calcium are leeched away, which may lead to a condition called **osteoporosis** (*oste/o* meaning "bone," *porosis* meaning "porous").

See Figure 8-9 for a schematic showing control of calcium in the bloodstream by the integration of the thyroid and parathyroid glands.

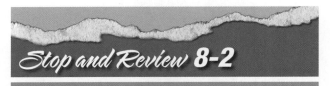

Stop and Review 8-2

a. What is the purpose of the pituitary gland?

b. Why is iodine added to salt?

c. What can result from low levels of calcium?

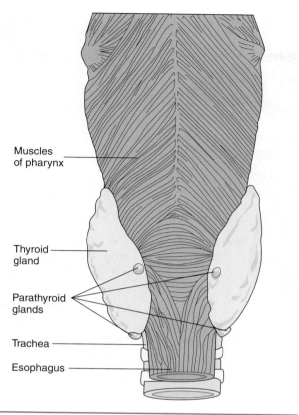

Figure 8-8   *The parathyroid glands.*

Source: Delmar/Cengage Learning

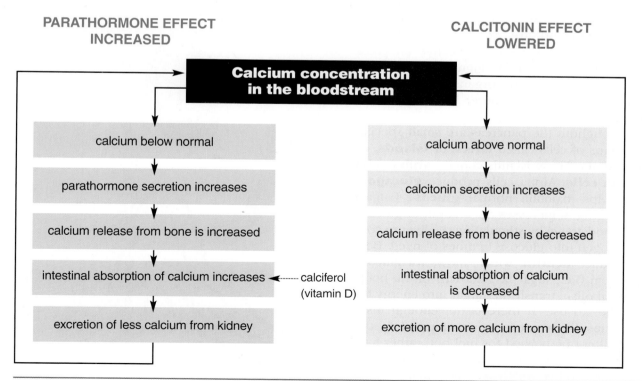

Figure 8-9   *Regulation of calcium in the bloodstream.*

Source: Delmar/Cengage Learning

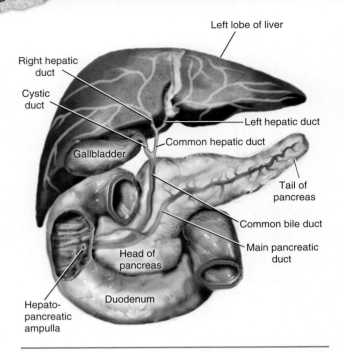

Figure 8-10   *Location of the pancreas.*

Source: Delmar/Cengage Learning

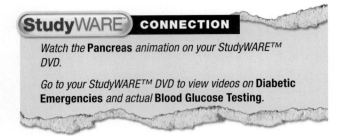

The Pancreas

The pancreas is both an exocrine gland and an endocrine gland. Its responsibilities as an exocrine gland are primarily digestive in nature through the various digestive enzymes it produces. You can see in Figure 8-10 its close proximity to the digestive organs (liver and gallbladder). We will focus here, however, on its endocrine functions.

Throughout the pancreas are small specialized groups of cells called **islets**, or **islands, of Langerhans**. These islands contain **alpha cells** and **beta cells**. Alpha cells produce **glucagon**, which helps maintain normal **glucose** (sugar) levels. Glucagon increases the amount of glucose in the bloodstream by stimulating the liver to convert glycogen into glucose in times of need. Beta cells produce **insulin**, which allows for glucose metabolism (i.e., sugar breakdown) in the body. This metabolism transforms sugar into energy for our bodies to use. If there is not enough insulin or if insulin is not functioning properly, the sugar will not be burned for fuel but, rather, will be excreted in the urine. This condition, which occurs in **diabetes mellitus**, leaves an individual with low levels of energy and excessive amounts of sugar in the urine.

The Adrenal Glands and Fight or Flight

The adrenal glands are small glands that sit atop each kidney (see Figure 8-11). Each adrenal gland has two parts that act as two separate glands. The outer portion of each gland is called the **adrenal cortex**. It secretes the following corticosteroids (more commonly known as steroids): **mineralcorticoids**, **glucocorticoids**, and **gonadocorticoids**, or **sex hormones**. The inner portion of each gland is called the **medulla**; it secretes epinephrine and **norepinephrine**.

The corticosteroids secreted by the adrenal cortex are essential to life. The mineralcorticoids regulate water and mineral salts, or electrolytes. A

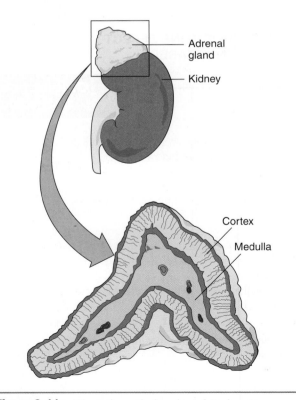

Figure 8-11   *The adrenal gland and its location.*

Source: Delmar/Cengage Learning

Clinical Relevancy

Diabetes

Diabetes is a common disease that affects many individuals. But what exactly is diabetes? As we've already discussed, there are two forms of diabetes: diabetes insipidus and diabetes mellitus. However, the form of diabetes with which most people are familiar is diabetes mellitus.

Diabetes mellitus is a condition whereby there is hyposecretion of insulin by the pancreas. This does not allow for breakdown of the carbohydrate sugar (glucose), which is needed for cellular energy. Because insulin does not break down glucose in the bloodstream, the glucose accumulates at high levels (a condition known as **hyperglycemia**), and the kidneys begin to excrete it in the urine. (A high sugar level found in the urine is called **glycosuria** [*glyc/o* meaning "sugar"].) So that the sugar content of the body does not rise dangerously high, the body also excretes large amounts of water. This causes the diabetic to be constantly thirsty (*polydipsia*).

Because the glucose can't be used for cellular energy, fats and protein must be broken down to make up for this energy need. This is why the diabetic may be constantly hungry (**polyphagia**), yet may not gain weight. Not only is burning fats for energy inefficient, this process also produces **ketones** as by-products. Ketones are toxic and can cause the diabetic to go into a coma or to die.

There are two types of diabetes mellitus. **Type 1** or *insulin-dependent (juvenile) diabetes* usually occurs in children or young adults. With this condition, the cells in the islets of the pancreas do not produce insulin. These diabetics must inject insulin into their bloodstreams and monitor glucose levels.

With **type 2** *(maturity-onset) diabetes,* insulin is present, but in insufficient amounts to meet the total needs of the body. This condition usually develops after age 40. Mild cases can be controlled by modifying the diet or taking certain oral drugs that are not insulin but stimulate the pancreas to produce more. In severe cases of type 2 diabetes, these noninsulin drugs are not enough and insulin must be injected into the body. Oral insulin is not used because it would be destroyed by the digestive juices of the stomach. See Table 8-1 for the clinical presentation of patients with insulin-dependent diabetes.

TABLE 8-1
Clinical Manifestations of Insulin-Dependent Diabetes (as Represented by the Acronym CAUTION)

Insulin-dependent diabetes is characterized by the sudden appearance of:

Constant urination (polyuria) and glycosuria

Abnormal thirst (polydipsia)

Unusual hunger (polyphagia)

The rapid loss of weight

Irritability

Obvious weakness and fatigue

Nausea and vomiting

Any one of these symptoms can signal diabetes.

Children usually exhibit dramatic, sudden symptoms and must receive prompt treatment.

(From the American Diabetes Association, New York)

---

major hormone in this grouping is **aldosterone**, which controls the levels of sodium and potassium within our bodies. This is crucial to body water balance. For example, if you were lost in the desert, your body would send signals to circulate aldosterone in the bloodstream, which would conserve sodium and water.

Glucocorticoids assist in the metabolism of carbohydrates, fats, and protein. The breakdown of these compounds for energy is especially needed in times of stress to the body. A major hormone in this group is **cortisol**, which aids in the metabolism of food products during stress. (The exact mechanism by which this is accomplished is further explained in the section on hormone secretion and regulation later in this chapter.)

Gonadocorticoids, or sex hormones, help develop secondary sexual characteristics. Their other functions are not clear, but they are believed to supplement male and female hormones from the ovaries and testes.

The hormones secreted by the medulla, epinephrine and norepinephrine, are the "fight-or-flight" hormones because they stimulate sympathetic nerves to raise blood pressure, increase heart rate and force, dilate airways, and increase the amount of energy available to the muscles.

Epinephrine is also known as *adrenaline;* this is why when we gear up and feel super-charged for a stressful event or athletic challenge, it is referred to as an "adrenalin rush."

The adrenal glands are essential because they respond to internal and external stresses (and we sure have enough of those!). Hypofunction of the adrenal glands causes **Addison's disease**, a condition whereby the body loses its ability to respond to stress and, as a result, the immune system's ability is impaired. Resistance, therefore, greatly decreases and chance of disease increases.

The Pineal Body, Thymus, and Placenta

The **pineal body** located deep within the brain is a small, pinecone-shaped structure; its function is not fully understood. It is theorized, however, that one of its functions is to produce **melatonin hormone**, which influences sleep-wake cycles and other circadian (daily) body rhythms. The pineal body has also been shown to have some effects on the female ovaries. This gland begins to degenerate at 7 years of age.

The thymus gland located in the center of the chest is believed to stimulate lymphocytes to help the immune system, especially early in life. This gland may be responsible for developing the immune response in newborns. The thymus gland grows until puberty. The **placenta**, or "lifeline from mom," produces several hormones during pregnancy and is, thus, classified as an endocrine gland.

The Sex Glands (Ovaries and Testes)

The sex glands are the ovaries, in the female, and the testes, in the male. These glands are important in the development of sexual characteristics,

especially during puberty. The testes produce the male hormone, testosterone, which is responsible for developing the deep voice, facial hair, and reproductive organs of the male. The ovaries produce the major female hormone, **estrogen**, which is responsible for developing the breasts and reproductive organs and regulating menstruation in the female. The ovaries also produce progesterone, which both helps prepare the mammary glands for milk production and aids in maintaining pregnancy. These will be discussed in more detail in the reproductive chapter.

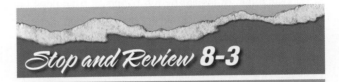

Stop and Review 8-3

a. What is diabetes mellitus?

b. What are the two divisions of the adrenal glands? What are the functions of each?

c. What is testosterone responsible for in the male?

Hormonal Secretion and Regulation

The Negative Feedback Loop

How does the body know when to release hormones into the bloodstream? How much should it release and when should it stop? Figure 8-12 shows the secretion and regulation of glucocorticoids during a period of stress.

First, some type of physical, mental, or environmental stress stimulates the hypothalamus, which sends signals to the pituitary gland to release adrenal corticotrophin hormone (ACTH) into the bloodstream. The ACTH circulates to the adrenal cortex, where it tells the cortex to release glucocorticoids to prepare the body for handling the stress.

The glucocorticoids, which regulate the metabolism of carbohydrates, fats, and proteins, begin to break down these compounds to increase the levels of glucose in the body. This extra energy is needed to handle and relieve the stress. As the stress is relieved, the level of signals sent to the hypothalamus decreases, thereby

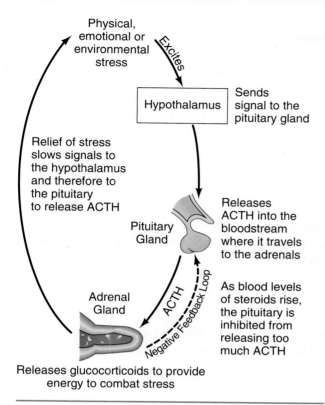

Figure 8-12 *Secretion and regulation of glucocorticoid hormones.*
Source: Delmar/Cengage Learning

lessening the amount of ACTH being released into the bloodstream. This, in turn, decreases the amount of glucocorticoids released to the adrenal cortex.

This homeostatic control of hormone levels utilizes the common **negative feedback loop** utilized in most homeostatic regulatory activities. This simply means that as the levels of glucocorticoids rise, the pituitary gland's release of ACTH is inhibited, or slowed down. This prevents excessive or continuous release of glucocorticoids. Without this negative feedback loop, the levels of glucocorticoids could rise dangerously high and begin to break down large amounts of the carbohydrates, fats, and proteins; in essence, the glucocorticoids would begin to break down the muscles and integrity of the body.

■ CHAPTER REVIEW

Exercises

1. Explain the differences between anabolic steroids and steroids normally found in your body.

2. Differentiate between endocrine glands and exocrine glands.

3. What does a diuretic do to the body to cause increased urination?

4. How are hormones regulated in the body?

5. Why are glucocorticoids important?

6. Which gland is responsible for the regulation of glucose levels via the production of glucagon?

7. List the side effects that can occur with the abuse of anabolic steroids.

8. Where are each of the following glands located?

   a. pineal

   b. thyroid

   c. pancreas

   d. pituitary

9. What is a goiter?

10. Define *polydipsia* and *polyuria*.

11. Contrast type I and type II diabetes.

Real Life Issues and Applications

What Is the Problem?

From a brief patient history you learn that a 50-year-old obese male presented to the Emergency Department (ED) with the following symptoms:

- polydipsia
- slight disorientation
- generalized weakness and malaise
- breath with a "Juicy Fruit gum type smell"
- polyuria

Furthermore, the patient stated that "he's been eating tons of food but not gaining any weight."

What would you expect the diagnosis to be? What would you expect the vital signs to be? What possible treatment modalities would you suggest for this patient?

Additional Activities

1. Contact a local hospital to obtain the name and phone number of an endocrinologist. Contact that physician and ask if he or she would speak to your class regarding the endocrine system.

2. What is your opinion regarding the use of anabolic steroids in athletics if it were done under a doctor's supervision and offered to all athletes?

3. Discuss the use of diuretics as a way to lose weight.

4. Discuss drugs that can cross the placental barrier and adversely affect the developing fetus.

Downloadable audio is available for selected medical terms in this chapter to enhance your learning of medical language.

StudyWARE CONNECTION

Go to your StudyWARE™ DVD and have fun learning as you play interactive games, view animations and videos, and take practice tests to help reinforce key concepts you learned in this chapter.

Workbook Practice   *Go to your Workbook for more practice questions and activities.*

CHAPTER 9

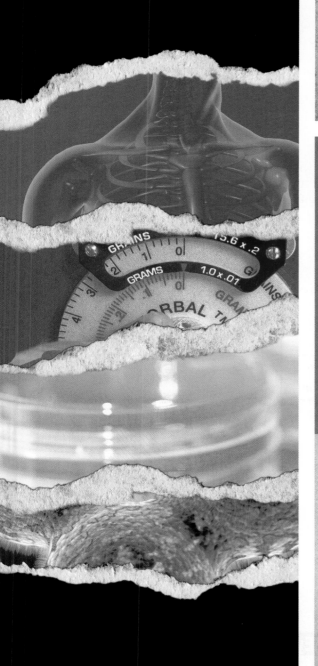

THE SPECIAL SENSES

Objectives

Upon completion of this chapter, you should be able to

■ List and describe the special senses of the body

■ Explain the structures and functions of the eye

■ Describe the process of vision

■ Explain the structures and functions of the ear

■ Describe the process of hearing and sound transmission

■ List and explain eye and ear disorders

Key Terms

adaptation

amblyopia
   (am-blee-**OH**-pee-ah)

anvil (**AN**-vil)

aqueous humor

auditory nerve

auricle (**AW**-reh-kul)

cataract (**KAT**-a-rack)

cerumen (see-**ROO**-men)

ceruminous glands
   (see-**ROO**-men-us)

choroid (**KOH**-roid)

ciliary muscles (**SILL**-ee-air ee)

cochlea (**KOCK**-lee-ah)

cones

conjunctiva
   (**KON**-junk-**TYE**-vah)

conjunctivitis
   (kon-**JUNK**-tih-**VYE**-tis)

eardrum

endolymph

eustachian tubes
   (you-**STAY**-she-un)

external auditory canal

external ear

extrasensory perception (**ESP**)

glaucoma (glaw-**KOH**-mah)

hammer

hyperopia
   (high-per-**OH**-pee-ah)

incus (**IN**-kus)

internal ear

iris

labyrinth (**LAB**-ih-rinth)

(continues)

labyrinthitis (**LAB**-ih-rin-**THIGH**-tis)
lacrimal glands (**LACK**-rih-mal)
lens
malleus (**MAL**-ee-us)
Ménière's disease (**MAIN**-ee-**AYRZ**)
middle ear
myopia (my-**OH**-pee-ah)
orbit
organ of Corti
ossicle (**AHS**-ih-kul)

otitis media (oh-**TYE**-tis **ME**-dee-ah)
oval window
perilymph (**PAIR**-eh-limf)
photopigments
pinna (**PIN**-nah)
pupil
retina (**RET**-ih-nah)
rods
sclera (**SKLAIR**-ah)
semicircular canals

stapes (**STAY**-peez)
stirrup
tactile corpuscles (**TACK**-tile)
taste buds
tinnitus (tin-**EYE**-tus)
tympanic cavity (tim-**PAN**-ick)
tympanic membrane
vertigo (**VER**-tih-go)
vestibule chamber (**VES**-tih-byule)
vitreous humor (**VIT**-ree-us)

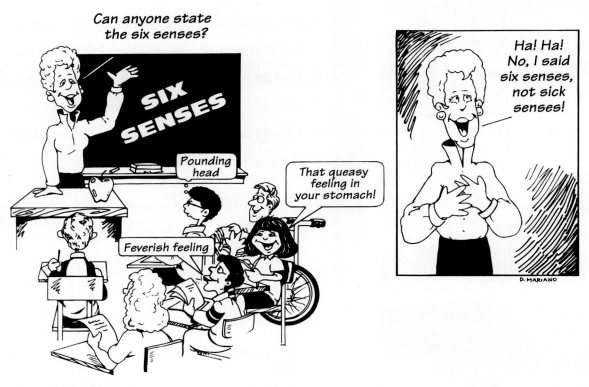

Source: Delmar/Cengage Learning

■ INTRODUCTION

Your senses allow you to detect changes in the environment and send this information from receptors to your brain via sensory, or afferent, neurons. Here the brain interprets the information and, in many circumstances, makes the appropriate motor, or efferent, response.

This chapter presents a basic overview of the structures and functions of two major sense organs—the eyes and the ears—along with some information about our other senses.

The Eye

The Layers of the Eye

The eye has many similarities to an older film camera. The light from the images you photograph with your camera passes through the small opening (pupil) and is focused on the photoreceptive film (retina). Hopefully, the autofocus on the camera (iris) is properly working, thus allowing the right amount of light to enter and focus properly on the film for a clear image.

Special Focus

More Than Just Five Senses

Traditionally, we have been taught that we possess the five senses of vision, hearing, smell, taste, and touch. There are more than five categories of sensory input to the brain, however. What about pain and pressure sensations? How do we "feel" hot and cold? How do our bodies sense position and balance (equilibrium)? What about feelings of hunger and thirst? These, too, are senses that are very important to survival. And what about common sense and intuition?

The senses of sight (eyes), sound and equilibrium (ears), taste (tongue), smell (nose), and touch (skin) are referred to as our *special senses.* These senses are found in well-defined regions of the body. However, we also have other senses scattered throughout our bodies in various regions. These are referred to as our *general senses,* and include the sensations of heat, cold, pain, nausea, hunger, thirst, and pressure, or deep touch.

The senses can be even further broken down. For example, the receptors of the skin are referred to as the *cutaneous senses,* and include touch, heat, cold, and pain. The *visceral (organ) senses* include nausea, hunger, thirst, and the need to urinate and defecate.

Before finishing this "enlightenment" of the senses, there is one more sense that many believe we possess. By "reading your mind," we see you have already identified this sense as **extrasensory perception (ESP)**, meaning senses outside (extra) the normal sensory perceptions. Although there is still debate over whether this phenomenon exists, we just know this chapter will be an *eye-opening* experience for you—and we hope the puns aren't making you *nauseous.*

The eye has three layers: the **sclera**, the **choroid**, and the **retina** (see Figure 9-1). The sclera is a tough, fibrous tissue that serves as the protective shield we commonly call the "white of the eye." The sclera contains a specialized portion called the *cornea.* The cornea is transparent, allowing for outside light to pass through the eye.

The second layer, or the choroid, is a highly vascularized region that provides nourishment to

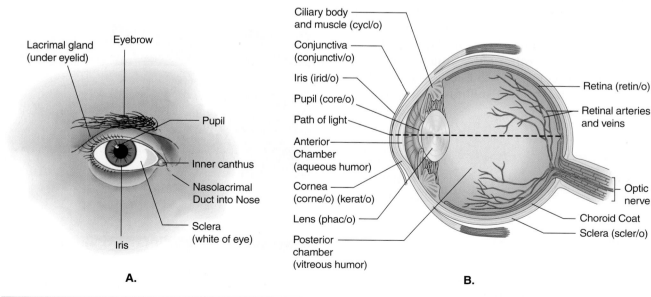

Figure 9-1 *(A) External view of eye. (B) Structures of the eye.*
Source: Delmar/Cengage Learning

the eye much in the same way as a battery pack "nourishes" a video camera. This layer contains the **iris** and the **pupil**. The iris is the colored portion of your eye. It controls the size of the pupil opening, through which light passes into the eye. The iris is a sphincter, meaning that it is able to relax, or contract, thereby making the pupil larger or smaller, depending on lighting conditions. In low light, the iris relaxes, allowing the pupil to dilate; this allows more light into the eye for a better image.

Located behind the pupil is the **lens**, which is surrounded by **ciliary muscles**. These muscles can alter the shape of the lens, making it thinner or thicker, to allow the incoming light rays to focus on the retinal area.

The third, or innermost, layer of the eye is the **retina**. This area contains the nerve endings that receive and interpret the rays of light into our vision. The retina is a delicate membrane, which continues posteriorly and joins to the optic nerve. It contains two types of light-sensing receptors, called **rods** and **cones**. These receptors contain **photopigments**, which cause a chemical change when light hits them. This change causes an impulse to be sent to the optic nerve, where the brain interprets it and we "see" an object. This interpretation occurs in the visual part of the cerebral cortex, located in the occipital lobe.

Why are there two types of photoreceptors? Just like a video camera, the eyes are exposed to different lighting conditions. In low-light conditions, video camera images are black and white, whereas in good lighting conditions, the images are fully colorized. The rods of our eyes are the photoreceptors for dim light; they provide us with black-and-white images in dark conditions. The cones, on the other hand, function in bright light and provide us with color vision. Each retina contains about 3 million cones and 100 million rods.

QUOTES & NOTES

The human eye can see about 7 million shades of color!

Protection of the Eye

The eye is protected by the skull bones that form the eye cavity, or **orbit**. Also protecting the eye are two movable folds of skin known as eyelids. The eyelids contain the eyelashes, which help prevent gross (i.e., large) particles

from entering the eye. A protective membrane called **conjunctiva** lines the cornea. In addition, the eye also contains **lacrimal glands**; these exocrine glands produce the tears needed for constant cleansing and lubrication. Tears are produced continuously and are spread throughout the eyes by blinking. Our eyes do not run under noncrying circumstances because the excess tear production drains into the nose via two small holes in the inner corner of each eye. When you cry, however, the excess tears run down your cheeks and more drain into your nose, causing it to run. The tears also act as an antiseptic to keep the eyeballs free of germs.

Two chambers of fluid within the eye also help to protect this structure. These "fluids of the eye" are referred to as *humors.* The **aqueous** (watery) **humor** bathes the iris, pupil, and lens and is the anterior chamber. The **vitreous humor** is a clear, jelly-like fluid that occupies the entire eye interior behind the lens; it is, therefore, the posterior chamber.

In summation, then, light enters the eye, passing through the conjunctival membrane, cornea, aqueous humor, pupil, lens, and vitreous humor and focusing on the retina. The photoreceptors in the retina cause a chemical impulse to be sent to the optic nerve, which carries the impulse to the brain for the interpretation we call *vision.* See if you can trace the pathway light takes in Figure 9-2.

Stop and Review 9-1

a. How is the eye like a camera?

b. List the three layers of the eye.

c. How does the size of the pupil change? Why is this necessary?

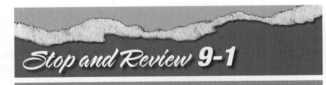

StudyWARE   **CONNECTION**

Go to your StudyWARE™ DVD to view an animation on the special sense of **Vision** *and a video on* **Applying Eye Medications**.

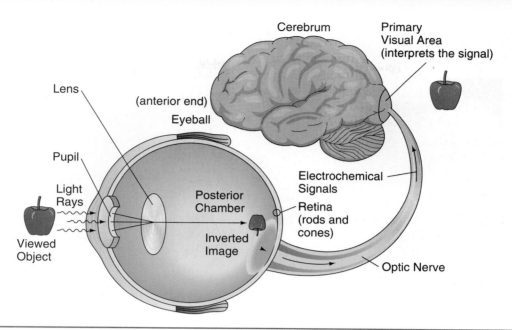

Figure 9-2 *The pathway of light through the eyes and how the brain interprets the signal.*
Source: Delmar/Cengage Learning

Clinical Relevancy

Eye Disorders

Conjunctivitis is an inflammation of the membrane that lines the eye. This condition can be either acute or chronic and is caused by a variety of irritants and pathogens. The acute form is commonly called *pinkeye,* is highly contagious, and is caused by a bacteria. A **cataract** is a condition whereby the lens loses its transparent nature, and light cannot easily pass through the clouded lens. It has been shown that increased exposure to sunlight may contribute to the development of cataracts. Left untreated, this condition can lead to blindness. The treatment is excising the clouded lens and replacing it with a new lens as shown in Figure 9-3.

Glaucoma can also lead to blindness. This disease is characterized by increased pressure in the fluid of the eye, which interferes with optic nerve functioning. Glaucoma

occurs in 20% of adults over age 40 and accounts for 15% of the cases of blindness in the United States. Given that this disease usually can be readily diagnosed and treated, this is truly a tragic loss.

Several imperfections of the eye can impair vision. The eyes may have difficulty focusing on near or far objects because light rays do not focus properly on the retina. **Hyperopia**, or farsightedness, results when the eye cannot focus properly on nearby objects, causing them to appear blurred. **Myopia**, or nearsightedness, results when the eye cannot focus properly on faraway objects, causing them to appear blurred. See Figure 9-4. **Amblyopia**, or lazy eye, usually occurs in childhood. With this condition, poor vision in one eye is caused by the dominance of the other eye, which does most of the work.

(continues)

(continued)

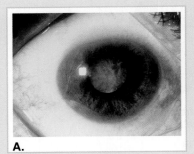

A.

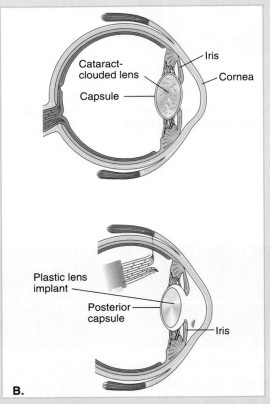

Iris

Cataract-clouded lens

Cornea

Capsule

Plastic lens implant

Posterior capsule

Iris

B.

Figure 9-3 *(A) An actual cataract. (Courtesy of The National Eye Institute) (B) Cataract extraction with replacement of intraocular lens.*

Source: Delmar/Cengage Learning

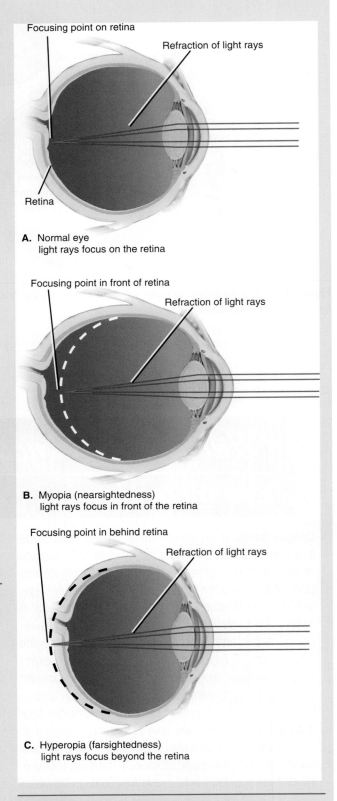

Focusing point on retina

Refraction of light rays

Retina

A. Normal eye
light rays focus on the retina

Focusing point in front of retina

Refraction of light rays

B. Myopia (nearsightedness)
light rays focus in front of the retina

Focusing point in behind retina

Refraction of light rays

C. Hyperopia (farsightedness)
light rays focus beyond the retina

Figure 9-4 *(A) Normal vision compared to (B) nearsightedness and (C) farsightedness.*

Source: Delmar/Cengage Learning

Special Focus

Fiber Optics in the Health Science Field

By utilizing the concept of light "piping," we are able to explore the inner workings of the body without making incisions. For example, the main airways of the lung can be observed via the use of a long, fiber-optic device called a *bronchoscope*. This device has a diameter slightly larger than that of a drinking straw. The lighted tip of the scope is flexible and can turn both left and right, which facilitates movement through the airways. After the patient has been sufficiently numbed (with a drug such as xylocaine), the bronchoscope is inserted through the patient's nose and gently pushed down the back of the throat, through the vocal cords, and into the lung.

A similar fiber-optic scope is used to examine the esophagus and stomach; this scope is called a *gastroscope*. And a *proctoscope* is used to examine the colon and large intestine.

One advantage of examining procedures using the aforementioned scopes is that general anesthesia is not required. In fact, patients are often offered a chance to look into the scopes—and into themselves!

Today, the use of fiber-optic scopes in some abdominal surgeries allows for smaller incisions and shorter hospital stays. Procedures such as gallbladder removal may now require only four small incisions that leave tiny scars. This is a great improvement over the older method, which left a scar several inches in length.

The Ear

Structures of the Ear

We hear by receiving vibrations via the air and translating them into interpretable sound. The ear is primarily responsible for hearing and equilibrium. The ear can be divided into three areas. Isn't it strange how almost everything can be divided into threes? Nevertheless, the three divisions are the **external ear**, the **middle ear**, or **tympanic cavity**, and the **internal ear**, or **labyrinth** (see Figure 9-5).

The external ear is the outer projection, or the part we can see (see Walt Disney's classic *Dumbo*). It also includes the canal (where we put the Q-tips, though we shouldn't) leading to the middle ear. The projecting part of the external ear, called the **pinna** or **auricle**, leads to the canal, or **external auditory canal**. The canal may contain earwax, called **cerumen**, which is secreted by the **ceruminous glands**. Cerumen helps to trap foreign particles and insects as well as helping to prevent the growth of microorganisms. At the end of the canal is the **eardrum**, or **tympanic membrane**. Here, the external ends, and the middle ear begins.

The middle ear, or tympanic cavity, is basically a space containing three small bones, or **ossicles**. These bones are joined in a manner so as to amplify (make louder) the sound waves that the tympanic membrane receives from the external ear. When amplified, the sound waves are then transmitted to the fluid contained in the internal ear.

The bones of the middle ear are named according to their shapes. The first ossicle attached to the tympanic membrane is the **hammer**, or **malleus**. The **incus**, or **anvil**, is attached to the hammer. Finally, the **stirrup**, or **stapes**, connects to a membrane called the **oval window**. The oval window is the beginning point of the internal ear and carries the amplified vibrations from the tympanic ossicles.

Also contained in the middle ear are the **eustachian tubes**. These structures allow air pressure on either side of the eardrum to be equalized. The tubes connect the nose and throat to the middle ear. In this way, they can sense the external atmospheric pressure (through the nose and throat openings) and the inner ear pressure (through their attachment to the middle ear). The equalization of pressure between the middle ear and external atmosphere allows the eardrum to freely vibrate with incoming sound waves. Sudden pressure changes, such as those experienced when flying in an airplane, can affect this area. This is why when flying, you are instructed

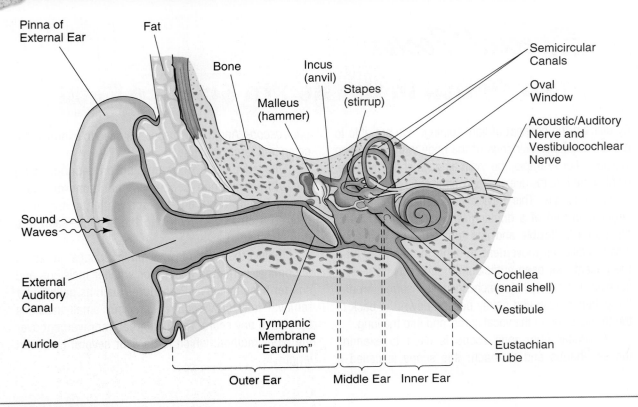

Figure 9-5   *The structures of the ear.*

Source: Delmar/Cengage Learning

to swallow or to chew gum—so that the inner ear can better adjust to the changing external atmosphere via the eustachian tubes.

The oval window membrane is now the starting point for the journey of sound into the internal ear or labyrinth. This area is composed of (guess what?) three separate hollow bony spaces that form a complex *maze.* Because another term for maze is *labyrinth,* this area is also referred to as the bony **labyrinth.** The three bony spaces are called the **cochlea,** the **vestibule chamber,** which houses the internal ear, and the **semicircular canals.** The labyrinth is responsible for maintaining our sense of balance. The semicircular canals contain sensory input related to equilibrium.

The cochlea is the bony, snail shell–shaped entrance to the internal ear, which is connected to the oval window membrane. The cochlea contains fluid called **perilymph,** which helps transmit sound through this area. The sound is then transmitted to the back of the maze which contains another fluid called **endolymph.** Here the sound is carried to tiny, hair-like receptors, which, in turn, are stimulated converting the vibrations to a signal that is conducted to the brain via the **auditory nerve.**

In summation, then, sound waves enter the external ear, travel through the canal, and vibrate the eardrum, or tympanic membrane. This is referred to as *sound conduction.* The middle ear then amplifies the sound via the ossicles. This is referred to as *bone conduction.* The last ossicle, the stapes, vibrates and causes a gentle pumping against the oval window membrane. This causes cochlear fluid, or perilymph, to move, thus transmitting the sound to the back of the labyrinth. Here, the sound is carried via endolymph to small, hair-like nerves found in the spiral structure lining the entire length of the cochlea called the **organ of Corti** and, eventually, reaches the hearing centers in the brain. This is referred to as sensorineural conduction. Figure 9-6 traces the pathway of sound waves.

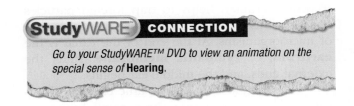

StudyWARE   **CONNECTION**

Go to your StudyWARE™ DVD to view an animation on the special sense of **Hearing.**

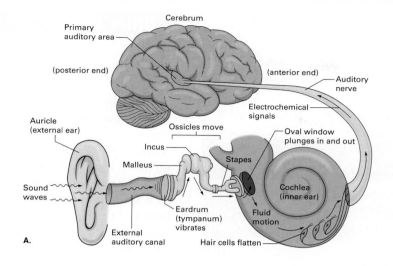

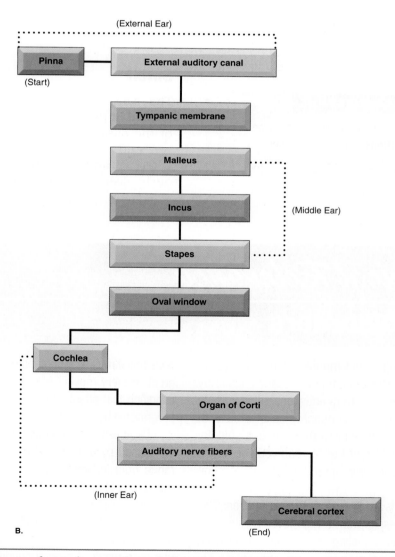

Figure 9-6 *(A) The pathway of sound waves through the ear structurally. (B) A schematic of the pathway of sound waves through the ear.*

Source: Delmar/Cengage Learning

Stop and Review 9-2

a. List and describe three structures found in the middle ear.

b. What structure of the ear is important for balance?

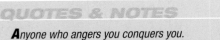

CONNECTION

Go to your StudyWARE™ DVD to view videos on the **Application of Ear Drops**, *and the use of* **Tympanic Thermometers**.

Other Senses

Taste

Taste receptors are located in the tongue and are called **taste buds** (see Figure 9-7). We have only five tastes: sweet, sour, salty, bitter, and umami (commonly called savory or the taste of glutanates). It was previously thought that there were respective receptors for these tastes each located in a specific region of the tongue. Currently it is believed that specific tastes can be detected over a wider area of the tongue than previously thought. Interestingly enough, the refinement of our taste for food is primarily dependent on our sense of smell.

Smell

The sense of smell arises from the receptors located in the olfactory region, or the upper part, of the nasal cavity (see Figure 9-8). This is why we "sniff": in order to bring smell up to this area where it can be interpreted. As mentioned previously, taste and smell are closely related; this is

Clinical Relevancy

Ear Disorders

Otitis (*ot/o* meaning "ear") **media** is an inflammation of the middle ear. This condition is usually caused by a bacteria or virus and frequently occurs in infants and young children. It is commonly associated with an upper respiratory infection (URI) such as a cold. By examining the structure of the ear, can you see how a cold or sinus infection can spread to an ear infection and vice versa?

Labyrinthitis is an inflammation of the inner ear. This condition usually results from a high fever. Labyrinthitis can cause **vertigo**, a feeling of dizziness or whirling in space. If you are not sure what vertigo is, watch the classic Alfred Hitchcock film of the same name. (Not only

does this film clearly demonstrate vertigo, but it is also a great mystery movie!) **Ménière's disease** is a chronic condition that affects the labyrinth and leads to tinnitus, progressive hearing loss, and vertigo.

Deafness can be either partial or complete and can be caused by a variety of conditions. These conditions range from inflammation and scarring of the tympanic membrane to auditory nerve damage, congenital defects, and brain damage. Finally, **tinnitus** is the medical term for a ringing sound in the ears, which according to superstition, means someone is talking about you. Actually, it can be a result of several conditions such as impacted cerumen, otitis media, and drug toxicity.

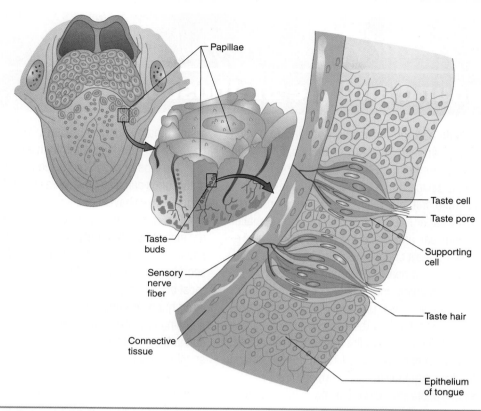

Figure 9-7 *The taste buds.*

Source: Delmar/Cengage Learning

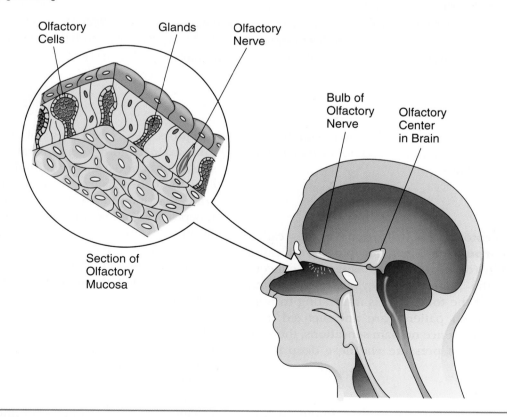

Figure 9-8 *The olfactory region.*

Source: Delmar/Cengage Learning

Clinical Relevancy

Sound and the Stethoscope

For many health care professionals, listening to a variety of sounds is an everyday part of the job. Lifesaving determinations often can be made through the use of a stethoscope, a device that enhances the ability to hear sounds. A simple stethoscope can be made by rolling a piece of heavy paper into a cone. If you hold the smaller opening to your ear and place the larger opening over the area of someone's chest where the heart is located, you should be able to hear the person's heartbeat.

With proper training and practice, a variety of information can be obtained via listening with a stethoscope, including the quality of a heartbeat, blood pressure, how well air is flowing in and out of the tracheobronchial tree, the amount and location of secretions in the lungs, and how well treatment modalities are working.

The volume of breath sounds can aid us in diagnosing disease. For example, lung diseases such as emphysema cause a higher than normal amount of air in the lungs. As a result, breath sounds decrease in volume because air does not transmit sound as well as does fluid or solid. Pneumonia, on the other hand, can cause the air sacs and airways of the lungs to fill with secretions and fluid. As a result, breath sounds increase in volume because sound travels better through liquid than air.

The type of sound produced by air moving in and out of the lungs can also provide valuable diagnostic information. Wheezes have a musical quality and result from constriction of the smooth muscles of the airways. Rhonchi are also somewhat musical in nature but have a "bubbly" sound and a lower pitch. Rhonchi often are caused by secretions in the larger airways. Wheezes and rhonchi are most often heard on exhalation. Crackles (or rales), on the other hand, are heard on inspiration. Crackles sound like cracking or popping and can result from fluid accumulation in the small airways or a sudden popping open of the small airways.

You will learn about many other breath and cardiac sounds as you continue your studies. Through practice, you will learn to differentiate these sounds and understand their meanings. Before you begin practicing on patients, however, we offer one general word of advice: *Always warm your stethoscope in your hands before placing it on a patient!* It is much easier to do this than it is to peel your patient off the ceiling!

why you cannot taste foods when you have a severe head cold. Pleasant food odors also initiate digestive enzymes.

Touch

Touch receptors are small, round bodies called **tactile corpuscles**. These receptors are located in the skin (dermis) and are especially concentrated in the fingertips. They are also located on the tip of the tongue. It is interesting to note that even when patients are anesthetized and, therefore, experience no pain sensations, they are still conscious of pressure via these deep touch sensors.

Temperature

Temperature sensors are also found within the skin. The body has separate heat and cold receptors. An interesting phenomenon called **adaptation** can be demonstrated via these sensors. Continued sensory stimulation causes the sensors to desensitize or adapt. For example, if you are continuously exposed to the cold, the receptors adjust so that you won't feel so cold. Another example is when you enter a hot bath. Initially, it may feel extremely hot. After a few seconds, however, it doesn't feel so hot, even though the actual temperature of the water has not changed.

Pain

Pain is a very important protective sense; it is the body's way of making us pay attention to particular dangers. It is the most widely distributed sense, being found in skin, muscles, joints, and internal organs. The pain receptors are merely a branching of nerve fibers called *free nerve endings*.

Special Focus

Loud Noises

"Turn down that loud music! You'll lose your hearing!" Have you heard that before? Believe it or not, we heard the same thing from our parents. Of course, that was back in the late 1960s and early 1970s—when there was *real* rock! We thought that neither rock nor our hearing would ever die. We were half right.

The negative effects of loud noises on hearing are well documented. Loud noises come not only from rock music, but also from chain saws, heavy machinery, airplanes, motorcycles, gunfire, mowers, and a variety of power tools.

Because we are individuals, we are susceptible to hearing loss in varying degrees. Exposure to loud noises usually causes a high-pitched ringing in the ears (called *tinnitus*). As the exposure to the noise continues, the microscopic hair cells in the organ of Corti are destroyed. Hearing loss usually begins in the upper frequencies (i.e., the higher pitches) and works its ways down through the lower ranges as the loss progresses.

How loud must noise be to do damage? It is generally thought that noises greater than 85 decibels will cause damage. It is important to note, however, that both *intensity* and *duration* of the noise affect hearing loss. Thus, it is important to limit exposure to louder noises.

How can you protect your hearing? *Turn down that loud music* and wear hearing protectors (ideally both the soft, foam plugs that fit in your ears and the fluid-filled cups that fit over your ears) when exposed to loud sounds. You may think you look like a dork, but remember this: When your hearing is gone, it is usually gone for good. If your friends make fun of you for protecting your hearing now, you will have the last laugh. Unfortunately, you may be the only one to hear it. Look at the following decibel scale which shows some common examples of noise sources.

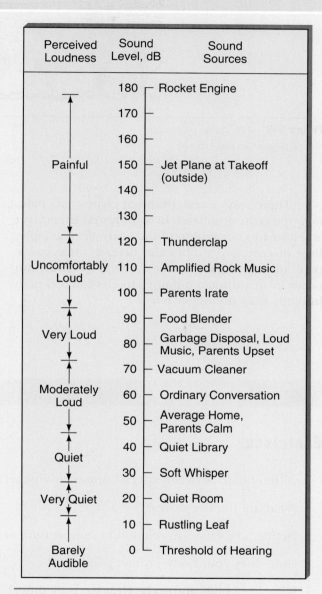

The decibel scale, including some common examples of decibel levels.

Source: Delmar/Cengage Learning

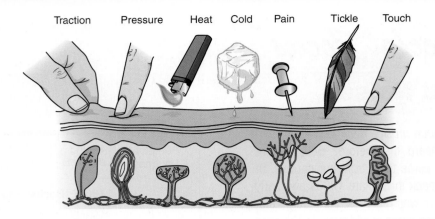

Traction   Pressure   Heat   Cold   Pain   Tickle   Touch

Figure 9-9   *The sense of touch.*

Source: Delmar/Cengage Learning

There are even different types of pain. *Referred pain* originates in an internal organ, yet is felt another region of the body. For example, liver disease and gallbladder disease often cause pain in the right shoulder. *Phantom pain* can occur in an amputated limb; patients can feel pain in limbs they no longer have.

Pain receptors do not adapt. Unless you are anesthetized, therefore, you feel pain as long as the pain-creating stimulus is present. Because pain receptors do not adapt, it is doubtful that people actually have different thresholds of pain. Rather, it is more likely that people just react in different degrees to pain. Figure 9-9 illustrates the sense of touch.

■ CHAPTER REVIEW

Exercises

1. Differentiate between special senses and general senses.

2. What are the five tastes?

3. Define adaptation in relation to temperature sensors.

4. How does your body protect your eyes?

5. What are cones and rods? How do they differ?

6. How does the brain receive sensory input from the eye?

7. How does the shape of the lens change?

8. List and describe the fluids of the eye.

9. List and describe three diseases of the eye.

10. List and describe two diseases of the ear.

11. Why can't you taste food very well when you have a sinus head cold?

Real Life Issues and Applications

Impairment of the Senses

A patient recently lost his eyesight and suffered extensive facial burns as a result of an industrial explosion. How do you think his other senses may compensate for this loss? How would you deal with this patient? What professions would be involved in this patient's care? Justify your choices.

Additional Activities

1. Pair off. Ask your partner to close his or her eyes. Using a sterile straight pin, a feather, a cotton ball, and an ice cube, test your partner's tactile senses. Ask your partner to describe the sensations.

2. What is ESP? Is it a true sense? Research ESP at a library and share your findings with the class.

Downloadable audio is available for selected medical terms in this chapter to enhance your learning of medical language.

StudyWARE™ CONNECTION

Go to your StudyWARE™ DVD and have fun learning as you play interactive games, view animations and videos, and take practice tests to help reinforce key concepts you learned in this chapter.

Workbook Practice *Go to your Workbook for more practice questions and activities.*

CHAPTER 10

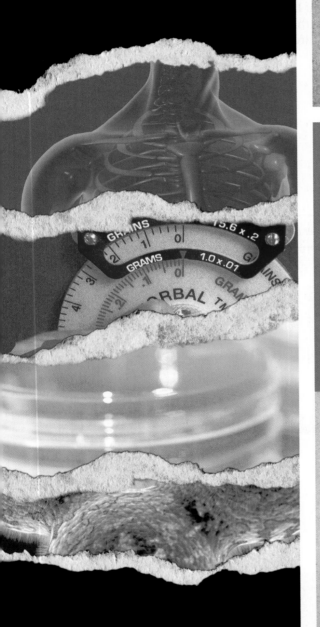

THE RESPIRATORY SYSTEM

Objectives

Upon completion of this chapter, you should be able to

- List and describe the major components of the respiratory system

- Describe the functions of the major structures in the respiratory system

- Describe how ventilation and respiration occur

- Discuss several diseases relating to the respiratory system

Key Terms

accessory muscles
adenoid (**AD**-eh-noid)
alveoli (al-**VEE**-oh-lye)
asthma (**AZ**-mah)
atelectasis (ah-tuh-**LEK**-tah-sis)
bronchi (**BRON**-kye)
bronchioles (**BRON**-kee-ohlz)
bronchitis (bron-**KYE**-tis)
bronchospasm
cardiopulmonary system
carina (kuh-**RINE**-uh)
chronic bronchitis
cilia (**SIL**-ee-ah)
conchae (**KON**-kay)
diaphragm (**DYE**-eh-fram)
emphysema (em-fih-**SEE**-mah)
empyema (em-pye-**EE**-mah)
epiglottis (ep-ih-**GLOT**-is)

erythropoiesis
(eh-**RITH**-roh-poy-**EE**-sis)
esophagus (eh-**SOF**-ah-gus)
Eustachian tubes
(you-**STAY**-kee-an)
hemoglobin
(**HE**-moh-**GLOW**-bin)
hemothorax
(**HE**-moh-**THOH**-racks)
hilum (**HIGH**-lim)
hydrothorax
(high-dro-**THOH**-racks)
laryngopharynx
(lah-**RING**-goh-**FAIR**-inks)
larynx (**LAIR**-inks)
lingula (**LING**-gu-lah)
lungs
medulla oblongata
(ob-long-**GAH**-tah)

(continues)

nasopharynx (**NAY**-zoh-**FAIR**-inks)
oropharynx (oh-roh-**FAIR**-inks)
pharynx (**FAIR**-inks)
pleural effusion
   (**PLOOR**-all eh-**FEW**-zhun)

pneumonia
pneumothorax
   (new-moh-**THOR**-racks)
respiration
sinus (**SIGN**-us)

sputum (**SPU**-tum)
trachea (**TRAY**-kee-ah)
tuberculosis (too-ber-kew-**LOH**-sis)
turbinates
ventilation

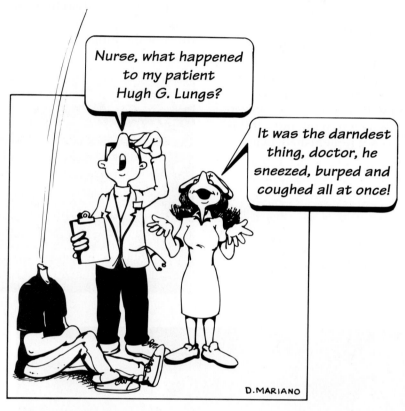

Source: Delmar/Cengage Learning

■ SYSTEM OVERVIEW

The respiratory system and the cardiovascular (heart and circulatory) system are closely interrelated. In fact, these two systems are sometimes considered one system called the **cardiopulmonary system**. The major components of the cardiopulmonary system are the heart; the vessels that transport blood from the heart, throughout the body, and back to the heart; and the lungs, which remove gaseous wastes from the blood and provide fresh oxygen for the body. The cardiovascular system is described in greater detail in Chapter 11; valuable information concerning the lymphatic system, which transports excess fluids from the tissues and is important in defending the body against infection, is also included.

These systems function without any conscious effort on your part. You probably didn't realize it, but in the time that it took you to read the preceding paragraph, your heart beat approximately 60 times and pumped approximately 4.2 liters of blood throughout your body. During this same time, you breathed approximately 12 times, moving more than 6,000 milliliters of air. And to think that some people believe reading isn't hard work!

It is hoped that you won't consider this chapter more work, but rather a journey into more amazing information about the human body.

StudyWARE CONNECTION

*View the proper way to assess the vital sign of breathing. Watch the **Respiration** video on your StudyWARE™ DVD.*

Major Structures of the Respiratory System

The respiratory system is responsible for providing all of the oxygen needed by the body and removing carbon dioxide. Oxygen is a needed component for cellular activity; carbon dioxide is a waste product resulting from the metabolic activity of cells in the body. Thus, oxygen is like the gasoline needed by your car, and carbon dioxide is like the exhaust fumes.

Unlike cars with large gas tanks, however, the human body has a very small reserve of oxygen. In fact, the body has an average oxygen reserve that lasts only about 4 to 6 minutes. If this reserve is used up and is not replenished, death is the inevitable outcome.

Simply stated, the respiratory system is a set of **lungs**, which contain small air sacs called **alveoli**. The alveoli are surrounded by networks of small blood vessels, called *capillaries*. In reality, however, the respiratory system is a little more complex than that. The major structures of the respiratory system are the **nose**, the **pharynx**, the **larynx**, the **trachea**, the **bronchi**, and the lungs. See Figure 10-1 that shows the major structures of the lung.

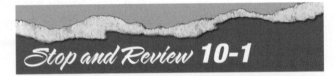

Stop and Review 10-1

a. What two systems combine to form the cardiopulmonary system?

b. List the major structures of the respiratory system.

c. What are the roles of oxygen and carbon dioxide in the body?

QUOTES & NOTES

If you could open your lungs and lay them down flat, they would cover an area the size of a tennis court. This provides a vast surface for gas exchange.

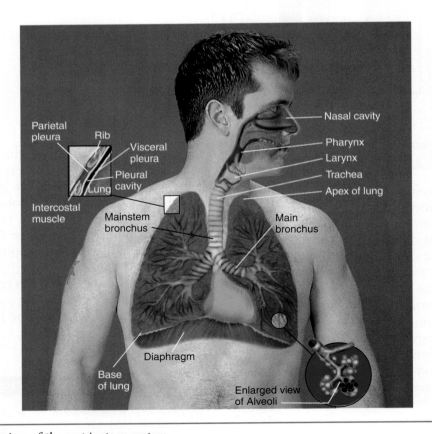

Figure 10-1   *Overview of the respiratory system.*

Source: Delmar/Cengage Learning

Divisions of the Respiratory System

The Upper Respiratory Tract

Figure 10-2 illustrates the upper respiratory system.

Your nose is the proud owner of two nostrils (also known as nares). Nares are the nose's openings to the outside world. As air enters the nose, the air must be warmed to body temperature and moistened so that the airways and the lungs do not dry out.

This warming and moisturizing process begins in the nasal cavities. Each of these cavities contains three scroll-like bones known as **turbinates**, or **conchae**. The conchae provide more surface area with which the incoming air can make contact. If you could unfold the turbinates, they would measure a surface area of 106 square centimeters! Thanks to the conchae, the nasal passageway is no longer straight. The air current thus becomes turbulent, thereby causing more air to make contact with those surfaces for better humidification.

The nasal cavities also are lined with sticky mucous membranes, which are richly supplied with blood. Incredibly, these mucous membranes each use 650 to 1,000 milliliters of water each day to humidify inspired air. Small particles such as dust and pathogens are usually trapped here before they are able to reach the lungs. Microscopic hair-like structures, called **cilia**, then act as tiny oars, pushing the debris-filled mucus toward the **esophagus** so that it can be swallowed. These little oars beat approximately 1,000 to 1,500 times per minute, moving the mucus approximately 2 centimeters (almost 1 inch) per minute. Cilia are also present in the airways of the lungs, where they work to push mucus up to the esophagus to be swallowed.

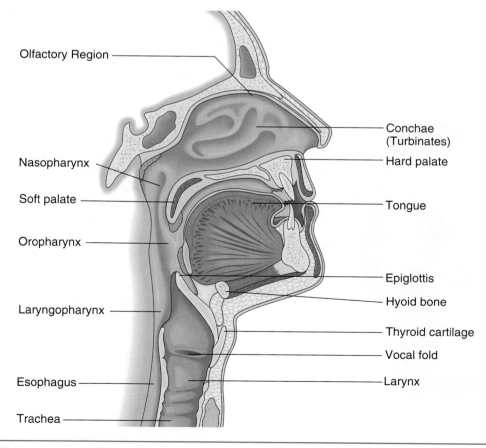

Figure 10-2 *The upper respiratory system.*
Source: Delmar/Cengage Learning

This *mucocilliary escalator* operates around the clock every day, and you don't even realize that it is happening.

Your sense of smell also originates in your nose. Sniffing noxious gas into the olfactory region makes you stop inhaling so the gas does not reach deeper into your lungs; thus, your nose provides a fairly safe way to sample noxious gas. It is interesting to note, as was mentioned in Chapter 9, that your ability to taste is related to your sense of smell. Next time you are eating, pinch your nose shut and see how well you can taste your food.

The next time someone calls you an airhead, don't be offended because they are absolutely correct! Your skull contains air-filled cavities, commonly called **sinuses**, which connect with the nasal cavities via small passageways (see Figure 10-3). Your sinuses don't exist when you are born. Rather they develop as you grow and help in making facial changes as you mature. Sinuses further warm and humidify the air that you breathe, reduce the weight of your skull (air-filled holes are lighter than solid bone), and provide resonance for your voice. The reduction in the weight of the skull is important, since it sits atop the cervical vertebrae like a stem of an apple. The weight reduction reduces the

chance of injury to the vital cervical region of the spinal cord.

Your throat, or pharynx, begins behind the nasal cavities. The pharynx can be divided into three sections: the **nasopharynx**, the **oropharynx**, and the **laryngopharynx** (refer back to Figure 10-2).

The nasopharynx (*naso* meaning "nose") is the uppermost section of the pharynx; it begins right behind the nasal cavities. Air that is breathed through the nose passes through the nasopharynx. This area contains lymphatic tissue, called **adenoids**, and passageways to the middle ear, called **Eustachian tubes**. Perhaps now you can see how an infection located in the nasal cavities can lead to a middle ear infection.

The oropharynx (*oro* meaning "mouth") is located right behind the mouth and below the nasopharynx. Air that is breathed in through the mouth as well as air that is breathed in through the nose passes through the oropharynx. The *palatine tonsils* are located in this area. Another set of tonsils known as the *lingual tonsils* can be found at the back of the tongue. In addition to air, anything that is swallowed also passes through this section.

The laryngopharynx (*laryngo* meaning "larynx") is the lowermost portion of the pharynx. Once again, any air that is breathed in as well as anything that is swallowed passes through this area. Swallowed materials usually pass through the esophagus on their way to the stomach, while air passes first through the larynx and then through the trachea on its way to the lungs.

What keeps food and liquids from going through the *glottis* (the opening that leads to the larynx) and into the lungs? Fortunately, a flap-like structure located above the glottis, called the **epiglottis** (*epi* meaning "above"), closes the opening to the larynx when you swallow and opens this entrance when you breathe (again, refer back to Figure 10-2).

From the laryngopharynx downward, the structures of the respiratory system resemble an upside-down tree. In fact, the airway that leads to the lungs and then branches out into the various lung segments is sometimes referred to as the *tracheobronchial tree.*

The Larynx: The Transition to Your Lower Airways

Your vocal cords can be considered the area of division between your upper and lower airways. Commonly known as the voice box, the larynx is a semirigid structure composed of numerous layers of cartilage. See Figure 10-4. The *Adam's apple,*

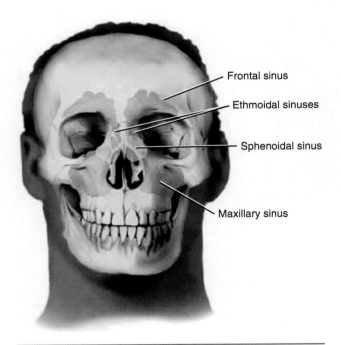

Frontal sinus

Ethmoidal sinuses

Sphenoidal sinus

Maxillary sinus

Figure 10-3   *The sinuses.*

Source: Delmar/Cengage Learning

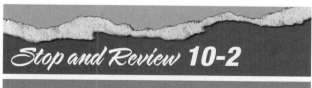

also known as the *thyroid cartilage,* is the largest of the cartilages found in the larynx. Cartilage is necessary to provide structure and support for your airways so they do not collapse and block the flow of air in and out of the lungs. As the airways branch out and get smaller in size, the need for cartilage becomes less important. Instead the airways are tethered to the lung tissue, or lung *parenchyma,* surrounding these airways. This tethering is known as *peribronchial radial traction.*

The Lower Respiratory Tract

The *windpipe* is a common nonmedical (lay) term used to describe the trachea, which extends from the larynx to approximately the center midpoint of your chest. As was mentioned previously, cartilage in the form of C-shaped structures is used in the anterior portion of the larynx to provide rigidity to the airway. The shape of these structures

serves an important purpose: It provides for some "give" in the posterior aspect of the larynx, thus allowing the esophagus to expand when you swallow larger chunks of food.

The esophagus and trachea, along with the thymus gland, superior and inferior vena cavas, and aorta, are positioned in a space located between the two lungs called the *mediastinum.*

The lower respiratory tract is protected by the *bony thorax,* which includes the rib cage and the sternum, or breast bone. When the trachea reaches the center of the chest, it divides (bifurcates) into two bronchi (bronchus, singular); the right mainstem, which is approximately 3 centimeters long, and the left mainstem, which is approximately 5 centimeters long. The site of bifurcation is called the **carina** (see Figure 10-5). One bronchus goes to the right lung and the other bronchus goes to the left lung.

The areas where the right and left mainstems attach to the lungs are known as *hila* (**hilum**, singular). The bronchi branch out into smaller and smaller airways as they spread into the lung segments until, finally, they divide into the smallest airways, known as **bronchioles**.

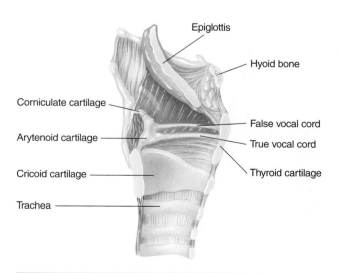

Figure 10-4 *Lateral view of the larynx.*
Source: Delmar/Cengage Learning

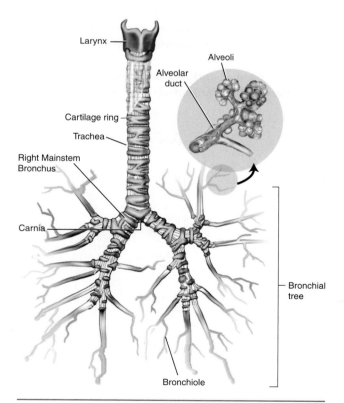

Figure 10-5 *Structures of the tracheobronchial tree.*
Source: Delmar/Cengage Learning

Clinical Relevancy
The Angle Makes a Difference

The branching angles of the main airways are not the same for both sides. The right mainstem branches off at a 20- to 30-degree angle from the midline of the chest, while the left mainstem branches off at a more pronounced 40- to 60-degree angle. The lesser angle of the right mainstem branching allows inhaled foreign bodies to more often lodge in the right lung. This is important to know if, for example, a child aspirates (inhales into the lung) an object, and a physician must enter the lung with a bronchoscope to remove the object. Time may be critical, and it may make a difference if the search is begun immediately in the right lung as opposed to the left lung.

Bronchioles have no cartilage and average about 1 millimeter in diameter.

Tiny air sacs, called alveoli, are located at the ends of the bronchioles. There are approximately 300 million alveoli in the average adult's lung. These terminal, or end, air sacs, shaped similarly to bunches of grapes, are surrounded by a network of blood-filled capillaries. This network allows for the exchange of gases between the blood and the fresh air of the lungs. Carbon dioxide is removed from the blood and exhaled out into the atmosphere, while oxygen is added to the blood to allow continued cellular function in the body.

Previously, we stated that the bronchi branch out into the lung segments, or lobes. Although the right lung possesses three segments, the superior, middle, and inferior lobes, the left lung possesses only a superior lobe and an inferior lobe (see Figure 10-6). Why only two segments in the left lung, you may ask? This is because the heart occupies a space in the left anterior area of the chest. The left lung does, however, have an area that corresponds to the right middle lobe: the **lingula**.

Breathing in and out causes the lungs to move. Over time, this could lead to irritation resulting from lungs rubbing against the inside of the thoracic cage. To prevent this, each lung is wrapped up in a sac, or membrane, called the *visceral pleura.* The thoracic cavity and the upper side of the diaphragm are lined with a similar membrane, called the *parietal pleura.* Between these two pleura is an extremely thin pleural space containing a slippery liquid called *pleural fluid.* This fluid greatly reduces friction as an individual breathes. Refer back to Figure 10-1.

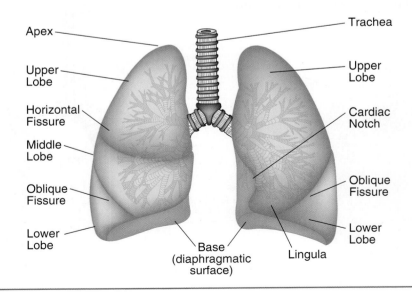

Figure 10-6 *Divisions of the lung.*

Source: Delmar/Cengage Learning

The Mechanics of the Respiratory System

How We Breathe

The control center that tells us to breathe is found in the brain in an area known as the **medulla oblongata**. Two terms associated with the breathing process are often used incorrectly. They are *ventilation* and *respiration*. **Ventilation** is the process of moving air in and out of your lungs, or more simply, breathing. **Respiration** describes the exchange of gases between the lungs and the blood. There are two steps to ventilation: *inspiration* (inhalation), or the act of breathing air into the lungs, and *expiration* (exhalation), or the act of taking air out of the lungs. You will probably breathe in 700 million lungsful of air during your lifetime.

Stop and Review 10-3

a. Where does the actual exchange of gas between your blood and the air you breathe in occur?

b. Why are the visceral pleura and the parietal pleura so important?

c. What is the purpose of cartilage in your airways?

Inspiration is the active step of ventilation. During inspiration, the main breathing muscle, the **diaphragm**, contracts, thus increasing the space in the thoracic cavity (see Figure 10-7).

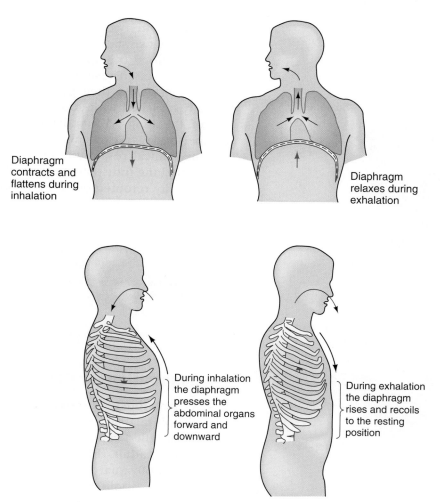

Diaphragm contracts and flattens during inhalation

Diaphragm relaxes during exhalation

During inhalation the diaphragm presses the abdominal organs forward and downward

During exhalation the diaphragm rises and recoils to the resting position

Figure 10-7 *Positions of the diaphragm during inspiration and expiration.*
Source: Delmar/Cengage Learning

This creates a lower-than-atmospheric pressure in the thoracic cavity, thus allowing air to rush into the lungs. In times of increased physical activity, **accessory muscles** help pull the rib cage up to make an even larger space in the thoracic cavity (see Figure 10-8).

Unlike inspiration, expiration is usually a passive act. As the diaphragm relaxes, it forms a dome-like shape, thus decreasing the amount of space in the thoracic cavity. As a result, pressure in the lungs becomes greater than the atmospheric pressure, and the air is pushed out of the lungs.

What makes the brain tell the lungs how quickly or slowly to breathe? Although we can consciously speed up or slow down our breathing, breathing rate is normally controlled by the level of carbon dioxide in the blood. If, when swimming, you have ever wanted to dive into deep water, you probably took several deep breaths and held the last one before diving in. You might have thought that taking those breaths

increased the amount of oxygen in your blood. In actuality, you were "blowing off" carbon dioxide. As a result, you had lower-than-normal levels of carbon dioxide in your blood, and your brain was fooled into believing that there was no need to breathe while you were underwater. Sometimes, accidental drowning occurs because the body doesn't think it is time to breathe, but the existing oxygen in the blood is being used up. In these cases, the individual "passes out" under water.

Here's another interesting fact. Since mosquitoes are too small to carry flashlights, how do they find you in the dark to bite you? They do it by using their carbon dioxide sensors. The sensors locate the increased concentrations of carbon dioxide emitted by you via your exhaled breath. As soon as these little creatures home in on you, they use their heat sensors to find an area of skin on which to begin their banquet!

Again, *respiration* is the term used to describe the exchange of gases between the lungs and the blood. Often you will hear news reports, or even physicians, stating that patients are placed on respirators to help them breathe. This, however, is incorrect. Those devices are actually mechanical *ventilators;* their purpose is to move air (usually enriched with additional oxygen) in and out of the lungs. Your alveoli and capillaries then perform gas exchange or respiration. However, mechanical respirators do exist and are used in heart/lung transplants where blood must be temporarily rerouted outside the body and mechanical gas exchange performed.

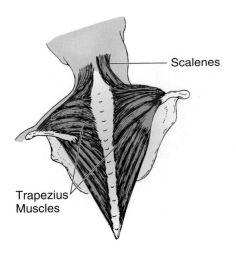

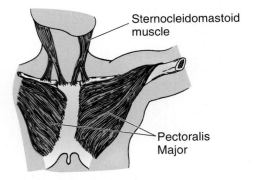

Figure 10-8 *Accessory muscles of inspiration.*
Source: Delmar/Cengage Learning

Respiration, or Gas Exchange

As previously discussed, each alveolar (alveoli, plural) sac is surrounded by a network of blood-filled capillaries (see Figure 10-9). In the average adult, this capillary network is approximately 60 square meters in size, or, put into perspective, about 80% the size of a tennis court. The membrane between the alveoli and the capillaries is quite thin. In fact, it is only 0.004 millimeter thick! The thinness of this membrane

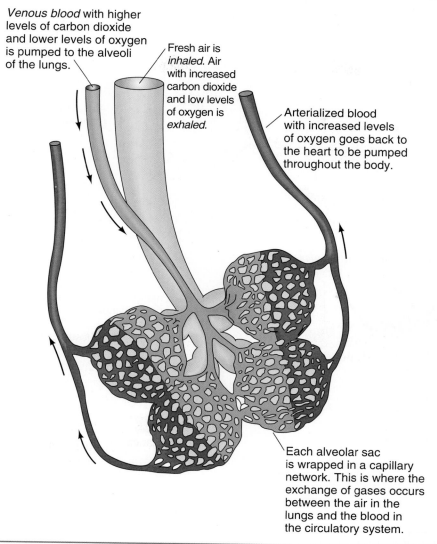

Venous blood with higher levels of carbon dioxide and lower levels of oxygen is pumped to the alveoli of the lungs.

Fresh air is *inhaled*. Air with increased carbon dioxide and low levels of oxygen is *exhaled*.

Arterialized blood with increased levels of oxygen goes back to the heart to be pumped throughout the body.

Each alveolar sac is wrapped in a capillary network. This is where the exchange of gases occurs between the air in the lungs and the blood in the circulatory system.

Figure 10-9 *Alveolar sacs and surrounding capillary network.*
Source: Delmar/Cengage Learning

aids in the diffusion of the gases between the lungs and the blood, wherein oxygen is brought into the blood and carbon dioxide is removed. This process is called *external respiration,* since it exchanges gas between the lungs and the outside (external) atmosphere.

Erythrocytes, or red blood cells (RBCs), are responsible for transporting most of the oxygen and a small amount of carbon dioxide in the blood. More specifically, within the erythrocytes, a protein molecule called *globin* and a compound of iron called *heme* combine to form **hemoglobin**, and hemoglobin performs the actual transportation. There are 25 to 30 trillion erythrocytes in the average adult human body, and it is estimated that there are about 280

million hemoglobin molecules on each erythrocyte! Furthermore, there are approximately 20 different types of hemoglobin in the body!

In general, if the hemoglobin is carrying large amounts of oxygen, as is the case with external respiration, the blood will be bright red. *Internal respiration* takes place at the various tissue sites where oxygen now flows into the tissues and carbon dioxide into the bloodstream. If the hemoglobin is carrying less oxygen and more carbon dioxide, as is the case with internal respiration, the blood will be darker red in color. (See Figure 10-10 for a simplified schematic of external and internal respiration.) This is evident when you look at the veins in your arm. Venous blood has lower levels of oxygen and higher levels of

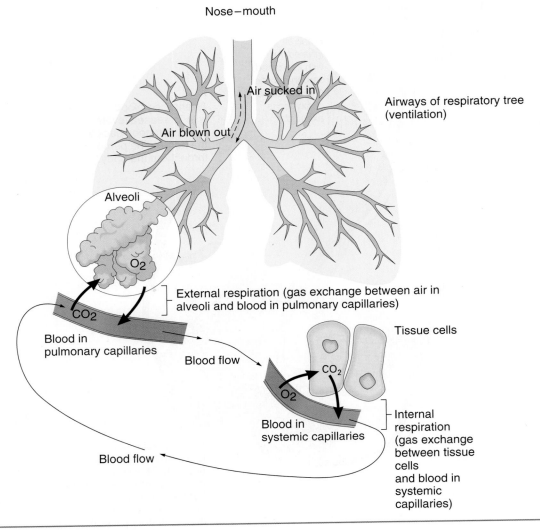

Nose – mouth

Air sucked in

Airways of respiratory tree (ventilation)

Air blown out

Alveoli

O_2

CO_2

External respiration (gas exchange between air in alveoli and blood in pulmonary capillaries)

Blood in pulmonary capillaries

Blood flow

Tissue cells

CO_2

O_2

Blood in systemic capillaries

Internal respiration (gas exchange between tissue cells and blood in systemic capillaries)

Blood flow

Figure 10-10 *External and internal respiration.*

Source: Delmar/Cengage Learning

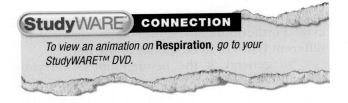

purpose; it provides more surface area. And more surface area translates into more contact area for the RBCs to pick up and leave off the gases they transport.

carbon dioxide. As a result, venous blood has a darker red tint, and those veins carrying venous blood appear bluish in color.

Red blood cells have an interesting shape. Believe it or not, you can actually make a large-scale replica of an RBC right in the privacy of your own home! Simply take a ball of dough and pinch it in the center. This shape may appear somewhat strange, but it serves an important

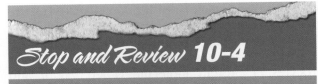

Stop and Review **10-4**

a. What is the main breathing muscle called?

b. What is an accessory muscle?

c. Why is hemoglobin important?

Special Focus

Compensating for Low Levels of Oxygen

It is amazing how the body can adapt to a variety of situations. For example, when increased exercise, high altitudes, high temperatures, or other circumstances require increased levels of oxygen and, thus, tax your body's ability to transport gases, your body can produce even more RBCs by a process called **erythropoiesis** (*erythr/o* meaning "red," *poiesis* meaning "to make"). This process begins when the kidneys detect low levels of oxygen coming to them from the blood. The kidneys then release a hormone called *erythropoietin* into the bloodstream. This hormone then travels through the blood and, eventually, reaches specialized cells found in the red bone marrow. When stimulated, these specialized cells increase their production of erythrocytes until the increased demand is met.

Clinical Relevancy

Disorders of the Respiratory System

As with any system of the body, the respiratory system is subject to a variety of diseases and problems. Following are descriptions of some of the more common respiratory ailments.

Atelectasis is a condition commonly encountered in the hospital setting. With atelectasis, the air sacs of the lungs are either partially or totally collapsed. This condition is typically caused by either a monotonous breathing pattern (i.e., a breathing pattern that doesn't include occasional deep breaths, or sighs) or a blockage of an air passage in the lung that prohibits air from entering a portion of the lung. Patients most susceptible to atelectasis are those who cannot or will not breathe deeply because of pain resulting from either surgery or an injury to the thoracic cage (e.g., broken ribs). Patients who generate large amounts of secretions and who are unable to cough up those secretions are also at risk for atelectasis. Quite often, if atelectasis is not corrected and secretions are retained, these patients can develop pneumonia within 72 hours. Pneumonia often can complicate a patient's recovery.

Pneumonia can be caused by a virus, a fungi, or a bacteria. This condition is characterized by inflammation of the infected areas with an accumulation of cell debris and fluid. In certain pneumonias, lung tissue is actually destroyed. Pneumonia, if severe enough, can lead to death.

Chronic obstructive pulmonary disease, or COPD, is a general term referring to either, or both, **emphysema** and **chronic bronchitis**. Emphysema is a nonreversible lung condition wherein the alveoli walls are destroyed, and the lung itself becomes weakened and "floppy" (see Figure 10-11). As the alveoli are destroyed, it becomes more difficult for gases to diffuse between the lungs and the blood. In addition, as the lung tissue becomes

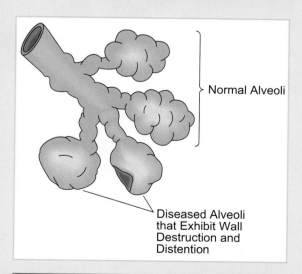

Normal Alveoli

Diseased Alveoli that Exhibit Wall Destruction and Distention

Figure 10-11 *Normal and emphysematous alveoli.*

Source: Delmar/Cengage Learning

(continues)

(continued)

weakened, not all of the air is expelled upon exhalation. Thus, air in the lung is breathed over and over.

Chronic bronchitis is a lung disease characterized by inflamed airways and large amounts of mucus (see Figure 10-12). As inflammation occurs, the airways swell, and the inner diameters of the airways get smaller in size. As they get smaller along with the large amounts of retained mucus, it becomes more difficult to move air in and out. This increases the work of breathing, resulting in the use of more oxygen and the production of more carbon dioxide.

Asthma is a potentially life-threatening lung condition wherein the body reacts to an allergy by constricting the airways of the lungs (see Figure 10-13). As a result of this constriction, which is also known as **bronchospasm**, it is difficult to get air into and even more difficult to get air out of the lungs. The inability

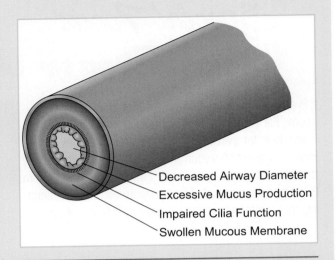

Decreased Airway Diameter
Excessive Mucus Production
Impaired Cilia Function
Swollen Mucous Membrane

Figure 10-12   *An airway of a patient with chronic bronchitis.*

Source: Delmar/Cengage Learning

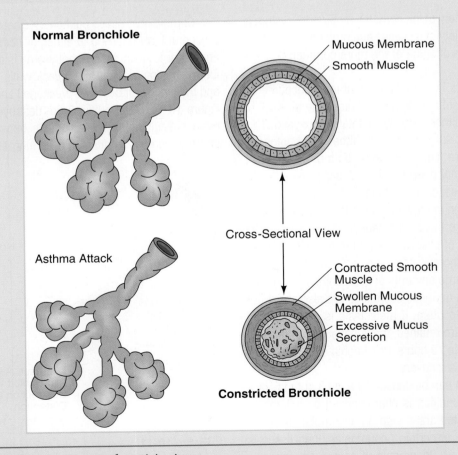

Normal Bronchiole

Mucous Membrane
Smooth Muscle

Cross-Sectional View

Asthma Attack

Contracted Smooth Muscle
Swollen Mucous Membrane
Excessive Mucus Secretion

Constricted Bronchiole

Figure 10-13   *Changes in an asthmatic's airway.*

Source: Delmar/Cengage Learning

(continues)

(continued)

to get air out of the lungs is known as gas trapping. As a result of gas trapping, fresh air cannot get into the lungs; thus the victim breathes the same air over and over. This decreases the amount of oxygen and increases the amount of carbon dioxide in the blood. Furthermore, because asthma is an inflammatory condition, the airways produce an increased amount of mucus secretions, or **sputum**. These secretions can block the airways, a phenomenon known as *mucus plugging.* Mucus plugging further reduces the flow of fresh air to the lungs. Although asthma can be a life-threatening disease, it can usually be reversed with the use of medication.

StudyWARE CONNECTION

To view an animations on **Asthma** *and* **Asthma in a Child,** *and a video on* **Asthma Emergencies,** *go to your StudyWARE*^TM *DVD.*

Tuberculosis (or TB, for short) is an infectious disease that was once a common disease but was virtually eradicated in the United States until recent years. Tuberculosis thrives in areas of the body having high oxygen content. One such area is the lung. Tuberculosis bacteria can lay dormant within the body for years before beginning to multiply. If tuberculosis continues unchecked, vast lung damage can occur. There has been growing concern recently about a multi-drug-resistant form of tuberculosis. This strain of the disease is highly resistant to the drugs normally used to treat TB and, thus, has a high mortality rate.

A **pneumothorax** is a condition wherein there is air inside the thoracic cavity but not in the lungs. Air can enter the thoracic cavity from two directions. It can rush into the thoracic cavity from the outside, as would

happen in the case of a stab or gunshot wound to the chest, or it can enter the thoracic cavity from the lungs, as would happen in the case of the lung developing a leak as a result of either a structural deformity or a disease process. In either case, if the gas cannot escape, it will continue to fill a space in the thoracic cavity, thus allowing less space for the lung or lungs to expand when breathing. If the lungs are too greatly restricted, a life-threatening situation may occur.

A **pleural effusion** is a condition wherein there is an excessive buildup of fluid in the pleural space between the parietal pleura and the visceral pleura. See Figure 10-14 which contrasts a pnuemothorax and a pleural effusion. This fluid may be pus, in which case the condition is known as an **empyema**; fluid, in which case the condition is known as a **hydrothorax**; or blood or bloody fluid, in which case the condition is known as a **hemothorax**. Because fluids are affected by gravity, pleural effusions tend to move toward the lowest point in the pleural space. If a pleural effusion is large enough, it can have the same effect as a large pneumothorax; that is, it can restrict the expansion of the lung or lungs. Because less air can flow in and out of the lungs, the patient must breathe in and out more rapidly to meet the body's demands for more oxygen and to remove carbon dioxide. This additional work can tire patients to the point where they can no longer breathe on their own.

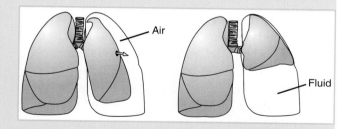

Figure 10-14 *Comparison of pneumothorax and pleural effusion.*

Source: Delmar/Cengage Learning

Professional Profile

Respiratory Care

The breath of life—that is what the respiratory therapist provides for those who either have difficulty breathing on their own or who have absolutely no ability to breathe.

Respiratory care practitioners work with patients of all ages. One minute they may be working with a baby that was born eight weeks too soon, and the next minute on a patient over 100 years of age!

This highly interesting profession requires vast knowledge of human anatomy and physiology, chemistry, physics, diseases and their effects on the respiratory and cardiovascular systems, as well as the types of respiratory medications and their effects on the human body. In addition, the respiratory care practitioner must be able to draw blood from arteries, perform CPR (cardiopulmonary resuscitation), and operate a myriad of advanced medical machinery such as breathing machines (also known as ventilators).

In bringing patients back from the precipice of death, the respiratory care practitioner experiences both excitement and a sense of accomplishment. This can provide these professionals with totally new views on life; things that once seemed extremely important often take on more realistic perspectives.

Communication skills are very important for the respiratory care practitioner. These professionals work with physicians in developing game plans for the recovery of patients. A respiratory care practitioner also is responsible for educating patients concerning their respiratory diseases and the most efficient ways to get better. They may also provide in-service education for other professions, such as nursing, in the proper application of oxygen therapy, drug delivery, or ventilator management.

Respiratory care practitioners don't only work in hospitals. These professionals also work in home-care settings, where they provide instruction to patients and patients' families. Areas of instruction can include the proper use of respiratory medical equipment, equipment cleaning procedures, respiratory drugs, and tips on exercise and ways to improve activities of daily living.

Respiratory practitioners also are very much involved in community service. They often go to elementary and secondary schools to lecture on a variety of subjects including lung disease, asthma management, and the effects of smoking and air pollution. Furthermore, these professionals are active in developing employee wellness programs for business and industry.

Educational requirements vary for respiratory care practitioners. There are one-year certificate programs, associate degree programs, usually offered by community colleges or universities; and baccalaureate programs, offered by universities. There are two levels of respiratory care practitioners. *Technicians* are usually graduates of the certificate, or entry-level, programs while therapists are graduates of the advanced-level programs. Both, however, can be called *respiratory care practitioners.*

For more information regarding this fascinating and rewarding profession, contact the American Association for Respiratory Care (AARC), 1720 Regal Row, Suite 122, Dallas, TX 75235, or visit www.aarc.org.

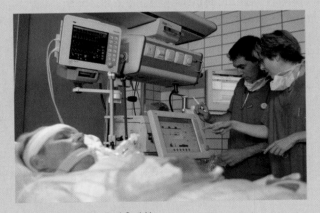

Courtesy Dräger Medical GmbH
Source: Delmar/Cengage Learning

StudyWARE CONNECTION

Oxygen therapy and inhaled medications are often used to treat respiratory disorders. To view videos on **Oxygen Therapy** *and* **How to Use a Medicated Inhaler**, *go to your StudyWARE™ DVD.*

■ CHAPTER REVIEW

Exercises

1. Differentiate between ventilation and respiration.

2. Explain what an RBC is and describe its function.

3. What are the microscopic, hair-like structures found in your airways called? Explain their purpose.

4. What are the purposes of the mucous membranes found in your airways?

5. Why is there cartilage in your larger airways?

6. Describe the pathway that oxygen takes from the outside atmosphere to the blood.

7. Approximately how much water do the mucous membranes in your airways use every day to moisten inspired air?

8. What is the general term used to describe a disease-producing organism?

9. Why are the visceral pleura and parietal pleura important?

10. What is the main breathing muscle called?

11. Why are gas trapping and mucus plugging potentially dangerous conditions in an asthmatic?

12. What is the name for the site of bifurcation where one bronchus goes to the right lung and the other bronchus goes to the left lung?

Real Life Issues and Applications

Respiratory Diagnosis

A teenage patient presented to the Emergency Department (ED) with the following symptoms:

- audible wheeze on inspiration and expiration
- shortness of breath (SOB)
- accessory muscle use
- increased chest diameter
- mild acrocyanosis
- tachypnea
- tachycardia

It was also noted that the patient has an allergy to cats and recently visited his aunt, who is a cat owner. What is the probable diagnosis based on the information given? How would you treat this patient? Imagine that you were an individual with this breathing disease. How would this condition change your lifestyle? How could your disease affect your family and friends?

Additional Activities

1. As a class, learn more about the respiratory diseases discussed in this text. Take turns describing an imaginary patient's disease symptoms and see who can correctly guess the disease.

2. Research how smoking or secondhand smoke can affect the lungs. Discuss your findings with the class.

3. Invite a respiratory care practitioner to class to discuss lung diseases and the respiratory care profession.

Downloadable audio is available for selected medical terms in this chapter to enhance your learning of medical language.

StudyWARE CONNECTION

Go to your StudyWARE™ DVD and have fun learning as you play interactive games, view animations and videos, and take practice tests to help reinforce key concepts you learned in this chapter.

Workbook Practice | *Go to your Workbook for more practice questions and activities.*

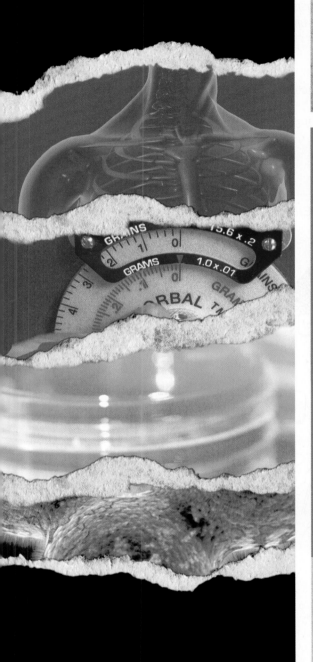

CHAPTER **11**

THE CARDIOVASCULAR AND LYMPHATIC SYSTEMS

Objectives

Upon completion of this chapter, you should be able to

- List the major components of the cardiovascular system

- Describe the functions of these components

- List the major components of blood and state their purposes

- Describe how the respiratory system and cardiovascular system are interrelated

- Describe factors that affect the exchange of gas at the alveolar-capillary membrane

- Describe factors that affect the exchange of gases at the tissue level

- State the functions of the lymphatic system

- Name the major structures of the lymphatic system

Key Terms

adenoids (**AD**-eh-noids)
angina pectoris (an-**JIGH**-nah-peck-**TORE**-is)
antibodies
aorta (ay-**OR**-tah)
aortic valve (ay-**OR**-tick)
arteries
arterioles (ar-**TEER**-ee-ohlz)
arteriosclerosis

atrioventricular node (**AY**-tree-oh-ven-**TRICK**-you-lahr)
atrium (**AY**-tree-um)
bundle of His (**HISS**)
capillaries
cardiac arrhythmias
cardiac cycle
cardiovascular (**KAR**-dee-oh-**VAS**-kyou-lar)
central chemoreceptors

(continues)

cerebrospinal fluid (**CSF**) (**SIR**-ee-broh-**SPY**-nal)
cholesterol (koh-**LESS**-ter-ol)
diastole (dye-**AH**-stol-ee)
dysrhythmias (dis-**RITH**-me-ahs)
endocarditis (**EN**-doh-kar-**DYE**-tis)
endocardium (**EN**-doh-**KAR**-dee-um)
erythrocytes (eh-**RITH**-roh-sites)
heart failure (**HF**)
ischemia (iss-**KEE**-me-ah)
lesion (**LEE**-zhun)
leukocytes (**LOO**-koh-sites)
lymph nodes (**LIMPF**)

lymphocytes (**LIM**-foh-sites)
mitral valve (**MY**-tral)
myocardial infarction
myocarditis (**MY**-oh-kar-**DYE**-tis)
myocardium (my-oh-**KAR**-dee-um)
occlusion (oh-**CLUE**-zhun)
palatine (**PAL**-ah-tine)
pericarditis (**PER**-ih-kar-**DYE**-tis)
pericardium (per-ih-**KAR**-dee-um)
peripheral chemoreceptors
phagocytosis (**FAG**-oh-sigh-**TOH**-sis)
plaque (**PLAK**)
plasma (**PLAZ**-mah)

prolapse
pulmonary valve
septum (**SEP**-tum)
sinoatrial node (**SIGN**-oh-**AY**-tree-ahl)
spleen
stenosis
systole (**SIS**-toll-lee)
thrombocytes (**THROM**-boh-sites)
tonsils (**TON**-sillz)
urea (you-**REE**-ah)
veins
ventricle (**VEN**-trih-kuhl)
venules (**VEN**-youls)

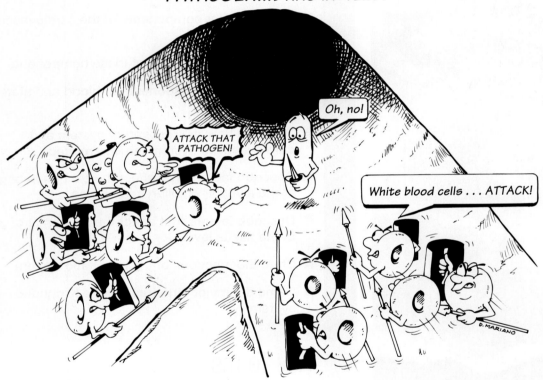

PATHOGEN...DYING IN "VEIN"!

Source: Delmar/Cengage Learning

■ SYSTEM OVERVIEW

When oxygen from the outside environment is brought into the lungs and blood, it must be transported (along with nutrients, blood cells, and other substances) throughout the body to areas where it is needed. That is where the **cardiovascular** system is needed.

This chapter provides general information regarding the circulatory, or cardiovascular (*cardio* meaning "heart," *vascular* meaning "vessels"), system. Remember that the cardiovascular system not only provides nutrients and oxygen for the body, but it also removes waste products resulting from cell metabolism. Another point to keep in mind is that the cardiovascular system is a closed, pressurized system, much like the radiator, hoses, and water pump in your car. Within this automotive system, a leak in any area, too little or too much water/antifreeze mixture, or a defective pump can lead to trouble. The trouble might be minor and require minimal maintenance (e.g., adding a little water/antifreeze mixture) or major and require extensive repair (e.g., corrective repair of the water pump). The same can be said for the cardiovascular system.

The major components of the cardiovascular system are the heart, which pumps the blood throughout the system; the blood, which is composed of a liquid portion called **plasma** and a variety of cells and is actually classified as a connective tissue; and the passageways through which the blood is transported. These passageways are: the **arteries**, which carry blood away from the heart; the **capillaries**, where the exchange of gases, nutrients, and waste products occurs at the cellular level and which act as connections between the arteries and **veins**; and veins, which bring blood *back* to the heart.

Also paralleling the cardiovascular system are the lymphatic vessels, lymph nodes, and spleen. These are important components of the immune system and also help transport fluids. This system will also be covered in this chapter.

The Cardiovascular System

The Heart

Let's begin at the heart of the cardiovascular system, which is, of course, the heart. The heart can be described as basically a muscle with a series of chambers located inside (see Figure 11-1). To get an idea of the approximate size of your heart, simply make a fist. Your heart is positioned slightly to the left of the center of your chest (using the sternum as the midline) and above your diaphragm.

The heart is composed of three layers of tissue. The smooth layer of tissue that lines both the heart and the blood vessels is called the **endocardium** (*end/o* meaning "inside," *cardium* meaning "heart"). This material also forms the valves of the heart. The next layer of tissue is the thickest layer; it is called the **myocardium** (*my/o* meaning "muscle"). This layer of muscle tissue does the work of pumping blood. The final layer of tissue is the **pericardium** (*peri* meaning "around"), a sac-like membrane that surrounds the heart.

Although the heart is one organ, it can actually be considered two pumps in one. The **septum** is a muscular wall that divides the right side of the heart from the left side. The right side is responsible for taking deoxygenated blood that has returned from the body and pumping it into the lungs. The left side of the heart is responsible for taking the now oxygenated blood from the lungs and pumping it throughout the body.

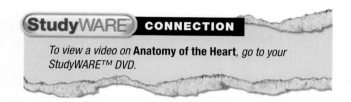

StudyWARE CONNECTION

To view a video on **Anatomy of the Heart**, *go to your StudyWARE™ DVD.*

Blood Flow

It is crucial to know how to trace the flow of blood through the heart (see Figure 11-1B). All of the blood that circulates in the body eventually returns to the heart through either the *superior vena cava,* if the blood is from the upper portion of the body, or the *inferior vena cava,* if the blood is from the lower part of the body. This blood essentially pours into the top chamber of the right side of the heart, called the right **atrium**. When the right atrium is filled, the heart begins to contract.

When deoxygenated blood is brought back into the right side of the heart, the electrical and muscular systems of the heart work together to pump the blood to the lungs (to become oxygenated) and to the rest of the body (for oxygen delivery to tissues see Figure 11-2).

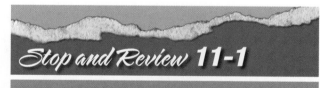

Stop and Review **11-1**

a. Trace the blood flow of the heart beginning in the venous system.

b. Can you relate the cardiovascular system to some everyday systems?

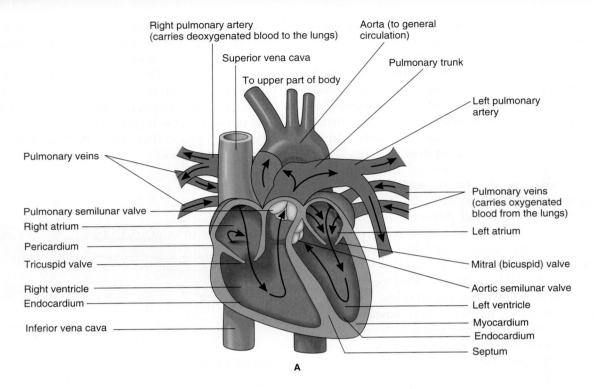

Right pulmonary artery
(carries deoxygenated blood to the lungs)

Superior vena cava

To upper part of body

Aorta (to general
circulation)

Pulmonary trunk

Left pulmonary
artery

Pulmonary veins

Pulmonary veins
(carries oxygenated
blood from the lungs)

Pulmonary semilunar valve

Right atrium

Left atrium

Pericardium

Tricuspid valve

Mitral (bicuspid) valve

Right ventricle

Aortic semilunar valve

Endocardium

Left ventricle

Inferior vena cava

Myocardium

Endocardium

Septum

A

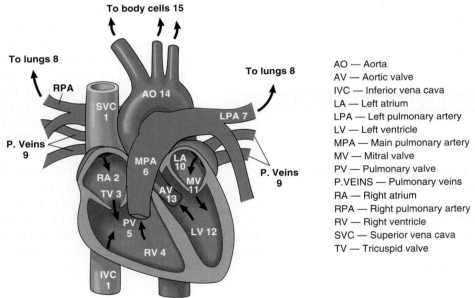

To body cells 15

To lungs 8

To lungs 8

RPA

SVC
1

AO 14

LPA 7

P. Veins
9

MPA
6

LA
10

MV
11

P. Veins
9

RA 2

TV 3

AV
13

PV
5

LV 12

RV 4

IVC
1

AO — Aorta
AV — Aortic valve
IVC — Inferior vena cava
LA — Left atrium
LPA — Left pulmonary artery
LV — Left ventricle
MPA — Main pulmonary artery
MV — Mitral valve
PV — Pulmonary valve
P.VEINS — Pulmonary veins
RA — Right atrium
RPA — Right pulmonary artery
RV — Right ventricle
SVC — Superior vena cava
TV — Tricuspid valve

1. Blood reaches heart through superior vena cava (SVC) and inferior vena cava (IVC)
2. To right atrium
3. To tricuspid valve
4. To right ventricle
5. To pulmonary valve (semilunar)
6. To main pulmonary artery
7. To left pulmonary artery and right pulmonary artery

8. To lungs—blood receives O_2
9. From lungs to pulmonary veins
10. To left atrium
11. To mitral (bicuspid) valve
12. To left ventricle
13. To aortic valve (semilunar veins)
14. To aorta (largest artery in the body)
15. Blood with oxygen then goes to all cells of the body

B

Figure 11-1   *(A) Structures of the heart. (B) Blood flow through the heart.*

Source: Delmar/Cengage Learning

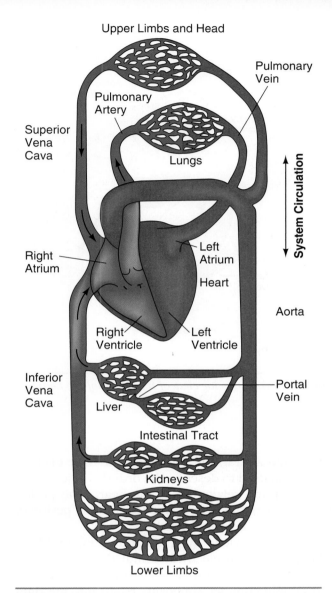

Figure 11-2 *Pulmonary and systemic blood flow.*
Source: Delmar/Cengage Learning

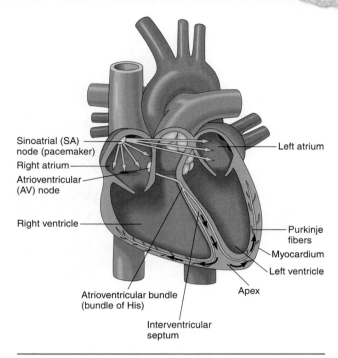

Figure 11-3 *The structures and path of cardiac conduction.*
Source: Delmar/Cengage Learning

Electrical Conduction in the Heart

Earlier in the book we discussed how cardiac muscle is different from other muscle tissue. Your heart is stimulated by an electrical charge from its pacemaker, called the **sinoatrial node** (or SA node, for short). The SA node can be found in the upper right wall of the right atrium (see Figure 11-3). When the cardiac muscle begins to contract, it forms a wave from the atrium downward, so that the blood is squeezed out from the right atrium and into the next chamber. This next chamber is called the right **ventricle**.

When the electrical charge passes the atrial chamber, the **atrioventricular node** (or AV

node, for short) is stimulated. The AV node, which is located in an area of the septum between the atria and the ventricles, then stimulates the bundle of HIS. The **bundle of HIS** (pronounced HISS) is located in the septal wall between the right and left ventricles; it branches out all over the walls of both ventricles, with the *right bundle branch* going to the right ventricle and the *left bundle branch* going to the left ventricle.

Blood that was already in the chamber of the right ventricle is squeezed into the pulmonary artery, which transports blood to the lungs. Remember, your heart is a two-pump system, wherein the right side pumps blood that is received from the body to the lungs for gas exchange, and the left side pumps oxygenated blood that is obtained from the lungs out to the body.

Being the questioning student you probably are, you may ask, "Why doesn't blood squirt back from the right ventricle into the right atrium?" The backflow of blood is normally prevented by the *tricuspid valve* (also called the *atrioventricular*

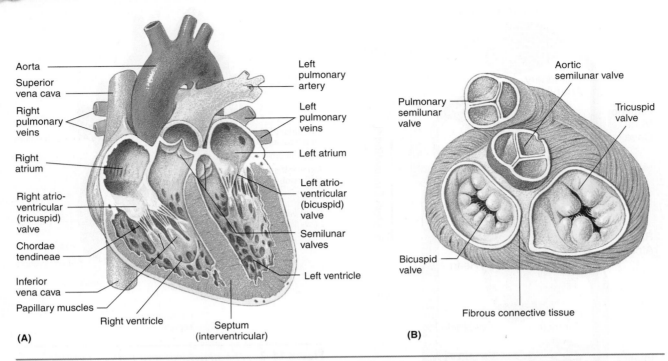

Figure 11-4   *(A) The interior structures of the heart. (B) Cross sectioned anterior view of the valves of the heart.*
Source: Delmar/Cengage Learning

valve because of its location), which is located in the opening between the right atrium and the right ventricle. This is a one-way valve that closes up as the pressure in the right ventricle increases during contraction, thus moving the blood toward the lungs via the pulmonary artery. The **pulmonary valve** (sometimes referred to as the *semilunar valve* because of its half-moon shape) functions the same way, so that blood in the pulmonary artery cannot flow back into the right ventricle at the end of the heart's contraction. See Figure 11-4 which shows an interior view of the heart structures and a cross section of the heart showing the valves.

After blood flows through the lungs, it travels back to the heart via the pulmonary vein. It now enters the top chamber in the left side of the heart, known as the *left atrium.* When this chamber is filled, the heart contracts, and the blood passes through the **mitral valve** (another atrioventricular valve) and into the left ventricle. The blood that was already in the left ventricle goes through the **aortic valve** (another semilunar valve) and out into the body's largest artery, the aorta.

While the heart is a two-pump organ, both sides pump at the same time—when the electrical charge causes that wave of contraction that travels

from the atria to the ventricles. **Cardiac cycle** is the term used to describe the orderly cycle of contraction and relaxation of the heart. The period of contraction is called **systole**, and the period of cardiac rest is called **diastole**.

As a review, then, the pumping of blood begins from an electrical stimulation, which sets up a wave-like contraction. The right and left atria both contract, squeezing blood into the right and left ventricles, respectively. The atria relax, as blood returning from the body fills the right atrium and blood returning from the lungs fills the left atrium. While the atria are filling, a wave-like contraction squeezes blood out of both ventricles. Blood from the right ventricle goes to the pulmonary artery and then to the lungs, while blood from the left ventricle goes out into the aorta and then into the body. When the ventricles are emptied, the atria begin filling the ventricles again.

Blood pressure is based on the cardiac cycle. The top number is the pressure generated by the pumping action of the heart during systole, which is generally 120 mm Hg (the force exerted by a column of mercury 120 millimeters high); the bottom number is the pressure that remains in the circulatory system when the heart is at rest (diastole). A normal value for diastolic pressure is considered to be 80 mm Hg.

The Electrocardiogram

The heart's contraction, termed *myocardial contraction*, is begun by an electrical impulse at the SA node, and this impulse spreads out and continues throughout the entire cardiac cycle. This electrical charge can actually be detected on the surface of the body. This surface detection of the electrical impulse traveling through the heart can be recorded by using an *electrocardiograph*, which records an *electrocardiogram* (ECG, or the German form EKG).

The normal EKG has three distinct waves that represent specific heart activities. See Figure 11-5. The *P wave* is the first wave on the EKG and represents the impulse generated by the SA node and depolarization of the atria right before they contract. The next wave is called the *QRS complex* (a combination of Q, R, and S waves). It represents the depolarization of the ventricles that occurs right before the ventricles contract. The ventricles begin contracting right after the peak of the R wave. Due to the greater muscle mass of the ventricles compared to the atria, this wave is greater in size than the P wave. The final wave is the *T wave*, which represents the repolarization of the ventricles where they are at rest before the next contraction. The repolarization of the atria and its charge appears to be missing in the tracing. It really isn't because it occurs during the QRS complex but is usually overshadowed by the ventricles' electrical activity! In the recording of a healthy heart, there are set ranges for the height, depth, and length of time for each of the waves and wave complexes. Changes in those parameters, or the addition of other abnormal types of waves, known as **cardiac arrhythmias** or **dysrhythmias**, can indicate health problems that involve the heart.

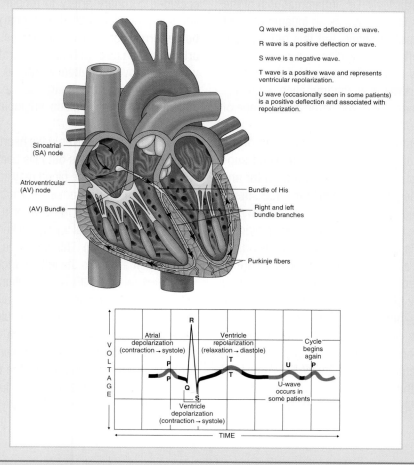

Q wave is a negative deflection or wave.

R wave is a positive deflection or wave.

S wave is a negative wave.

T wave is a positive wave and represents ventricular repolarization.

U wave (occasionally seen in some patients) is a positive deflection and associated with repolarization.

Sinoatrial (SA) node

Atrioventricular (AV) node

(AV) Bundle

Bundle of His

Right and left bundle branches

Purkinje fibers

Figure 11-5 *The EKG or ECG tracing.*

Source: Delmar/Cengage Learning

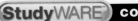

StudyWARE® CONNECTION

To view an animation on **The Heart** *and a video on* **The Cardiac Cycle and ECG**, *go to your StudyWARE™ DVD.*

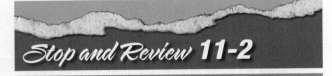

Stop and Review 11-2

Relate the electrical conduction system in the heart to the mechanical action that it produces.

Clinical Relevancy

Disorders of the Heart

Even though the heart is a wonderfully durable organ of the body, it can fall prey to disease. Following are descriptions of a few of the heart infirmities that you may encounter during your career.

There are several *itises* (i.e., inflammations) of the heart. **Endocarditis** literally means an inflammation of the lining of the heart's cavities, but this term is also used to refer to inflammatory diseases of the heart valves. **Myocarditis** is an inflammation of the muscle of the heart. **Pericarditis** is an inflammation of the sac that surrounds the heart or of the serous membrane of the heart's outer surface.

There may be times when cardiac muscle of the heart itself does not receive a sufficient blood supply. *Coronary artery disease* is a general term for any disease that adversely affects the arteries that supply blood to heart tissue, thus decreasing blood flow. As a result of this decreased blood flow, an individual may feel pain in his or her chest, which can radiate to the left shoulder and arm. This is known as **angina pectoris**. If the closure, or **occlusion**, of the coronary arteries that supply blood to the heart muscle is not severe, tissue may become injured because of low oxygen levels. This condition is called **ischemia**. If the decrease in blood flow is severe enough, however, heart tissue may actually die, or *infarct.* This may lead to a reduction in the heart's ability to pump blood, or even to death. **Myocardial infarction**, or MI, is a

term used to describe death of heart tissue—or, in lay terms, a heart attack.

Coronary artery disease can be treated with a procedure in which a tiny balloon is inflated in an occluded coronary artery to reopen the blood flow. A surgical procedure called a coronary bypass can also be performed on serious blockages. Here the blocked artery is bypassed with another grafted healthy blood vessel to provide a detour for blood to flow through to deliver oxygen to the heart muscle. See Figure 11-6 which shows both balloon angioplasty and coronary bypass surgery.

Sometimes the valves in the heart become diseased. If the mitral valve closes but falls backward, a tight seal will not occur, and some blood may squirt backward into the left atrium. This is known as a mitral valve **prolapse**. When either additional material or a **lesion** causes an obstruction in the mitral valve, it is known as mitral valve **stenosis** (narrowing). This condition affects blood flow from the left atrium to the left ventricle.

Heart failure (HF) is a condition wherein the heart fails as an effective pump. When it fails, the body retains abnormal amounts of fluid. Since fluid is gravity dependent, it is common to see edema of the lower legs, ankles, and feet. If severe enough, some of this fluid may wind up in the lungs and make the exchange of gases between the bloodstream and the lungs more difficult. As a result, oxygen levels in the body may decrease.

(continues)

(continued)

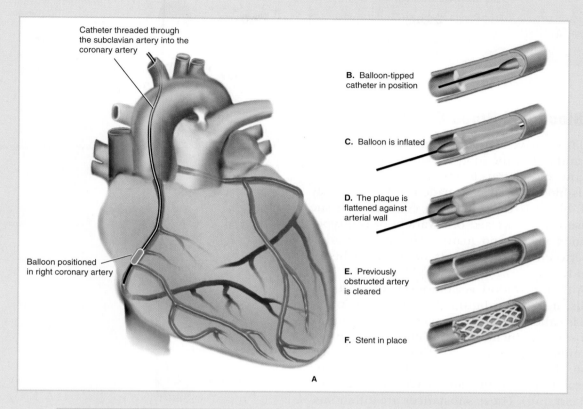

Catheter threaded through the subclavian artery into the coronary artery

B. Balloon-tipped catheter in position

C. Balloon is inflated

D. The plaque is flattened against arterial wall

Balloon positioned in right coronary artery

E. Previously obstructed artery is cleared

F. Stent in place

A

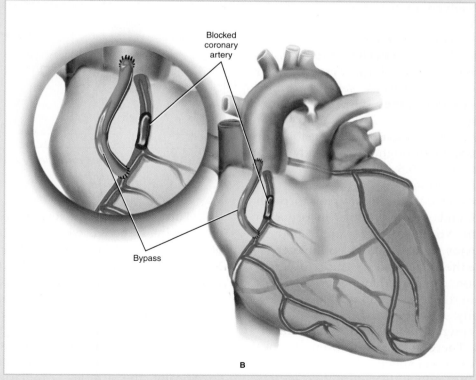

Blocked coronary artery

Bypass

B

Figure 11-6 *(A) Balloon angioplasty. (B) Coronary bypass.*

Source: Delmar/Cengage Learning

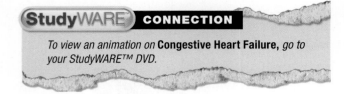

To view an animation on **Congestive Heart Failure,** *go to your StudyWARE™ DVD.*

The Blood and Blood Vessels

Thus far we have learned about the movement of air in and out of the lungs, how the heart works, and how blood travels through the heart. But what is blood? What is it made of? As previously stated, blood is classified as a connective tissue because it is composed of a variety of cell types contained in a liquid matrix. The average adult has between 5 and 6 quarts of blood in his or her body.

Although blood is composed of a variety of cells, it is still a liquid. The fluid portion of blood is called *plasma.* Plasma contains a variety of substances, including nutrients, waste products, mineral salts (e.g., calcium and sodium), carbon dioxide, oxygen, and fibrinogen and prothrombin (two substances needed for proper blood clotting). These substances are either suspended or dissolved in the plasma, which is about 90% water.

Blood also contains three main kinds of specialized blood cells: **erythrocytes** (*RBCs,* meaning "red blood cells"), **leukocytes** (known as *WBCs* for "white blood cells," *leuk/o* meaning "white"), and **thrombocytes** (also called platelets). See Figure 11-7.

Erythrocytes are primarily responsible for transporting oxygen throughout the body. Normally, there are 4.5 to 5.5 million RBCs in each cubic millimeter of blood.

Leukocytes have the ability to pass through capillary walls and go into tissues in order to fight infection. Normally there are 5,000 to 10,000 leukocytes in each cubic millimeter of blood. Because the body produces more WBCs to combat infection, a higher-than-normal number of leukocytes in the blood can indicate an infection in the body. **Phagocytosis** is the process wherein WBCs engulf, ingest, and destroy infecting organisms. There are several different types of WBCs and each has specific immune responsibilities. The WBCs include *neutrophils, eosinophils, basophils, monocytes,* and *lymphocytes.*

Blood cell		Function
Erythrocyte		O_2 and CO_2 transport
Neutrophil		Immune defenses (Phagocytosis)
Eosinophil		Defense against allergens and parasites
Basophil		Inflammatory response
Monocyte		Immune surveillance
B Lymphocyte		Antibody production
T Lymphocyte		Cellular immune response
Platelets		Blood clotting

Figure 11-7   *Blood cells and their function.*
Source: Delmar/Cengage Learning

Thrombocytes (platelets) are responsible for the clotting process, which prevents you from bleeding to death as a result of a small wound. Normally there are 250,000 to 400,000 thrombocytes in each cubic millimeter of blood.

The important roles that blood plays in the body are evident from the preceding discussion. But how does blood get where it needs to go in the body? The answer is via a network of passageways known as the blood vessels, or, more specifically, the arteries, capillaries, and veins (see Figure 11-8).

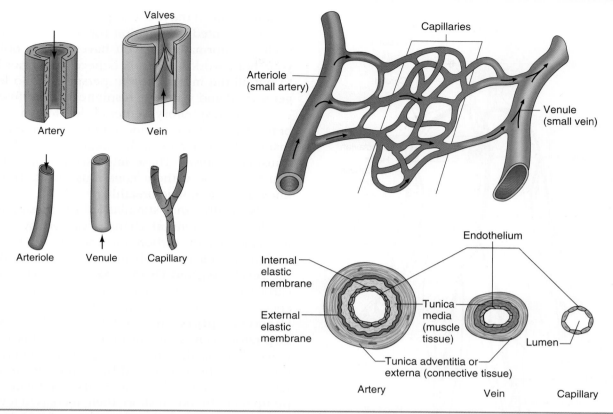

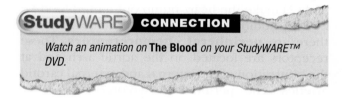

Figure 11-8 *Types of blood vessels.*

Source: Delmar/Cengage Learning

StudyWARE CONNECTION

*Watch an animation on **The Blood** on your StudyWARE™ DVD.*

As was mentioned previously, arteries are the vessels that carry blood away from the heart. Arteries generally carry blood that is higher in oxygen and lower in carbon dioxide. The *exception* is the pulmonary artery. This artery, which comes from the right ventricle, carries blood from the body to the lungs so that carbon dioxide can be dropped off and additional oxygen can be picked up. Arteries have thick, muscular, elastic walls, which enable them to receive blood as it is pumped under high pressure from the heart.

As blood continues its journey to the tissues, the arteries branch out into smaller and smaller pathways, the smallest of which are called **arterioles**. Arterioles, in turn, connect with capillaries. Capillaries possess very thin walls; in fact, the walls are only one cell layer thick. This is

necessary because the diffusion of gases and the transfer of nutrients and waste products at the cellular level occur in the capillaries. A thicker barrier would pose insurmountable problems. When diffusion and transfer are complete, the blood must be able to get back to the heart and lungs. For this reason, capillaries are attached to **venules**, the smallest form of veins. Here, the blood begins its return journey.

As venules continue, they combine into bigger and bigger veins until they form the two major veins of the body: the superior vena cava and the inferior vena cava. The superior vena cava collects blood from the upper portion of the body, while the inferior vena cava collects blood from the lower portion of the body. Note that veins have thinner walls than arteries; veins don't need as much muscle tissue because they are located on the low-pressure side of the circulatory system.

It is also interesting to note that there are one-way valves in veins to keep blood from flowing backward. No matter where the blood comes from, it all ends up going into the right atrium of the heart to begin the cycle. See Figure 11-9 which shows the major arteries and veins of the body.

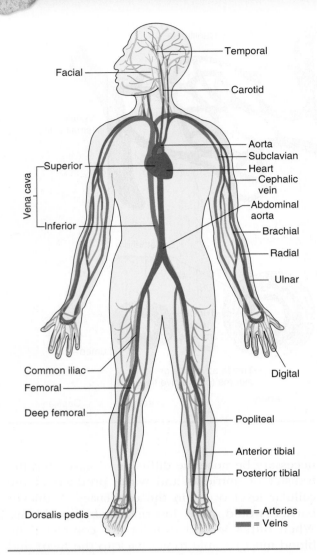

Figure 11-9   *Major arteries and veins of the body.*
Source: Delmar/Cengage Learning

StudyWARE®   CONNECTION

To view videos on **Assessing Pulses and Blood Pressure**, *go to your StudyWARE™ DVD.*

Putting It All Together: The Cardiopulmonary System

Now that we have covered the basics of the heart, lungs, and blood, we can put this information together to understand the cardiopulmonary system. Some of the following is a review of previously presented information (or totally new and exciting information, if you haven't been doing your homework!); but this is necessary in order to put all the information in perspective. So let's get started and ventilate, respirate, and perfuse!

Your respiratory center is located in your brain. The center is composed of a group of cells that cause the nerves of the breathing muscles to transmit impulses. These impulses usually allow you to breathe without conscious effort. This is known as autonomic breathing.

Normally, the stimulation of these cells results from chemical changes caused by varying amounts of carbon dioxide in the blood. Carbon dioxide can easily move from the blood to the **cerebrospinal fluid** (**CSF**, for short). When carbon dioxide levels increase in the CSF, those specialized brain cells (also known as **central chemoreceptors**) respond by stimulating the inspiratory center of the brain. When this happens, there is first an increase in the depth of the breath; this is followed by an increase in the rate of breathing. The heart is also stimulated to pump more blood. In short, then, increased levels of carbon dioxide in the blood cause the brain to: (1) make the lungs breathe more deeply and more rapidly in order to expel excess carbon dioxide and (2) make the heart pump out more blood.

In addition to the central chemoreceptors, there are **peripheral chemoreceptors**. These receptors are located on the aortic arch and at the bifurcation of the internal and external carotid arteries. The peripheral chemoreceptors have very high oxygen needs and are very sensitive to dips in blood oxygen levels. If the oxygen level in the blood decreases, these receptors send messages to the central respiratory receptors to increase both the depth of breathing (known as tidal volume) and the rate of breathing. In addition, the heart rate is increased, thus increasing the amount of blood being pumped.

During times of increased oxygen need, the capillaries surrounding each alveolar sac constrict. This is done in order to line up the RBCs and slow their passage by the alveoli. This allows each RBC more time to pick up oxygen and drop off carbon dioxide before once again beginning its journey through the body. If the need for more oxygen is chronic or long term, your body can attempt to alleviate the problem by increasing the number of RBCs; in this way there are more carriers to transport the limited amount of oxygen.

Clinical Relevancy

Clogged Pipes and Arteries

A common problem with blood vessels occurs to some degree for all of us as we age. Arteriosclerosis, also known as *hardening of the arteries,* is a result of the thickening of the internal diameter of the artery, which causes the involved vessels to become less flexible or even brittle. Blood vessels in this condition have a tendency to rupture. Since these vessels are less flexible and can't readily accommodate increases in blood volume, the body is more susceptible to high blood pressure.

Normally, blood vessels have a smooth inner lining, which promotes efficient blood flow by decreasing resistance. *Atherosclerosis* is a potentially life-threatening condition in which fatty deposits, called plaque, build up on the inner lining of blood vessels. As a result, blood flow can become greatly restricted or totally blocked. The fatty material that makes up plaque is composed mostly of cholesterol. Interestingly, all blood vessels are susceptible to atherosclerosis, but the aorta and coronary arteries seem particularly susceptible to developing this condition. See Figure 11-10 which shows atherosclerosis.

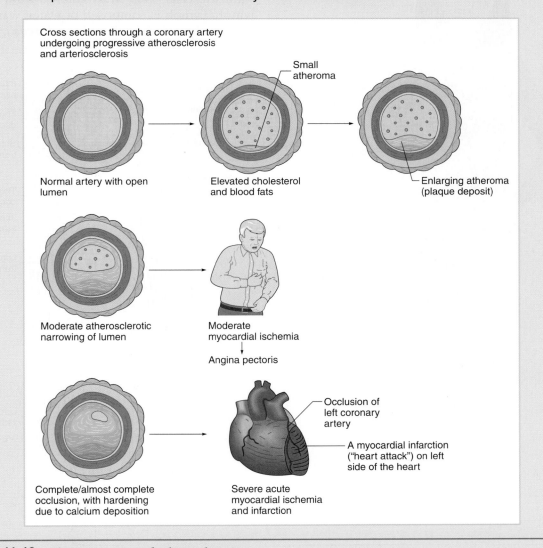

Cross sections through a coronary artery undergoing progressive atherosclerosis and arteriosclerosis

Small atheroma

Normal artery with open lumen

Elevated cholesterol and blood fats

Enlarging atheroma (plaque deposit)

Moderate atherosclerotic narrowing of lumen

Moderate myocardial ischemia

Angina pectoris

Complete/almost complete occlusion, with hardening due to calcium deposition

Severe acute myocardial ischemia and infarction

Occlusion of left coronary artery

A myocardial infarction ("heart attack") on left side of the heart

Figure 11-10 *The progression of atherosclerosis.*

Source: Delmar/Cengage Learning

Note that these attempts on the part of the body to improve oxygenation are double-edged swords. As the capillaries in the lungs decrease in diameter, resistance to the blood passing through them increases. As a result, pressure increases throughout the pulmonary system, including in the heart. As the number of RBCs increases, the blood becomes thicker, or more viscous. This makes the blood harder to pump, thereby increasing the workload for the heart. If you constantly work any muscle, in time it usually becomes larger; the heart is no exception. Thus, with this increased work-load, the heart may enlarge. If the heart becomes too large, it may actually become less effective at pumping. This can lead to even more problems, including, possibly, right-sided heart failure.

The Lymphatic System: Transporting Immunity

Thus far we have looked at the cardiovascular sys-tem as being a transportation system, wherein the heart pumps blood, and the blood vessels transport blood. There is also another very important trans-portation system in the body. This system helps to maintain the fluid balance of the body, remove waste products of cellular activity, and fight infections. This is the lymphatic system (see Figure 11-11).

Lymphatic vessels are very similar in design to blood vessels. Lymphatic capillaries take fluid from the cells. This straw-colored fluid is called lymph. Lymph is composed of water, waste prod-ucts (such as carbon dioxide and **urea**), digested

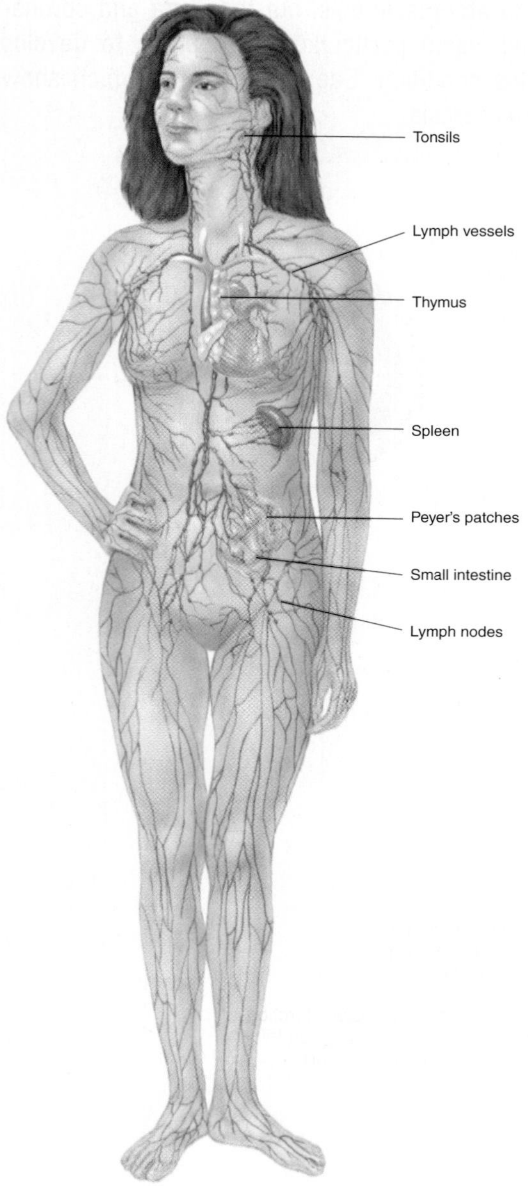

Figure 11-11A   *The organs and vessels of the lymphatic system.*

Source: Delmar/Cengage Learning

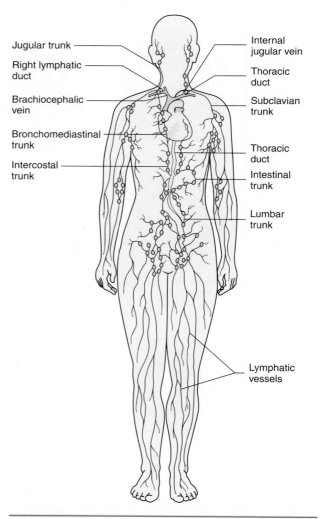

Figure 11-11B   *The nodes of the lymphatic system.*

Source: Delmar/Cengage Learning

nutrients, hormones, salts, lymphocytes, and a few granulocytes.

Lymphatic capillaries then combine to form larger lymphatic vessels. These vessels all eventually empty into one of two main lymphatic ducts: the left lymphatic duct, or thoracic duct, or the right thoracic duct. Lymph vessels from the left side of the body (including the left side of the head, neck, chest, and abdomen, and the left leg) empty into the thoracic duct, while lymph vessels from the right side of the head, neck, and upper trunk, and the right arm, drain into the right lymphatic duct. The right lymphatic duct is approximately 1/2 inch long, and the thoracic duct is approximately 16 inches long. Regardless of the side on which the lymph drains, this fluid travels first to the superior vena cava via either the left or right subclavian veins and then to the right atrium of the heart.

As the lymph passes through these vessels, it is filtered by oval-shaped, specialized tissues called **lymph nodes** (see Figure 11-11B). Previously, we compared the cardiovascular system to the cooling system in a car. Similarly, the lymph nodes are much like the oil filter in a car; they remove various solid particles from the lymph fluid. Lymph nodes are rounded structures and generally range in size from that of a pinhead to approximately 1 inch in diameter. Lymph nodes are usually found in groups throughout the body. The number of lymph nodes per group can range from 2 to more than 100. Lymph nodes are composed of lymphoid tissue, which is a specialized tissue that can remove substances such as cancer cells, pathogenic organisms, and dead blood cells found in the blood. This tissue also helps protect the body from infection by producing **lymphocytes** (which compose between one-fifth and one-quarter of the body's WBCs), which produce specific **antibodies** to protect us from allergens and pathogens. See Figure 11-12 for a depiction of a lymph node.

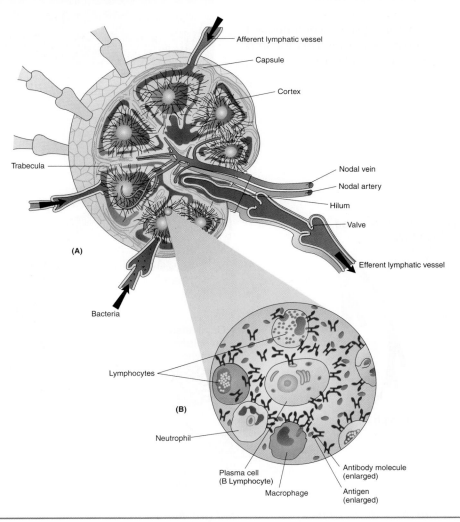

Figure 11-12 *(A) Cross section of a lymph node. (B) Lymph node fighting antigen/pathogens.*

Source: Delmar/Cengage Learning

Lymphoid tissue is found in other structures besides the lymph nodes, including the **tonsils** (also known as **palatine** tonsils), the **adenoids** (also known as pharyngeal tonsils), and the **spleen**. The spleen is different from lymph nodes in the sense that it filters blood instead of lymph fluid. This organ is located in the upper left area of your abdomen just under the diaphragm; here, it is protected by your rib cage. Under normal circumstances, this slightly flattened organ is approximately 5 to 6 inches long and 2 to 3 inches wide. The spleen performs several functions, including:

- removing old, worn-out RBCs
- removing iron from hemoglobin for reuse by bone marrow (to make new RBCs)
- creating RBCs before you are born
- producing lymphocytes, monocytes (another type of WBC), and antibodies to help the body fight disease
- acting as a filter for foreign bodies
- acting as a reservoir for blood, which can be added to the circulatory system when needed

Figure 11-13 illustrates the relationship between the lymphatic and circulatory systems.

You have been blessed with a large amount and variety of lymphatic tissue in your body. This is important because certain diseases such as tonsillitis and cancer may require the removal of varying amounts of this tissue. Even so, your body usually can still protect you from infection with whatever lymphatic tissue is left.

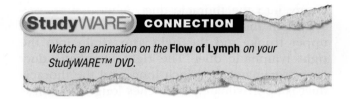

StudyWARE CONNECTION

Watch an animation on the **Flow of Lymph** *on your StudyWARE™ DVD.*

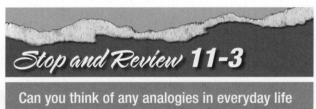

Stop and Review **11-3**

Can you think of any analogies in everyday life to the lymphatic system?

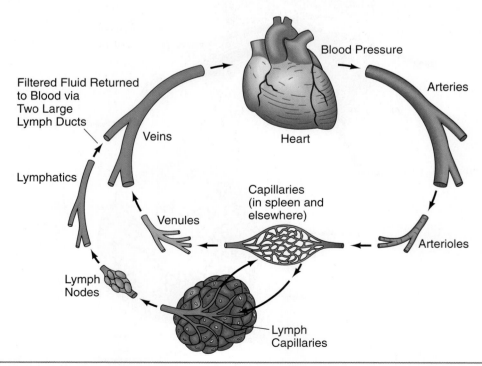

Figure 11-13   *The relationship between the circulatory and lymphatic systems.*

Source: Delmar/Cengage Learning

Professional Profile
Cardiovascular Technologist

Blood is the living river: coursing through your veins to all parts of your body, providing fuel and nutrients, and removing the waste products of metabolism. Without this river, its channels (the blood vessels), and its pump (the heart), your life would cease.

Cardiovascular technologists are involved in diagnosing and treating patients who are suspected of having a problem with their pumps (cardiac disease) or channels (peripheral vascular disease). More formally stated, the cardiovascular technologist performs three general areas of diagnostic evaluation:

- *Invasive cardiology,* which requires entering the body to perform diagnostics of the heart;
- *Noninvasive cardiology,* which involves observing heart function from outside the body without penetrating or entering the body; and
- *Noninvasive peripheral vascular studies,* which involve observing the blood pathways of the body without penetrating or entering the body.

Cardiovascular technologists aid physicians in determining what is wrong with patients by performing a variety of tests. These tests may be something as simple and noninvasive as an electrocardiogram (EKG or ECG) or an echocardiogram (wherein sound waves are used to produce an image of the heart), or they may be as complex and invasive as a cardiac catheterization.

An understanding of anatomy and physiology is obviously important for the cardiovascular technologist; equally important, however, is an understanding of math (which is the subject of Section Two). For example, math is required when reading an ECG tracing, as the measurements of heights and distances between certain patterns on the tracing give you the heart rate and indicate any irregularities. Measuring and interpreting various blood pressures in different areas of the heart, pulmonary artery, and **aorta** (known as *hemodynamic studies*) would be almost impossible without some math background. Finally, statistics and managing patient data collected daily require math proficiency.

Educational requirements include a high school diploma usually followed by a course of study that lasts for two years. The first year includes basic core courses, and the second year comprises areas of specialization. Cardiovascular schools can be found at postsecondary vocational/technical schools, hospitals, colleges, or universities.

If you are interested in the heart and its function as well as in the function of the circulatory system and how disease affects it, this may be the allied health profession for you! For more information on this fascinating field, contact the Alliance of Cardiovascular Professionals, P.O. Box 2007, Midlothian, VA 23113, or go to www.acp-online.org.

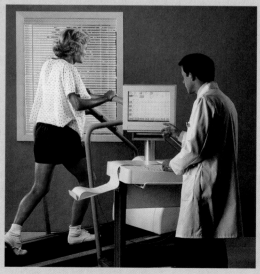

Courtesy of Spacelabs Medical, Inc.
Source: Delmar/Cengage Learning

■ CHAPTER REVIEW

Exercises

1. Describe how the respiratory system and the cardiovascular system interrelate to form the cardio-pulmonary system.

2. How can heart disease affect breathing?

3. How does the arterial system differ from the venous system in the cardiovascular system?

4. How can lung disease affect the heart?

5. How does the lymphatic system differ from the cardiovascular system?

6. What organ is composed of lymphoid tissue and serves as both a filter to remove worn-out RBCs from the blood and a reservoir for blood?

7. What color is lymph?

8. What is another term for thrombocytes, and why are thrombocytes needed by the body?

9. What is the difference between ischemia and infarction?

10. What is the difference between systole and diastole?

Real Life Issues and Applications

Setting Up a Cardiopulmonary Rehabilitation Program

Suppose you have been chosen by your department supervisor to set up a cardiopulmonary rehabilitation program. You have some background as a staff respiratory therapist, and are totally on your own and solely responsible for its creation. How would you find information concerning cardiopulmonary rehabilitation? What kinds of patients would you target? How would you get word out to those patients? How would you persuade physicians to send patients to you? What would you include in your program? How would you evaluate the effectiveness of your program? Share this information with your class.

Additional Activities

1. Create a simple drawing that traces the flow of blood through the cardiopulmonary system.

2. Research the relationship between diet and heart disease. Discuss your findings with the class.

3. Invite a physician to class to discuss what happens during a cardiac arrest that occurs in the hospital setting.

Downloadable audio is available for selected medical terms in this chapter to enhance your learning of medical language.

StudyWARE **CONNECTION**

Go to your StudyWARE™ DVD and have fun learning as you play interactive games, view animations and videos, and take practice tests to help reinforce key concepts you learned in this chapter.

CHAPTER 12

THE GASTROINTESTINAL SYSTEM

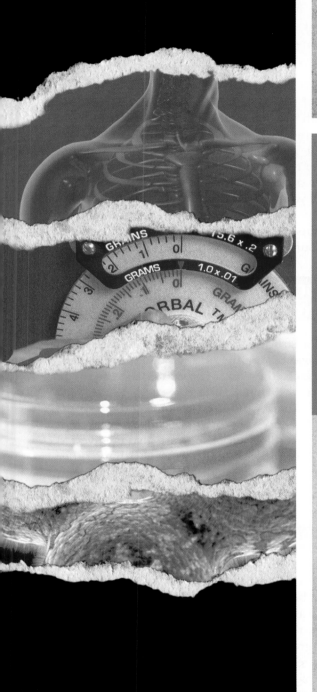

Objectives

Upon completion of this chapter, you should be able to

- Explain the purposes of the gastrointestinal system
- List the various structures of the gastrointestinal system and their functions
- Describe the process of digestion
- State the importance of good nutrition
- Describe a number of diseases of the gastrointestinal system

Key Terms

alimentary canal
  (al-ih-**MEN**-tair-ee)
amino acids (ah-**ME**-no)
appendix (ah-**PEN**-dix)
atherosclerosis
  (**ATH**-er-**OH**-skleh-**ROH**-sis)
bile
bolus
carbohydrates
chyme (**KYM**)
duodenum (**DEW**-oh-**DEE**-num)
enzymes
esophagus (eh-**SOF**-ah-gus)
fructose
gallbladder
gastric juice
gastrointestinal
glucose (**GLOO**-kohs)

glycerol (**GLISS**-er-all)
gullet
hypertension
incisors (in-**SIGH**-zorz)
lacteals (**LACK**-tee-ahls)
large intestine
lipids
liver
lower esophageal sphincter
  (**LES**)
molars
mumps
oral cavity
osteoporosis
  (**OSS**-tee-oh-por-**OH**-sis)
pancreas (**PAN**-kree-ass)
pancreatic juice
  (pan-kree-**AT**-tick)

(continues)

papilla (pah-**PILL**-ah)
parotid glands (pah-**ROT**-id)
pepsin
peristalsis (per-ih-**STAL**-sis)
pharynx (**FAIR**-inks)
premolars

proteins
prothrombin (pro-**THROM**-bin)
pyloric sphincter (py-**LOR**-ick)
saliva (suh-**LIE**-vuh)
salivary glands (**SAL**-ih-vair-ee)
small intestine

soft palate (**PAL**-at)
stomach
stool
sublingual
uvula (**YOU**-view-lah)
villi (**VILL**-eye)

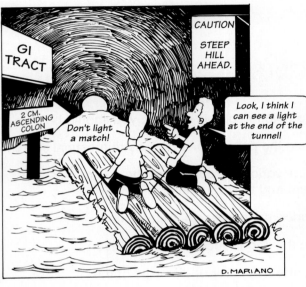

Source: Delmar/Cengage Learning

■ SYSTEM OVERVIEW

You have come a long way in understanding the human body since beginning this book. As you studied the body systems covered thus far, you may have wondered what powers them. In the respiratory chapter, we alluded to the fact that oxygen was needed to help fuel the body and maintain life. Unless you are an air fern, however, a variety of substances are needed in order to sustain life. This is one of the reasons why we need the **gastrointestinal** (*gastr/o* meaning "stomach," *intestin/o* meaning "intestines"), or digestive, system.

The gastrointestinal system can be compared to a factory. In a factory, raw materials (food) are taken in and processed (broken down and digested) into usable materials (e.g., nutrients and water), and excess materials by-products (wastes) are removed (excreted). Some excess materials can be warehoused throughout the body for future use.

Here is an interesting concept: The food you eat travels through a hollow tube and never truly enters your body! To demonstrate this, take

a piece of paper and write the word *body* on one side. With the side that says *body* on the outside, roll the piece of paper into a tube. Pretending that your pencil is food, drop it down through the paper tube. Your pencil was never truly inside the layer of paper, which represented your body. Similarly your food travels through a 30-foot tube, known as the **alimentary canal**. Although this tube is inside your body, food is never actually *inside* your body.

Major Structures of the Gastrointestinal System

The major structures of the gastrointestinal system are: the **oral cavity**, the **pharynx**, the **esophagus**, the **stomach**, the **small intestine**, and the **large intestine** (see Figure 12-1).

The **liver**, **pancreas**, and **gallbladder**, often called *accessory organs* because they are not a part of the alimentary canal, are also involved in the digestive process. As is the case with the other body systems, each of these structures serves a specific purpose.

The Digestive Process

Before discussing these structures and their functions, several aspects of the digestive process need to be explained. Digestion requires both mechanical and chemical activity. *Mechanical digestion* refers to the breaking down of food into progressively smaller and smaller particles through tearing, cutting, and grinding, and the moving of food along the digestive tract. As part of this mechanical process, food is also liquefied to allow it to travel more easily through the tract.

While mechanical digestion does serve to grind up and liquefy food, the process does not convert food to substances usable by the body. This is where *chemical digestion* comes into play. Substances called **enzymes** speed up the process of breaking down food. Without enzymes, it would take approximately 25 years to digest

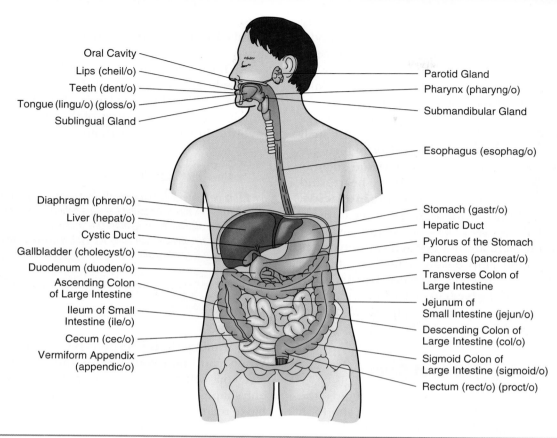

Oral Cavity
Lips (cheil/o)
Teeth (dent/o)
Tongue (lingu/o) (gloss/o)
Sublingual Gland

Parotid Gland
Pharynx (pharyng/o)
Submandibular Gland

Esophagus (esophag/o)

Diaphragm (phren/o)
Liver (hepat/o)
Cystic Duct
Gallbladder (cholecyst/o)
Duodenum (duoden/o)
Ascending Colon of Large Intestine
Ileum of Small Intestine (ile/o)
Cecum (cec/o)
Vermiform Appendix (appendic/o)

Stomach (gastr/o)
Hepatic Duct
Pylorus of the Stomach
Pancreas (pancreat/o)
Transverse Colon of Large Intestine
Jejunum of Small Intestine (jejun/o)
Descending Colon of Large Intestine (col/o)
Sigmoid Colon of Large Intestine (sigmoid/o)
Rectum (rect/o) (proct/o)

Figure 12-1   *The major structures of the GI system.*
Source: Delmar/Cengage Learning

Special Focus

A Friendly Word of Advice Concerning Dieting

In our society, there is continuing pressure to be thin. As a result, a multimillion-dollar diet industry exists, and people often go to ridiculous lengths to lose weight. Some try diets of only one food; some fast regularly; others stuff themselves and then vomit. This is all done in the pursuit of the mythical "perfect body." But remember—your muscles and bones are still growing, and you need a balanced diet to stay healthy now and later in life.

If you are considering dieting, keep two important words in mind: *balance* and *moderation*. If you really feel you need to lose weight, contact your doctor or personnel at a hospital-based diet program for information. They will most likely instruct you to eat smaller portions of all the nutritional groups, and to develop a regular exercise plan. By making this a lifestyle, chances are you will not have to worry about dieting in the future.

For those of you who feel you are too thin and need to gain weight, balance and moderation also come into play. Do not take the easy, and potentially dangerous, way out by increasing your fat intake while decreasing your activity level. Instead, gradually increase your food intake for all of the nutritional groups and develop an exercise routine. This way, you gain healthy weight. Visit mypyramid.gov for both the latest food and activity pyramids, which can serve as excellent guides for a healthy lifestyle.

And for each of you who are questioning the need to gain or lose weight, take a good long look at yourself and think, "Am I comfortable with my weight?" Chances are, if you ignore societal pressures (from peers and the media), you can find the right balance for yourself. Be happy with that, and go on and enjoy your life! After all, you're only young once!

a single meal! (While there are approximately 10,000 different types of enzymes in your body, not all of them are used in the digestive process; some are used for other activities of the body.)

Through the use of enzymes, the body breaks down **carbohydrates** (which are quick sources of energy most often found in sugars and starches such as pasta) into usable energy substances such as **glucose** and **fructose**. **Proteins** (which are needed to create and repair body tissue such as muscles and organs like your liver, heart, and kidneys) are broken down into **amino acids**. Proteins are found in foods such as meat, eggs, milk, and fish. Proteins also serve as sources of energy when there are not enough carbohydrates in the body and help ensure a healthy immune system. Finally, enzymes convert **lipids** (fats) into fatty acids and **glycerol**. After food is broken down into these simpler substances, *absorption* can take place. See Figure 12-2.

The Beginning: The Oral Cavity

The oral cavity receives food and begins the preparation of food for digestion. Here, the food is torn and ground into smaller pieces through *mastication* (chewing). Saliva, from the salivary glands, is added to the food as it is being broken down.

The main parts of the oral cavity that are involved with digestion of food are the teeth, tongue, and salivary glands. See Figure 12-3 which shows the structures of the mouth, muscles involved in chewing, teeth and salivary glands.

> **QUOTES & NOTES**
>
> *More people experience tooth decay than any other disease. A strong link has been found between poor dental hygiene and heart disease and diabetes. One of the reasons is periodontal infections can enter the systemic bloodstream and cause cardiovascular damage.*
>
> *A small percentage of people lose their second set of teeth and grow a third set.*

Your teeth are responsible for mastication. When you open your mouth and look in a mirror, you will notice that your teeth have different shapes. The front teeth, known as **incisors**, have relatively thin, almost sharp edges. Their function is to tear and cut chunks of food away

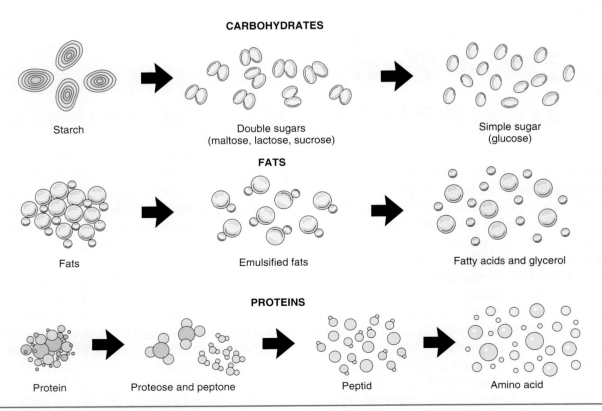

CARBOHYDRATES

Starch   Double sugars
(maltose, lactose, sucrose)   Simple sugar
(glucose)

FATS

Fats   Emulsified fats   Fatty acids and glycerol

PROTEINS

Protein   Proteose and peptone   Peptid   Amino acid

Figure 12-2   *Breaking down starch, fat, and protein in foodstuffs into usable substances.*

Source: Delmar/Cengage Learning

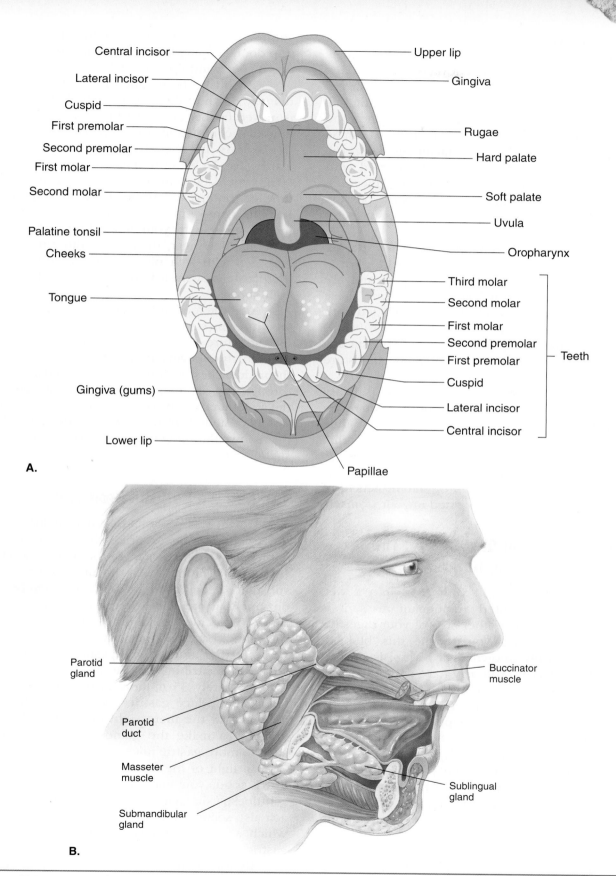

Figure 12-3 *(A) Structures of the oral cavity. (B) Muscles involved in chewing, and teeth and salivary glands.*
Source: Delmar/Cengage Learning

from the main portion, such as when you bite into a slice of pizza. After that piece of food is in your mouth, your **premolars** and **molars** grind the food into even smaller pieces. This is why those teeth have flatter surfaces. During this phase of digestion, your tongue moves the food around your oral cavity so that all the food can be ground up. The tongue also facilitates *deglutination* (swallowing). Your tongue is covered with tiny projectiles called **papilla**. These projectiles, more commonly known as *taste buds,* possess cells that serve as the receptors of taste (refer again to Figure 12-3).

You possess three pairs of **salivary glands** as shown in Figure 12-3. The **parotid glands** are the largest pair of salivary glands and are located anterior and inferior to your ears. These are the glands that swell up when infected with the **mumps** virus. The *submaxillary,* or *submandibular,* glands are found near the inner surface of your lower jaw, while **sublingual** glands are located under your tongue.

As was previously stated, your salivary glands produce **saliva**. Saliva aids in liquefying food, thus making the food easier to digest. While saliva is 99% water, it also contains enzymes that begin breaking down food while you are chewing. Specifically, the enzyme *ptyalin,* or *salivary amylase,* begins the breakdown of starch, which, of course, continues to be digested in your stomach.

Life Beyond the Oral Cavity: The Pharynx and Esophagus

After you have chewed your food into a wet, nondescript, and utterly repugnant mass, it is time to move it to another area of your digestive tract. With the aid of your tongue, this "blob" of food, technically known as a **bolus**, is pushed into your pharynx. You may have wondered why the food *usually* goes down your throat instead of up your nose. The answer is because the **uvula** (that soft, punching-bag-shaped mass attached to the **soft palate** and hanging down in the back of your throat) blocks the passageway between your nasal and oral cavities when you swallow. This, however, is not foolproof. You may have experienced the embarrassing phenomena of laughing or sneezing at the same time you were attempting to swallow something and having liquid or food come out your nose.

You may also have wondered (especially if you didn't read the chapter on the respiratory system) how food is kept out of the lungs when you swallow. In review, the epiglottis acts as a trap door, keeping food and liquid from traveling down your windpipe, or trachea.

Obviously, the tongue cannot push food all the way down to the stomach. The bolus of food is moved further downward by way of rhythmic, muscular contractions of the pharynx, known as **peristalsis**. These contractions occur in a downward wave. To better understand this motion, the effect would be similar to holding an uncapped tube of toothpaste upside down in your hand. Imagine gently squeezing the tube in a smooth motion—first with your index finger, then with your middle finger, then with your ring finger, and then with your pinky. This should force the toothpaste downward and onto the floor—or your shoes!

After the food bolus passes through the pharynx, it reaches a 9- to 10-inch-long flexible, tube-like structure called the *esophagus* (or **gullet**). This structure begins in the throat, travels through the middle chest region (that is, the mediastinum), through the diaphragm, and, eventually, ends in the abdominal cavity. Here it attaches to and empties its contents into the stomach. See Figure 12-4 that shows the sequence of swallowing and peristaltic action.

The Sac We Call the Stomach

The stomach is a sac-like structure located in the upper left quadrant of the abdomen (see Figure 12-5). This organ is filled with **gastric juices** and mucus. Gastric juice is an acidic substance composed mainly of **pepsin**, an enzyme that breaks down the proteins found in food. Hydrochloric acid in the stomach destroys unwanted bacteria and other microorganisms while further aiding the digestion of food. This acid also contributes to the absorption of iron. Approximately 35 million gastric glands in the stomach produce gastric juice. It is interesting to note that the mere sight or smell of food is enough to make the glands in your stomach secrete more gastric juices.

In light of the fact that gastric juices break down food, you may wonder why your stomach doesn't dissolve itself. Fortunately, the stomach also secretes and maintains a mucous lining, which acts as a protective barrier between the gastric juices and the stomach lining.

By way of muscle contractions, the stomach makes a churning action. This action increases the effectiveness of the gastric juices. If this

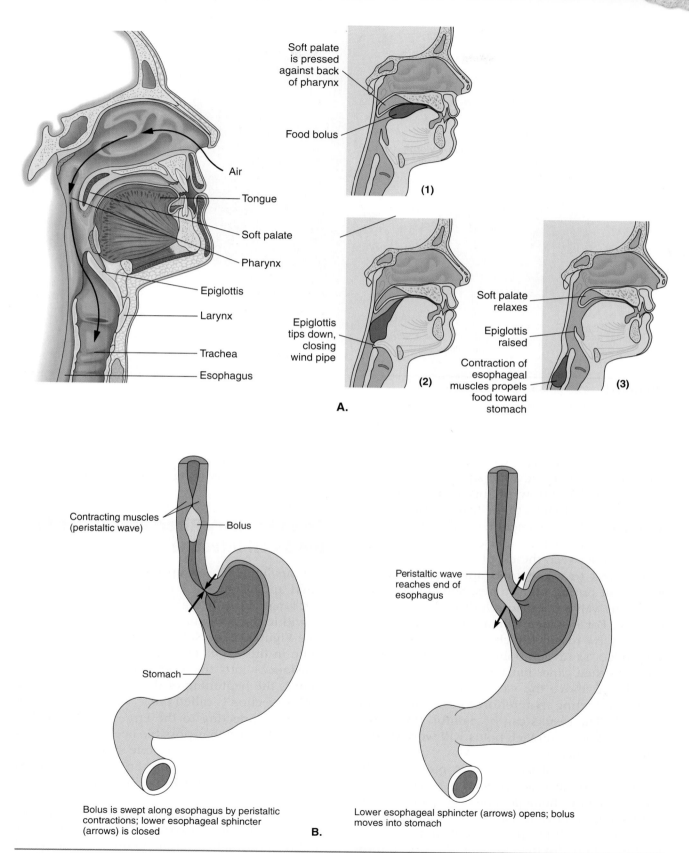

Figure 12-4   *(A) The sequence of swallowing. (B) Peristaltic action.*

Source: Delmar/Cengage Learning

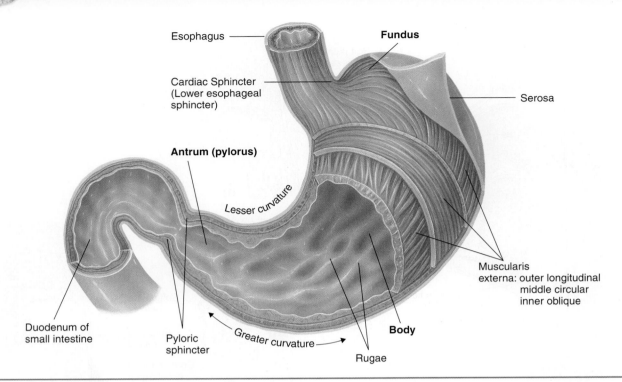

Figure 12-5 *The stomach.*

Source: Delmar/Cengage Learning

churning action occurs, why don't gastric juices and partially digested food squirt back up into your throat? Backflow of this nature normally does not occur thanks to the **lower esophageal sphincter (LES)**, sometimes called the *cardiac sphincter.* This ring-like muscle structure, which is located between the esophagus and the stomach, opens to allow food and liquids in and stays shut during other times. Sometimes, however, this valve does not work quite efficiently enough. For instance, when you are in a hurry, you may try to quickly chew up and swallow a very large "sandwich bolus." That ball of bread, meat, lettuce, and mustard (hold the mayo!) may lodge above the valve, while the muscles keep contracting in an effort to force it into the stomach. The results can be painful. Eventually, however, your sandwich bolus will work its way into your stomach.

As a result of the digestive process in the stomach, partially digested food becomes a semi-liquid, creamy, homogeneous substance called **chyme**. After chyme leaves the bottom of the stomach through the **pyloric sphincter**, it travels for a short distance through the **duodenum** on its way to the small intestine. In the duodenum, a 9- to 10-inch structure, **bile** from the liver

and **pancreatic juice** (from the pancreas, of course) are added along with intestinal juice.

Down the Lazy River: Adventures in the Small Intestine

The small intestine is a portion of the alimentary canal approximately 1 inch in diameter and 23 feet long! The only logical way this structure can fit within the abdominal cavity is to be coiled up (see Figure 12-6). Not only does digestion continue in this segment, but *absorption* of needed substances into the body occurs. The duodenum is the beginning of the small intestine, the middle section is called the *jejunum,* and the last section connecting to the large intestine is the *ileum.* Absorption is possible because the food is now broken down into usable substances at the tissue level and these substances are absorbed by the millions of **villi** that line the wall of the small intestine.

Villi are microscopic, finger-like projections containing networks of blood capillaries and lymph capillaries, called **lacteals**. The blood capillaries absorb and transport digested nutrients into general circulation for use by the body's

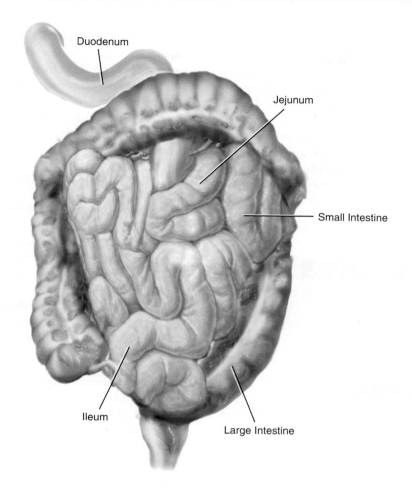

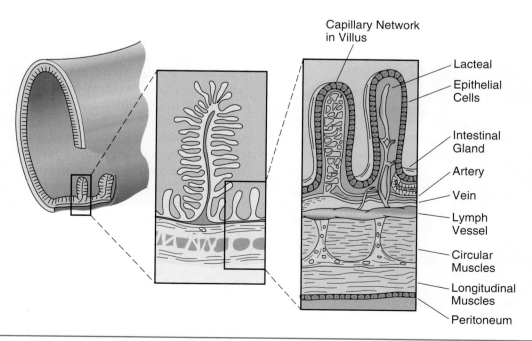

Figure 12-6 *The small intestine and a magnified view of the inner lining of the small intestine.*
Source: Delmar/Cengage Learning

cells, or send the nutrients to storage. The lacteals pick up the majority of the fat that is digested and transport it to the lymphatic system, where it is then released into the circulatory system. Water is also absorbed by the small intestine. On the average, about 10 liters of water are absorbed each day. If necessary, however, your small intestine can absorb at least 1 liter of water every hour! After food has made its way through the small intestine, normally only indigestible substances, waste material, and excess water are left (refer back to Figure 12-6).

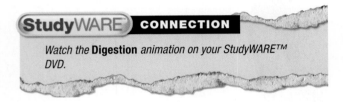

Watch the **Digestion** animation on your StudyWARE™ DVD.

The Accessory Organs

As was mentioned earlier, the liver, pancreas, and gallbladder are termed *accessory organs* because, although they are involved with digestion, they are not part of the alimentary canal (see Figure 12-7).

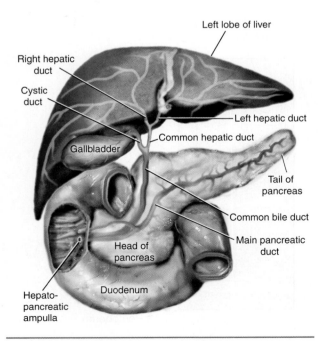

Figure 12-7   *The accessory digestive organs.*
Source: Delmar/Cengage Learning

The liver is a 3- to 4-pound organ located in the upper right quadrant of the abdomen under the diaphragm. Under normal conditions, you cannot feel the liver by palpating your abdomen. The color of your liver is very much like that of the fresh liver you see at the grocery store. Your liver is responsible for a variety of vital functions, and you could not survive without it. Among other things, the liver:

- maintains correct blood sugar (glucose) levels;
- filters out and destroys old red blood cells (RBCs) and saves the iron to be used again;
- produces bile, which is necessary for the digestion and utilization of fats;
- acts as a storehouse for a variety of vitamins such as vitamins K, A, D, E, and B12;
- produces **prothrombin**, which is necessary for blood clotting; and
- filters out harmful toxins that may be ingested.

Bile manufactured by the liver goes to the gallbladder. The gallbladder can store and concentrate about 50 milliliters of bile. When fatty foods are eaten, this 7- to 10-centimeter-long, pear-shaped organ is signaled to release bile to the duodenum via the common bile duct. Some of the bile used comes directly from the liver via the hepatic ducts. The action of bile on fats is similar to how soap dissolves grease. Bile breaks down fat sufficiently so that the fat can be absorbed by the lacteals of the villi in the intestinal wall and utilized by the body.

The pancreas is located behind the stomach. This oblong, flattened organ is about 15 centimeters long. It is responsible for producing pancreatic juice, which contains more digestive enzymes. This juice travels first through the pancreatic duct, and then through the common bile duct to get to the duodenum. The enzymes in this juice help in the digestion of proteins and fats. Although not directly related to digestion, the pancreas also contributes to the control of blood sugar levels via its production of insulin.

The End of the Trail: The Large Intestine

The large intestine is the final portion of the digestive system (see Figure 12-8). This structure is approximately 5 feet long and 2 inches in

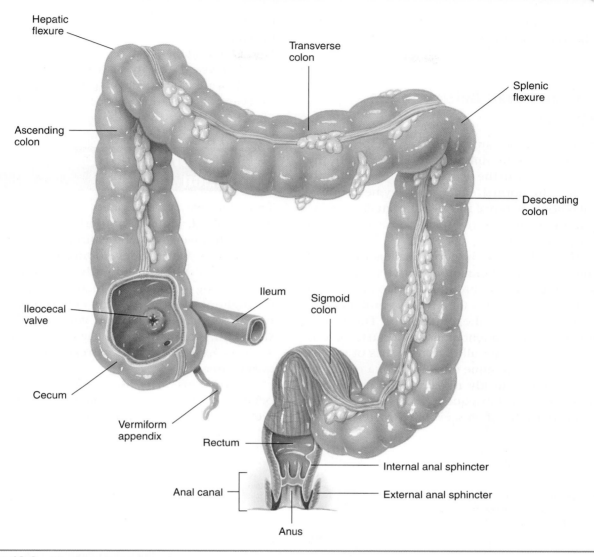

Figure 12-8 *The large intestine.*
Source: Delmar/Cengage Learning

diameter. Like the small intestine, the large intestine is curled up within the abdominal area.

The large intestine serves several purposes. Some of the water that remains in the indigestible waste products is absorbed. You may not know this, but your large intestine contains a colony of bacteria vital to your good health. This bacteria works on undigested substances and is needed to synthesize vitamin K as well as some of the B-complex vitamins. Vitamin K is very important; without it, your liver would not be able to produce prothrombin, which, as was mentioned previously, causes the blood to clot. The large intestine also serves as the storage and elimination structure for indigestible substances.

An interesting structure attached to the large intestine is the **appendix**. This narrow, approximately 3-inch-long tube is open to the large intestine and closed on the other end, and is poorly perfused. If this structure becomes plugged for

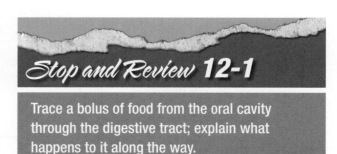

Stop and Review **12-1**

Trace a bolus of food from the oral cavity through the digestive tract; explain what happens to it along the way.

any reason, infection can occur, and the appendix can become inflamed. If not treated, *appendicitis* can be a life-threatening condition.

Waste Removal: Getting to the Bottom of It

Although the time can vary greatly, the process of digestion, from the time you eat a meal until the time you eliminate the waste, takes approximately 12 hours. In normal situations, chyme requires about 6 hours to travel through the small intestine and approximately 3 to 4 hours to travel through the large intestine.

The makeup of the food dictates the speed of digestion and elimination of the waste products. Liquid passes through the stomach most quickly, carbohydrates take longer, proteins longer yet, and fats take the longest time. This results in an interesting phenomenon. Because of this variation in time, not all digested parts of a meal are excreted at the same time. Parts of a meal that aren't excreted quickly remain to be mixed and excreted with a subsequent meal or meals. As a result, portions of this excreted material (also

known as feces, or **stool**) may have come from meals that were eaten days earlier.

Other factors such as hydration of the body, stress, physical activity or inactivity, and disease can also affect the rate of digestion. To see an overview of the entire process of digestion, see Figure 12-9.

The Importance of Good Nutrition

Thus far, we have looked at how the body digests food. Equally important is to understand what we *should* be eating. Understanding nutrition as well as developing healthy eating habits should be started early in life. Doing so goes a long way toward maintaining wellness throughout life. In fact, it is believed that good nutritional habits combined with a healthy lifestyle can eliminate or at least delay diseases such as **hypertension**, **atherosclerosis**, and **osteoporosis**.

Hypertension is high blood pressure. It is believed that an excessive intake of salt in the diet may be a factor in the development of this

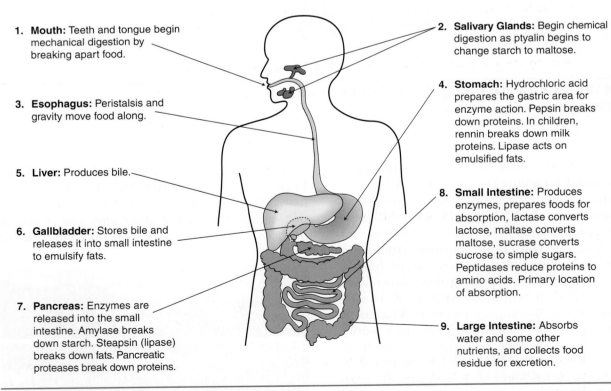

1. **Mouth:** Teeth and tongue begin mechanical digestion by breaking apart food.

2. **Salivary Glands:** Begin chemical digestion as ptyalin begins to change starch to maltose.

3. **Esophagus:** Peristalsis and gravity move food along.

4. **Stomach:** Hydrochloric acid prepares the gastric area for enzyme action. Pepsin breaks down proteins. In children, rennin breaks down milk proteins. Lipase acts on emulsified fats.

5. **Liver:** Produces bile.

6. **Gallbladder:** Stores bile and releases it into small intestine to emulsify fats.

7. **Pancreas:** Enzymes are released into the small intestine. Amylase breaks down starch. Steapsin (lipase) breaks down fats. Pancreatic proteases break down proteins.

8. **Small Intestine:** Produces enzymes, prepares foods for absorption, lactase converts lactose, maltase converts maltose, sucrase converts sucrose to simple sugars. Peptidases reduce proteins to amino acids. Primary location of absorption.

9. **Large Intestine:** Absorbs water and some other nutrients, and collects food residue for excretion.

Figure 12-9 *An overview of the process of digestion.*

Source: Delmar/Cengage Learning

condition. Hypertension can predispose an individual to heart disease, renal (kidney) disease, or circulatory problems.

Atherosclerosis results from the buildup of fatty material on the inside walls of the arteries. As this layer builds up, the inner diameters of the arteries decrease, making it harder for blood to flow through. Limiting fats and certain kinds of cholesterol in the diet is believed to aid in the prevention of this disease. Atherosclerosis can lead to stroke and/or heart attack.

Osteoporosis occurs when the bones lose their density and become porous (that is, full of holes). As a result, these bones become brittle and can be easily broken. Osteoporosis can be caused by a lack of calcium, magnesium, and vitamin D in the diet. It is believed that exercise along with a good diet can not only halt osteoporosis, but may even reverse the process.

Good nutrition is not only physically beneficial; it also improves mental ability, as well as emotional and psychological well-being.

If you take away anything from this section on nutrition, let it be two words: *moderation* and *balance.* In other words, eat the right amount (moderation) from *all* the food groups (balance).

In order to maintain a healthy body, you must ensure that you consume foods from all of the nutritional groups (not to be confused with food groups). Failure to do so can cause deficiencies in your body. The nutritional groups are carbohydrates, fats, proteins, vitamins, minerals, and water.

Carbohydrates (found in foods such as pastas, breads, cereals, and potatoes) provide quick energy. Carbohydrates are also called *starches* or *sugars. Cellulose,* commonly called *fiber,* is the indigestible part of the carbohydrate group. Fiber provides *bulk* for the digestive system, which allows for regular bowel movements. These foods are easily digested.

Fats, often referred to as *lipids,* are more concentrated forms of energy than are carbohydrates. Fat provides insulation to aid in maintaining body temperature, acts as a cushion to protect bones and organs, and aids in the absorption of certain vitamins. Fats can be obtained from fatty meats, dairy products, oils, and egg yolks. Cholesterol is a part of the fats group and is important for body function. Only small amounts of this substance are needed, however. This group is, generally, more difficult to digest than are carbohydrates.

Proteins, which possess the "building blocks" of life, are needed to build tissue and repair cells. Proteins can be utilized by the body as a source of energy and to produce heat. Proteins are also necessary to maintain a healthy immune system. Animal food sources such as meat, fish, eggs, and dairy products provide complete proteins. Proteins that do not contain all of the necessary building blocks of life, known as *incomplete proteins,* can be found in vegetable sources such as peas, beans, nuts, and cereals.

Vitamins can be called the regulators of the body. Without vitamins, energy from the foods we eat could not be utilized. Vitamins also aid in the building and repair of cells and in keeping the nervous system functioning properly.

Minerals are nonliving compounds that contribute to regulating the body and aid in cell growth and repair.

Water, of course, is necessary for life. It is found in every cell of the body. Indeed, your body is approximately two-thirds water. Without water, nutrients and waste by-products could not be transported. Water is needed for practically all functions of the body. The food pyramid (Figure 12-10) illustrates the recommended food groups and servings for each per day.

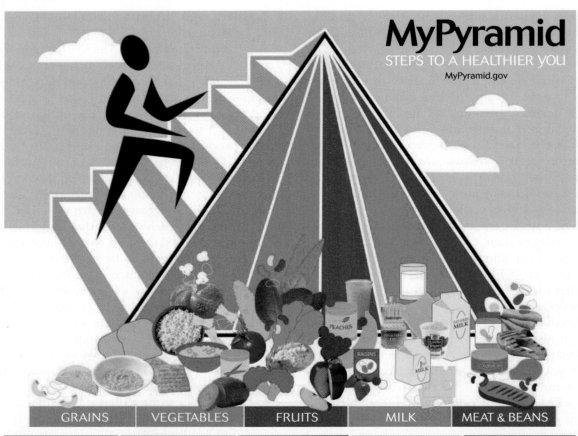

MyPyramid
STEPS TO A HEALTHIER YOU
MyPyramid.gov

GRAINS	VEGETABLES	FRUITS	MILK	MEAT & BEANS

GRAINS Make half your grains whole	**VEGETABLES** Vary your veggies	**FRUITS** Focus on fruits	**MILK** Get your calcium-rich foods	**MEAT & BEANS** Go lean with protein
Eat at least 3 oz. of whole-grain cereals, breads, crackers, rice, or pasta every day 1 oz. is about 1 slice of bread, about 1 cup of breakfast cereal, or ½ cup of cooked rice, cereal, or pasta	Eat more dark-green veggies like broccoli, spinach, and other dark leafy greens Eat more orange vegetables like carrots and sweetpotatoes Eat more dry beans and peas like pinto beans, kidney beans, and lentils	Eat a variety of fruit Choose fresh, frozen, canned, or dried fruit Go easy on fruit juices	Go low-fat or fat-free when you choose milk, yogurt, and other milk products If you don't or can't consume milk, choose lactose-free products or other calcium sources such as fortified foods and beverages	Choose low-fat or lean meats and poultry Bake it, broil it, or grill it Vary your protein routine — choose more fish, beans, peas, nuts, and seeds

For a 2,000-calorie diet, you need the amounts below from each food group. To find the amounts that are right for you, go to MyPyramid.gov.

Eat 6 oz. every day	Eat 2½ cups every day	Eat 2 cups every day	Get 3 cups every day; for kids aged 2 to 8, it's 2	Eat 5½ oz. every day

Find your balance between food and physical activity
- Be sure to stay within your daily calorie needs.
- Be physically active for at least 30 minutes most days of the week.
- About 60 minutes a day of physical activity may be needed to prevent weight gain.
- For sustaining weight loss, at least 60 to 90 minutes a day of physical activity may be required.
- Children and teenagers should be physically active for 60 minutes every day, or most days.

Know the limits on fats, sugars, and salt (sodium)
- Make most of your fat sources from fish, nuts, and vegetable oils.
- Limit solid fats like butter, margarine, shortening, and lard, as well as foods that contain these.
- Check the Nutrition Facts label to keep saturated fats, *trans* fats, and sodium low.
- Choose food and beverages low in added sugars. Added sugars contribute calories with few, if any, nutrients.

MyPyramid.gov
STEPS TO A HEALTHIER YOU

U.S. Department of Agriculture
Center for Nutrition Policy and Promotion
April 2005
CNPP-15

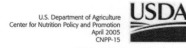

USDA is an equal opportunity provider and employer.

Figure 12-10   *MyPyramid*.

Source: Courtesy U.S. Department of Agriculture

Clinical Relevancy

Colostomy

Certain diseases of the large intestine require surgical repair and time for healing. As a result, a new opening needs to be made in the large intestine to reroute the fecal matter. This procedure is called a colostomy and can be either temporary or permanent depending upon the situation. This opening leads to the outside of the body where a bag is attached and the feces collected. For examples of the standard sites that are utilized for these openings, see Figure 12-11.

Disorders of the Gastrointestinal System

Following are descriptions of some of the more common diseases of the gastrointestinal system that you may encounter in your career.

Heartburn is when gastric juices back up into the lower portion of the esophagus. Unlike the stomach, the esophagus is not protected with a mucous lining. The

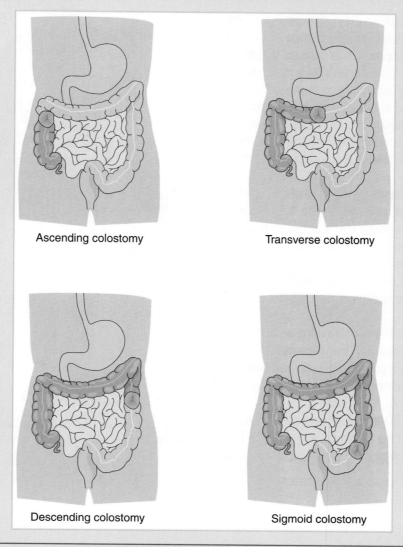

Ascending colostomy

Transverse colostomy

Descending colostomy

Sigmoid colostomy

Figure 12-11 *Locations for colostomies. The blue sections may be surgically removed if the colostomy is permanent.*

Source: Delmar/Cengage Learning

(continues)

(continued)

tissue of the esophagus, therefore, becomes irritated, and a burning sensation results. While antacids can be used to relieve the symptoms, it is important to discover the underlying cause and correct it.

Gastritis is a condition wherein the lining of the stomach becomes inflamed. This condition can be either acute or chronic and can be caused by a variety of things, such as certain infectious diseases, spicy foods, and drugs.

A *peptic ulcer* can occur in the stomach or duodenum. This is a painful condition wherein *lesions* form as a result of either overproduction of gastric juices or an insufficient production of mucus for the stomach lining. Peptic ulcers are believed to result from stress or certain pathogens.

Colitis is a disease wherein the large intestine becomes inflamed. Patients with this disease may exhibit either diarrhea or constipation. It is believed that stress and dietary habits are contributing factors to this condition.

Cholecystitis is an inflammation of the gallbladder. This condition can lead to blockage of the common bile duct, which stops the flow of bile. Related to cholecystitis is the formation of gallstones (*cholelithiasis*) from bile of crystallized cholesterol. These can cause blockage of the bile ducts.

Cirrhosis is a disease wherein there is chronic destruction of the liver cells, which are then replaced with fibrous connective tissue and scar tissue. Normally associated with chronic alcoholism, cirrhosis is also linked with hepatitis, excessive use of over-the-counter and prescription drugs, toxins, and bile duct disease. See Figure 12-12 that illustrates the various signs of cirrhosis throughout the body.

Peritonitis is a condition wherein the serous membrane that lines the abdominal cavity becomes inflamed. This can result from a ruptured appendix, gallbladder, or intestine, where the contents of the organ are released into the abdominal cavity.

Ascites is a general term used to describe an abnormal amount of fluid in the peritoneal cavity. As the situation worsens, abdominal girth increases. Ascites can result from cirrhosis, cancer, and advanced congestive heart failure.

Hepatitis B is a potentially life-threatening disease caused by a virus. This virus is found only in blood; it can therefore be transmitted via both accidental needle sticks and inadequately sterilized medical equipment. As a health care professional, you will obviously be at higher risk for contracting hepatitis B. Consequently, you should consider obtaining a vaccine to protect yourself from this disease.

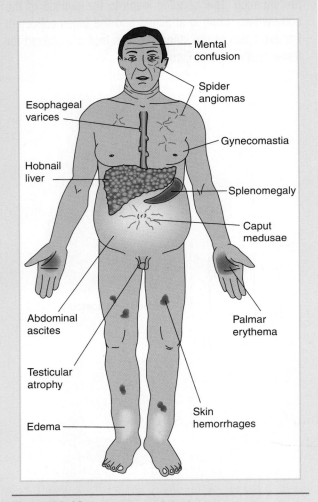

Figure 12-12 *Cirrhosis of the liver.*
Source: Delmar/Cengage Learning

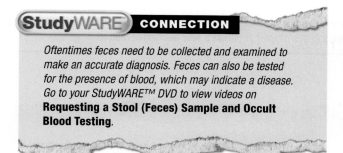

StudyWARE CONNECTION

Oftentimes feces need to be collected and examined to make an accurate diagnosis. Feces can also be tested for the presence of blood, which may indicate a disease. Go to your StudyWARE™ DVD to view videos on **Requesting a Stool (Feces) Sample and Occult Blood Testing.**

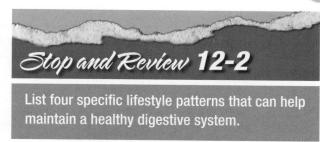

Stop and Review **12-2**

List four specific lifestyle patterns that can help maintain a healthy digestive system.

■ CHAPTER REVIEW

Exercises

1. List the basic nutritional groups and explain the importance of each.

2. List and describe three diseases of the gastrointestinal system.

3. Approximately how long is the small intestine, and what are its functions?

4. List four functions of the liver.

5. What is the function of pancreatic juice?

6. What factors alter the body's rate of digestion?

7. What is the main responsibility of the villi in your small intestine?

8. What are the wave-like muscular contractions that move food downward through the digestive system called?

9. Why are enzymes important in the gastrointestinal system?

10. Why is hydrochloric acid important for digestion? What keeps it from dissolving the stomach?

Real Life Issues and Applications

Plan of Action for Obesity and Smoking

One of your patients is a 60-year-old overweight female. She has a 30-year history of smoking. This patient complains of SOB and diaphoresis on minimal exertion. Tachycardia is also noted. What body systems are affected by these conditions? As a member of the hospital's patient care team, what plans would you suggest for the care of this patient, both during her hospital stay and after she goes home?

Additional Activities

1. Bring in examples of advertisements and articles on dieting. Discuss in class how society views overweight people.

2. Research the differences between nutritional groups and the basic food groups, which were discussed in this chapter. Discuss your findings with the class.

3. Devise a one-week balanced meal plan for your family. Cost-wise, how much different is it to eat a healthy versus an unhealthy diet?

Downloadable audio is available for selected medical terms in this chapter to enhance your learning of medical language.

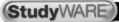

StudyWARE CONNECTION

Go to your StudyWARE™ DVD and have fun learning as you play interactive games, view animations and videos, and take practice tests to help reinforce key concepts you learned in this chapter.

Workbook Practice   Go to your Workbook for more practice questions and activities.

CHAPTER 13

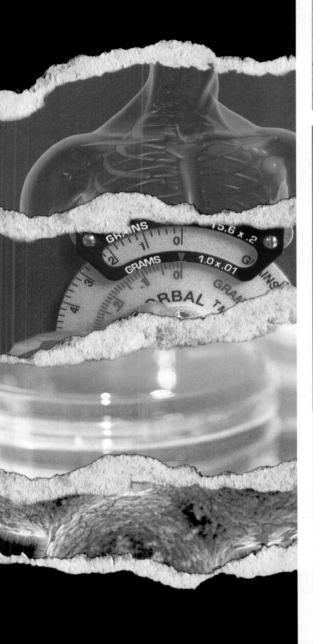

THE URINARY AND REPRODUCTIVE SYSTEMS

Objectives

Upon completion of this chapter, you should be able to

■ List the major structures of the urinary system and describe their functions

■ Describe the functions of the kidneys

■ List the structures of the male and female reproductive systems and describe the functions of these structures

■ Describe several diseases of the genitourinary system

Key Terms

acute kidney failure
anuria (an-**YOU**-ree-ah)
Bartholin's glands
benign prostatic hypertrophy (**BPH**) (bee-**NINE PRO**-stat-ic high-**PER**-troh-fee)
bulbourethral glands (**BOL**-boh-you-**REE**-thral)
calculi (**KAL**-q-lye)
chronic renal failure
clitoris (**KLIT**-oh-ris)
Cowper's glands
ejaculation (ee-**JACK**-you-**LAY**-shun)
ejaculatory duct (ee-**JACK**-you-lah-**TOR**-ree)
embryo (**EM**-bree-oh)

endometriosis (**EN**-doh-**ME**-tree-oh-sis)
estrogen (**ES**-troh-jin)
fallopian tubes (fal-**LOH**-pee-on)
fertilization
fetus (**FEE**-tus)
filtrate
genitourinary (**JIN**-eh-toh-**YUR**-ih-nair-ee)
graafian follicles (**GRAF**-ee-an **FOL**-lick-kulz)
incontinence
kidney
labia majora (**LAY**-be-ah)
labia minora
motility

(continues)

nephrolithiasis
    (**NEF**-row-lith-**EYE**-ah-sis)
nephron (**NEF**-ron)
oliguria (ol-ig-**YOU**-ree-ah)
ovaries (**OH**-vah-reez)
pelvic inflammatory disease (**PID**)
penis (**PEE**-nis)
progesterone (pro-**JES**-ter-own)
prostate gland (**PRAWS**-tate)
retroperitoneal
    (**RET**-roh-**PAIR**-eh-toe-**NEE**-all)

scrotum (**SKROH**-tum)
semen (**SEE**-men)
seminal vesicles
    (**SEM**-ih-nal **VES**-ih-kulz)
sexually transmitted disease (**STD**)
sperm
spermatozoa
    (**SPER**-mat- oh-**ZOH**-ah)
testes (**TESS**-teez)
testicles
urea (you-**REE**-ah)

ureter (you-**REE**-ter)
urethra (you-**REE**-thrah)
urinary bladder
urine (**YOU**-rine)
uterus (**YOU**-ter-us)
vagina (vah-**JYE**-nah)
vas deferens (vas-**DEF**-er-enz)
voiding
womb
zygote (**ZYE**-goht)

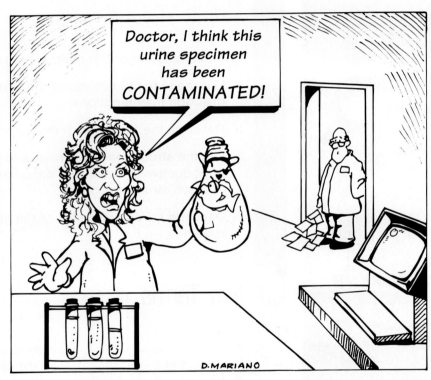

Source: Delmar/Cengage Learning

■ SYSTEM OVERVIEW

In Chapter 12 we discovered that one of the functions of the intestines is to absorb water. But what happens when you have too much water in your body? How is it removed? How are the waste products of cellular metabolism removed from your body? The two main functions of the urinary system are to remove waste products from the bloodstream and maintain proper fluid balance in the body. The function of the reproductive system may be obvious; it allows for the continuation of our species. Often, these two systems are considered as one system known as the **genitourinary** system.

The Urinary System

There are many structures in the urinary system needed for filtration, secretion, absorption, and elimination of fluids in our bodies. These structures form an intricate filtration and tubular system that is vital to maintain pH and proper fluid and electrolyte balance.

Structures of the Urinary System

The majority of the body's excretory function is performed by the urinary system. The elimination of waste products resulting from cellular metabolism and of other wastes from the blood is necessary in order to sustain life. If this cleansing did not occur, there would be an initial buildup of toxins at the cellular level followed by a poisoning of the entire body and, eventually, death.

The major structures of the urinary system are the **kidneys**, the **ureters**, the **urinary bladder**, and the **urethra**.

The Kidneys

Your kidneys are bean-shaped organs approximately 13 centimeters long, 8 centimeters wide, and 5 centimeters thick. They are located one on either side of the spinal column, posterior to the abdominal cavity and inferior to the thoracic diaphragm (see Figure 13-1). Because both kidneys sit behind the digestive organs in the *peritoneal*

space, they are considered **retroperitoneal** in location.

Kidneys eventually create a waste-filled liquid called **urine**. Urine is formed via the filtering of blood plasma by the kidneys. Kidneys are truly amazing filters. Each kidney has 600 milliliters of blood flow through it *every minute*! And this is just an average blood flow; it can be greater or reduced, depending on the situation. The kidneys work together to filter a total of 125 milliliters of blood every minute.

Filtration in the kidneys is performed by microscopic structures called **nephrons**. See Figure 13-2. There are over 1 million nephrons in each kidney. Nephrons possess hollow tubes; these tubes are used in the filtration process. If

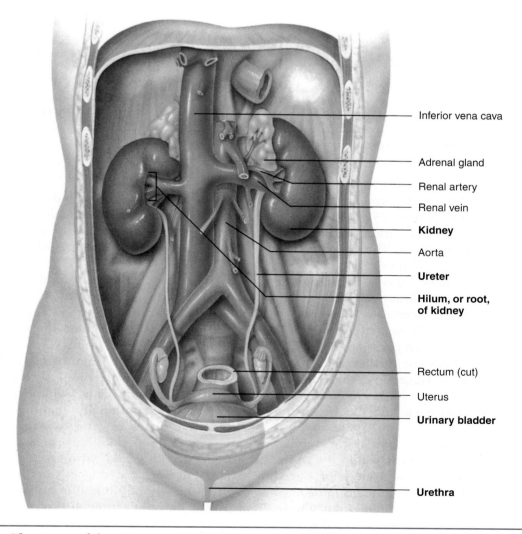

Inferior vena cava

Adrenal gland

Renal artery

Renal vein

Kidney

Aorta

Ureter

Hilum, or root, of kidney

Rectum (cut)

Uterus

Urinary bladder

Urethra

Figure 13-1 *The organs of the urinary system.*

Source: Delmar/Cengage Learning

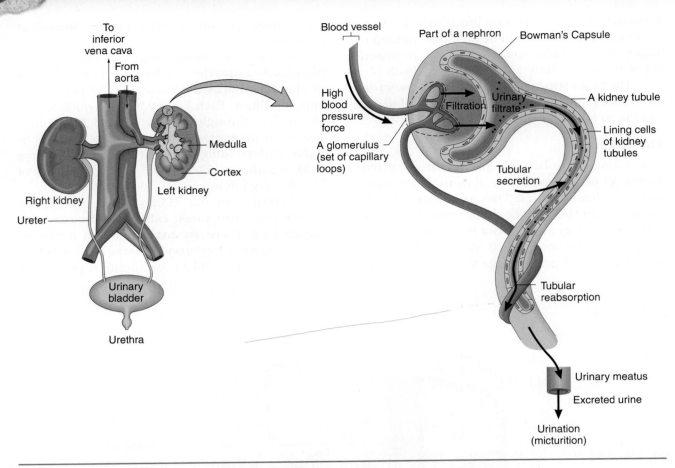

Figure 13-2   *The nephron and the process of urine formation.*

Source: Delmar/Cengage Learning

you could unravel these tubes and lay them in a line, the line would stretch for 75 miles!

Filtration of the blood occurs in the Bowman's capsule area of the nephron. The **filtrate** (i.e., the plasma that has been filtered) contains water; metabolic wastes; glucose; ions such as sodium, potassium, calcium, and bicarbonate; and a variety of other materials essential to life. Much of this fluid, including the essential materials, is selectively *reabsorbed* (taken back into the bloodstream) by the kidneys for further use by the body. As you can see in Figure 13-2, the materials that need to be kept in the body are reabsorbed (tubular reabsorption) back into the circulating blood vessels.

The materials that remain in the tubular system are eventually secreted within the urine. Normally, about 1 milliliter of urine is produced every minute, for a total of about 1.5 liters each day. Urine is a liquid solution composed mainly of water (approximately 95%) and other substances such as nitrogenous wastes (**urea**) and inorganic salts. The color of urine can vary from clear to

deep amber. The color depends on the amount of liquid consumed and the amount of urine created by the kidneys. Clear urine or urine the color of lemon juice is desirable; this is why it is important to stay well hydrated.

The blood flow to the kidneys determines how much urine is produced. Blood flow to the kidneys can be affected by a variety of things such as heart disease, variations in blood pressure, drugs, and fluid and salt intake.

By varying the amount of urine created, the kidneys provide the correct fluid balance for the body. This is important because the body is continually gaining and losing water. For instance, the average adult male consumes 2,500 milliliters of water daily by way of drinking and eating foods that contain water. Furthermore, the cells in the body create approximately 300 milliliters of water daily as a result of cellular metabolism. Counteracting this is the loss of water by the body when we perspire, which happens in cool as well as in hot weather. Even breathing allows water to escape—when we exhale. To illustrate this point, watch your breath when you exhale outside in cold weather and notice the cloud of water vapor. The kidneys, indeed, have to maintain a balancing act between water coming in and going out of the body!

Not only do the kidneys control fluid balance in the body, they also regulate the acid-base balance, thus ensuring correct pH for proper body functioning. The kidneys control acid-base balance by secreting varying amounts of hydrogen ions and ammonia. This occurs during the final phase of urine formation in the kidneys.

It is interesting to note that despite all the work your kidneys do, they do not work at full capacity. In fact, under normal conditions, you can survive quite well with only one kidney.

The Ureters

After urine is formed by the kidneys, it is transported to the urinary bladder through narrow, 10- to 12-inch-long tubes called ureters. Each kidney has one ureter to perform this function.

The Urinary Bladder

The urinary bladder can be considered the holding tank for urine. The urinary bladder is a hollow organ with elastic fibers and involuntary muscles. It can hold approximately 500 milliliters of urine. Emptying the bladder (called **voiding**) occurs as a result of muscular contraction. Although the urinary bladder contains involuntary muscles, the nervous system can control muscular contraction to a degree to cause emptying.

The Urethra

Urine from the bladder travels through a sphincter, which controls urine flow to the urethra. The urethra is a hollow tube that transports urine to the outside of the body. The female urethra is 1 to 1.5 inches long, while the male urethra is approximately 8 inches long. The male urethra serves the dual purposes of urine elimination and **semen** delivery. See Figure 13-3 that shows the ureters, urinary bladder, and urethra.

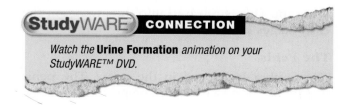

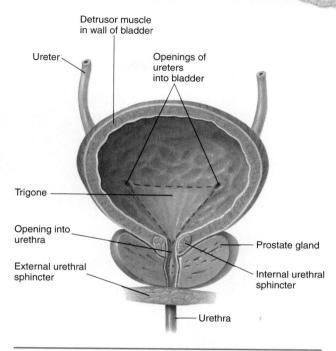

Figure 13-3 *The ureters, urinary bladder, and urethra.*

Source: Delmar/Cengage Learning

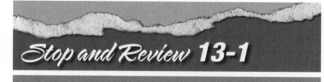

Stop and Review 13-1

a. Describe the process of urine formation.

b. Describe the structure and function of the urinary bladder.

The Reproductive Systems

Regardless of the level of development, all living organisms must reproduce in order to carry on their species; reproduction, therefore, is one of the most fundamental functions of all living organisms.

Reproductive Structures of the Male

The reproductive organs of the male are the **testes** (also known as **testicles**), the **seminal vesicles**, and the **penis** (see Figure 13-4).

The Testes

The testicles are enclosed in a sac-like structure called the **scrotum**. Testicles manufacture **sperm** (or **spermatozoa**), which is the male sex

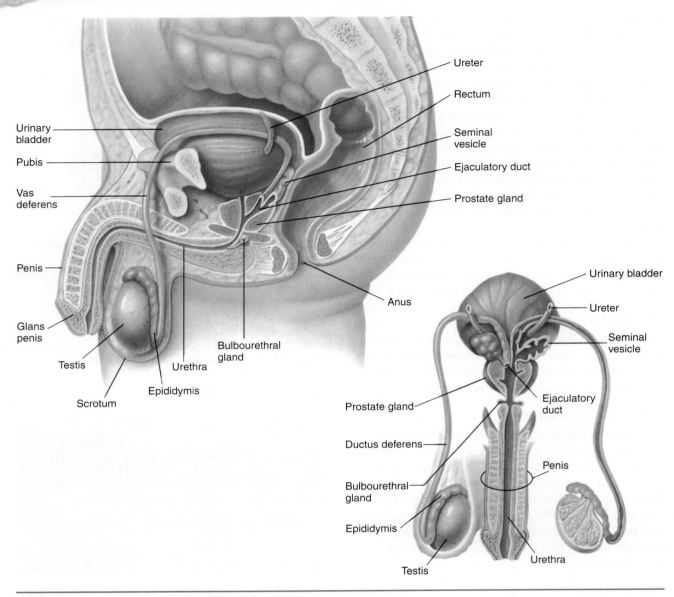

Figure 13-4 *The male reproductive system.*

Source: Delmar/Cengage Learning

cell. It is interesting to note that the reproductive organs of the male are all located outside the body. This is because sperm are very sensitive to heat and can be killed by body temperature.

After sperm are manufactured, they are transported through a narrow tube called the **vas deferens**. This tube travels up into the pelvic region, around the urinary bladder, and back down to join with the urethra.

Seminal Vesicles and Prostate Gland

Glands called seminal vesicles join with the final portion of the vas deferens to form the **ejaculatory duct**. These glands produce a thick, yellowish secretion that provides nourishment for the sperm. Before reaching the urethra, the ejaculatory duct passes through the **prostate gland**. The purpose of this gland is to provide additional fluid to aid in the movement of sperm (known as **motility**).

Bulbourethral, or **Cowper's**, **glands** produce a thick, mucous secretion that acts as a lubricant. This is released into the urethra in the early stages of sexual arousal.

The Penis

The urethra is housed in the penis. The penis is a highly perfused organ composed of erectile

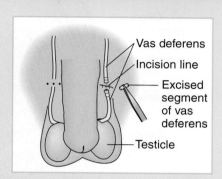

Clinical Relevancy

Male Sterilization

Without sperm reaching the female sex cell (egg), pregnancy cannot occur. One way of preventing pregnancy is through the surgical procedure called a vasectomy. The vas deferens are the transport tubes for sperm. By removing a segment from both vas deferens, the flow of sperm will then be prohibited from leaving the body. See Figure 13-5 for an illustration of this procedure.

Figure 13-5 *The vasectomy procedure.*
Source: Delmar/Cengage Learning

tissue. During arousal, the penis fills with blood and becomes erect.

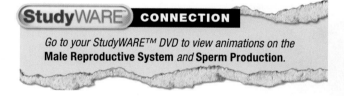

Go to your StudyWARE™ DVD to view animations on the **Male Reproductive System** *and* **Sperm Production.**

Reproductive Structures of the Female

The internal female reproductive organs are the **ovaries**, the **fallopian tubes**, the **uterus**, and the **vagina**. The external female reproductive organs (*genitalia*) are the **labia majora**, the **labia minora**, the **clitoris**, and the **Bartholin's glands**. See Figure 13-6 for a view of the internal and external structures of the female reproductive system.

The Ovaries

The ovaries are the primary female reproductive organs. They are almond-shaped structures approximately 4 to 5 centimeters in length located in the lower abdomen, one on either side of the uterus. The ovaries produce the hormones **estrogen** (which gives women their sexual characteristics, such as breasts and body contour) and **progesterone** (which is involved in preparing the uterus for pregnancy). Within each ovary are thousands of tiny sacs called **graafian follicles**, each of which contains one ovum (plural, ova), or egg.

The Fallopian Tubes

The fallopian tubes rise from the upper portion of the uterus. These structures come close, but do not attach, to the ovaries. The fallopian tubes serve two purposes. First, they provide passageways for ova to travel from the ovaries to the uterus. Second, they allow sperm to fertilize the ovum. The sperm and ovum meet in the fallopian tube; thus, **fertilization** actually occurs within the fallopian tubes. Once the ovum is fertilized, it then enters the uterus where it may implant for further development.

The Uterus

The uterus is the organ where the fertilized egg grows and develops into a **fetus**. Also known as the **womb**, the uterus is normally about 3 inches long, 2 inches wide, and 1 inch thick. During pregnancy, however, it will increase in size as the fetus grows. The shape of the uterus is somewhat like that of an upside down, slightly flattened pear.

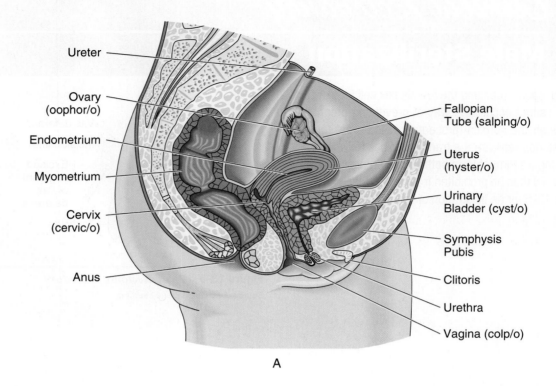

Ureter

Ovary
(oophor/o)

Endometrium

Myometrium

Cervix
(cervic/o)

Anus

Fallopian
Tube (salping/o)

Uterus
(hyster/o)

Urinary
Bladder (cyst/o)

Symphysis
Pubis

Clitoris

Urethra

Vagina (colp/o)

A

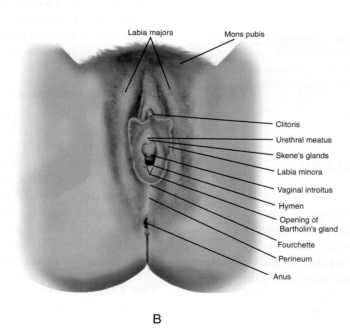

Labia majora   Mons pubis

Clitoris

Urethral meatus

Skene's glands

Labia minora

Vaginal introitus

Hymen

Opening of
Bartholin's gland

Fourchette

Perineum

Anus

B

Figure 13-6   *(A) Internal structures of the female reproductive system. (B) External structures of the female reproductive system.*

Source: Delmar/Cengage Learning

The Vagina

The vagina is the opening from the uterus to the outside of the body. It is composed of smooth muscle and contains a mucous membrane lining. The muscles of the vagina can contract and expand to allow for both insertion of the penis during intercourse and passage of the child during birth.

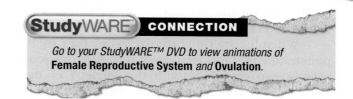
QUOTES & NOTES

The breath of a newborn can smell like garlic! This happens when the garlic digested by the mother travels through her blood to the placenta and into the baby's system!

The Labia Majora and the Labia Minora

The labia majora and the labia minora are fleshy folds of skin that protect the opening of the external female genitalia.

The Clitoris

The clitoris is a highly sensitive organ composed of erectile tissue similar to that of the male penis. It does not, however, contain the urethra. The female urethra has its own orifice, located posteriorly to the clitoris.

Bartholin's Glands

The Bartholin's glands are located on either side of the external opening to the vagina. These glands produce mucus secretions, which serve to lubricate the vagina.

Reproduction

Under normal conditions, one ovum in the female matures each month. The mature ovum is released by the ovary and travels to the fallopian tube. The journey through the fallopian tube takes approximately 5 days.

During sexual intercourse, sperm is deposited by the male into the female's vagina. Sperm will remain viable in the female's reproductive tract for only 1 to 2 days. They can, however, remain there for up to 2 weeks before degenerating. The sperm (which possess a shape similar to that of a tadpole) then begin swimming toward the ovum in the fallopian tube. See Figure 13-7 which shows the route of sperm and ovum, and the structures of the sperm cell.

Because they are subject to a number of hostile conditions, including secretion acidity in the vagina and high temperatures in the female's abdomen, an extremely large number of sperm are released by the male during **ejaculation**. There are approximately 100 million spermatozoa in every milliliter of seminal

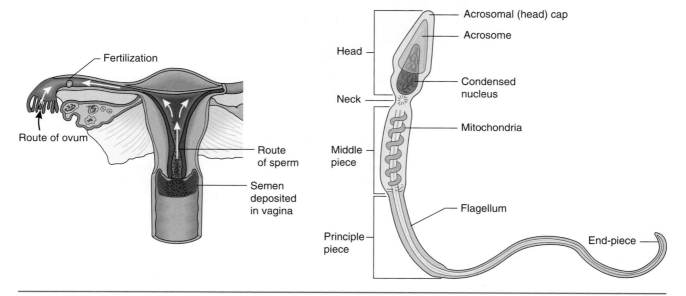

Figure 13-7 *The routes of sperm and ovum, and structures of the sperm cell.*
Source: Delmar/Cengage Learning

fluid, and, on the average, 2 to 4 milliliters of ejaculate is delivered by the male.

When the sperm reach the ovum, they try to penetrate and, thus, fertilize it. When the nucleus of a sperm combines with the nucleus of the ovum, fertilization occurs. The fertilized egg is then referred to as a **zygote**. If fertilization does not occur, the ovum dies and is eliminated during menstruation.

The zygote travels to the uterus, where it embeds in the lining of the uterus. At this point and for the next three months, the zygote is considered an **embryo**. After three months, this unborn, continually growing organism is called a *fetus*. Within approximately 40 weeks, a fertilized egg fully develops into a child. See Figure 13-8 which shows the development of a fetus and the stages of delivery of an infant.

Prenatal Developmental Sequence

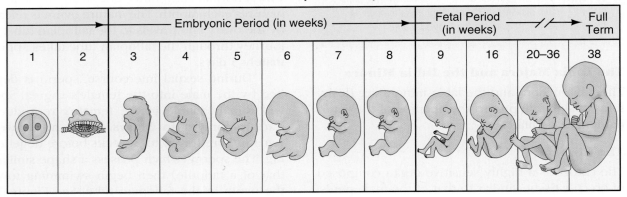

Figure 13-8   *(A) The development of a fetus. (B) The stages of delivery of an infant.*

Source: Delmar/Cengage Learning

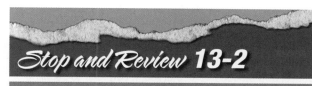

Stop and Review 13-2

a. Describe the surgical procedure performed on males to prevent pregnancy.

b. What is the purpose of Cowper's and Bartholin's glands?

c. List and describe the function of the structure in the female reproductive system.

QUOTES & NOTES

*H*ow big is a newborn baby?

A full-term baby (i.e., one that is carried the whole nine months) is usually approximately 20 inches in length and between 6 and 9 pounds in weight.

StudyWARE™ CONNECTION

Go to your StudyWARE™ DVD to view a video on an **Infant Examination**.

Clinical Relevancy

Disorders of the Genitourinary System

Following are descriptions of some of the diseases of the genitourinary system that you may encounter during your health care career.

Acute kidney failure is a condition wherein there is either a decrease in urine production (known as **oliguria**) or no urine production (**anuria**). This condition can be caused by heart disease, shock, poison, bleeding, and injury. If not reversed, toxins can remain in the blood and build up to life-threatening levels. **Chronic renal failure** occurs when there is a loss of nephron function over a period of time.

Nephrolithiasis (also known as kidney stones, or **calculi**) occurs when salts that normally dissolve in urine become solidified. As these stones increase in size, they may block passageways in the urinary system, thus causing a backup of urine. If they cannot be dissolved or dislodged, surgical removal of calculi may be necessary. Ultrasonic waves may be used in a noninvasive attempt to pulverize the stones so that they can be passed easier during urination.

Incontinence is a condition wherein an individual loses voluntary control over the ability to urinate. This is common in children who have not yet been toilet trained and in those individuals who have lost bladder control as a result of strokes or spinal cord injuries.

Pelvic inflammatory disease (PID) is a general term used to describe any inflammation of the female reproductive system. Pelvic inflammatory disease can result directly from an infection of the female reproductive organs that spreads through the fallopian tubes and the peritoneal cavity or can be secondary to a primary infection such as gonorrhea. If left untreated, PID can lead to infertility and even death.

Prostate cancer is the most common cancer among males age 50 and older. This disease causes enlargement of the prostate gland. Surgical removal of the cancerous growth is done though the penis and requires no incision in the abdomen.

Sexually transmitted disease (STD) is a general term used to describe a disease transmitted usually as a result of unsafe sex (i.e., not using or improperly using a condom). Sexually transmitted diseases include but are not limited to the bacterial diseases of gonorrhea, syphilis, and chlamydia (the latter of which is one of the most rapidly spreading STDs in the United States) and the viral infection called genital herpes (i.e., herpes simplex II). At this time, there is no known cure for herpes simplex II. Human immunodeficiency virus/acquired immune deficiency syndrome (HIV/AIDS) is another disease that can be sexually transmitted and for which there is currently no known cure.

Two common conditions are **benign prostatic hypertrophy (BPH)** in the male and **endometriosis** in the female. BPH is a slow-growing enlargement of the prostate gland found commonly in males over 50 years of age. As the prostate swells in size, it narrows the urethra, decreasing the flow of urine. As a result, the flow is lessened and the individual urinates more frequently

(continues)

(continued)

throughout the day and night. Endometrial tissue is the tissue that proliferates and sloughs off every menstrual cycle (period). Endometriosis occurs in females when endometrial tissue escapes the uterus and implants itself in the abdominal and/or pelvic cavities instead of normally being discharged monthly from the body. Herein lies the problem; because the newly implanted tissue proliferates, decays, and bleeds in these areas, it can lead to scarring and potential damage to the organs in these areas. See Figure 13-9 which shows BPH and endometriosis.

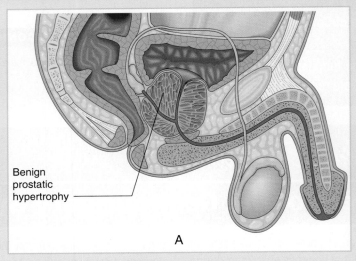

Benign prostatic hypertrophy

A

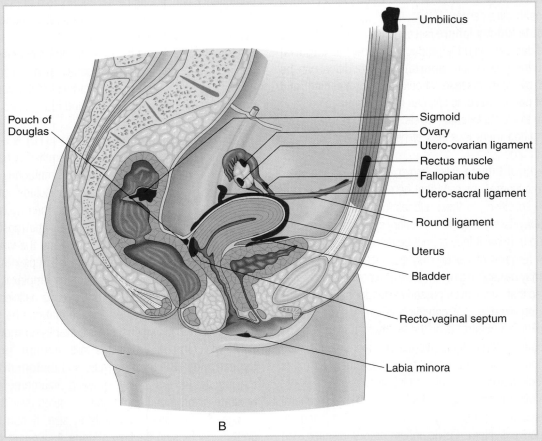

Umbilicus

Pouch of Douglas

Sigmoid
Ovary
Utero-ovarian ligament
Rectus muscle
Fallopian tube
Utero-sacral ligament

Round ligament

Uterus

Bladder

Recto-vaginal septum

Labia minora

B

Figure 13-9   *(A) Benign prostatic hypertrophy (BPH). (B) Endometriosis. Dark red areas represent implantation.*

Source: Delmar/Cengage Learning

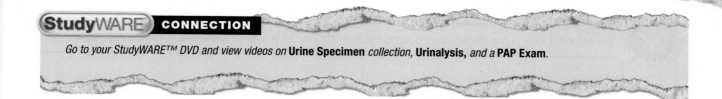

StudyWARE™ CONNECTION

Go to your StudyWARE™ DVD and view videos on **Urine Specimen** *collection,* **Urinalysis,** *and a* **PAP Exam.**

■ CHAPTER REVIEW

Exercises

1. List two functions of the kidneys.

2. What organ produces urine, and what rate of urine production per minute is considered normal?

3. What is considered normal daily urine production?

4. What are the narrow tubes that lead from the kidneys to the urinary bladder called?

5. What is the average capacity of the urinary bladder?

6. Name two bacterial STDs.

7. What is the term *voiding* used to describe?

8. List two female hormones and describe their functions.

9. List a male hormone and describe its function.

10. How long will sperm remain viable in the female's reproductive tract?

Real Life Issues and Applications

Fluid Balance

Your patient has been moved to the intensive care unit as a result of the following signs and symptoms:

- profound peripheral edema
- concentrated urine
- fluid intake of 2,000 mL/day
- fluid output of 50 mL/day
- coarse crackles in the base of each lung

What do you predict the diagnosis to be? How would you treat this patient?

Additional Activities

1. In this chapter you learned that you can live with only one kidney. Discuss in class the concept of selling extra organs for use in transplants instead of donating them upon death. What could be some of the ethical and legal implications of such an activity?

2. Discuss how you would battle the growing national incidence of STDs.

Downloadable audio is available for selected medical terms in this chapter to enhance your learning of medical language.

StudyWARE **CONNECTION**

Go to your StudyWARE™ DVD and have fun learning as you play interactive games, view animations and videos, and take practice tests to help reinforce key concepts you learned in this chapter.

Workbook Practice　　*Go to your Workbook for more practice questions and activities.*

SECTION TWO

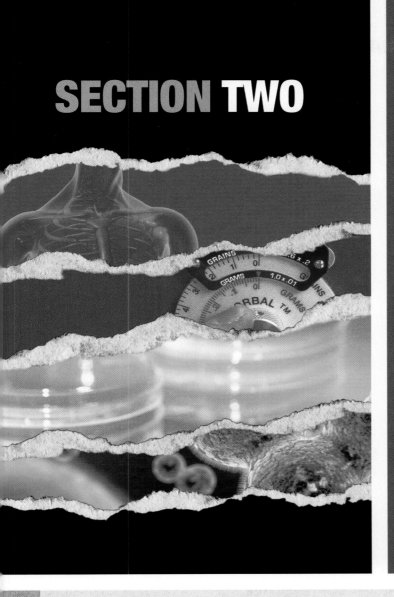

Fundamentals of Mathematics

SECTION OVERVIEW

You may wonder why there is a math section in a textbook about health sciences. That is because math is used extensively to solve problems and equations in the various health professions. Thus, a thorough understanding of mathematics will be required as you pursue your chosen health field. In addition, this section will help prepare you for the upcoming Chemistry section where math will be applied to understand concepts and principles.

This section will apply math to clinical anatomy and physiology concepts you have already learned such as solving for physiologic variables like cardiac output, stroke volume, and mean arterial pressure. Math is also needed in everyday life to perform such mundane yet important functions as balancing your checkbook, planning a budget, cooking, and determining sale prices, taxes, and, of course, batting averages. So batter up!

CHAPTER 14

BASIC MATHEMATICAL DEFINITIONS AND FRACTIONS

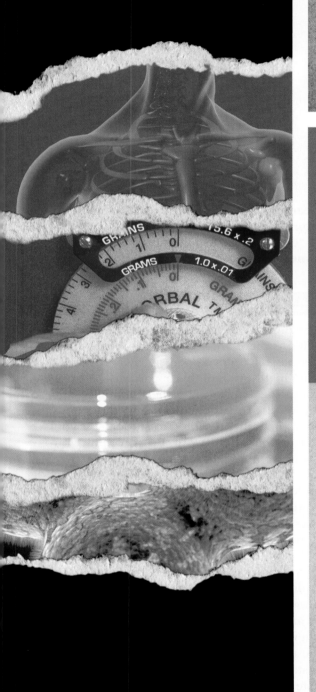

Objectives

Upon completion of this chapter, you should be able to

- Relate mathematics to everyday activities in the health sciences and state the importance of a thorough understanding of mathematics to a successful career in the health professions

- Define basic numerical terms and types of numbers

- Define and perform various operations with fractional numbers

Key Terms

common denominator

common fraction

denominator

gram (g)

improper fraction

least, or lowest, common
    denominator (LCD)

liter (L)

meter (m)

metric system

mixed numbers

numerator

ophthalmometer (off-thal-
    MOM-et-er)

proper fractions

reciprocal

respirometer (res-per-**OM**-et-er)

thermometer

DEFINING FRACTIONS THROUGH PERSONALITY TRAITS

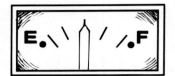

An optimist would
say this gas tank
is 1/2 full.

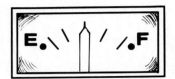

A pessimist would
say the gas tank
is 1/2 empty.

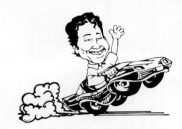

A teenager would just
get in and drive!

Source: Delmar/Cengage Learning

■ INTRODUCTION

What is mathematics? You may think of mathematics as a tool used to solve problems; and this is partially correct. It is true that one of the purposes of mathematics is in classroom problem solving. But mathematics is more than just a tool used in school. The average individual uses mathematics for a variety of everyday purposes including balancing a checkbook, estimating a dinner bill before the waitress brings the check (unless you like to do dishes), and calculating a batting average. Percentages and decimals are used in calculations from taxes to tips. Fractions are used in everything from cooking to building houses.

Mathematics is used daily in the health field, as well. For example, the ability to correctly calculate the dosage of a drug for a patient may mean the difference between life and death. The vital signs of blood pressure, pulse, temperature, and respiration all relate in some way to mathematics. Many measurements taken in the health professions require mathematical calculations. For example, by measuring the amount of air a patient is breathing over a period of time, you can determine whether the patient needs to be placed on a breathing machine (commonly called a *ventilator*). Many medical instruments are used to measure patient parameters and, thus, require the user to understand some mathematics. For example, the **thermometer** (*thermos* meaning "temperature,"

meter meaning "to measure") is used to measure temperature; the **ophthalmometer** (*ophthalmus* meaning "eyes") is used to measure eyes; and the **respirometer** is used to measure breathing.

Basic Definitions

Before beginning with some basic mathematical definitions, here are some words to the wise. Many people have developed a "mental block" concerning math. We feel this is partially because of the language barrier (i.e., the unfamiliar terminology used in mathematics), and the sterile way math is initially presented to students. If you develop a phobia about math, do you think you can do well in the other sciences that require math? What about life in general? Balancing checkbooks, maintaining family budgets, and making sure you're not being overcharged for bills or services are some real-life uses of math.

Try not to view math as an obstacle to "get through" but, rather, as a much-needed friend that will help you in both school and "real life." How can you do this? The first step is to understand and acknowledge how important math is to your personal and professional lives. The second step is to believe in your ability to solve math problems. The third and final step is to take the time to understand math. We can help you only with the last step; you must take the first two steps on your own.

The mathematics section, like all the individual science sections, contains *Stop and Review* features. These are included to check your understanding of each concept being presented. Because many concepts build on each other, it is important to ensure that you understand each step along the way.

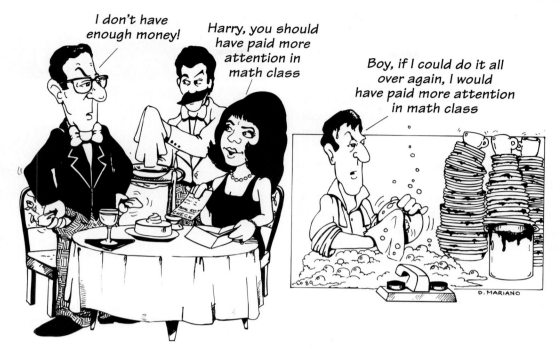

Source: Delmar/Cengage Learning

Basic Units of Measurement

Several systems are used for measuring. The one we commonly use in the United States is the *English system*. In the English system, distance is measured in inches, feet, yards, and miles; weight is measured in ounces, pounds, and tons; and volume is measured in pints, quarts, and gallons. Although this system of measurement may be the one with which you are most familiar, it is not the system of choice used throughout the world and within the health professions. The reason is that the English system is very cumbersome to use because it has no common conversions within the system. There are 12 inches in a foot, 3 feet or 36 inches in a yard, and 63,360 inches or 5,280 feet in a mile.

Most scientific and medical measurements utilize what is commonly referred to as the **metric system**. Although more than one system has been developed wherein metric units are used, the system accepted as "the" metric system is the International System of Units.

As illustrated in Table 14-1, the metric system uses only three basic units of measure: the **meter (m)** for length, the **liter (L)** for volume, and the **gram (g)** for weight. The metric system has only one basic unit of measure for each type of measurement. Compare this to the English system, which has many units of measure for distance, volume, and weight. In our English system, for example, with the unit of measure of distance,

TABLE 14-1 Basic Units of Measurement in the Metric System		
TYPE	**UNIT**	**APPROXIMATE ENGLISH SYSTEM EQUIVALENT**
Distance (length)	meter	39 inches
Volume	liter	1 quart
Weight (mass)	gram	$\frac{1}{40}$ ounce

we have inches, feet, yards, and miles, versus the single unit of a meter in the metric system.

In the metric system, the prefixes are used to indicate the different lengths, volumes, and weights. The conversion is the same for each type of measurement. There are 1,000 meters in a kilometer, 1,000 grams in a kilogram, and 1,000 liters in a kiloliter. Further discussion on the metric system will be forthcoming in Chapter 16. For now, just be aware that a milliliter (mL) is a unit of volume, a centimeter (cm) a unit of length, and a kilogram (kg) a unit of weight.

Many times in health care we are dealing with parts of a whole. For example, we may have a large bottle of medicine but the dosage requires only a portion or *fraction* of the bottle to be given. When assessing the severity and extent of burns on a patient, we use percentages of damaged tissue to determine treatment. Therefore, this chapter will begin with a discussion of fractions, and Chapter 15 will carry it further with decimals and percentages.

Fractions

A **common fraction** is a comparison of two numbers. Fractions usually are written $\frac{a}{b}$, where a is called the **numerator** and b the **denominator**. The denominator, or bottom number, tells how many total parts it takes to make the whole. The numerator, or top number, is the actual number of parts of a whole being considered.

Remember that a fraction is a comparison of a part (or parts) to a whole. Consider, for example, the circle in Figure 14-1, which is separated into 10 sections, 3 of which are removed. In the fraction "three-tenths," the numerator (3) tells how many equal parts are represented, while the denominator (10) tells into how many parts the whole is divided.

> **QUOTES & NOTES**
>
> **F**ractions have been used for more than 3,600 years. They appear in an Egyptian handbook of mathematics called the *Rhind papyrus*, written around the year 1650 B.C.

Example:

If 17 pills have been used from a bottle originally containing 50, then $\frac{17}{50}$ of the bottle have been used. We can also look at this in a different way: 33 pills out of the 50 are left, or $\frac{33}{50}$.

Simplifying Fractions to Lowest Terms

Being able to simplify a fraction to the lowest equivalent fraction (i.e., to the lowest terms) is extremely important. In *Stop and Review 14-1b*,

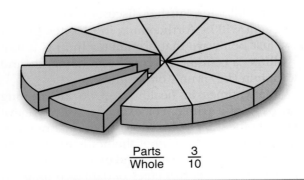

$$\frac{\text{Parts}}{\text{Whole}} \quad \frac{3}{10}$$

Figure 14-1   *A fraction is a comparison of parts (numerator) to a whole (denominator).*

Source: Delmar/Cengage Learning

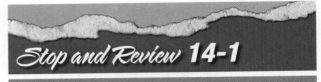

Stop and Review 14-1

a. If 13 pills remain in a bottle originally containing 40 pills, what fraction would apply?

b. If you gave a patient 20 mL of a 100-mL bolus (a concentrated amount of a drug) of Lidocaine, what fraction of the drug have you given to the patient? What fraction of the drug is left?

the fractions $\frac{20}{100}$ and $\frac{80}{100}$ can be simplified to $\frac{1}{5}$ and $\frac{4}{5}$, respectively. But what process is used to simplify fractions?

A most fundamental rule of fractions states that the numerator (the top number) and the denominator (the bottom number) can be divided or multiplied by the same nonzero number without changing the value of the fraction. More simply put, if the top and bottom numbers of a fraction are multiplied or divided by the same number, it's still the same fraction—only now in another form.

The technique of dividing the numerator and denominator of a fraction is used to simplify the fraction. Lowest terms have the smallest possible denominator. When simplifying fractions to lowest terms, it is therefore important to first find the largest number that will divide equally into both the numerator and the denominator.

Example:

$$\frac{6}{8} = \frac{6 \div 2}{8 \div 2} = \frac{3}{4}$$
$$\frac{6}{9} = \frac{6 \div 3}{9 \div 3} = \frac{2}{3}$$

Fractions can be simplified by "mentally" dividing the numerator and denominator by the same number. This is sometimes referred to as *canceling*.

Example:

$$\frac{\cancel{6}^{3}}{\cancel{8}_{4}} = \frac{3}{4} \qquad\qquad \frac{\cancel{6}^{2}}{\cancel{9}_{3}} = \frac{2}{3}$$

Mentally divide the numerator and denominator by 2

Mentally divide the numerator and denominator by 3

In the preceding example, the numbers 2 and 3 were chosen because they are the largest numbers that divide evenly into both the numerators and denominators of the respective fractions. Although it is not necessary to divide the numerator and denominator by the largest number, it saves steps to do so. For example, to simplify $\frac{15}{30}$, the numerator and denominator could be divided by 5 to get $\frac{3}{6}$ and then by 2 to get the simplest form, $\frac{1}{2}$. Or $\frac{15}{30}$ could have been simplified by dividing the numerator and denominator by 15 to get the same answer.

Example:

A bottle of medicine contains 400 mL of a liquid. If 150 mL is used as one dose, what fraction of the bottle was used? The fraction $\frac{150}{400}$ simplifies to $\frac{3}{8}$ by dividing both the numerator and denominator by 50. So $\frac{3}{8}$ of the bottle was used.

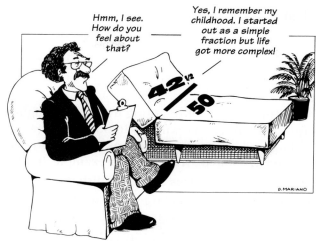

UNRAVELING OF A COMPLEX FRACTION

Source: Delmar/Cengage Learning

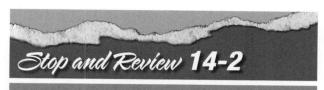

Stop and Review **14-2**

Write each of the following fractions in lowest terms.

a. $\frac{18}{24}$

b. $\frac{16}{28}$

c. A bottle contains 300 mL of liquid. If 200 mL were given to a patient, what fraction does this represent? What fraction remains?

d. A bottle contains 800 tablets. The pharmacist asks that 350 tablets be sent to the nurses' station. What fraction of the bottle was sent?

Rewriting Fractions to Higher Terms

Fractions can also be rewritten to higher terms. This often must be done in order to add or subtract fractions, which must have the same denominator before the addition or subtraction can be done. Although this means that the numbers in the fractions will be higher, the fractions themselves will be of the same value. In other words,

equivalent fractions can be produced by rewriting two fractions so that they have higher numbers in the numerator and denominator. This is done by simply multiplying the numerator and denominator by the same number.

Example:

$$\frac{3}{4} = \frac{?}{20}$$

Multiply both the numerator and denominator by 5.

$$= \frac{3 \times 5}{4 \times 5} \qquad = \frac{7 \times 6}{8 \times 6}$$

denominator by 6.

In the previous example, the first decision that had to be made was to decide what number you should use to multiply the numerator and denominator of the fractions. In the first example, the 4 would need to be multiplied by 5 to get the new denominator of 20, and therefore the numerator and denominator were multiplied by 5.

An alternate solution is to divide the original denominator into the new denominator plus multiply the numerator by the result.

Example:

$$\frac{3}{4} = \frac{?}{20}$$

Think $20 \div 4 = 5$

$$\frac{3}{4} = \frac{?}{20}$$

Then $5 \times 3 = 15$

$$\frac{3}{4} \searrow \frac{?}{20}$$

$$\frac{3}{4} = \frac{15}{20}$$

This process of rewriting fractions to higher equivalent fractions will be important later for adding and subtracting fractions, but it also can be used to compare fractions. For example, instruments of various sizes might be listed as $\frac{4}{5}$, $\frac{7}{10}$, and $\frac{11}{15}$. List them from largest to smallest.

Since $\frac{4}{5} = \frac{24}{30}$, $\frac{7}{10} = \frac{21}{30}$ and $\frac{11}{15} = \frac{22}{30}$, then from largest to smallest they are: $\frac{4}{5}$, $\frac{11}{15}$, and then $\frac{7}{10}$.

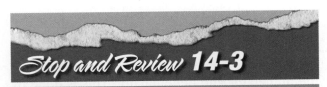

Stop and Review 14-3

a. Rewrite each of the following fractions:

$$\frac{4}{5} = \frac{?}{15} \qquad \frac{5}{6} = \frac{?}{36} \qquad \frac{7}{8} = \frac{?}{32}$$

b. A patient has a bottle of medication that originally contained 80 pills. If $\frac{1}{4}$ of the pills has been used, how many pills have been taken?

Improper Fractions

So far, we have focused on fractions where the numerator is less than the denominator; these are called **proper fractions**. (To remember this, think of things that are proper as things that are the way we expect them to be.) But what about the fraction $\frac{3}{2}$? This fraction may seem unusual because the top number is larger than the bottom number. When the numerator in a fraction is as large as, or larger than, the denominator, the fraction is known as an **improper fraction**.

For example, if you bought 3 half-gallon containers of milk, this could be written as $\frac{3}{2}$ gallons. But this is the same as $1\frac{1}{2}$ gallons. Notice that $\frac{3}{2}$ is an improper fraction, whereas its equivalent $1\frac{1}{2}$ has both a whole number and a proper fraction. Numbers that contain both whole numbers and fractions, such as $1\frac{1}{2}$, are called **mixed numbers**.

To change an improper fraction into a whole number or mixed number, simply divide the denominator into the numerator.

Example:

$\frac{3}{2}$ is the same as
$$2\overline{\smash{\big)}3} \quad \begin{array}{c} 1\frac{1}{2} \\ \underline{2} \\ 1 \end{array}$$

As shown in the preceding example, the fractional portion of the answer is derived by placing the *remainder* (1) over the denominator (2).

Example:

$$\frac{7}{3} = 3\overline{\smash{\big)}7} \quad \begin{array}{c} 2\frac{1}{3} \\ \underline{6} \\ 1 \end{array}$$

$$\frac{17}{5} = 5\overline{\smash{\big)}17} \quad \begin{array}{c} 3\frac{2}{5} \\ \underline{15} \\ 2 \end{array}$$

$$\frac{12}{3} = 3\overline{\smash{\big)}12} \quad \begin{array}{c} 4 \\ \underline{12} \\ 0 \end{array}$$

$$\frac{10}{4} = 4\overline{\smash{\big)}10} \quad \begin{array}{c} 2\frac{2}{4} \\ \underline{8} \\ 2 \end{array}$$

In the last part of the preceding example, remember to simplify $\frac{2}{4}$ to $\frac{1}{2}$ so that $2\frac{2}{4} = 2\frac{1}{2}$.

Changing Mixed Numbers to Improper Fractions

The mixed number $1\frac{1}{2}$ can be changed to the improper fraction $\frac{3}{2}$. To change a mixed number to an improper fraction, determine the total number of parts in the whole number. Next, add the number of parts represented by the fraction.

Example:

$$2\frac{5}{8} = \frac{?}{8}$$
$$2 = \frac{16}{8}, \text{ then } \frac{16}{8} \text{ and } \frac{5}{8} \text{ totals } \frac{21}{8}$$

Clinical Relevancy

Fractions as They Relate to Determining Drug Effectiveness

In determining how effective a drug is in treating a patient, certain drug tests or trials are performed. One such test determines the Therapeutic Index (TI) of a particular medication. This tells how effective (therapeutic) the drug is in relationship to how toxic (poisonous) it can be. The formula for determining the TI of a particular drug is $TI = LD_{50}/ED_{50}$. The LD_{50} represents the lethal dose required to kill 50% of an animal population, while the ED_{50} represents the dose needed to be therapeutically effective in 50% of the tested animal population. The TI is the comparison of the lethal dose to the effective dose, and a desirable TI is an improper fraction. The reason for this is if the $TI = 1$, the same amount of drug needed to cure a patient would also kill the patient. Therefore, the lower the TI, the more dangerous the drug.

For example, a drug that has an LD_{50} of 8 grams and an ED_{50} of 2 grams would yield a TI of $\frac{8}{2}$. This improper fraction simplifies to 4. Another drug may have an LD_{50} of 200 grams and an ED_{50} of 2 grams. The TI for this drug would be $\frac{200}{2}$, or 100. Which drug is safer to administer? Because the lower the TI, the more dangerous the drug, the answer to this question is the second drug.

Unless a patient is allergic to it, penicillin, with a TI of 100, is a relatively safe drug to administer, because the lethal dose is 100 times the amount needed to effectively treat the patient. Digitalis, on the other hand, must be used more cautiously because it has a TI of 2. A patient taking digitalis, therefore, must be monitored carefully and have blood levels drawn frequently to prevent toxicity. Toxicity can lead to headaches, nausea, heart irregularities, coma, and eventually death.

Stop and Review 14-4

Write each of the following fractions as a mixed or whole number.

a. $\frac{12}{7}$

b. $\frac{15}{3}$

c. $\frac{19}{6}$

Write each of the following fractions as a mixed number and simplify.

d. $\frac{15}{6}$

e. $\frac{24}{16}$

f. A health care professional was asked to administer 500 units of a medication. However, all that is in stock are bottles containing 150 units. To determine how many bottles must be administered, find $\frac{500}{150}$. Express the answer as a mixed number, in simplest form.

Many times you can take shortcuts in math to make performing the problems easier. Here is one that will help in changing mixed numbers to improper fractions. To find the new numerator, mentally multiply the denominator by the whole number; then add the result to the numerator. For example, to change the mixed number $2\frac{5}{8}$ to an improper fraction, first multiply 2×8; this gives you 16. Next, add $16 + 5$ (the numerator in the fraction of the mixed number); this gives you the new numerator, or 21. Finally, write the new numerator over the denominator; this gives you the improper fraction of $\frac{21}{8}$.

Example:

$$7\frac{2}{3} \ (3 \times 7 = 21) = \frac{21 + 2}{3} = \frac{23}{3}$$

$$4\frac{5}{6} \ (4 \times 6 = 24) = \frac{24 + 5}{6} = \frac{29}{6}$$

Mathematical Operations on Fractions

Throughout this text, you will see the importance of a thorough understanding of fractions in the health care field, especially addition, subtraction, multiplication, and division.

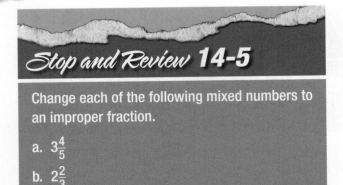

Stop and Review 14-5

Change each of the following mixed numbers to an improper fraction.

a. $3\frac{4}{5}$

b. $2\frac{2}{3}$

c. $6\frac{1}{4}$

Adding and Subtracting Fractions

To add fractions having the same denominator, write the sum of the numerators and keep the same denominator. Be sure to simplify and write the fraction in lowest terms, as necessary.

Example:

$$\frac{2}{5} + \frac{1}{5} = \frac{2+1}{5} = \frac{3}{5}$$

Note: Be careful—*DO NOT* add the denominators.

To subtract fractions having the same denominator, write the difference between the numerators and keep the same denominator. Again, remember to simplify if necessary.

Example:

$$\frac{5}{6} - \frac{1}{6} = \frac{4}{6} = \frac{2}{3}$$

$$\frac{7}{15} + \frac{8}{15} = \frac{15}{15} = 1$$

To add or subtract fractions having different denominators, you first need to rewrite the fractions

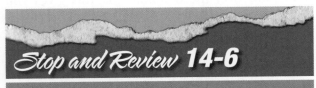

Stop and Review 14-6

Add or subtract each of the following fractions and simplify.

a. $\frac{3}{5} + \frac{3}{5}$

b. $\frac{4}{9} - \frac{1}{9}$

c. $\frac{11}{12} + \frac{5}{12}$

so that they have the same denominator (called a **common denominator**). More specifically, you should rewrite the fractions so that they each have the smallest common denominator (called the **least, or lowest, common denominator [LCD]**); then add or subtract the numerator as noted previously. To do this, you first determine the smallest number into which both denominators will evenly divide. You then rewrite each fraction to a higher equivalent fraction having that denominator. Finally, add the renamed fractions, remembering to simplify, as necessary.

Example:

$$\frac{2}{3} + \frac{1}{7}$$

The smallest number into which both denominators (3 and 7) can evenly divide is 21. So, 21 is the LCD. And since the LCD is 21, multiply the numerator and denominator of the first fraction by 7, and the numerator and denominator of the second fraction by 3, so that each fraction is rewritten to a higher equivalent fraction having a denominator of 21.

$$\frac{2 \times 7}{3 \times 7} + \frac{1 \times 3}{7 \times 3} = \frac{14}{21} + \frac{3}{21}$$

Finally, we have like fractions (i.e., fractions having the same denominator) that can be added together.

$$\frac{14}{21} + \frac{3}{21} = \frac{17}{21}$$

Example:

$$\frac{4}{5} - \frac{3}{10}$$

Note that the second fraction already has the LCD; therefore, there is no need to rewrite this fraction.

$$\frac{4}{5} - \frac{3}{10} = \frac{4 \times 2}{5 \times 2} - \frac{3}{10} = \frac{5}{10} = \frac{1}{2}$$

Multiplying Fractions

To multiply fractions, you don't need to have the same denominator in all of the fractions. Instead, you simply multiply the numerators and multiply the denominators, and rewrite the answer in lowest terms, as necessary.

Example:

$$\frac{4}{5} \times \frac{5}{8} = \frac{20}{40} = \frac{1}{2}$$

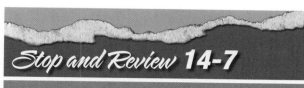

Add or subtract the following fractions and simplify.

a. $\frac{2}{3} + \frac{3}{4}$

b. $\frac{14}{15} - \frac{3}{5}$

c. $\frac{9}{10} - \frac{7}{15}$

d. A bottle is $\frac{4}{5}$ full. One dose calls for $\frac{2}{3}$ of a bottle. How much of the original bottle remains?

e. Three bottles of the same medication have been opened. They are $\frac{3}{4}$, $\frac{7}{8}$, and $\frac{3}{8}$ of their original amounts. If added together, how many bottles would this represent?

Remember: To rewrite (simplify) the answer to the lowest terms, mentally divide the numerator and denominator by the same number, making sure that you choose the largest number that can divide evenly into both numbers.

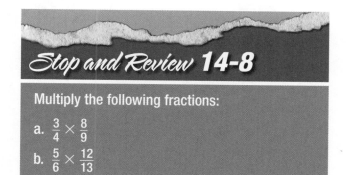

Multiply the following fractions:

a. $\frac{3}{4} \times \frac{8}{9}$

b. $\frac{5}{6} \times \frac{12}{13}$

A common application of multiplication of fractions is to find a fractional part of a whole.

Example:

a. To find four-fifths of 200, multiply $\frac{4}{5} \times 200 = \frac{4}{5} \times \frac{200}{1} = \frac{800}{5} = 160$.

b. If a bottle contains 750 units of liquid, how many units are in two-thirds of the bottle? That is, what is $\frac{2}{3}$ of 750?

$$\frac{2}{3} \times 750 = \frac{2}{3} \times \frac{750}{1} = \frac{1500}{3} = 500$$

This method works just as well for fractional parts of a fraction. For example, if $\frac{1}{6}$ of all emergency room visits to a hospital are related to injuries, and $\frac{2}{3}$ of those were involved in motor vehicle accidents, what fraction of all emergency room visits are due to motor vehicle accidents? That is, find $\frac{1}{6} \times \frac{2}{3} = \frac{1}{9}$. So one-ninth of all emergency room visits are motor vehicle related.

Stop and Review 14-9

a. A patient has a bottle of medication that originally contained 80 pills. If $\frac{1}{4}$ of the pills have been taken, how many pills have been used? How many remain in the bottle?

b. In a nursing class, $\frac{2}{3}$ of the students are women and $\frac{1}{4}$ of those are mothers. What fraction of the entire class are mothers?

Dividing Fractions

Before discussing division of fractions, we must define the term **reciprocal**. Two numbers are reciprocals if their product is 1. For instance, $\frac{2}{3} \times \frac{3}{2} = \frac{6}{6} = 1$; therefore, $\frac{2}{3}$ and $\frac{3}{2}$ are reciprocals. The easiest way to determine a fraction's reciprocal is to invert the fraction (i.e., write it upside down).

To find the reciprocal of a whole number, first write the whole number as a fraction by simply dividing the number by 1. For instance, to rewrite the whole number 6 as a fraction, divide it by 1 to get $\frac{6}{1}$. Then invert the fraction form of the whole number. For instance, the reciprocal of $\frac{6}{1}$ (or 6) is $\frac{1}{6}$.

Example:

$$\frac{3}{4} \times \; ? = 1 \qquad \frac{3}{4} \times \frac{4}{3} = 1$$

and

$$12 \times \; ? = 1 \qquad 12 \times \frac{1}{12} = 1$$

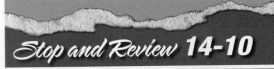

Stop and Review 14-10

Find the reciprocal for each of the following.

a. $\frac{1}{4}$

b. $\frac{7}{8}$

c. 3

Stop and Review 14-11

a. $\frac{2}{3} \div 6$

b. $\frac{3}{4} \div \frac{7}{8}$

c. Suppose you have $\frac{3}{4}$ of a bottle of medication left. If each dose is $\frac{1}{8}$ of a bottle, to find the number of doses remaining in the bottle, find $\frac{3}{4} \div \frac{1}{8}$.

To divide a fraction, simply multiply the fraction by the reciprocal of the second fraction or number.

Example:

$$\frac{5}{6} \div \frac{2}{3} = \frac{5}{6} \times \frac{3}{2} = \frac{15}{12} = \frac{5}{4} = 1\frac{1}{4}$$

$$\frac{4}{5} \div \frac{4}{15} = \frac{4}{5} \times \frac{15}{4} = \frac{60}{20} = \frac{3}{1} = 3$$

An application of division is to find the number of doses remaining in a container. For example, if one dose is 3 mL and 12 mL are available, since $\frac{12}{3} = 4$, there are 4 doses remaining. That is, 4 doses of 3 mL each would equal 12 mL. Similarly with fractions, suppose you have $\frac{1}{2}$ of a bottle of medication left. If each dose is $\frac{1}{16}$ of a bottle, to find the number of doses remaining in the bottle, find $\frac{1}{2} \div \frac{1}{16} = \frac{1}{2} \times \frac{16}{1} = 8$. There are 8 doses remaining. As a check, $8 \times \frac{1}{16} = \frac{1}{2}$. That is, 8 doses that are each $\frac{1}{16}$ of the bottle represent $\frac{1}{2}$ of the bottle.

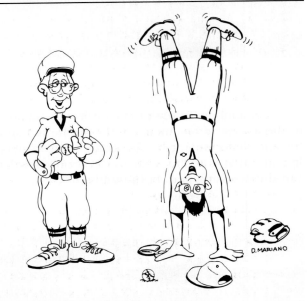

FRED IS A RECIPROCAL TO HIMSELF.

Source: Delmar/Cengage Learning

■ CHAPTER REVIEW

Exercises

1. A person eats 5 donuts out of a box originally containing 12. What fraction of the donuts has been eaten? What fraction remains for the next person?

2. A nurse worked 50 hours in one week. If 10 of those hours were overtime hours, what fraction of the total were overtime hours? What fraction were not overtime hours?

3. Write each of the following fractions in lowest terms.

   a. $\dfrac{10}{30}$ f. $\dfrac{9}{36}$

   b. $\dfrac{15}{20}$ g. $\dfrac{95}{125}$

   c. $\dfrac{6}{14}$ h. $\dfrac{64}{72}$

   d. $\dfrac{36}{54}$ i. $\dfrac{24}{56}$

   e. $\dfrac{48}{120}$ j. $\dfrac{140}{420}$

4. Rewrite each of the following fractions to a higher equivalent fraction.

   a. $\dfrac{3}{4} = \dfrac{}{12}$ f. $\dfrac{9}{16} = \dfrac{}{32}$

   b. $\dfrac{9}{10} = \dfrac{}{40}$ g. $\dfrac{1}{2} = \dfrac{}{360}$

   c. $\dfrac{5}{12} = \dfrac{}{36}$ h. $\dfrac{7}{8} = \dfrac{}{48}$

   d. $\dfrac{5}{9} = \dfrac{}{36}$ i. $\dfrac{7}{9} = \dfrac{}{81}$

   e. $\dfrac{3}{4} = \dfrac{}{16}$ j. $\dfrac{2}{3} = \dfrac{}{312}$

5. Write each of the following fractions as a mixed or whole number; simplify as necessary.

   a. $\dfrac{11}{8}$ f. $\dfrac{16}{5}$

   b. $\dfrac{23}{6}$ g. $\dfrac{14}{2}$

   c. $\dfrac{16}{4}$ h. $\dfrac{78}{6}$

   d. $\dfrac{18}{10}$ i. $\dfrac{84}{8}$

   e. $\dfrac{44}{14}$ j. $\dfrac{92}{6}$

6. Write each of the following mixed numbers as an improper fraction.

   a. $3\dfrac{2}{3}$ f. $9\dfrac{2}{3}$

   b. $6\dfrac{1}{3}$ g. $7\dfrac{1}{4}$

   c. $7\dfrac{1}{2}$ h. $2\dfrac{5}{12}$

   d. $4\dfrac{5}{6}$ i. $3\dfrac{9}{10}$

   e. $3\dfrac{1}{5}$ j. $12\dfrac{4}{5}$

7. A health care professional was asked to administer 500 units of a medication. However, all that is in stock are bottles containing 200 units. How many bottles must be administered? Express the answer as a common mixed number.

8. A health care professional was asked to administer 650 units of a medication. However, all that is in stock are bottles containing 150 units. How many bottles must be administered? Express the answer as a mixed number.

9. Add or subtract each of the following, and simplify.

    a. $\frac{3}{8} + \frac{3}{8}$

    b. $\frac{2}{7} + \frac{5}{7}$

    c. $\frac{5}{16} + \frac{9}{16}$

    d. $\frac{1}{2} + \frac{2}{3}$

    e. $\frac{3}{4} + \frac{1}{5}$

    f. $\frac{2}{15} + \frac{3}{10}$

    g. $\frac{3}{4} - \frac{1}{2}$

    h. $\frac{7}{8} - \frac{1}{3}$

    i. $\frac{7}{16} - \frac{1}{4}$

10. A patient is given $\frac{1}{2}$ tablespoon of medication before lunch and $\frac{1}{4}$ tablespoon after lunch. How much total medication did the patient receive?

11. A patient is given $\frac{3}{4}$ tablespoon of medication in the morning and $\frac{5}{8}$ tablespoon in the afternoon. How much total medication did the patient receive? Express the answer as a mixed number.

12. Two bottles of the same medication have been opened. They are $\frac{15}{16}$ and $\frac{1}{2}$ of their original amounts. If added together, how many bottles would this represent?

13. Three bottles of the same medication have been opened. They are $\frac{3}{4}$, $\frac{2}{3}$, and $\frac{1}{2}$ of their original amounts. If added together, will they fit into 2 bottles?

14. Multiply each of the following.

    a. $\frac{2}{3} \times \frac{3}{5}$

    b. $\frac{5}{6} \times \frac{4}{15}$

    c. $\frac{7}{8} \times \frac{16}{21}$

    d. $\frac{3}{7} \times \frac{35}{39}$

    e. $\frac{2}{27} \times \frac{9}{10}$

15. A bottle is only half full. A health care provider is to give $\frac{2}{3}$ of the remaining bottle. To determine how much of the original bottle this represents, find $\frac{1}{2} \times \frac{2}{3}$.

16. A bottle is three quarters full. A health care provider is to give $\frac{1}{3}$ of the remaining bottle. How much of the original bottle does this represent?

17. What is $\frac{2}{5}$ of $\frac{3}{8}$?

18. What is $\frac{1}{6}$ of $\frac{2}{3}$?

19. In a class of 36 nursing students, $\frac{2}{3}$ are female. How many students are male?

20. A bottle contains 1,000 tablets. A pharmacy technician is asked to supply three-fourths of them to the nurses' station. How many should be sent?

21. A bottle contains 3,000 units of a medication. A pharmacy technician is asked to withdraw two-fifths of it for use in a solution. How much should be withdrawn?

22. Approximately one-half of the 206 bones in the human skeleton are in the hands and feet. About how many are not in the hands and feet?

23. Find the reciprocals for each of the following.

    a. $\frac{1}{3}$

    b. $\frac{2}{3}$

    c. 5

    d. 7

    e. $\frac{12}{5}$

24. Divide each of the following.

    a. $\frac{3}{4} \div \frac{6}{7}$

    b. $\frac{2}{3} \div \frac{5}{3}$

    c. $\frac{7}{8} \div \frac{21}{16}$

    d. $\frac{3}{8} \div \frac{5}{8}$

    e. $\frac{21}{10} \div \frac{7}{30}$

    f. $\frac{3}{7} \div \frac{7}{3}$

    g. $\frac{15}{16} \div \frac{1}{32}$

    h. $12 \div \frac{6}{5}$

    i. $8 \div \frac{8}{25}$

    j. $27 \div \frac{9}{5}$

25. Suppose you have $\frac{3}{4}$ of a bottle of medication left. If each dose is $\frac{1}{16}$ of a bottle, to find the number of doses remaining in the bottle, find $\frac{3}{4} \div \frac{1}{16}$.

26. Suppose you have $\frac{7}{8}$ of a bottle of medication left. If each dose is $\frac{1}{24}$ of a bottle, to find the number of doses remaining in the bottle, find $\frac{7}{8} \div \frac{1}{24}$.

27. Suppose you have $\frac{4}{5}$ of a bottle of medication left. If each dose is $\frac{1}{10}$ of a bottle, find the number of doses remaining in the bottle.

28. A surgical technologist is opening boxes of instruments of various sizes. The sizes listed are $\frac{1}{2}, \frac{1}{4}, \frac{3}{8}, \frac{3}{4}$, and $\frac{5}{8}$. If they are to be arranged in order from smallest to largest, how should they be arranged?

29. One hour of break time was to be split between three residents. The first took a break of $\frac{5}{12}$ of an hour, and the second took a $\frac{1}{4}$ hour break. How much time remained for the third resident? Did she get her fair share?

Real Life Issues and Applications

Hard Decisions with Fractions

Suppose for the sake of argument that you were chosen from the total population of the United States to dole out $100 billion for health care. This $100 billion would be the total health care budget for our nation for 1 year. What fraction of this amount would you spend on new equipment for research or on new equipment for diagnostics and treatment of disease? What fraction would you spend to find a cure for AIDS or a cure for cancer? What about prenatal care or the care of premature infants? How would you justify giving to one group and not to another? Would giving an equal amount to each group be a good idea, or would the resulting lower amount of money given to each group prevent any one group from accomplishing anything?

Using what you have learned about fractions, devise a simple budget showing the actual amount of money to be given to each area of health care that you think is important. Then, explain the reasons for your decisions. If you have difficulty deciding to whom to give the money or even how to divide up the money, you are not alone. State and federal governmental agencies have to make these tough decisions on a regular basis.

Additional Activity

Invite a pharmacist to class to discuss drug dosage calculations, medication errors, and pharmacy-related safeguards in the health care system.

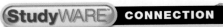 **CONNECTION**

Go to your StudyWARE™ DVD and have fun learning as you play interactive games, view animations and videos, and take practice tests to help reinforce key concepts you learned in this chapter.

Workbook Practice   *Go to your Workbook for more practice questions and activities.*

CHAPTER 15

DECIMALS, PERCENTS, AND RATIOS

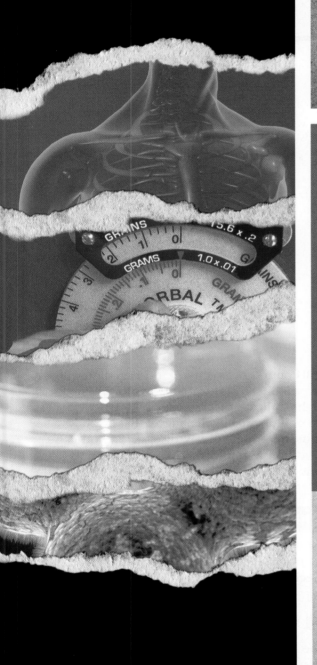

Objectives

Upon completion of this chapter, you should be able to

- Write decimals in word form

- Estimate values for operations involving decimals and use a calculator to find the results

- Write equivalent numbers as percents, fractions, and decimals

- Represent fractions as ratios in simplest form

- Differentiate the terms *solute, solvent*, and *solution*

- Differentiate between W/V solutions and V/V solutions and express each as percent solutions and ratio solutions

- Calculate unit price and rate of flow

Key Terms

decimals
intake and output (I&O)
percents
percent solution
ratios
solute

solution
solvent
unit price
V/V solution
W/V solution

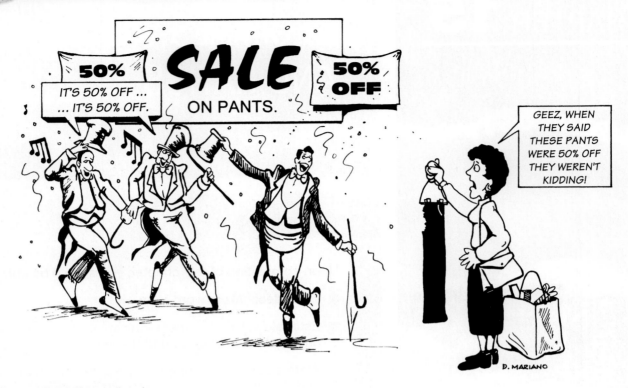

Source: Delmar/Cengage Learning

■ INTRODUCTION

In the previous chapter, we learned about fractions. There are, however, other ways to represent parts of a whole. These include **decimals**, **ratios**, and **percents**. In the health field, these representations tend to be used more often than fractions are used.

For example, blood tests can reveal information about a patient's health. These tests are typically performed in laboratories by medical laboratory technicians and the results are analyzed by clinicians. Many of the levels are reported in decimal form. The presence of abnormal values can often be of diagnostic significance for specific disease states.

An analysis of red blood cells, which carry oxygen to the tissues, would typically show a value within the range of 4.5 to 6.3 million cells per milliliter. If the number of red blood cells is too low, the patient may have a condition called anemia where the body's tissues may not get enough oxygen. This can be the result of a deficiency in iron or certain vitamins.

Another type of cell found in the blood is the white blood cell. This type of cell is important for the body to fight infections. A normal white

blood cell count is between 4.5 and 11.0 thousand cells per milliliter (thou/mL). A level that is too high might indicate diseases such as a bacterial infection or leukemia, while a level that is too low might indicate bone marrow disease. So you can see why a thorough understanding of decimals is important.

Decimals

In addition to fractions, another way of looking at numbers that are part of a whole is through the use of decimals.

Writing Decimals in Word Form

Given the widespread use of calculators, a complete understanding of decimals has never been more important. Using a calculator, it can easily be seen that $\frac{3}{4}$, which equals $3 \div 4$, can be written as 0.75. The decimal 0.75 is read "seventy-five hundredths," which can be written as the fraction $\frac{75}{100}$. This, of course, simplifies to $\frac{3}{4}$.

In math, the symbol {…} means "and so forth." Any fraction having a denominator of {10, 100, 1,000, 10,000 …} can easily be written as a decimal.

Example:

$$\frac{3}{10} = 0.3, \text{ read "three-tenths"}$$

$$\frac{25}{100} = 0.25, \text{ read "twenty-five hundredths"}$$

$$\frac{375}{1000} = 0.375, \text{ read "three hundred seventy-five thousandths"}$$

In each of the preceding examples, notice that the number of zeros in the denominator of the fraction is the same as the number of places to the *right* of the decimal point, which, in turn, corresponds to the way the fraction is read (see Figure 15-1).

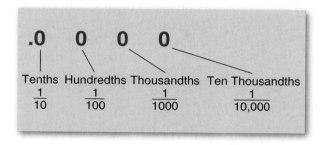

Figure 15-1 *The decimal system (showing corresponding place values).*
Source: Delmar/Cengage Learning

Another important use of the decimal point is to separate the whole number from the portion that is less than 1. The decimal point is read as the word *and*. For example, 10.23 is read "ten and twenty-three hundredths."

Example:

0.104   is read "one hundred four thousandths"

100.004   is read "one hundred and four thousandths"

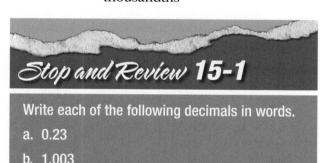

Stop and Review 15-1

Write each of the following decimals in words.

a. 0.23

b. 1.003

c. 104.2

Decimal Operations and Estimation

Because you will likely use a calculator to perform most ordinary problems involving decimals, there is no need to spend much time discussing mathematical operations involving decimals. You should learn enough, however, to determine whether the answers obtained via the use of a calculator are "reasonable." This will help you catch errors that result from hitting wrong calculator keys.

For example, if you use a calculator to add 2.1 + 5.06 and the result is 52.7, you should be able to draw the conclusion that an error has occurred. You do this through estimation. Given that 2.1 is approximately 2 and 5.06 is approximately 5, the sum of these two numbers should be approximately 7. Estimation, thus, gives you an idea of the "reasonableness" of an answer.

Examples:

Estimate the value of 16.03 + 7.9 + 162.011, and then use a calculator to find the exact value.

16.03   is approximately 16

7.9   is approximately 8

162.011   is approximately 162

The answer, therefore, should be approximately 186. The calculator gives the exact answer as 185.941.

Estimate the value of 45.591 ÷ 5.01, and then use a calculator to find the exact value.

$$\frac{45.591}{5.01} \text{ is approximately } \frac{45}{5} = 9$$

The answer, therefore, should be approximately 9. The calculator gives the exact answer as 9.1.

Percents

Percents are used frequently in the health field. For instance, drug concentrations often are represented as percents (e.g., 2% [two percent]

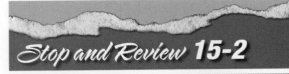

Stop and Review 15-2

a. Estimate the value of each of the following, and then use a calculator to determine the exact value.

$$\frac{20.3}{1.9}$$

$$2.01 + 3.66 + 15.1$$

$$4.02 \times 16.03$$

b. Over an 8-hour period, a pediatric patient's fluid intake and urinary output (intake and output, or I&O) were measured. The child ingested 200.2 mL, 150.0 mL, and 25.1 mL of fluid; the child's urine output was 130.5 mL and 170.5 mL. What was the child's fluid balance (the difference between the I&O) for that 8-hour period?

solutions), and percentages are often used with burn patients to describe how much of the patient's body has been burned (e.g., 5% of body surface).

Changing Percents to Fractions

Nearly everyone knows the importance of oxygen; if there were no oxygen, we would not exist. But do you know how much of our atmosphere is composed of oxygen? The answer is approximately 21%, or 21 parts out of 100 parts. Carbon dioxide makes up 0.03% of our atmosphere, or 0.03 parts out of 100 parts. The most abundant gas is nitrogen, which composes approximately 79% of our atmosphere, or 79 parts out of 100 parts. See Figure 15-2.

As you already may have determined from the preceding two paragraphs, the symbol %

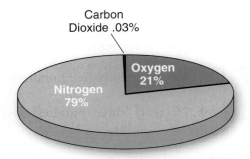

Figure 15-2 *Pie graph representing the approximate percentages of gases in our atmosphere.*
Source: Delmar/Cengage Learning

represents the word *percent*, which means "out of 100." A percent is a simple means of writing any fraction having a denominator of 100. For example, 50% means $\frac{50}{100}$ or 50 (parts) out of 100 (parts).

To change a percent to a fraction, simply write the percent as a fraction having a denominator of 100; remember to simplify the fraction.

Example:

$$25\% = \frac{25}{100} = \frac{1}{4}$$

$$150\% = \frac{150}{100} = \frac{3}{2} = 1\frac{1}{2}$$

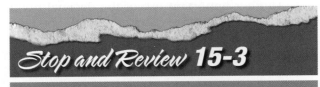

Stop and Review 15-3

Write each of the following percents as fractions in the simplest form.

a. 40%

b. 200%

c. 75%

Changing Percents to Decimals

To change a percent to a decimal, move the decimal point two places to the left. Remember, a whole number is considered to have a decimal point to the right of it.

Example:

$$25\% = 0.25$$

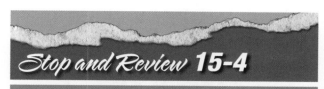

Change each of the following percents to decimals.

a. 15%

b. 300%

c. 37.5%

Changing Decimals to Percents

To change a decimal to a percent, move the decimal point two places to the right, for example, 35% = 0.35. Note that it may be necessary to add zeros, for example, 0.6 = 60%.

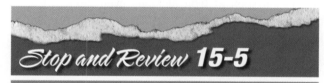

Change each of the following decimals to a percent.

a. 0.15

b. 0.2

c. 1.25

Changing Fractions to Percents

To change a fraction to a percent, first change the fraction to a decimal, and then change the decimal to a percent. Use a calculator when appropriate.

Example:

$$\frac{2}{5} = \frac{4}{10} = 0.4 = 40\%$$

$$\frac{4}{5} = \frac{8}{10} = 0.8 = 80\%$$

$$\frac{7}{20} = \frac{35}{100} = 0.35 = 35\%$$

Just as with fractions, since $\frac{1}{4}$ = 25% = 0.25, use multiplication to find 25% of 200. That is, $0.25 \times 200 = 50$ is equivalent to $\frac{1}{4} \times 200 = 50$. Similarly, to find 75% of 500, multiply $0.75 \times 500 = 375$ or $\frac{3}{4} \times 500 = 375$.

> **QUOTES & NOTES**
>
> **P**ractical Application. Did you ever wonder if there is an easy way to figure out a 15% tip at a restaurant? Just move the decimal point on the bill one place to the left to find 10%. Then take half of that 10% to arrive at the remaining 5%. Add those two numbers, and you've got 15%!

Changing Mixed-Number Percents to Simple Fractions

Sometimes percents are written using mixed numbers (i.e., whole numbers along with fractions),

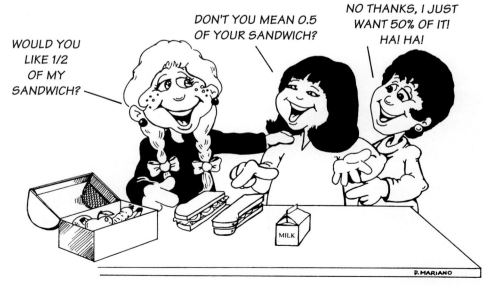

Source: Delmar/Cengage Learning

Special Focus

Effects of Oxygen Therapy and High Altitudes

One of the most common therapies is oxygen therapy. As you breathe now, you are breathing room air which contains 21% oxygen. However, certain disease states and environmental conditions may necessitate increasing the amount of oxygen delivered to your body tissues. For example, at sea level the atmospheric pressure (P_B) is 760 mm Hg (millimeters of mercury). We can find the available oxygen by multiplying the atmospheric pressure by the oxygen percent. To perform the calculation, you must convert the percentage into the decimal form. Therefore, the answer becomes:

760 mm Hg $\times$ .21 (decimal form of 21% oxygen) = 159.6 mm Hg of oxygen

If we want to increase the amount of available oxygen, we can place the patient on a higher-percentage device such as an oxygen mask set at 50%. This patient would now have more oxygen available as follows:

760 mm Hg $\times$ .50 = 380 mm Hg of oxygen

An environmental example is mountain climbing. As you climb above sea level, the atmospheric pressure becomes less. Let's assume you have reached a height where it has dropped to 600 mm Hg. The oxygen now available is:

600 mm Hg $\times$ .21 = 126 mm Hg of oxygen

As we further develop and build this equation in future chapters, you will see that other factors reduce the available oxygen at high altitudes even more. Thus, mountain climbers often need supplemental oxygen, just as patients with lung disease do.

---

such as $66\frac{2}{3}\%$. To change a mixed-number percent to a simple fraction, first change the mixed number to an improper fraction, $66\frac{2}{3}\% = \frac{200}{3}\%$. Next, divide by 100 and simplify. (Remember, *percent* means "out of 100.")

$$66\frac{2}{3}\% = \frac{200}{3}\% = \frac{200}{3} \div 100 = \frac{200}{3} \times \frac{1}{100} = \frac{2}{3}$$

Thus, $66\frac{2}{3}\%$ is the same as the fraction $\frac{2}{3}$.

Ratios

Another way to show the relationship between numbers is to use ratios. A ratio is simply a comparison between two numbers. For example, the fraction $\frac{1}{2}$ can be written as the ratio 1:2. Thus, the fraction $\frac{1}{2}$ is the same as the ratio 1:2, the decimal 0.50, and the percent 50%. All of these are different ways of expressing the same value (see Figure 15-3).

As is the case with fractions, ratios can be simplified. As with fractions, simply divide both numbers in the ratio by the largest number that divides evenly into both.

Stop and Review 15-6

Change each of the following mixed-number percents first to a fraction and then to a decimal.

a. $16\frac{2}{3}\%$

b. $83\frac{1}{3}\%$

$$\frac{1}{2} = \begin{array}{l} \text{1:2} \\ \text{0.50} \\ \text{50\%} \end{array}$$

Figure 15-3   *Equivalent expressions for fractions, ratios, decimals, and percentages.*

Source: Delmar/Cengage Learning

Example:

For the ratio of 50:2, the largest number that will divide evenly into both 2 and 50 is 2. Dividing both numbers in the original ratio by 2 yields a simplified ratio of 25:1.

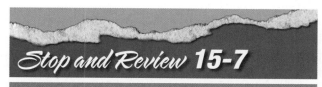

Stop and Review 15-7

Simplify each of the following ratios.

a. 50:5

b. 30:15

c. 100:1

Another use of ratios is to find the individual cost or **unit price** of an item—that is, the price of one item. To find the unit price, set up a fraction,

$$Unit\ price = \frac{total\ price}{number\ of\ items},$$

Example:

A bottle of 100 aspirins sells for $7.50, while a bottle of 150 aspirins of the same brand sells for $12.00. Which is the better buy?

The unit price for each is $\frac{7.50}{100} = 0.075$ and $\frac{12.00}{150} = 0.080$.

Since each aspirin in the 100-tablet bottle costs less, it is the better buy.

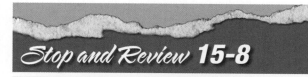

Stop and Review 15-8

a. An IV dispenses fluid at a rate of 750 mL in 5 hours. How much liquid is dispensed in 1 hour? How much in 3 hours?

b. Which can of coffee is the better buy, a 42-ounce can for $13.00 or a 12-ounce can for $4.00?

Clinical Relevancy

The Importance of Percents and Ratios in Drug Calculations

Percents and ratios are especially important in drug dosage calculation problems because many times a drug is ordered in a dosage that is not premixed. How would you mix a medicine to ensure that the **solution** is of the right amount and the right strength?

The term *solution* means a uniform (homogenous) mixture of two or more substances. The part of the solution that is dissolved into a liquid is known as the **solute**. A solute can be either a solid or a liquid. The liquid that does the dissolving is called a **solvent**. As an illustration, in making a cup of hot chocolate, the powdered mix is the

solute, and the hot water or milk that dissolves the mix is the solvent.

It is important to know whether the solute is a solid or liquid. If the solute is a solid (as in the hot chocolate example), the solution concentration can be defined as a ratio of the *weight* of the solute in relation to the *volume* of the solution. This is called the **W/V solution**, where the weight of the solute (W) is usually expressed in grams. Hot chocolate can also be made using a liquid chocolate solute. If the solute is a liquid, the solution concentration can be defined by the ratio that compares the *volume* of

(continues)

(continued)

the liquid solute in relation to the *volume* of the solution. This is called a **V/V solution**, where a volume (V) of solute is added to a volume (V) of solvent to reach the desired volume of solution, and where volume is usually expressed in milliliters (mL).

The strength of a solution can be determined by comparing the parts of solute to the parts of the total solution. For example, the more hot chocolate mix (solute) used, the stronger the hot chocolate will be; likewise, the less water or milk (solvent) used to dilute the hot chocolate mix, the more concentrated (stronger) the hot chocolate will be.

The strength of a solution can also be expressed as a **percent solution**. A percent solution compares the solute to 100 milliliters of the total solution. Thus, a 10% solution contains either 10 mL (V/V solution) or 10 grams (W/V solution) of solute per 100 mL of solution. The percent solution works well for both V/V solutions and W/V solutions.

The strength of the solution can also be expressed in terms of a ratio. The first number of the ratio represents parts of solute, whereas the second number represents the total parts of solution. Thus a 1:100 solution contains one part solute for every one hundred parts of total solution. You will use this knowledge of percents and ratios to express solution strength when you learn to calculate drug dosages in the problems in Chapter 19.

QUOTES & NOTES

The following quotes have been attributed to baseball legend Yogi Berra. Can you now appreciate the humor in them?

"You better cut the pizza in four pieces; I'm not hungry enough to eat six pieces."

"You give 100 percent in the first half of the game, and if that isn't enough, in the second half you give what's left."

"Baseball is 90% mental—the other half is physical."

"Ninety percent of the putts that are short don't go in."

■ CHAPTER REVIEW

Exercises

1. Write each of the following decimals in word form.
   a. 0.35
   b. 1.021
   c. 16.1
   d. 102.102
   e. 104.401

2. Write each of the following in decimal form.
   a. four-tenths
   b. two and sixteen hundredths
   c. two hundred four and one hundred three ten-thousandths
   d. three hundred and four thousandths

3. For each of the following, first estimate the answer, and then use a calculator to obtain a more precise answer.

   a. $\dfrac{31.25}{16.4}$

   b. 17.2 + 3.011 + 104.21

   c. 2.3 × 102.65

   d. 231.612 − 105.7

   e. 124.6 ÷ 5

4. To prevent anemia, a doctor advises a patient to eat foods that provide at least 12 milligrams (mg) of iron each day. In one day, the patient ate the following foods with the amount of iron in parentheses: oatmeal with raisins (2.9 mg), tomato juice (1.25 mg), peanut butter crackers (1.95 mg), fish (1.3 mg), potatoes (1.2 mg), and peas (1.7 mg). Did the patient get enough iron? If not, how much more will the patient need?

5. Write each of the following percents as a fraction; remember to simplify.

   a. 47%

   b. 20%

   c. 175%

   d. 6%

   e. 30%

6. Write each of the following percents in decimal form.

   a. 3%

   b. 79%

   c. 67.5%

   d. 250%

   e. 62.5%

7. Write each of the following decimals as a percent.

   a. 0.5

   b. 0.15

   c. 2.5

   d. 3.45

   e. 0.355

   f. 3

8. What is 30% of 120?

9. What is 37% of 200?

10. About 32% of a paycheck goes toward taxes. How much tax is paid on a $1,000 paycheck? If 10% of the paycheck is put toward retirement, how much remains as take-home pay?

11. A full bottle of liquid medicine has 400 units. If a doctor orders that 30% be administered, how many units were used? How much remains?

12. There are 2,400 tablets in a bottle. A pharmacist wants 75% of them to be packaged into smaller containers. How many must be repackaged? If there are 100 in each smaller package, how many smaller packages will there be?

13. A physician ordered 120 syringes for his office. However, when they were delivered, she found that $12\frac{1}{2}$% were broken. How many syringes were usable?

14. The length of a person's thigh bone is about 27% of the person's height. How long is the thigh bone if the person is 80 inches tall?

15. Write each of the following fractions as a percent.

   a. $\dfrac{3}{5}$

   b. $\dfrac{7}{8}$

   c. $\dfrac{3}{4}$

   d. $\dfrac{4}{7}$

   e. $\dfrac{1}{3}$

16. Approximately one out of every ten Americans is left-handed. What percent is this?

17. A scientific study considers people who are 20% above their ideal body weight to be overweight. If you weigh 150 pounds and have an ideal body weight of 120 pounds, are you considered overweight according to this study?

18. Jonas Salk developed a vaccine for polio in 1954. The following year, the number of reported polio cases dropped from 29,000 to 15,000. What was the percent drop, to the nearest whole percent?

19. Complete the following table:

fraction	decimal	percent
a. $\frac{1}{4}$	_____	_____
b. _____	_____	$87\frac{1}{2}\%$
c. _____	_____	40%
d. _____	0.7	_____
e. _____	_____	$33\frac{1}{3}\%$
f. _____	0.625	_____
g. $\frac{1}{8}$	_____	_____

20. Simplify each of the following ratios.

a. 30:10

b. 20:15

c. 14:6

d. 54:36

21. If the average adult heart beats about 8 times every 6 seconds, and a baby's heart beats about 7 times every 3 seconds, which heartbeat is faster?

22. A student at a local college pays tuition of $3,000 for 12 credits. How much does the student pay per credit?

23. If 24 cans of a beverage cost $16.00, while 30 cans cost $21.00, which is the better buy?

24. For a W/V solution of a drug, describe what each of the following percent solutions means in terms of the solute and solution.

a. 30%

b. 50%

c. 2%

25. For a V/V solution of a drug, describe what each of the following ratio solutions means in terms of the solute and solution.

a. 1:100

b. 1:50

c. 1:1,000

Real Life Issues and Applications

Ratios in Medicine

With normal breathing, it takes twice as long to exhale as it does to inhale. This can be expressed by the ratio 1:2. Certain disease states of the lungs can alter this ratio. Patient A has a 2-second inspiratory (I) time and a 4-second expiratory (E) time. Patient B has a 2-second I time and a 1-second E time. What are their respective I:E ratios? Which patient has a normal ratio?

Additional Activity

What is normal saline? Go to a pharmacy and identify the various products that contain normal saline solution. Share your information with the class.

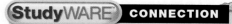

CONNECTION

Go to your StudyWARE™ DVD and have fun learning as you play interactive games, view animations and videos, and take practice tests to help reinforce key concepts you learned in this chapter.

Workbook Practice | *Go to your Workbook for more practice questions and activities.*

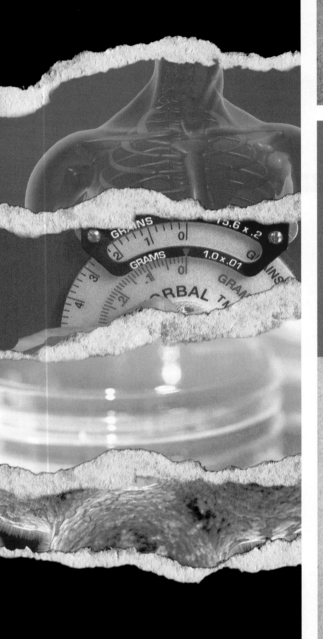

CHAPTER 16

EXPONENTS, SCIENTIFIC NOTATION, AND THE METRIC SYSTEM

Objectives

Upon completion of this chapter, you should be able to

- Evaluate numbers having positive and negative exponents
- Represent numbers in scientific notation
- Change units within the metric system
- Convert units between systems of measurement

Key Terms

base
centi
deca (da)
deci (d)
English system of measurement
exponent
factor-label method
giga (G)
gram (g)
hecto (h)
kilo (k)

liter (L)
mega (M)
meter (m)
metric system of measurement
micro (mc)
milli (m)
nano (n)
pico (p)
scientific notation
units

PROFOUND MATHEMATIC SAYINGS TO REMEMBER

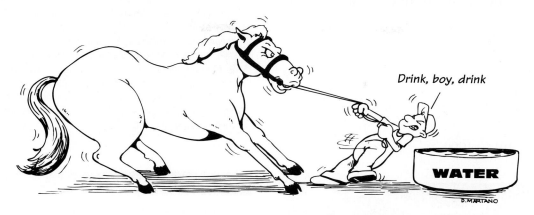

Drink, boy, drink

You can liter a horse to water but you can't make it drink.

Source: Delmar/Cengage Learning

■ INTRODUCTION

In health care we deal with very large numbers, such as the number of cells in your body, or very small numbers, such as the microscopic size of the cell. In addition, health care professionals regularly use the *metric system* of measurement in their clinical practice. Therefore, this chapter focuses on **scientific notation** and the **metric system of measurement**, both of which are based on the power of 10, and therefore can be related to the decimal system, discussed in Chapter 15.

Working with scientific notation and the metric system requires a basic understanding of the powers of 10 and of where to move the decimal point. This is especially true for conversions within the metric system. Also discussed in this chapter are conversions between the **English system of measurement**, which is used predominately in the United States, and the *metric system of measurement,* which is used worldwide and in the health professions.

Exponents and Base

The health professions often require the use of both extremely large numbers and extremely small numbers. For instance, there are about 25,000,000,000 blood cells circulating in an average adult's body, and many organisms found in the body are microscopic in size. It is, therefore, often convenient to write these numbers in an abbreviated form known as *scientific notation.*

Doing this requires an understanding of certain terminology.

Consider the expression b^n, where b is called the **base** and n the **exponent**. The n represents the number of times that b is multiplied by itself: b^n is read "the nth power of b." Exponents of 2 and 3 are read "squared" and "cubed." That is, 3^2 is read "3 squared," while 4^3 is read "4 cubed."

Examples:

$$3^4 = 3 \times 3 \times 3 \times 3 = 81$$
$$5^3 = 5 \times 5 \times 5 = 125$$

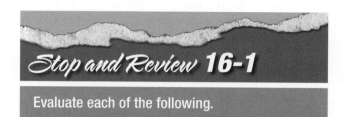

Stop and Review 16-1

Evaluate each of the following.

a. 3^2

b. 4^3

c. 2^5

d. 10^3

e. 10^5

When the exponent is positive, the resulting number is relatively large. Small numbers less than 1 can also be represented in scientific notation, however. In these cases, negative exponents are used. A negative exponent can be thought of as a fraction. To do this, you simply put b in the denominator and the positive version of n in the numerator. For example, $2^{-3} = \frac{1}{2^3} = \frac{1}{8}$. So, in general, $b^{-n} = \frac{1}{b^n}$.

Examples:

$$3^{-2} = \frac{1}{3^2} = \frac{1}{9}$$

$$10^{-3} = \frac{1}{10^3} = \frac{1}{1000}$$

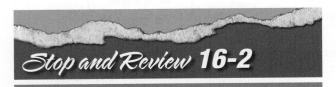

Stop and Review 16-2

Write each of the following using a positive exponent, and then change each to a fractional form.

a. 4^{-3}

b. 3^{-4}

c. 10^{-1}

d. 10^{-2}

e. 10^{-4}

The Power of 10—Base 10

Of special interest are the powers of 10, or base 10. When b is 10, the number of zeros in the answer equals the exponent.

Example:

$$10^2 = 10 \times 10 = 100$$

$$10^3 = 10 \times 10 \times 10 = 1,000$$

$$10^4 = 10 \times 10 \times 10 \times 10 = 10,000$$

$$10^5 = 10 \times 10 \times 10 \times 10 \times 10 = 1,000,000$$

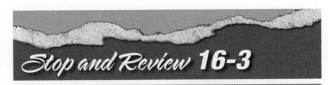

Stop and Review 16-3

Evaluate each of the following.

a. 10^6

b. 10^7

Scientific Notation

Now that you are familiar with the concepts of exponents and bases, you are ready to take on scientific notation. To write a number in scientific notation, write it as a product of a number greater than or equal to 1 and less than 10, with a corresponding power of 10. In other words, only one number should be to the left of the decimal point.

As an example, consider those 25,000,000,000 blood cells in your body. We can shorten this number to 2.5×10^{10}. The exponent is 10 because in order to ensure that only one number is to the left of the decimal point, we need to move the decimal point 10 places—from the end of the number to between the 2 and 5. See Figure 16-1 that illustrates this concept.

Examples:

$$201,000 = 2.01 \times 100,000 = 2.01 \times 10^5$$

$$0.00062 = 6.2 \times 0.0001 = 6.2 \times 10^{-4}$$

25,000,000,000. ← Begin here

Move to the left 10 places so you have:

$$2.5 \times 10^{10}$$

Begin here → **.0000000025**

Move to the right 10 places so you have:

$$2.5 \times 10^{-10}$$

Figure 16-1 *The process of scientific notation.*
Source: Delmar/Cengage Learning

So, in scientific notation, the decimal point is moved so that only one nonzero digit is to the left of the decimal; the number of places that the decimal is moved is the exponent.

Further, as is illustrated in the preceding example and Figure 16-1, if the decimal point is moved to the left, the exponent is positive; if the decimal point is moved to the right, the exponent is negative. Notice also that the exponent is positive if the number is large and negative if the number is small (less than 1).

Examples:

$$201{,}000 = 2.01 \times 10^5$$

The decimal is moved 5 places to the left, the exponent is positive, and the number is large.

$$0.00062 = 6.2 \times 10^{-4}$$

The decimal is moved 4 places to the right, the exponent is negative, and the number is small.

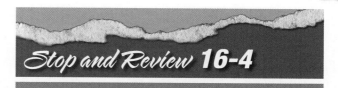

Stop and Review 16-4

Write each of the following in scientific notation.
a. 41,000
b. 601,000
c. 80,000,000
d. 0.0012
e. 0.0000101
f. 0.000003

The Metric System

As discussed previously, there are several measurement systems. The one we commonly use is the *English system*, which uses measurements in inches, feet, yards, and miles; ounces, pounds, and tons; and pints, quarts, and gallons.

However, this system is not the system of choice used throughout the world and within the health professions.

Most scientific and medical measurements utilize what is commonly referred to as the *metric system*. Although more than one system has been developed wherein metric units are used, the system accepted as *the* metric system is the International System of Units.

As illustrated in Table 16-1, there are only three basic units of measure in the metric system:

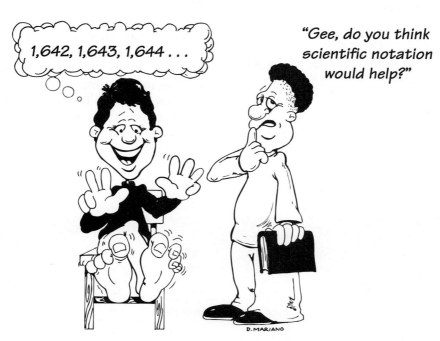

1,642, 1,643, 1,644 . . .

"Gee, do you think scientific notation would help?"

D. MARIANO

Source: Delmar/Cengage Learning

TABLE 16-1
Measurement in the Metric System

TYPE	UNIT	APPROXIMATE ENGLISH SYSTEM EQUIVALENT
Distance (length)	meter	39 inches
Volume	liter	1 quart
Weight (mass)	gram	$\frac{1}{40}$ ounce

the **meter**, the **liter**, and the **gram**. In the metric system, the prefixes are used to indicate the different powers of 10. Table 16-2 shows the common prefixes used in the metric system and their respective powers of 10.

As can be seen from Table 16-2, a kilometer is 1,000 (or 10^3) meters, and a centigram is one-hundredth (or 10^{-2}) gram. The ease of working with the metric system is that to convert within the system, you simply move the decimal point the proper number of places and change to the appropriate prefix. This is done because changing units is a multiplication or division by 10. For example, 2 kilometers is 2 × 1000 = 2000 meters.

Examples:

22,340 *m* = 22.340 *km*

Move the decimal point 3 places to the left, and change from *m* to *km*.

43 *cl* = 0.0043 *hl*

Move the decimal point 4 places to the left, and change from *cl* to *hl*.

160 *mg* = 0.16 *g*

Move the decimal point 3 places to the left, and change from *mg* to *g*.

Stop and Review **16-5**

Convert each of the following to the units noted.

a. 62 m to kilometers (km)
b. 107 L to decaliters (daL)
c. 0.4 kg to milligrams (mg)
d. 20 cm to millimeters (mm)

Notice that this is similar to what is done in scientific notation. This is because the metric system, like scientific notation, is based on the powers of 10.

Refer to Table 16-3 for a more complete listing of prefixes used in the metric system.

Conversion of Units

The importance of changing from one form of a number to another, as in changing from fractions to decimals to percents, has already been demonstrated. But what about changing between **units** such as hours, minutes, and seconds? How many minutes are there in 8 hours? Being able to convert between units is just as important as being able to convert between forms of numbers. We have already discussed some conversions of this

TABLE 16-2
Common Prefixes of the Metrix System

	THOUSANDS	HUNDREDS	TENS	UNIT	TENTH	HUNDREDTH	THOUSANDTH
Prefix	kilo	hecto	deca	*liter* (L)	deci	centi	milli
Abbreviation	(k)	(h)	(da)	*meter (m)*	(d)	(c)	(m)
Powers	10^3	10^2	10^1	*gram* (g)	10^{21}	10^{22}	10^{23}

TABLE 16-3
Metric System Prefixes and Abbreviations

PREFIX	POWER OF TEN	ABBREVIATION
Giga	10^9	G
Mega	10^6	M
Kilo	10^3	k
Hecto	10^2	h
Deca	10^1	da
Deci	10^{-1}	d
Centi	10^{-2}	c
Milli	10^{-3}	m
Micro	10^{-6}	mc or
Nano	10^{-9}	n
Pico	10^{-12}	p

QUOTES & NOTES

No man may be so great that he cannot be proven wrong.

—Aristotle

nature within the metric system; for example, we know that 20 cm is equal to 200 mm. But how many centimeters are there in a foot?

Factor-Label Method

The **factor-label method** works for all conversions of units, even outside of the metric system. To use this method, simply write the original quantity as a fraction, and then treat the units as is done in the multiplication of fractions. In other words, "cancel" the units.

For example, to change from hours to seconds, first write hours as a fraction over 1. Now you may not know how many seconds are in one hour, but you do know how many minutes are in one hour, so you can first convert to minutes by making a fraction that represents this. Since we are solving for seconds, we need to determine how many seconds are in a minute by making a representative fraction. The next step is to cancel the like units that divide out. The final conversion should look like this:

$$\frac{\cancel{hours}}{1} \times \frac{\cancel{minutes}}{\cancel{hours}} \times \frac{seconds}{\cancel{minutes}} = seconds$$

Notice that by carefully placing the units so that canceling is possible, the units can be changed. In changing from one unit to another, remember that

Clinical Relevancy

Scientific Notation and the Metric System in the Health Professions

Red blood cells (also known as RBCs, or erythrocytes) play a very important role as the main oxygen transporter in our blood. These cells are relatively small; approximately 7.5 microns (0.0075 mc) in diameter and 2.5 microns (0.0025 mc) thick. (These and other cells are discussed in the Anatomy and Physiology and the Microbiology sections of this text.)

What if you were reading an article in a scientific journal concerning RBCs and it stated that RBCs were 7.5 $\times 10^{-6}$ in diameter. Would you know what that means? And what about cellular counts? Some are in the 100,000 range and, many times, are listed on the patient's chart in scientific notation. Obviously, a working knowledge of scientific notation and the metric system is needed.

Other examples abound. For instance, when a breathing tube is placed in a patient's airway (intubation), the tip of that tube should ideally remain at least 2.5 cm

above the area where the airway branches into the right and left lungs (carina). This distance is approximately the length from the tip of your thumb to the first joint. But if you did not know this, what would you do if you had an order to pull the tube back 2 cm? You would either need to have a ruler marked in centimeters or be able to convert centimeters to inches and use a ruler marked only in inches.

There are also many times when health professionals must convert a patient's weight from pounds to kilograms—for proper drug dosage and certain treatment modalities, for example. If health professionals didn't know how to convert between the English and metric systems, patients would be at a marked disadvantage.

Perhaps now you can see how lost health professionals would be without a working knowledge of scientific notation and the metric system.

multiplication by 1 does not change the value of a quantity. That is, the ratios of 60 min/1 hr and 60 sec/1 min are both equal to 1.

Example:

How many seconds are there in 8 hours?

$$\frac{8 \ hours}{1} \times \frac{60 \ min}{1 \ hour} \times \frac{60 \ sec}{1 \ min} = 28{,}800 \ sec.$$

The same method is used with quantities involving more units.

Example:

Convert 7,200 feet per hour to feet per second.

$$\frac{7200 \ feet}{1 \ hour} \times \frac{1 \ hour}{60 \ min} \times \frac{1 \ min}{60 \ sec} = 2 \ \frac{ft}{sec}$$

This method works for any units, including those within the metric system. All that needs to be known are such conversions as

$$1000 \ m = 1 \ km, \ 100 \ g = 1 \ kg,$$
and 1000 mL = 1 L.

Example:

Convert 14.2 kilograms to milligrams.

$$\frac{14.2 \ kg}{1} \times \frac{1000 \ g}{1 \ kg} \times \frac{1000 \ mg}{1 \ g} = 14{,}200{,}000 \ mg$$
$$= 1.42 \times 10^7 \ mg$$

With the factor-label method, it is no longer necessary to remember which way to move the decimal point; we need only to know the conversions. Because conversion within the metric system requires only simple movement of the decimal point, the factor-label method is not traditionally used for conversions within the metric system. This method *must* be used, however, when converting between the metric and English systems. All that is needed is to memorize one conversion in each of the three types of measure. This allows a "bridging" of the systems.

TABLE 16-4	
Conversion Table	
For units of length	1 inch = 2.54 centimeters (cm)
For units of weight	2.2 pounds (lbs) = 1 kilogram (kg)
For units of volume	1.06 quart = 1 liter (L)

Examples:

How many centimeters are in 1 foot?

$$\frac{1 \ ft}{1} \times \frac{12 \ in}{1 \ ft} \times \frac{2.54 \ cm}{1 \ in} = 30.48 \ cm$$

Convert 2 gallons to liters.

$$\frac{2 \ gal}{1} \times \frac{4 \ qt}{1 \ gal} \times \frac{1 \ L}{1.06 \ qt} = 7.55 \ L$$

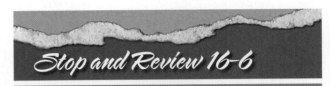

Stop and Review 16-6

Convert each of the following.

a. 1,350 g to pounds (lb)

b. 2.5 yd to meters (m)

Thus, by knowing just a few equivalent values, conversion between any units is made relatively simple. It is not difficult to see how valuable the factor-label method can be in the health professions. For instance, consider this frequently occurring situation. A 150-pound patient is brought into the emergency department. The patient requires the proper amount of a certain drug in order to save his life. This drug is to be given 10 mg/kg of body weight; too little of the drug would not be effective, and too much may be toxic. How would you figure out how much of the drug to give the patient? Begin by converting the patient's weight in pounds to kilograms. Then, because the drug is ordered 10 mg/kg, multiply the result by 10. (The answer to this problem is found in the *Real Life Issues and Applications* section at the end of this chapter.)

Professional Profile
Medical Assisting

Perhaps you are an individual who likes the medical field but are not sure that patient care is what you want to do all the time. You may be an individual who also likes office managing and administration, but not to the level of doing it all day long. If you fit this description, then you may want to consider the allied health profession of medical assisting.

Medical assistants have a wide range of responsibilities. They often are the individuals responsible for the efficient operation of a physician's office. In fact, more medical assistants are hired for work in a doctor's office than are any other allied health professionals.

Office administration and business skills that may be required include managing personnel; scheduling patient appointments; maintaining accurate patient medical records; typing physician dictation; handling various correspondence (which may include phone calls, reports, test results, and manuscripts); handling patients' accounts, billing, and insurance matters; keeping accurate financial records; dealing with sales representatives; and ordering equipment and supplies (both office and medical).

If you choose this profession, you may be responsible for any or all of the following clinical duties: preparing patients for examination (and, possibly, assisting with examinations); taking and recording vital signs; taking accurate medical histories; performing basic treatments; instructing patients on the proper uses of medications or on diagnostic or therapeutic procedures; performing basic lab tests and EKGs; and sterilizing and preparing equipment and instruments used for examinations and procedures. It sounds almost like being a junior doctor with a business degree!

It would be a good idea for you to become familiar with computers and word processing, as well as some basic accounting. A thorough understanding of medical terminology and the metric system along with solid basic math skills are a must. Educational programs for medical assistants are either 1 year (for a certificate or diploma) or 2 years (for an associate degree) in duration.

When you consider that there are more than 300,000 (that's 3.0×10^5 !) doctors in the United States, employment opportunities look very good for medical assistants. Salary will vary depending on level of education, geographic region, and amount of responsibility.

For more information concerning this highly diverse profession, visit the American Association of Medical Assistants at http://www.aama-ntl.org/.

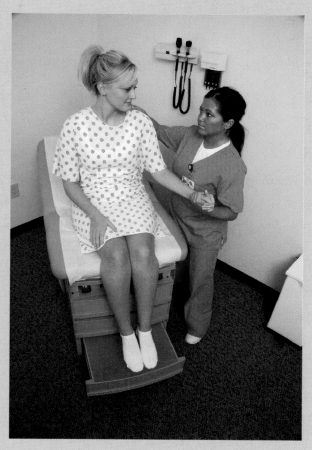

Source: Delmar/Cengage Learning

■ CHAPTER REVIEW

Exercises

1. Evaluate each of the following.
   a. 2^3 d. 2^5
   b. 5^2 e. 5^3
   c. 3^3

2. Evaluate each of the following.
   a. 10^2 d. 10^8
   b. 10^3 e. 10^7
   c. 10^4

3. Write each of the following with a positive exponent.
   a. 3^{-1} d. 4^{-2}
   b. 5^{-2} e. 3^{-3}
   c. 2^{-3}

4. Write each of the following with a positive exponent.
   a. 10^{-3} d. 10^{-7}
   b. 10^{-5} e. 10^{-10}
   c. 10^{-6}

5. Write each of the problems in exercise number 4 in decimal form.

6. Write each of the following in scientific notation.
   a. 450,000   f. 0.00012
   b. 602,000   g. 2,010,000
   c. 0.0011   h. 32,401,000
   d. 0.0000522   i. 0.0010001
   e. 26,200,000   j. 0.00000009

7. A red blood cell count is typically about 5,000,000 per mm^3. Express this in scientific notation.

8. Platelets are the mechanism in the blood that assists the blood in clotting. A normal count is 300,000,000,000 per mm^3. Express this in scientific notation.

9. The walls of a human heart are made of muscles that contract about 99,000 times each day. Express this in scientific notation.

10. The human brain has about one hundred billion nerve cells. Write this in both decimal and scientific notation.

11. Each pair of lungs has about three hundred million air sacs. Write this in both decimal and scientific notation.

12. Mitochondria are the "power-generating" portion of a cell. Their typical size is $5 \times 10^{-6}\, m$. Express this as a decimal.

13. X-rays vary in length. Write the length of the X-ray $1 \times 10^{-10}\,m$ in decimal notation.

14. The planet mercury is about 57,900,000 kilometers from the sun. Express this distance in scientific notation.

15. Convert each of the following to the units noted.

   a. 5 m to millimeters (mm)

   b. 5,000 m to kilometers (km)

   c. 3,025 cm to meters (m)

   d. 6.2 m to centimeters (cm)

   e. 4.7 km to centimeters (cm)

16. Convert each of the following to the units noted.

   a. 2.55 mL to liters (L)

   b. 200 mL to liters (L)

   c. 2.6 kL to milliliters (mL)

   d. 4,000 mL to kiloliters (kL)

   e. 17.1 L to milliliters (mL)

17. Convert each of the following to the units noted.

   a. 50,000 mg to kilograms (kg)

   b. 100,000 ng to milligrams (mg)

   c. 7.66 kg to decigrams (dg)

   d. 2.1 kg to grams (g)

   e. 3,000 g to centigrams (cg)

18. The daily value (DV) is a reference point that suggests guidelines for a healthy diet. If the DV for fiber is 24 grams, express this in milligrams.

19. A teaspoon of common table salt contains about 1,900 mg of sodium. How many grams of sodium is this?

20. An athletic trainer recommends that an athlete drink 1,750 mL of water during a 3-hour workout. Express this in liters per hour.

21. Convert each of the following to the units noted.

   a. 4 hr to minutes (min)

   b. 6 weeks to hours (hr)

   c. 4 ft to inches (in.)

   d. 5 m to millimeters (mm)

   e. 2.6 kL to milliliters (mL)

   f. 100,000 ng to milligrams (mg)

   g. 3 mi to feet (ft)

   h. 16 lb to ounces (oz)

   i. 3.2 gal to quarts (qt)

22. Convert each of the following to the units noted.

   a. $88\,\dfrac{ft}{sec}$ to $\dfrac{miles}{hour}\left(\dfrac{mi}{hr}\text{ or } mph\right)$

   b. 500 g to ounces (oz)

   c. 4.1 km to miles (mi)

   d. 16 lb to kilograms (kg)

   e. 7,000 g to pounds (lb)

   f. 16 in. to centimeters (cm)

   g. 15 lb to grams (g)

   h. 7 gal to milliliters (mL)

23. The length of a building lot is 33 yards. How long is the lot in feet?

24. There are about 6 quarts of blood in the average-sized man. Express this to the nearest tenth of a liter.

25. The cholesterol level for a patient was listed as 175 mg per 100 mL of blood. Express this in grams per liter.

26. John has 10 qt of soda for his punch. According to his recipe, he needs 4 L of soda. Does he have enough?

27. Which is longer, 20 cm or 9 in.?

28. If you drove 15 km, how many miles did you drive?

29. If your heart beats about once per second, how many times would it beat in one day?

Real Life Issues and Applications

Dosage Calculation

The answer to the dosage-based-on-body-weight problem is 682 mg. Now try one more. Assume a 200-pound patient presents to the Emergency Department (ED) and requires a drug with a dosage of 0.5 mg/kg of body weight. What is the correct dosage of this drug for this patient?

Additional Activity

Relate the metric terms *deci*, *centi*, and *milli* to our monetary system.

StudyWARE CONNECTION

Go to your StudyWARE™ DVD and have fun learning as you play interactive games, view animations and videos, and take practice tests to help reinforce key concepts you learned in this chapter.

Workbook Practice   *Go to your Workbook for more practice questions and activities.*

CHAPTER 17

AN INTRODUCTION TO ALGEBRA

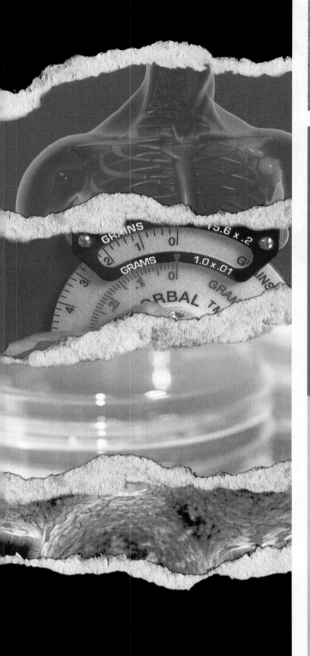

Objectives

Upon completion of this chapter, you should be able to

■ Perform proper order of operations

■ Perform addition, subtraction, multiplication, and division of signed (i.e., positive and negative) numbers

■ Identify terms within, and evaluate and simplify variable expressions

■ Relate words to algebraic expressions

Key Terms

Celsius temperature scale
coefficient
counting numbers
distributive law
factors
Fahrenheit temperature scale
integers
irrational numbers
order of operations

rational numbers
real number line
signed numbers
similar terms
terms
T-score
variables
whole numbers

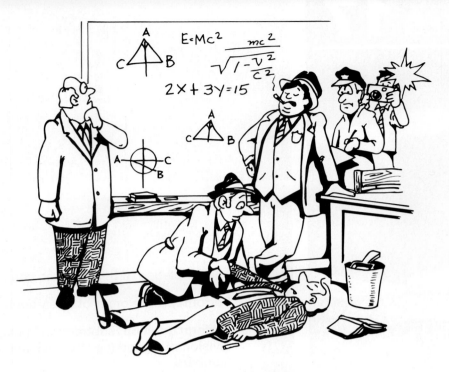

MAYBE HE KNEW TOO MUCH.

Source: Delmar/Cengage Learning

■ INTRODUCTION

Now that we have covered some of the math basics, we need to learn how to manipulate these values to solve clinical problems for diagnosis and treatment. Certain fundamental concepts underlie the study of algebra and algebraic manipulations. The first and most important of these is a thorough understanding of basic arithmetic. Also necessary for the study of algebra is the ability to answer certain questions, including: How do you know whether to perform addition or multiplication first? What do parentheses mean? What happens when you multiply, subtract, divide, or add numbers having positive and negative signs? What are variables and variable expressions? This chapter provides the answers to these questions and, thus, sets the stage for solving equations (which is the subject of Chapter 19).

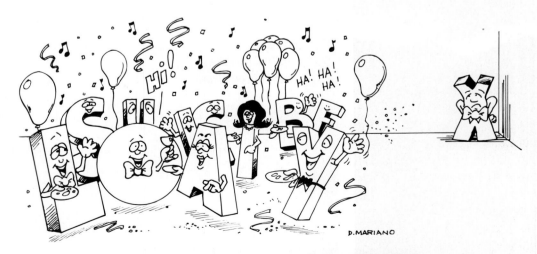

CAN YOU SPOT THE ISOLATED VARIABLE?

Source: Delmar/Cengage Learning

Order of Operations

What is the correct value of $2 + 3 \times 4$? Is it $2 + 3 \times 4 = 5 \times 4 = 20$? OR is it $2 + 3 \times 4 = 2 + 12 = 14$? There can be only one correct answer for these types of math problems. The correct answer to this problem is 14, because the multiplication, 3×4, must be performed before the addition. This example shows the need for a specific order when solving math problems to ensure that everyone gets the same answer every time.

In general, mathematicians do not like ambiguity; they want one and only one answer. This is especially important in the health care field. Imagine solving a formula to determine the correct dosage of a medication. If two practitioners used the same numbers but used different rules to solve the problem, they could arrive at two different dosages. Which is correct? Which could cure? Which may kill?

To prevent the possibility of achieving more than one answer, there is an agreed-upon **order of operations** for solving arithmetical problems. The order of operations is as follows:

Step 1. Perform all operations inside **p**arentheses or grouping symbols. Some grouping symbols are: parentheses ( ), brackets [ ], and the fraction bar.

Step 2. Evaluate **e**xponents.

Step 3. Perform **m**ultiplications and **d**ivisions from left to right as they occur.

Step 4. Perform **a**dditions and **s**ubtractions from left to right as they occur.

Because this order can be confusing to remember, a mnemonic (i.e., a code or saying that aids in memory) has been developed to help you remember. The mnemonic is "**P**atients **E**xpect **M**eals, **D**elicious **A**nd **S**atisfying." Notice that the first letter in each word indicates the order of operations:

Patients, P = parentheses
Expect, E = exponents
Meals, M = multiplication
Delicious, D = division
And, A = addition
Satisfying, S = subtraction

Special Focus

Order of Operations: Why Is It Important?

Consider the following scenario as it relates to the importance of order of operations in the health care professions.

A physician gave strict orders for a patient on fluid restriction to consume 2,500 mL of water over a four-day period. The first day, the patient consumed 400 mL of water. For the next three days, the patient consumed 700 mL of water each day. Nurse Smith was pleased that the nursing staff had followed the doctor's orders.

"What do you mean?" exploded Nurse Jones. "We've *overhydrated* that poor patient. We'll all lose our jobs. Look," Nurse Jones exclaimed as he wrote the following on a piece of paper:

$400 + 3 \times 700 =$

$403 \times 700 =$

$282,100$

"I'm afraid to go into his room," wailed Nurse Jones. "He may look like a water balloon!"

"Nonsense," sneered Nurse Smith, and grabbing a pencil and paper, she wrote:

$400 + (3 \times 700) = 2500$

Who is right and why?

Notice that if you do not know the proper order of operations, different answers might result from this important formula used to treat patients.

Using this mnemonic will help you to remember the order of arithmetical operations.

Thus, in the previously mentioned example, $2 + 3 \times 4$, if the addition were meant to be done first, the problem would be written $(2 + 3) \times 4$, and the correct answer would indeed be 20. But without the parentheses, the multiplication must be done first.

Examples:

$2 \times (8 - 2)$ First subtract $8 - 2 = 6$ since it is inside the ( );

2×6 then multiply.

The answer is 12.

$13 - 6 \times 2 \div 4$ First multiply 6×2;

$13 - 12 \div 4$ Then divide $12 \div 4$.

$13 - 3$ And finally, subtract.

The answer is 10.

Be sure to do *all* the steps!! The solution to the second problem in the previous example should look like this:

$13 - 6 \times 2 \div 4$

$13 - 12 \div 4$

$13 - 3$

10

Note that each line is equivalent to the previous one; in other words, the numerical value does not change in spite of the manipulations you are performing. It is important that each line of your expression be equal to the previous one. You cannot be lazy; you must rewrite each part of the expression, even if no calculation is performed on all parts.

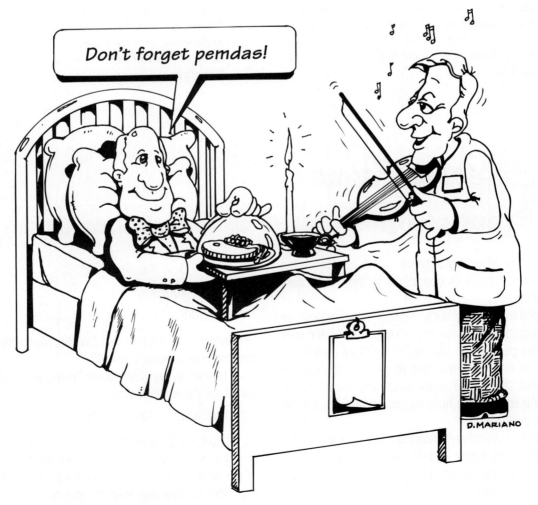

Source: Delmar/Cengage Learning

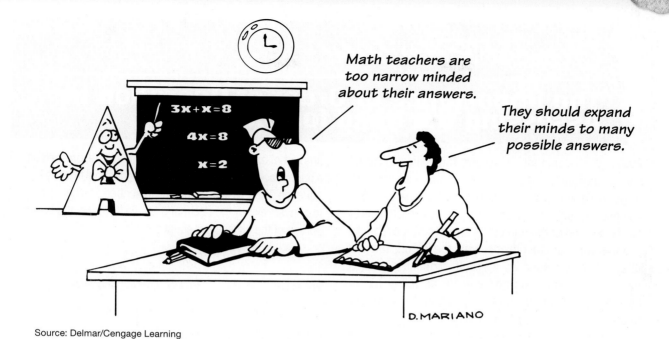

Math teachers are too narrow minded about their answers.

They should expand their minds to many possible answers.

D. MARIANO

Source: Delmar/Cengage Learning

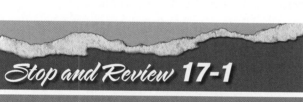

Stop and Review 17-1

Evaluate each of the following.

a. $4 \times 3 - 5$

b. $7 - 4 \div 2$

c. $(3 \times 2)^2 - 2^2$

d. $(5 \times 2) - 3^2 + 1$

e. $3 \times (16 - 4^2) + 25$

Operations on Signed Numbers

Before discussing the use of algebra in the health professions, just as with arithmetic, we need to first define some basic terminology.

Types of Numbers

The **counting numbers** are those which are used to count $\{1, 2, 3, 4, ...\}$. The $\{\ \}$ means the set or group of numbers, and the .... at the end means much the same as "etc.," or to continue on in the same manner. The **whole numbers** are $\{0, 1, 2, 3, ...\}$. Whole numbers include zero, while counting numbers do not.

Integers are the positives and negatives of whole numbers, that is $\{...., -2, -1, 0, 1, 2, ...\}$. We include negative numbers because we will be using some of the concepts of algebra to solve health-related problems.

The Real Number Line

The integers can be represented as points on a number line:

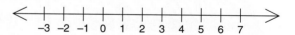

This number line is often referred to as the **real number line**, because any real number can be located as a point on this line. Simply put, real numbers (as opposed to imaginary numbers) are numbers that can be found or approximated with a calculator and located as a point on the number line.

Example:

We have located some real numbers on the following real number line.

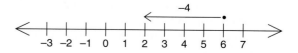

Real numbers can be categorized as either **rational numbers** or **irrational numbers**.

Clinical Relevancy

The Importance of Order of Operation in Assessing the Need for Oxygen

Although the amount of oxygen found in the atmosphere (normally 21%, or 0.21) is sufficient for most of us to survive, many patients having heart or lung diseases require additional oxygen. Alveoli, the little air sacs found at the end of the airways that exchange oxygen and carbon dioxide with the blood, may be affected or damaged as a result of these diseases. Because too much oxygen can be as lethal as too little, it is important to know exactly how much oxygen to provide.

The alveolar air equation aids health professionals in determining proper oxygen therapy. Simply put, the level or **p**ressure of **o**xygen in the **a**lveoli (PAO_2) is related to the barometric pressure (P_B) minus the water vapor in the air (P_{H_2O}). Because water vapor takes up space in the lungs and exerts a force or pressure, it must be subtracted. The resulting difference is then multiplied by the amount of oxygen being provided to the patient (FIO_2). Although the amount of oxygen delivered to the patient is expressed as a percentage, it must be converted to a decimal to solve the equation. Thus, if 50% oxygen is prescribed, it is necessary to convert this to the decimal 0.50. Following is the basic portion of the alveolar air equation:

$$PAO_2 = (P_B - P_{H_2O}) \times FIO_2$$

For example, if $P_B = 730$, $P_{H_2O} = 47$, and $FIO_2 = 0.40$, the result found by *incorrectly* subtracting P_B from the product of $P_{H_2O} \times FIO_2$ would be 711.20. Whereas the *correct answer*, which is found by subtracting $P_B - P_{H_2O}$ inside the parentheses first and then multiplying FIO_2, is 273.20. As is demonstrated by this clinical example, it is important to understand the order of operations. (The alveolar air equation and how to work with and solve equations are discussed later in this book.)

Clinical Relevancy

The Number Line in the Health Care Field

A bone density test is used to determine whether a person has a "brittle bone disease" known as osteoporosis. As you might know, this condition becomes increasingly more common as we age. To measure bone density, a score called a **T-score** is used. A T-score below –2.5 indicates osteoporosis. Use the number line to determine if a patient whose score is –1.9 has the disease.

Rational numbers can be written as a fraction with an integer numerator and a counting number denominator. When you think of a rational number, think of a fraction. An irrational number is a number that when written as a decimal, never ends or repeats. This is similar to some irrational people who can go on and on forever without ever repeating themselves.

Example:

Rational Numbers: $\frac{2}{3}$, $4 = \frac{4}{1}$, $\frac{-9}{2}$, $-\frac{145}{16}$

Irrational Numbers*: $\sqrt{3}$, π

* Although you should be aware that they exist, we will not focus on irrational numbers because they are seldom used by practicing health care

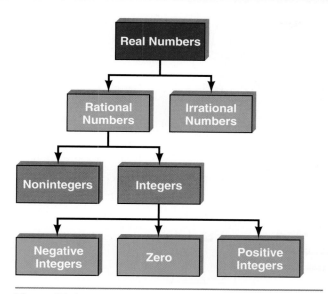

Figure 17-1 *A schematic diagram of the real number system.*

Source: Delmar/Cengage Learning

professionals. For example, while the exact value of $\sqrt{3}$, which doesn't have an exact decimal value, may be important to a mathematician or an engineer, health care providers can use the fact that $\sqrt{3}$ is *approximately* equal to 1.732.

Figure 17-1 is a schematic diagram showing all categories of real numbers and how these numbers relate to each other. Real numbers can be broken down into two main groups, rational and irrational numbers. A good way to remember this concept is to relate it to people. People are real, and it just so happens that some are rational and some are irrational. Now, the rational group of numbers can be further divided into integers and nonintegers. The integers are the positive and negative whole numbers and zero. The nonintegers include numbers such as fractions, decimals, and square roots.

Addition of Signed Numbers

The main concept distinguishing arithmetic from algebra is the concept of negative numbers. Health care professionals often deal with negative values. Many equations used in the health professions do contain negative numbers or variables. Thus, when you begin to solve equations, you will need to have a thorough understanding of negative numbers.

As mentioned, all real numbers can be represented as points on the number line. Addition of **signed numbers** can be thought of as movement along the number line. Movement to the right indicates addition of a positive number, and movement to the left indicates addition of a negative number.

Examples:

$(+3) + (+2)$

Begin with $+3$ on the number line and move 2 units to the right.

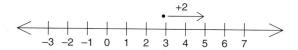

The result is $+5$, or 5.

$(+6) + (-4)$

Begin with $+6$ on the number line and move 4 units to the left.

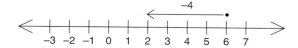

The result is $+2$, or 2.

When a number is written without a sign, it is thought of as a positive number. For example, $(+3) + (+2) = +5$ is the same as $3 + 2 = 5$.

Also, no two signs are ever written together without parentheses. For example, $6 + -4$ must be written $6 + (-4)$.

Example:

$(-3) + (-2)$

Begin with -3 on the number line and move 2 units to the left.

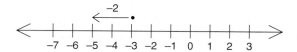

The result is -5.

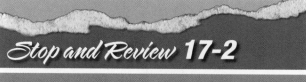

Stop and Review **17-2**

Add each of the following.

a. $(+2) + (+5)$

b. $(-2) + (-3)$

c. $(-3) + (-1)$

d. $(-3) + (+3)$

e. $(+2) + (-2)$

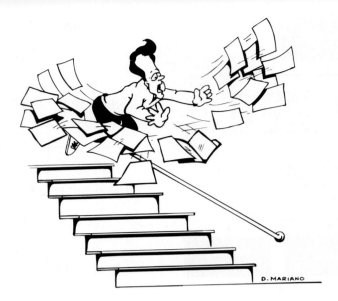

"In math, as in life, make sure you do all the steps."

Source: Delmar/Cengage Learning

Following, then, are rules for adding signed numbers:

- If the signs are the same, add the numbers and use the same sign.
- If the signs are opposite, subtract the numbers and use the sign of the larger number.

Examples:

$$(+3) + (+2) = +5$$
$$(+6) + (-4) = +(6 - 4) = +2 = 2$$
$$(-3) + (+2) = -(3 - 2) = -1$$

Subtraction of Signed Numbers

To subtract signed numbers, change to addition. All subtraction problems can be changed to addition problems. Subtraction can be thought of as addition of the opposite; that is, simply add the opposite of the number you would have subtracted. But what are opposite numbers? They are simply the same numbers with opposite signs.

Examples:

The opposite of $+2$ is -2.

The opposite of -3 is $+3$.

Remember, addition of opposite numbers always results in 0.

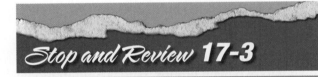

Stop and Review **17-3**

Find the opposite of each of the following.

a. -2

b. $+4$

So, to subtract signed numbers, add the opposite:

1st number $-$ 2nd number = 1st number $+$ opposite of 2nd number

Examples:

$$(+2) - (+4) = (+2) + (-4) = -2$$
$$(-3) - (-2) = (-3) + (+2) = -1$$
$$(+3) - (-4) = (+3) + (+4) = +7 = 7$$
$$(-1) - (+2) = (-1) + (-2) = -3$$
$$(-1) - (-3) = (-1) + (+3) = +2 = 2$$

Remember, no two signs are written together, so that $3 - -4$ should be written $(+3) - (-4)$.

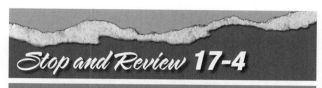

Stop and Review 17-4

Subtract each of the following.
a. $(+1) - (-3)$
b. $(-3) - (+2)$
c. $(-5) - (-1)$
d. $(+3) - (-2)$
e. $(-4) - (+1)$

Addition and Subtraction of Three or More Terms

To solve problems involving more than one addition or subtraction, remember to follow the order of operations and work from left to right.

Examples:

$(+2) - (+4) + (-3) - (-5)$

Subtract the first two terms $(+2) + (-4) = -2$;

The equation becomes $(-2) + (-3) - (-5)$;

Add the terms $(-2) + (-3) = -5$;

The equation becomes $(-5) - (-5)$;

Rewrite as $(-5) + (+5)$;

The answer is 0.

Now consider $2 - 3 + 5 - 6$.

$$-1 + 5 - 6$$
$$4 - 6$$
$$-2$$

Remember to write out all the steps so that you can check the solution! Use of this step-by-step system ensures that the problem is done quickly and correctly. It is necessary to develop and use this system on the simpler problems, so that when you encounter more complicated problems, you will already have a system in place.

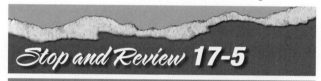

Stop and Review 17-5

Solve each of the following.
a. $(+2) - (-3) - (+2) + (-4)$
b. $3 - 6 + 2 - 1 + 7$

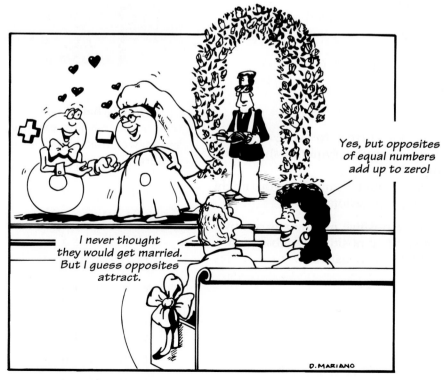

I never thought they would get married. But I guess opposites attract.

Yes, but opposites of equal numbers add up to zero!

D. MARIANO

Source: Delmar/Cengage Learning

Special Focus

Signed Numbers in the Health Care Field

Another reason why an understanding of signed numbers is important is because they are used in solving various equations in the health professions. For example, conversions between the Celsius and Fahrenheit temperature scales are often necessary in the health care field. The formulas for these conversions are as follows:

$$°C = \frac{5}{9}(F - 32) \quad °F = \frac{9}{5}C + 32$$

Suppose that you needed to convert $-20°C$ to degrees F. Performing this conversion requires addition and multiplication of signed numbers along with proper order of operations, in order to achieve the correct solution.

$$°F = \frac{9}{5}(-20) + 32$$
$$°F = -36 + 32 \quad °F = -4$$

To convert in the opposite direction (from Fahrenheit to Celsius), you would use the first equation. As with the first conversion, you must perform correct order of operations (i.e., simplify inside the parentheses first) to avoid getting the wrong temperature conversion.

Multiplication of Signed Numbers

Multiplication is actually repeated addition of the same number. Some different notations for the multiplication of the numbers 2 and 3 are as follows:

$$2 \times 3 \quad 2 \cdot 3 \quad (2)(3)$$

But what happens when a negative number is multiplied by a positive number? In light of the fact that multiplication is repeated addition, consider the following:

$$2 \times (-3) = (2)(-3) = (-3) + (-3) = -6$$

$$5 \times (-2) = (5)(-2)$$

$$= (-2) + (-2) + (-2) + (-2) + (-2) = -10$$

Remember, it is not correct to write 5×-2 because no two operation symbols should be written together.

From the preceding examples, you might draw the following conclusions:

- The product of positive numbers is positive.
- The product of a positive number and a negative number is negative.

Examples:

$$(2)(4) = 8$$
$$(-2)(5) = -10$$
$$(5)(-6) = -30$$
$$(-1)(6) = -6$$

Stop and Review 17-6

Multiply each of the following.

a. $(4)(-1)$

b. $(3)(6)$

c. $(-3)(4)$

d. $(5)(2)$

Now, what about the product of two negative numbers? For example, what is $(-2)(-3)$? To answer that question, consider the following pattern:

$$(3)(-3) = -9$$
$$(2)(-3) = -6$$
$$(1)(-3) = -3$$
$$(0)(-3) = 0$$

Notice that the product increases by 3 each time. Now consider the following pattern:

$$(-1)(-3) = 3$$
$$(-2)(-3) = 6$$
$$(-3)(-3) = 9$$

As the preceding pattern suggests, the product of two negative numbers is positive.

In summary, then, the rules for multiplication of signed numbers are as follows:

- If the signs are the same, the product is positive.
- If the signs are opposite, the product is negative.

It is important to remember not to confuse the rules for multiplication with the rules for addition and subtraction.

Examples:

$$(4)(-5) = -20$$
$$(-6)(-2) = 12$$
$$(5)(-5) = -25$$
$$(-3)(-1) = 3$$
$$(4)(-2) = -8$$

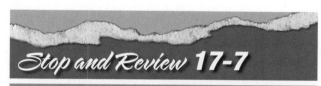

Stop and Review **17-7**

Multiply each of the following.

a. $(-1)(3)$
b. $(-5)(-2)$
c. $(3)(9)$
d. $(6)(-5)$
e. $(-7)(-3)$

Multiplication of Three or More Terms

To perform problems involving more than one multiplication, remember to follow the order of operations and work from left to right.

Example:

$$(2)(3)(-4)$$

Multiply the first two terms $(2)(3) = 6$;

The equation becomes $(6)(-4) = -24$;

The answer is -24.

$$(-2)(5)(-2)(-1)$$

Multiply the first two terms $(-2)(5) = -10$;

The equation becomes $(-10)(-2)(-1)$;

Multiply the second two terms $(-10)(-2) = 20$;

The equation becomes $(20)(-1) = -20$;

The answer is -20.

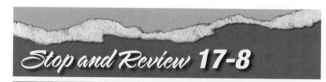

Stop and Review **17-8**

Multiply each of the following.

a. $(5)(-2)(-3)$
b. $(-6)(-4)(-1)(-2)$

Division of Signed Numbers

Division of signed numbers has rules the same as those for multiplication, namely:

- If the signs are the same, the answer is positive.
- If the signs are opposite, the answer is negative.

This is because division can be thought of as multiplication of the reciprocal.

Examples:

$$\frac{-4}{2} = -2$$
$$\frac{-6}{-3} = 2$$
$$\frac{10}{-2} = -5$$

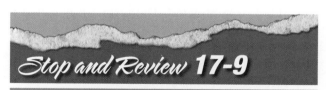

Stop and Review **17-9**

Divide each of the following.

a. $\dfrac{-6}{-2}$
b. $\dfrac{-16}{4}$
c. $\dfrac{9}{-3}$
d. $\dfrac{12}{2}$

Multiple Operations with Signed Numbers

The rules for signed numbers can be used along with the rules for order of operations to perform more complicated problems.

Example:

$$(-1)(-3) + \left(\frac{-8}{4}\right) - (-3)(4)$$
$$(+3) + (-2) - (-12)$$
$$1 - (-12)$$
$$1 + (+12) = 13$$

Problem Solving

Probably the most useful purpose of algebra is to solve problems wherein a quantity is allowed to vary.

Variable Expressions

In the formula $A = \frac{1}{2}bh$, A represents the area of a triangle, b represents the base, and h the height. Knowing the numerical values of two of these **variables**, the value of the unknown variable can be determined.

When letters are used to represent unknown quantities, they are called *variables*. Any expression containing variables is called a variable expression. For example,

$$3x - 2y + 7xy - 6$$

is called a variable expression containing variables x and y. This expression contains four quantities, which are added together: $3x$, $-2y$, $7xy$, and -6. These are called **terms**. *Terms* are quantities that are added or subtracted. The term -6 is called a *constant term*, or simply a *constant*, because it contains no variables and, therefore, cannot vary. The term $3x$ represents the product 3 times x, where the quantities 3 and x are called **factors**. *Factors* are quantities that are multiplied. The factor 3 is a special factor called a numerical coefficient, or simply **coefficient**.

Note: To represent the product of 3 times x, there is no need to use parentheses because $(3)(x) = 3x$. When using numbers such as 3 times 2, however, there is no choice but to use parentheses $(3)(2)$; otherwise, 32 would be written, which is not a product but, instead, represents the number thirty-two.

Example:

For the expression $4xy + y - 3$, identify the terms, the constant term, the factors of each variable term, and the coefficient of each variable term.

terms:	$4xy$, y, and -3
constant term:	-3
factors of $4xy$:	4, x, and y, with 4 the coefficient
factors of y:	y is the only factor, with 1 the coefficient

Note: When the coefficient is 1 or -1, it is not usually written because $1y = y$ and $-1y = -y$.

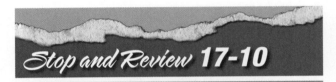

Stop and Review **17-10**

For the expression $4xy - x + 2y - 1$, identify the terms, the constant terms, the factors of each variable term, and the coefficient of each variable term.

Evaluating Variable Expressions

To evaluate variable expressions, replace the variables with the numbers they stand for. As always, be sure to use the proper order of operations.

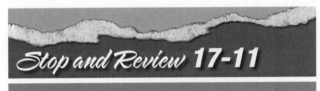

Stop and Review **17-11**

Evaluate $3(x + y) - 4x$ if $x = -2$ and $y = 1$.

Example:

Find $3(a - b) + 2ab$ if $a = -2$ and $b = 3$

$$3(-2 - 3) + 2(-2)(3)$$
$$3(-5) + 2(-2)(3)$$
$$-15 + 2(-2)(3)$$
$$-15 + (-4)(3)$$
$$-15 + (-12)$$
$$-27$$

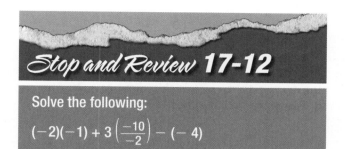

Stop and Review 17-12

Solve the following:

$$(-2)(-1) + 3\left(\frac{-10}{-2}\right) - (-4)$$

QUOTES & NOTES

René Descartes, a seventeenth-century mathematician, was the first to use letters to represent variables. A very sickly person, he spent much of his time in bed. He said that he did his most productive mathematical thinking in bed.

Diophantus, a Greek mathematician, developed the foundation of algebra in about the year 200. He is considered by many to be the father of algebra.

StudyWARE) CONNECTION

Go to your StudyWARE™ DVD to view a video on **Pulse and Pulse Rates**.

Clinical Relevancy

Variables in the Health Care Field

The vital sign of pulse, or heart rate, can be a very important variable in many equations used in the health professions. Just what is a pulse? Each time the heart pumps, it generates a "wave" of pressure within the arterial system of blood vessels. This wave of pressure is what we palpate, or feel, when we take someone's pulse.

A pulse should be taken either for 30 seconds and multiplied by 2, or for 1 full minute. The normal pulse for an adult ranges from 60 to 100 beats per minute.

Not only can you quantify a pulse, but you can also qualify, or describe, it. You can describe the force, or quality, of a pulse. Is it very weak and hard to find? This sometimes is called a *thready pulse*. Is it bounding, or very forceful? Is it present at all? If not, the situation may call for cardiopulmonary resuscitation (CPR).

Many factors affect pulse rate, including physical activity, emotion, fever, disease, and drugs. Some clinical conditions may cause the heart to beat more quickly than is normal (*tachycardia*). These include fever and severe anemia. Anemia means low hemoglobin (Hb) levels. Hemoglobin is the material needed to transport oxygen to the tissues. You can think of Hb as buses that transport oxygen to the tissues, muscles, brain, and elsewhere throughout the body. If we have fewer buses (anemia), we need to get the buses we do have moving faster in order to maintain the delivery system. (Hemoglobin is discussed in greater detail in the Chemistry section.)

There are also conditions that can cause the heart to beat more slowly than is normal (*bradycardia*), such as when the heart muscle is not receiving proper electrical signals to beat, or when there is insufficient oxygen in the blood to fuel the heart to be able to beat normally. This latter condition is called severe hypoxemia. Breaking this word down means less than normal (*hypo*) levels of oxygen (*oxy*) in the blood (*emia*).

After you have determined a patient's pulse, you can use this "variable" to ascertain other valuable information. One such piece of information is cardiac output (CO), or the total amount of blood pumped from the heart per minute. Cardiac output can be determined using a simple equation. Two factors that affect CO are how fast the heart is beating (i.e., heart rate, or pulse) and the amount of blood the heart ejects each time it beats (known as *stroke volume*). The equation that relates these variables, then, is:

$$C.O. = rate \times stroke\ volume$$

The normal cardiac output is 6 liters/minute.

Simplifying Variable Expressions

In algebra, variable expressions that can be written in simpler forms are often encountered. For example, can $2x + 3x$ be added and, thus, simplified? The answer is "yes," as long as they are similar. In mathematics, **similar terms** are terms that have the exact same variables, so that $2x + 3x = 5x$ is much like 2 apples plus 3 apples equals 5 apples. And as everyone knows, an apple a day keeps the doctor away. However, $2x + 3y$ cannot be added because they are not similar terms; it would be like trying to add 2 apples and 3 oranges.

Examples:

In each of the three variable expressions following, which terms are similar to 3x?

$$4x - 6y - 3x + 4y$$

$4x$ and $-3x$ are similar to $3x$

$$3x - 6x + 2x + y$$

$3x$, $-6x$ and $2x$ are similar to $3x$

$$3xy + 4y - 6x + 7$$

only $-6x$ is similar to 3x

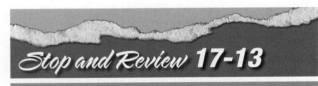

Stop and Review **17-13**

In each of the following variable expressions, which terms are similar to 4y?

a. $3x - 7y + 6x + 2y$

b. $3xy + 4y - 3$

Addition of Variable Terms

To add variable terms, use the rules for addition of signed numbers, add the coefficients, and keep the same variable factor.

Examples:

$$4x - 3x = (4 - 3)x = 1x = x$$
$$-6y + 4y = (-6 + 4)y = -2y$$
$$3x - 6x + 2x = (3 - 6 + 2)x =$$
$$(-3 + 2)x = -1x = -x$$

$$4x - 6y - 3x + 4y = (4 - 3)x + (-6 + 4)y$$
$$= x - 2y$$

The order in which two numbers are added does not matter, so x − 2y is the same as −2y + x.

Example:

$$3x - 6x + 2x + y = (3 - 6 + 2)x + y$$
$$= (-3 + 2)x$$
$$= -1x + y$$
$$= -x + y, \text{ or } y - x$$

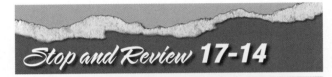

Stop and Review **17-14**

Add each of the following variable expressions.

a. $2x - 3y + 7x + 3y$

b. $2x - 4x + 7y + 2y$

c. $2a - 2b - 6ab + 7a$

Distributive Law

One last rule often used in simplifying variable expressions is the **distributive law** of multiplication over addition. As an illustration, to simplify $2(3 + 4)$, you would use the order of operations (parentheses first) to get $2(7) = 14$. Notice, however, that

$$2(\overset{\frown}{3 + 4}) = (2 \times 3) + (2 \times 4) = 6 + 8 = 14$$

The result is no coincidence. The 3 and the 4 inside the parentheses can each be multiplied by the 2 in front and the results added.

Thus, the distributive law is

$$a(\overset{\frown}{b + c}) = ab + ac$$

Example:

Evaluate $2(\overset{\frown}{4 - 5})$

Using the order of operations:

$$2(4 - 5) = 2(-1) = -2$$

Which is the same result using the distributive law:

$$2(4 - 5) = (2)(4) - (2)(5) = 8 - 10 = -2$$

The distributive law is especially helpful in working with variable expressions.

Example:

Rewrite $2(x - 3)$

$2(x - 3) = 2x - 6$

To remove parentheses when immediately preceded by a negative sign, change the sign of each term inside the parentheses.

Example:

$-(3x - 4)$

$-(3x - 4) = -1(3x - 4)$

$-3x + 4 \; or \; 4 - 3x$

In the preceding example, notice that the coefficient of -1 is not written. Remember, the order in which two numbers are added does not matter.

Example:

$-(2x - 4) = -2x + 4 \; or \; 4 - 2x$

$-(1 - x) = -1 + x \; or \; x - 1$

$-(a - 2) = -a + 2 \; or \; 2 - a$

When the parentheses are preceded by a $+1$, there is no change in sign because multiplying by 1 does not change the value of a quantity.

Example:

$(2x - 4) = 2x - 4$

$(-x + 1) = -x + 1$

As can be seen in the preceding example, when the coefficient is $+1$, there is no change, so the parentheses are simply removed.

From Words to Algebra

The main reason for introducing variable expressions is to solve problems written in words. Years ago, these were called *statement problems* and were generally considered to be extremely challenging. More recently, they have been called *word problems*, which makes it sound like they are not as difficult. To make them sound really easy, they might be called *story problems*. But don't be

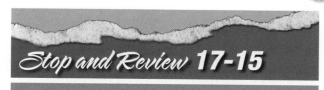

Stop and Review 17-15

Remove the parentheses on each of the following variable expressions.

a. $2(x - 2)$

b. $4(2x + 1)$

c. $-2(3a - 5)$

d. $-(x + 1)$

e. $-(2 - a)$

f. $(t + 3)$

fooled; they are the same no matter what they are called.

In the health care professions, word or story problems are solved daily. Many make use of given formulas, where patients are assessed and data is collected and substituted as variables in the formulas. The resulting answers may help to properly diagnose or treat the patients.

The most difficult part of solving word problems is to translate the words into variable expressions. Table 17-1 lists some phrases with corresponding operations and variable expressions to help you in this process. As you will note

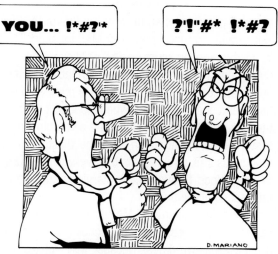

Can you translate these words and expressions?

TABLE 17-1

Phrases with Corresponding Operations and Variable Expressions

OPERATION	PHRASE	VARIABLE EXPRESSION
Addition	3 *added to x*	$3 + x$ or $x + 3$
	4 *more than y*	$4 + y$ or $y + 4$
	t *increased by 3*	$t + 3$
	the total of a and b	$a + b$
Subtraction	2 *less than x*	$x - 2$
	4 *subtracted from y*	$y - 4$
	t *decreased by 1*	$t - 1$
Multiplication	3 *times x*	$3x$
	6 *multiplied by y*	$6y$
	the product of 2 and w	$2w$
Division	*x divided by 3*	$\dfrac{x}{3}$
	the quotient of a and 2	$\dfrac{a}{2}$
	the ratio of w and 5	$\dfrac{w}{5}$

Stop and Review **17-16**

Write a variable expression for each of the following phrases.

a. 3 more than x

b. the product of 2 and y

c. 7 less than w

d. x divided by 7

e. a patient's temperature, t, increased by 4

f. 15 less than a pressure, p

g. double the rate of flow, r, increased by 2

while studying this table, similar phrasing is used over and over in word problems. For this reason, the more word problems you do, the better you will get at doing them!

Clinical Relevancy

Mean Arterial Pressure (MAP)

Blood pressure is a very important vital sign. A variation of blood pressure often used in the Intensive Care Unit is the mean arterial pressure, or MAP for short. The MAP is an average pressure in the cardiovascular system during one full cardiac cycle. A cardiac cycle includes one heart contraction (when blood is pumped out of the heart) and one rest period (when blood fills the heart for the next cycle). The MAP reading is a combination of the systolic (heart contraction) and the diastolic (heart at rest) pressures. It represents the average pressure used to drive blood through the systemic circulation and to the tissues of the body.

Physicians often use MAP to determine whether a patient's blood pressure is responding to administered drugs (vasoactive drugs). Because MAP relates to blood flow to the tissues, the patient's oxygen delivery status can be monitored. How do you determine MAP? The equation uses variables and order of operations that we previously discussed and is as follows:

$$MAP = \frac{(2 \times \text{diastolic pressure}) + \text{systolic pressure}}{3}$$

This equation can be shortened using variables to the following form:

$$MAP = \frac{2d + s}{3}$$

If a patient's systolic pressure is 125 mm Hg (millimeters of mercury) and his diastolic pressure is 80 mm Hg, what is his MAP? Substituting these variables into the equation, you get:

$$MAP = \frac{2(80) + 125}{3}$$

The solution: 95 mm Hg is the mean arterial pressure.

■ CHAPTER REVIEW

Exercises

1. Simplify each of the following.

a. $5 - 8 \div 2$

b. $16 + 3 \times 5$

c. $21 - (3 + 4) + 4^2$

d. $(2 + 6)^2 - 6^2$

2. Simplify each of the following.

a. $4(8) + (3 - 2)^3$

b. $(4 - 7)^2 + (2)^3$

c. $\dfrac{16 + 2}{12 - 3} + (5)^2$

3. Find the MAP for each of the following patient pressures.

a. systolic 120 mm Hg, diastolic 70 mm Hg

b. systolic 160 mm Hg, diastolic 95 mm Hg

4. Add each of the following.

a. $(+2) + (-7)$

b. $(+3) + (+5)$

c. $(7) + (-4)$

d. $(-6) + (+9)$

e. $(-3) + (-8)$

f. $(-2) + (-4)$

5. Subtract each of the following.

a. $(+2) - (-7)$

b. $(+3) - (+5)$

c. $(7) - (-4)$

d. $(-6) - (+9)$

e. $(-3) - (-8)$

f. $(-2) - (-4)$

6. Simplify each of the following.

a. $3 - 2 + 1$

b. $7 - 10 - 5$

c. $5 - 6 - 2$

d. $3 - (-1) + 6$

e. $4 - 7 - 3$

f. $-2 + (-6) - 1$

7. A dieter had the following weight gains and losses for 6 months: gained 2.3 lb, lost 1.2 lb, lost 2.2 lb, lost 0.2 lb, gained 1.1 lb, and lost 1.0 lb. Does this dieter weigh more or less than when he or she began the diet?

8. Multiply each of the following.

a. $(-3)(3)$

b. $(6)(2)$

c. $(-4)(-1)$

d. $(-2)(-10)$

e. $(-7)(2)$

f. $(-1)(17)$

9. Divide each of the following.

   a. $\dfrac{16}{-4}$

   b. $\dfrac{-12}{-3}$

   c. $\dfrac{-25}{5}$

   d. $\dfrac{18}{-9}$

   e. $\dfrac{12}{-6}$

   f. $\dfrac{-14}{-7}$

10. Simplify each of the following.

    a. $3 - 4(-2) + (-3)$

    b. $(-7)(2) - (6 - 2) - (-1)$

    c. $(6 - 12)^2 - \left(\dfrac{12}{-3}\right)$

11. Identify the terms, factors, and coefficients for each of the following variable terms.

    a. $3xy + 2x$

    b. $6x - 7y + 2$

    c. $3xy + x - 1$

12. Evaluate each of the following variable expressions using the given values.

    a. $2(a - b) + 3a$, if $a = 2$ and $b = 1$

    b. $7(x + y - 1) - 2xy$, if $x = 5$ and $y = 1$

    c. $x - 2(x + y) - 2y$, if $x = -1$ and $y = 3$

13. In each of the following variable expressions, identify the terms that are similar to $6x$.

    a. $4x + 7y - 6$

    b. $3xy + 2x - 4y - 3x + 2$

    c. $x + 3a - 3x + 7$

14. In each of the following variable expressions, identify the terms that are similar to $-7y$.

    a. $4x + 7y - 6$

    b. $3xy + 2x - 4y + 2y - 3$

    c. $x + 3y - y + 7$

15. Simplify each of the following variable expressions.

    a. $6x + 4x + 7y - 6$

    b. $6x + 3xy + 2x$

    c. $6x + x - 3x + 3a + 7$

16. Use the distributive law to remove the parentheses in each of the following variable expressions.

    a. $2(x + y)$

    b. $-2(x + 1)$

    c. $-3(x - 5)$

    d. $-4(3x + 2)$

    e. $-2(x - 4)$

17. Remove the parentheses and simplify each of the following variable expressions.

    a. $2(x + y) + 6x$

    b. $-2(x + 1) - 5$

    c. $-(3x + 2) + 4x$

    d. $-2(x - 4) + 7x - 1$

18. Write a variable expression for each of the following.

    a. x added to 5

    b. 7 more than y

    c. p increased by 10

    d. 4 less than m

    e. x decreased by 1

    f. the product of 3 and x

    g. 7 times x

    h. y divided by 2

    i. the ratio of z and 7

19. Write a variable expression for each of the following:

    a. 40% of a number, n

    b. 25% of a temperature, t

    c. one-half of a length, l

    d. a normal temperature of 98.6 degrees, increased by x

    e. the number of calories in p packets, if each packet has 200 calories

20. A patient's temperature was taken at the beginning of the day. The initial temperature was 99 degrees and throughout the day it: increased by 3 degrees, decreased by 4 degrees, increased by 6 degrees, decreased by 2 degrees, and decreased by 4 degrees. What was the temperature at the end of the day?

21. A patient's temperature was taken at the beginning of the day. The initial temperature was 98 degrees and throughout the day it: increased by 1 degree, decreased by 3 degrees, increased by 4 degrees, decreased by 2 degrees, and increased by 3 degrees. What was the temperature at the end of the day?

Real Life Issues and Applications

A Medical Equation

A pulmonologist has asked you to determine the amount of oxygen a patient is receiving at the alveolar level. This value is known as the PAO_2 (pressure of alveolar oxygen). The equation to determine the PAO_2 is:

$$(P_B - P_{H_2O})\, FIO_2 - PaCO_2\,(1.25), \text{ where}$$

P_B = the barometric pressure

P_{H_2O} = the pressure of water vapor in the air

FIO_2 = the amount of oxygen inspired

$PaCO_2$ = the pressure of carbon dioxide in the artery

You obtain the following data:

P_B = 760 mm Hg

P_{H_2O} = 47 mm Hg

FIO_2 = 0.50

$PaCO_2$ = 40 mm Hg

Determine the patient's PAO_2.

Additional Activity

A major factor in the efficient diagnosis and treatment of disease is obtaining a good patient history to determine the many variables that can affect patient health. A patient history can be obtained via a formal or informal interview with the patient and should include pertinent variables such as:

- age
- height
- gender
- the reason the patient is seeking medical help
- weight
- history of past illness
- family history of illness
- current medical complaint
- allergies
- smoking history
- work history

Sometimes this information is offered freely by the patient; other times you need to do your detective work.

For best results, it is important to try to put the patient at ease. A proper introduction and statement of purpose (e.g., "Hello, Mr. Smith, I'm John Doe from the _____ department and I'm here to talk with you about your medical past"), along with a pleasant tone of voice and positive nonverbal communication (eye contact, posture, hand gestures), can help you get a useful patient history. The only way to get good at this is to practice, practice, practice!

In order to learn this technique, practice with a partner. One of you will be the patient and the other will be the health care professional. First, the "patient" creates a patient history, writing it down on a piece of paper. Then, the "health care professional" conducts an interview to obtain the patient's history. When the interview is over, compare notes with your partner. How close did the interviewer come to obtaining complete and correct information? What could the interviewer have done to obtain a better patient history? Now switch roles and see how the new interviewer does. Discuss your findings with the class.

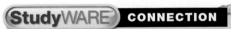

StudyWARE CONNECTION

Go to your StudyWARE™ DVD and have fun learning as you play interactive games, view animations and videos, and take practice tests to help reinforce key concepts you learned in this chapter.

Workbook Practice   *Go to your Workbook for more practice questions and activities.*

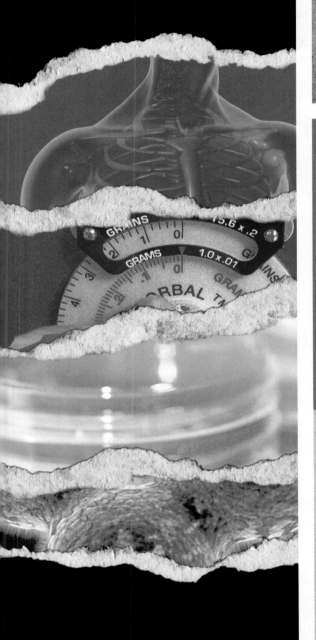

CHAPTER 18

AN INTRODUCTION TO EQUATIONS

Objectives

Upon completion of this chapter, you should be able to

- Determine whether a given value is a solution to an equation

- Solve equations of the form $x + a = b$

- Solve equations of the form $cx = b$

- Solve equations of the form $cx + a = b$

- Solve equations of the form $ax + b = cx + d$

- Solve equations having parentheses

Key Terms

constant
equation
solutions to equations

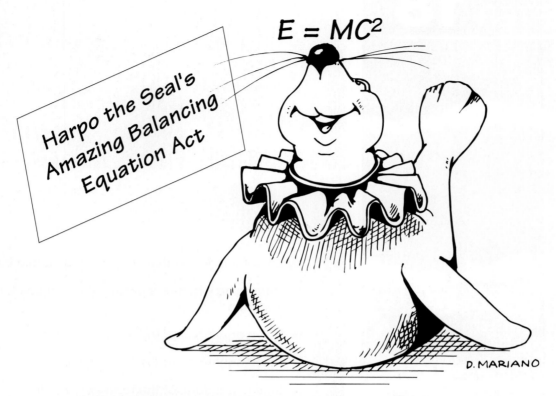

$$E = MC^2$$

Harpo the Seal's Amazing Balancing Equation Act

D. MARIANO

EINSTEIN'S MATHEMATICAL CIRCUS.

Source: Delmar/Cengage Learning

■ INTRODUCTION

In the health care field, there are many types of **equations** that must be solved and understood in order to diagnose and treat patients. Many students have difficulty in the health professions because they do not understand what an equation is or how to solve it. Obviously, attempting to apply a concept you do not understand can be overwhelming. The purpose of this chapter, therefore, is to take the mystery out of solving basic equations.

Equations

One of the main reasons for a discussion of algebraic expressions is to reach the next step, which is solving equations.

Testing Solutions

An equation is a statement that two expressions are equal on either side of the "equal sign." For example,

$$x - 2 = 6$$

$$3x = 12$$

$$F = ma$$

Think back to Chapter 17 and the mean arterial pressure equation: $MAP = \dfrac{(2 \times diasolic) + systolic}{3}$

The preceding may seem like, and indeed are, different types of equations. Yet, they are all solved using the same basic techniques. When you become comfortable in solving basic equations, you will be able to find the correct answer no matter what form the equation takes.

By the end of the next two chapters you should realize that the equations where MAP = M, diastolic pressure = d, and systolic pressure = s

$$M = \frac{2d + s}{3}, \ d = \frac{3M - s}{2}, \ and \ s = 3M - 2d$$

are equivalent to one another, and all represent relationships between mean arterial, diastolic, and systolic pressures.

In other words, you can isolate and solve for any variable.

There is an old adage that questions, "Is it better to give a poor man a fish, or teach him how to fish?" Of course, simply giving him the fish will satisfy his immediate hunger; but he will soon again be hungry. If you teach him how to fish, on the other hand, he will never be hungry again. Similarly, it is better to understand how to solve equations in a general sense, and thereby "feed yourself," than it is to be dependent on someone else should an unfamiliar equation come along. If you learn the basics of solving equations, they will all become familiar.

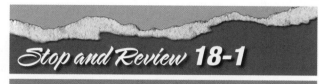

Stop and Review **18-1**

For each of the following, determine whether the given value is a solution.

a. Is 2 a solution to $x + 6 = 8$?

b. Is -3 a solution to $4t = -12$?

c. Is 5 a solution to $2y + 4 = 10$?

QUOTES & NOTES

In the sixteenth century, Robert Recorde introduced the equal sign that we use today. He used two parallel lines because he felt that no two things can be more equal than a pair of parallel line segments.

A **solution to an equation** is a value which when substituted into the equation results in a true statement. A solution, then, is a value that "satisfies" the equation. For example, is 8 a solution to $x - 2 = 6$? When 8 is substituted in for x, the equation $8 - 2 = 6$ results. This is obviously a true statement; that is, 8 "satisfies" the equation. Remember, if the resulting statement is true, then the value substituted is a solution.

Examples:

Is -2 a solution to $3x = 6$? The answer is no, because $3(-2)$ is equal to -6 not $+6$; the value of -2 does not "satisfy" the equation.

Is 1 a solution to $3t + 2 = 4(t + 1)$? Substituting 1 for t gives you

$$3(1) + 2 = 4(1 + 1), \text{ or}$$
$$3 + 2 = 4(2), \text{ or}$$
$$5 = 8$$

This statement is not true; therefore, 1 is not a solution to this equation.

Equations of the Form $x + a = b$

In the preceding section, we saw that 8 is a solution to the equation $x - 2 = 6$. The equations $x - 2 = 6$ and $x = 8$ have the same solution; that is, 8. These equations are said to be equivalent because they have the same solution. The form $x = 8$ is the simplest form of the equation; that is

the *variable = constant* form. In this form of equation, the solution is the **constant**; the variable is always isolated on one side. In fact, solving an equation always requires rewriting the equation to yield the *variable = constant* form. This isolates the variable and gives it a constant value.

Now, how can you solve for this *variable = constant* form? An equation is much like the seesaw found on a playground. In order for it to balance, the same weight must be placed on each side. If the seesaw is to remain balanced, the weight on both sides must always be equal. If a weight is added to one side, the same weight must be added to the other side. If the same weights are added to both sides the seesaw will remain balanced. An equation has a similar property, in that it is meant to be balanced. Adding (or subtracting) the same number to both sides of an equation produces an equivalent equation; in this way, the equation remains balanced.

In the problem $x - 2 = 6$, if you add 2 to both sides, you get:

$$x - 2 + 2 = 6 + 2$$

The number 2, the opposite of -2, was chosen so that $-2 + 2 = 0$. Notice that this allows the variable x to be all by itself on one side. Now the equation reads $x = 8$. Thus, to solve an equation of this form, always choose the opposite constant term.

Example:

Solve the equation $x - 3 = 4$

Because $+3$ is the opposite of -3, add $+3$ to both sides.

$$x - 3 + 3 = 4 + 3$$
$$x = 7$$

The solution is 7.

Always be sure to substitute your solution into the original equation to check whether it yields a true statement. In the preceding example, $7 - 3 = 4$; so the solution is correct.

Example:

Solve the equation $t + 5 = 7$

Because -5 is the opposite of $+5$, add -5 to both sides.

$$t + 5 - 5 = 7 - 5$$
$$t = 2$$

The solution is 2. Be sure to check the solution.

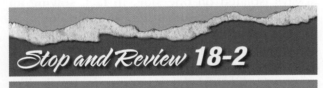

Stop and Review **18-2**

Solve each of the following equations.

a. $x - 2 = 3$

b. $x + 5 = 3$

c. $y - 4 = 1$

d. $a + 3 = -1$

Equations of the Form $cx = b$

As was previously mentioned, equations can take various forms; but they can all be solved using the same principles, or rules. From the previous discussion, you know that an equation is like a balanced seesaw. If three students of equal size were sitting on one side of the seesaw, and three weights of 100 pounds each (i.e., 300 pounds total) were on the other side, then each student must weigh 100 pounds in order for the seesaw to balance. Again, an equation is similar to a seesaw. The equations $3x = 300$ and $x = 100$ are equivalent equations because they each have the solution 100.

The second rule for solving equations states that multiplying or dividing an equation by the same nonzero number produces an equivalent equation.

Example:

Solve the equation $3x = 300$

Divide both sides by 3
$$\frac{3x}{3} = \frac{300}{3}$$
$$x = 100$$

The solution is 100.

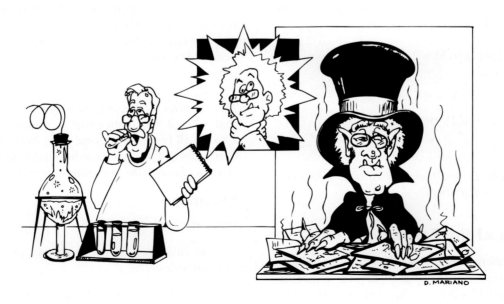

D. MARIANO

Always be sure to check your solution!

Source: Delmar/Cengage Learning

Clinical Relevancy

Equations in the Health Care Field

Tidal volume (V_T) is the normal amount of air you breathe in when you are at rest. Not all of this air is involved in the gas exchange in your lungs, however. Gas exchange means adding oxygen to your blood and removing excess carbon dioxide from your system. The amount of gas utilized during gas exchange is known as *alveolar volume* (V_A), because true gas exchange occurs in the little lung sacs called *alveoli*.

Not all of the air that is breathed in at the end of an inspiration makes it down to the alveoli. A portion of this air remains in the large conducting airways such as the trachea and right and left mainstem bronchi. Because this volume of gas is not involved in gas exchange, it is called *deadspace volume* (V_D).

From the preceding definitions, then, we can infer that the total volume of air breathed in at rest (V_T) is equal to the sum of the volume of air that remains in the airways (V_D) and the volume of the air in the alveoli (V_A), which exchanges gas with your blood. Mathematically, this is represented as follows:

$$V_T = V_D + V_A$$

Understanding this formula allows us to determine any of the unknown values as long as we know the other two.

As an example, consider the following: Patient Smith has a tidal volume (V_T) of 800 cc, and we know his deadspace volume (V_D) is 150 cc. What is the volume of gas that is involved in gas exchange at the alveolar level (V_A) during each breath?

Given: $V_T = 800$ *cc*

$$V_D = 150 \text{ } cc$$
$$V_A = \text{ ?}$$

If $V_T = V_D + V_A$ then $800 = 150 + V_A$
Add -150 cc to both sides:

$$800 - 150 = 150 - 150 + V_A$$

$$650 = V_A$$

The solution: 650 cc
Checking: $800 = 150 + 650$
So, 650 cc of each 800 cc breath is involved with gas exchange.

Remember, the objective is *always* to get the equation to the *variable = constant* form. In the preceding example, x is the variable and 100 the constant, so the objective is achieved.

Examples:

Solve the equation $7x = 35$

Divide both sides by 7

$$\frac{7x}{7} = \frac{35}{7}$$
$$x = 5$$

The solution is 5. Be sure to check the solution.

Solve the equation $\frac{y}{5} = 2$

Multiply both sides by 5

$$\frac{y}{5} \times 5 = 2 \times 5$$
$$y = 10$$

The solution is 10. Be sure to check the solution.

Solve the equation $\frac{3x}{2} = 9$

Multiply both sides by 2 to eliminate the fractions

$$\frac{3x}{2} \times 2 = 9 \times 2$$

Divide both sides by 3

$$3x = 18$$
$$x = 6$$

The solution is 6. Be sure to check the solution.

The formula $F = ma$ occurs in physics. If $F = 128$ and $a = -32$, find m.

Substitute the values for F and a

$$128 = m\,(-32)$$

Divide both sides by -32

$$\frac{128}{-32} = \frac{m(-32)}{-32}$$

$$-4 = m$$

The solution is -4. Be sure to check the solution.

    While the solution to the last equation in the preceding example may not mean anything to you, and the units for F, m, and a were not provided, none of these things matter at this point. The important thing right now is to see how easy it is to solve equations. To understand the relationship between F, m, and a, and what each represents, it is important to be able to solve equations.

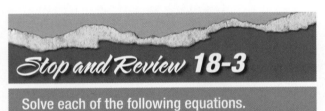

Stop and Review 18-3

Solve each of the following equations.

a. $4x = -8$

b. $3t = 15$

c. $\frac{x}{3} = 2$

d. $\frac{3z}{4} = 6$

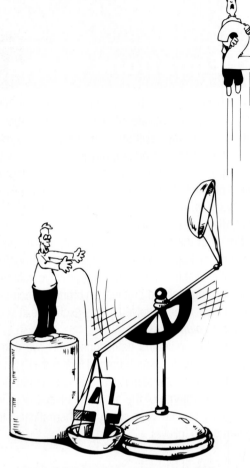

THE CONSEQUENCES OF AN UNBALANCED EQUATION.

Source: Delmar/Cengage Learning

Special Focus

Health Care Equations of the Form $cx = b$

The equation for determining cardiac output (CO) is one example of the $cx = b$ equation form. Taking a patient's pulse can provide another example. We normally determine a patient's pulse by counting the number of heartbeats (HB) during a 60-second period. Let's assume that patient Smith had 75 HB during a 60-second period. It would then be said that patient Smith had a pulse, or heart rate (HR), of 75 bpm (beats per minute). If a patient has a normal, regular pulse, you may count the number of HB during a 30-second time period and multiply that number by 2 to get your patient's HR. The equation would look like this:

$$HB \ (per \ 30 \ seconds) \times 2 = HR$$

So, if patient Brown had an HR of 70 beats per minute, what was her HR for a 30-second time period?

$$HB \times 2 = HR$$

So, substituting for HR, the equation becomes $HB \times 2 = 70$. Dividing both sides by 2

$$\frac{HB \times 2}{2} = \frac{70}{2}$$

Her HB was 35 beats per 30-second time period.

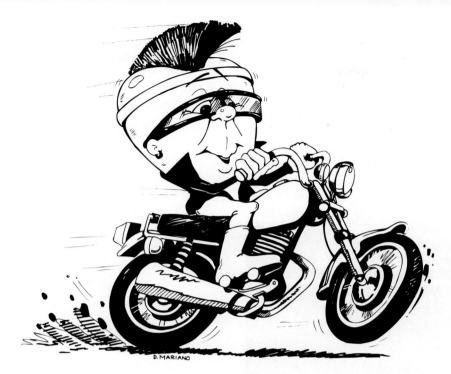

This is not the cardiac cycle we're talking about.

Source: Delmar/Cengage Learning

Equations of the Form $cx + a = b$

The next step in learning to solve equations is to consider equations of the form $cx + a = b$. Remember, as always, the objective is to isolate the variable so that the equation takes the *variable = constant* form.

The first step is to isolate the variable by adding the opposite of a to both sides. Then, solve for the variable as is done in solving equations of the form $cx = b$.

Examples:

Solve the equation $2x + 3 = 5$

Because -3 is the opposite of $+3$, add -3 to both sides.

$$2x + 3 + (-3) = 5 + (-3)$$
$$2x = 2$$

Divide both sides by 2

$$\frac{2x}{2} = 2$$
$$x = 1$$

The solution is 1. Be sure to check the solution.

Solve the equation $4x - 7 = 5$

Because $+7$ is the opposite of -7, add $+7$ to both sides.

$$4x - 7 + 7 = 5 + 7$$
$$4x = 12$$

Divide both sides by 4

$$\frac{4x}{4} = \frac{12}{4}$$
$$x = 3$$

The solution is 3. Be sure to check the solution.

In physics you might encounter the equation $v = 32t + 10$. The v represents the velocity of an object thrown into the air under certain conditions. Find t when $v = 106$.

Substitute the value of 106 for v

$$106 = 32t + 10$$

Because -10 is the opposite of $+10$, add -10 to both sides.

$$106 + (-10) = 32t + 10 + (-10)$$
$$96 = 32t$$

Divide both sides by 32 to isolate t

$$\frac{96}{32} = \frac{32t}{32}$$

$3 = t$ or $t = 3$

The solution is 3. Be sure to check the solution.

Although continually saying "check the solution" may sound like a broken record, this is a crucial habit to develop—it may someday save a life.

Stop and Review 18-4

Solve each of the following equations.

a. $3x + 5 = 11$

b. $4z + 9 = -1$

c. $3 - 2x = 7$

d. $2 - 7x = -5$

Equations of the Form $ax + b = cx + d$

To solve an equation of the form $ax + b = cx + d$, rewrite the equation in the *variable* = *constant* form. Once again, begin with the process of isolating the variable by adding the variable term to both sides of the equation; then, combine the variable terms and solve as for other equation forms.

Examples:

Solve the equation $4x - 3 = 2x + 5$

Add $-2x$ to both sides

$$4x - 3 - 2x = 2x - 2x + 5$$

$$2x - 3 = 5$$

Add $+3$ to both sides

$$2x - 3 + 3 = 5 + 3$$

$$2x = 8$$

Divide both sides by 2

$$\frac{2x}{2} = \frac{8}{2}$$

$$x = 4$$

The solution is 4. Be sure to check the solution.

Solve the equation $6d - 5 = 2d + 3$

Add $-2d$ to both sides

$$6d - 2d - 5 = 2d - 2d + 3$$

$$4d - 5 = 3$$

Special Focus

Health Care Equations of the Form $cx = b$

People come in all sizes. Even for a given height, you will find underweight people, average-weight people, and overweight people. There may come a time in your career when you need to know the ideal body weight (IBW) of a patient. For example, IBW is used in determining drug dosages and determining many types of individualized settings for medical equipment and treatments. The following formula is used to calculate the IBW for a female:

$IBW = 105 + ($*height in inches* $- 60)(5)$

Find the IBW for a woman who is 65 in. tall.

$IBW = 105 + (65 - 60)(5)$

$IBW = 105 + (5)(5)$

$IBW = 105 + 25$

$IBW = 130$

To find the IBW for a male, use the following equation:

$IBW = 106 + ($*height in inches* $- 60)(6)$

If a male patient is 65 in. tall, what is his IBW? The correct answer is 136 lb.

Add +5 to both sides

$$4d - 5 + 5 = 3 + 5$$
$$4d = 8$$

Divide both sides by 4

$$\frac{4d}{4} = \frac{8}{4}$$
$$d = 2$$

The solution is 2, which will check upon substitution.

Equations with Parentheses

If an equation involves parentheses, first remove the parentheses, and then solve as before. Use the distributive law to remove parentheses. Remember that, for example, $2(x + 5) = 2x + 10$

Example:

Solve the equation $2(x + 5) = 14$

Distribute the 2

$$2x + 10 = 14$$

Add −10 to both sides

$$2x + 10 + (-10) = 14 + (-10)$$
$$2x = 4$$
$$x = 2$$

The solution is 2. Be sure to check the solution.

Stop and Review 18-5

Solve each of the following equations.

a. $4x + 3 = 3x + 4$

b. $7x - 10 = 3x + 8$

c. $9x + 2 = 8x - 1$

Clinical Relevancy

Revisiting Mean Arterial Pressure (MAP)

In Chapter 17 you learned about mean arterial pressure, or MAP for short. Again, mean arterial pressure is nothing more than the average pressure in the cardiovascular system during one full cardiac cycle. A cardiac cycle includes one heart contraction (when blood is pumped out of the heart and into the body) and one rest period for the heart (when blood fills the heart for the next cycle).

The MAP reading is a combination of the systolic (heart-at-work) and the diastolic (heart-at-rest) pressures. It represents the average pressure used to drive blood to the systemic circulation and to the tissues of the body. (Mean stands for "average"; this is discussed further in Chapter 20.)

Here again is the formula for determining MAP:

$$MAP = \frac{(2 \times diasolic) + systolic}{3}$$

This equation can be shortened to the following form:

$$M = \frac{2d + s}{3}$$

To show you that you can solve for any variable in this equation, what if you know the MAP is 95 mm Hg, and the systolic pressure is 125 mm Hg, and you are asked to determine the diastolic pressure? Because an equation must be balanced, the result should be 80 mm Hg. The equation becomes

$$95 = \frac{2d + 125}{3}$$

Multiply both sides by 3 to eliminate the fraction

$$2d + 125 = 285$$

Add −125 to both sides to get

$$2d = 160$$

Divide by 2 in order to isolate the variable

$$d = 80$$

Thus, the diastolic pressure is 80 mm Hg.

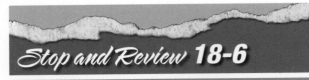

Stop and Review 18-6

Solve each of the following equations.

a. $3(t + 4) = 27$

b. $3(x - 3) = x - 1$

Professional Profile

Nursing

One of the well-known health professions is undoubtedly nursing. There are several levels of nurses. The licensed practical nurse (LPN) deals directly in the care of sick people. These nurses possess technical knowledge but have limited education and training. Their focus is mainly bedside care: They take patients' temperatures and other vital signs; check and change dressings on wounds or injured areas; assist in feedings; and, depending on the state, administer prescribed medication, assist in diagnostic and laboratory procedures, give injections, and start intravenous fluids. Education programs for LPNs take from 12 to 24 months to complete.

The registered nurse (RN) also provides care for patients; but these nurses are more involved with the "total person." This means that they care for patients on a psychological and emotional as well as physiological level. In addition, RNs often are involved in the supervisory and administrative aspects of health care organizations, which means that they have more responsibilities. Educational requirements for RNs are more extensive than are those for LPNs. Registered nurse programs vary in length from 2 to 5 years. Associate degrees in nursing (ADN) take approximately 2 years to complete and are usually offered at community or junior colleges. Diploma programs take 2 to 3 years to complete. This type of program is usually offered by hospitals. Baccalaureate programs (BSN) allow you to obtain a bachelor of science degree in nursing. This type of degree takes approximately 4 to 5 years to complete and is usually offered by colleges or universities.

Nurses who are interested can continue their educations beyond these degrees into areas of specialization. Such specialty areas include anesthesia, nurse practitioner, and nurse midwivery, among other specialties.

Although hospitals currently offer the majority of employment opportunities for nurses, there are other career paths open to this profession. Outpatient facilities, nursing homes or personal care facilities, physicians' offices, industry and schools, the government, and the Armed Forces are just a few of the institutions that have a need for nurses.

For further information regarding opportunities and educational programs in the challenging field of nursing, contact the National League for Nursing's website at www.nln.org.

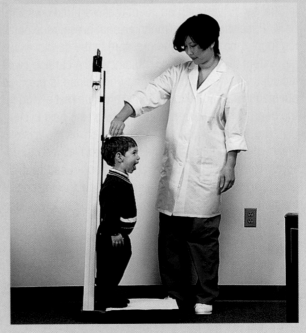

Source: Delmar/Cengage Learning

■ CHAPTER REVIEW

Exercises

1. Determine whether each of the following is a solution.

a. Is 1 a solution to $3x = 4$?

b. Is 2 a solution to $7 - 3x = 1$?

c. Is -10 a solution to $\frac{x}{10} = 17$?

d. Is 0 a solution to $5x + 10 = 10$?

2. Determine whether each of the following is a solution.

a. Is 2 a solution to $2(x + 3) = 9$?

b. Is -1 a solution to $-(x - 4) = 5$?

c. Is 3 a solution to $5(x - 4) = 6$?

d. Is 4 a solution to $4(x + 1) = 3x + 7$?

3. Solve each of the following equations.

a. $x - 3 = 7$

b. $x + 2 = 4$

c. $x - 7 = 3$

d. $x + 4 = 1$

e. $y + 2 = 3$

f. $t - 6 = 6$

4. A chemistry experiment requires students to find the mass of liquid in a flask. Write an equation to find the mass of water, w, for a flask with a mass of 8.4 g empty and 23.6 g when filled with water.

5. Write an equation which represents a patient's temperature before the patient was given medication if the temperature, t, decreases by 5 degrees to a normal temperature of 98.6 degrees.

6. Solve each of the following using the $V_T = V_D + V_A$ equation.

a. A patient's $V_D = 250$ *cc* and her $V_A = 500$ *cc*. What is her V_T?

b. A patient has a tidal volume of 400 cc and an alveolar volume of 200 cc. What is his deadspace volume?

7. Solve each of the following equations.

a. $2x = 14$

b. $6x = 36$

c. $2x = -40$

d. $7x = -28$

8. Solve each of the following equations.

a. $\frac{x}{2} = 1$

b. $\frac{t}{9} = 3$

c. $\frac{y}{4} = -2$

d. $\frac{m}{3} = 4$

9. Solve each of the following equations.

a. $\frac{2x}{5} = 4$

b. $\frac{3x}{7} = 6$

c. $\frac{-3x}{4} = 3$

10. The density of an object is a measure of its compactness. For example, equal-sized pieces of Styrofoam and steel will not weigh the same. That's because steel is much more dense than Styrofoam. The relationship between density, d, mass, m, and volume, v, is given by $m = dv$. Find the mass of a piece of

a. wood with a density of 0.95 g/cc and a volume of 7.2 cc.

b. ice with a density of 0.93 g/cc and a volume of 5.3 cc.

c. metal with a density of 3.6 g/cc and a volume of 2.4 cc.

11. Consider the formula given in the previous problem for the relationship between density, d, mass, m, and volume, v: $m = dv$. An object will float in water if its density is less than 1.0 g/cc and sink if its density is larger than 1.0 g/cc. Rewrite the formula to determine if the following will float or sink if immersed in water.

   a. mass of 24 grams and a volume of 21.2 cc

   b. mass of 16 grams and a volume of 17.2 cc

12. Sound waves are caused by vibrating objects. They cause a disturbance in the air that travels through the air. The speed of a sound wave, s, is given by the frequency, f, multiplied by the wavelength, w: $s = fw$. Find the wavelength of a sound wave with a frequency of 1,000 vibrations per second and a speed of 330 meters per second.

13. Find the patient's HR (in bpm) for each of the following.

   a. 50 HB per 30 seconds   c. 25 HB per 15 seconds

   b. 68 HB per 30 seconds

14. Solve each of the following equations.

   a. $3x - 7 = 1$ d. $4 - 3x = 1$

   b. $4x + 3 = 11$ e. $6 + 5x = -4$

   c. $3x - 7 = 8$

15. Find the IBW for each of the following.

   a. male measuring 72 inches in height   c. male measuring 170 centimeters in height

   b. female measuring 5 feet 4 inches in height   (remember to first convert to inches)

16. Solve each of the following equations.

   a. $2x - 5 = 1 - x$ c. $6x + 1 = 5x + 2$

   b. $2 - 3x = -2 - 2x$ d. $3 - 5x = 9 - 7x$

17. Solve each of the following equations.

   a. $4(3 - 2x) = -2x$ c. $2a - 5 = 2(2a + 4)$

   b. $5(3 - 2y) = 3 - 4y$ d. $4(x - 7) = 2(4x - 6)$

18. A principle dealing with levers states that $F_1x = F_2(d - x)$. If $F_1 = 50$, $F_2 = 100$, and $d = 15$, solve for x.

19. Find the MAP for each of the following.

   a. systolic pressure of 160 mm Hg and diastolic pressure of 65 mm Hg

   b. diastolic pressure of 50 mm Hg and systolic pressure of 110 mm Hg

20. Forensic scientists use many equations to predict characteristics of the human skeleton. If police discover a human thigh bone, the formula used might be $h = 2.4t + 61.4$, where h represents the height of the skeleton and t the length of the thigh bone, each measured in centimeters.

   a. How tall would a person have been if the thigh bone measured 40 cm?

   b. What is the length of the thigh bone for a person who is 160 cm tall?

Real Life Issues and Applications

An Emergency Medical Equation

A 5'2", 180-pound female was brought into the Emergency Department. She suffered severe, crushing chest injuries in an automobile accident and needs to be placed on a mechanical ventilator in order to survive. As the respiratory therapist, you must determine the correct tidal volume (V_T) for this patient. The formula to determine correct V_T volume is the following:

$$V_T = IBW \times 10$$

What is the correct V_T for this patient?

Additional Activity

Contact someone in the medical profession and ask them to provide you with at least one formula that they use in common practice. Share your findings with your class.

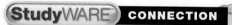

StudyWARE CONNECTION

Go to your StudyWARE™ DVD and have fun learning as you play interactive games, view animations and videos, and take practice tests to help reinforce key concepts you learned in this chapter.

Workbook Practice   *Go to your Workbook for more practice questions and activities.*

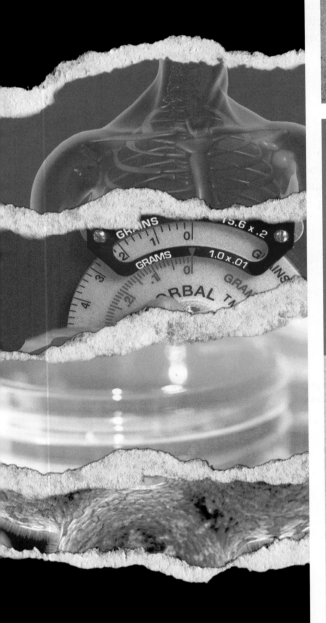

CHAPTER 19

MORE EQUATION FORMS

Objectives

Upon completion of this chapter, you should be able to

- Evaluate and determine solutions to various equation forms

- Relate equations in word form

- Set up and solve proportions

- Perform drug dosage calculations

Key Terms

cross-multiplying
formulas

proportion
story problems

THE ONE EQUATION THAT NO ONE HAS BALANCED.

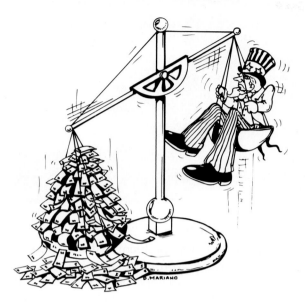

The balanced budget.

Source: Delmar/Cengage Learning

■ INTRODUCTION

As mentioned in the previous chapter, the main reason for introducing you to variable expressions is to enable you to solve problems written in words. These **story problems** can take many forms, as will be seen in this chapter.

The discussion in this chapter begins with the simplest of these problems—those involving **formulas**. A formula is simply an equation wherein the variables represent some recognized quantity. There are many formulas used within the health care field, and some are included here. Again, the major focus at this time is understanding the concept of solving equations.

Equation Forms

While equations can take on many forms, we will consider some of the most basic forms used in the health care field.

Formulas

As an example of a formula, consider the familiar formula to find the area of a rectangle, $A = l \times w$, or usually written $A = lw$. In this formula, A represents the area, l the length, and w the width of the rectangle.

Example:

Find the width of a rectangle with an area of 50 sq ft and a length of 10 ft.

$$A = lw$$

Substitute 50 for A and 10 for l

$$50 = 10w$$

Divide both sides by 10

$$\frac{50}{10} = \frac{10w}{10}$$

$$5 = w$$

or $w = 5$

The width is 5 feet.

As illustrated in the preceding example, always be sure to answer the question in sentence form. This ensures that you are answering the question which was asked.

Special Focus

The Temperature Scales

In the health care field, the Celsius temperature scale is often used. What if you needed to convert a Fahrenheit value to a Celsius value? The formula to change from Fahrenheit to Celsius is $C = \frac{5}{9}(F - 32)$.

Example:
Find the temperature of 212° *F* on the Celsius scale.

Substitute 212 for *F*

$$C = \frac{5}{9}(212 - 32)$$

$$C = \frac{5}{9}(180)$$

$$C = 100°$$

The temperature of 212° *F* is equivalent to 100° *C*.

QUOTES & NOTES

The hottest temperature recorded on earth was 136 degrees F in Azizia, Tripolitania, in northern Africa on September 13, 1922. Compare this to the temperature on the surface of the sun, which is approximately 10,000 degrees F! The highest temperature on record in the United States is 134 degrees F recorded in Death Valley, California, on July 10, 1913.

The coldest temperature recorded on earth was −128.6 degrees F in Soviet Antarctica at the Vostok Station on July 21, 1983. The coldest temperature on record in the United States is −80 degrees F recorded in Prospect Creek, Alaska, on January 23, 1971.

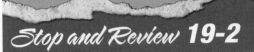

Stop and Review 19-2

Write each of the following as an equation and then solve each equation.

a. 4 more than *y* results in 9

b. the product of 2 and *w* is 16

c. 4 subtracted from *y* equals −3

d. the quotient (answer in a division problem) of *b* and 2 is 8

Stop and Review 19-1

Let's review the concept of cardiac output (CO) that we mentioned in the previous chapters, and then use the formula. It is very important to determine how efficiently the heart is pumping blood to the various parts of the body. How well the heart is performing is a function of how fast it beats (*f* = frequency) and how much blood the left ventricle ejects into the aorta (*SV* = stroke volume) each time the heart beats. This relationship is known as the cardiac output, and the formula is as follows:

$$CO = SV \times f$$

If the cardiac output for a given patient is 6 L/min, and the frequency is 70 beats per minute (bpm), what is the stroke volume?

From Words to Equations

In Chapter 18 we explained how words can be translated to variable expressions. Those same variable expressions can be used to develop equations.

Examples:

Words   *Equations*

3 added to *x* is 7 $x + 3 = 7$

2 less than *y* equals 5 $y - 2 = 5$

3 times *m* is 6 $3m = 6$

The ratio of *w* to 5 is 10 $w/5 = 10$

After you have formed the equations, the "fun" begins; just solve as noted in previous sections.

Choosing a Variable

More often than not, story problems will not give you the variable; therefore, you must choose a variable. When possible, choose an appropriate variable, such as *n* for number, *a* for age, *w* for width, and so on.

Examples:

Seven added to some number is 8; find the number.

Let *n* represent the unknown number

$$n + 7 = 8$$

Add −7 to both sides

$$n + 7 + (-7) = 8 + (-7)$$
$$n = 1$$

The unknown number is 1.

Five times a girl's age is 40; find her age.

Let *a* represent the girl's age

$$5a = 40$$

Divide both sides by 5

$$\frac{5a}{5} = \frac{40}{5}$$
$$a = 8$$

The girl's age is 8.

Elvis bought 3 cartons of jelly donuts. There were 72 donuts altogether. How many donuts were in each carton?

Let *n* be the number of donuts in each carton. Because there were 3 cartons

$$3n = 72$$

Divide both sides by 3

$$\frac{3n}{3} = \frac{72}{3}$$
$$n = 24$$

There were 24 donuts in each carton.

Forty percent of some number is 120. What is the number?

Remember to first convert 40% to the decimal form 0.40

$$0.40n = 120$$
$$n = \frac{120}{0.40}$$
$$n = 300$$

The number is 300.

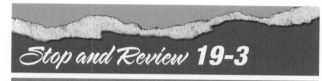

Stop and Review 19-3

If 30% of the food needs at a refugee camp were met by 50 tons of food, what amount would be needed to adequately supply the entire camp?

Proportions

In the health care field, one of the most useful areas of solving equations is with proportions.

Equating Ratios

In previous chapters, we saw that the comparison of two numbers can take many different forms. For example, the comparison of 3 to 4 can be written as a

fraction: $\frac{3}{4}$,

quotient: $3 \div 4$, or

ratio: 3:4.

We will now consider an equation that equates two ratios.

A **proportion** is a statement that two ratios are equal. For example, we saw previously that $\frac{3}{4} = \frac{6}{8}$; this is a proportion. This proportion can also be written 3:4 = 6:8, as a comparison of ratios. However, since the rules of algebra can be more easily applied to the fractional form $\frac{3}{4} = \frac{6}{8}$, we will write these proportions as fractions.

In general, the proportion $\frac{a}{b} = \frac{c}{d}$ is equivalent to the equation $ad = bc$. Sometimes it is said that the product of the means (b and c) equals the product of the extremes (a and d). This is also known as **cross-multiplying**, where $\frac{a}{b} \diagdown \frac{c}{d}$.

Once again consider the proportion $\frac{3}{4} = \frac{6}{8}$. If we cross-multiply, we get $3 \times 8 = 4 \times 6$, or $24 = 24$, which is certainly a true statement.

In our discussion of renaming fractions as higher equivalent fractions, we encountered problems such as $\frac{3}{4} = \frac{?}{8}$, or, equivalently, $\frac{3}{4} = \frac{x}{8}$. Cross-multiplying yields:

$$4x = 24$$

Divide both sides by 4

$$\frac{4x}{4} = \frac{24}{4}$$

Thus, $\frac{3}{4} = \frac{6}{8}$.

GREAT MOMENTS IN MATH
The conversion of a percentage to a decimal

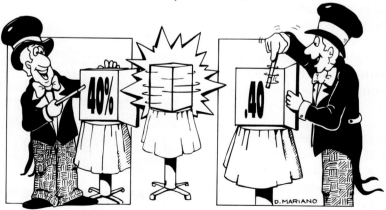

To convert from percentages to decimals
move the decimal point two places to the left.

Examples:

Solve for x if $\dfrac{x}{10} = \dfrac{9}{30}$

Cross-multiply

$30x = 90$

Divide both sides by 30

$\dfrac{30x}{30} = \dfrac{90}{30}$

$x = 3$

Thus, $\dfrac{3}{10} = \dfrac{9}{30}$.

Solve for T if $\dfrac{300}{T} = \dfrac{500}{25}$

Cross-multiply

$500T = 7500$

Divide both sides by 500

$\dfrac{500T}{500} = \dfrac{7500}{500}$

$T = 15$

As a check: $\dfrac{300}{15} = \dfrac{500}{25}$

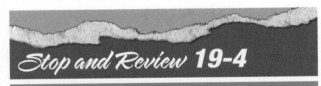

Stop and Review 19-4

While studying the gas laws, you will encounter problems such as $\dfrac{P}{100} = \dfrac{750}{250}$. Find the value of P.

Setting Up Proportions

Of course, before proportions can be solved, they must first be set up. Problems involving proportions are some of the most common word problems encountered in the health professions. Specifically, they are utilized in determining correct drug dosages.

Following are examples of some story problems involving proportions, each of which is solved by setting up equal ratios.

Examples:

An architect wishes to make a scale drawing of a house that is 60 ft tall. If each block on the graph paper corresponds to a 2-ft distance, how many blocks high will the scale drawing be? So if one block equals 2 feet, then x blocks equal 60 ft.

Set up equal ratios

$\dfrac{1\ block}{2\ feet} = \dfrac{x\ blocks}{60\ feet}$

Cross-multiply

$2x = 60$

Divide both sides by 2

$x = 30$

The scale drawing will be 30 blocks high.

If a quarterback throws 9 touchdowns in 8 games, how many touchdowns would you expect him to throw in 16 games?

Set up equal ratios

$\dfrac{9\ touchdowns}{8\ games} = \dfrac{t\ touchdowns}{16\ games}$

Cross-multiply

$8t = 144$

Divide both sides by 8 to get

$t = 18$

He would be expected to throw 18 touchdowns.

If 1 *kg* equals 2.2 *lb*, how many kilograms is 8.8 *lb*?

Set up equal ratios

$\dfrac{1\ kg}{2.2\ lb} = \dfrac{w\ kg}{8.8\ lb}$

Cross-multiply

$2.2w = 8.8$

Divide both sides by 2.2

$w = 4$

Thus, 8.8 lb equals 4 kg.

The last problem can also be done using the factor-label method from Chapter 16. Perform the problem using that method and see if the same answer results.

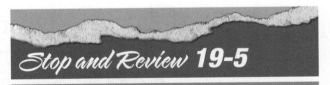

Stop and Review 19-5

A doctor's office used 45 needles in 1 month. How many needles would you expect the office to use in 1 year (i.e., 12 months)?

Drug Dosage Calculations

While there are many methods for expressing the strength of a drug, here we will discuss a few that use proportions.

Percent Solutions

An area where equations and proportions are frequently used in health care is in determining proper drug dosages. The majority of these problems can be solved by setting up simple proportions.

One way the potency of a drug can be described is by stating its *percentage of solution*. This tells the strength of the solution as parts of the solute (drug) per 100 mL of solution. After all, that is what a percent is—some number related to 100. As we discussed earlier in the text, a solute can be either a solid or a liquid. If the solute is a solid, it is expressed in grams as a $\frac{W}{V}$ solution. If the solute is liquid, it is expressed in milliliters as a $\frac{V}{V}$ solution.

For example, a 20% salt water, or saline, solution contains 20 g of salt (a solid solute) dissolved in enough water (solvent) to yield 100 mL of solution. The following example uses this information in the context of a problem.

Example:

How much salt is needed to make 1,000 mL of a 20% solution?

First, write down what you know

$$20\% \ solution = \frac{20 \ g \ salt}{100 \ mL \ of \ solution}$$

Next, place this into a proportion of what you need to determine

$$\frac{20 \ g \ salt}{100 \ mL \ of \ solution} = \frac{x \ g \ salt}{1000 \ mL \ of \ solution}$$

The *x* grams represents the "how much salt is needed"; thus, the left side of the equation represents what is known, and the right side represents the unknown amount of the solute (in this case, salt) needed to make the final solution.

Solving by cross-multiplying

$$\frac{20}{100} = \frac{x}{1000}$$
$$20000 = 100x$$
$$x = 200$$

Thus, to make 1,000 mL of a 20% salt solution, you would combine 200 g of salt with enough water to fill a container to the 1,000 mL mark.

In the preceding example, 1,000 mL could have been given as the equivalent 1 L. If that had been the case, you would have needed to make sure that all units in the numerators and denominators were the same before cross-multiplying.

Example:

What is the percent strength of a salt solution containing 5 g of salt in 1 L?

Write down what is known

$$\frac{5 \ g \ salt}{1 \ L \ of \ solution}$$

Set up as a proportion to what is needed:

$$\frac{5 \ g \ salt}{1 \ L \ of \ solution} = \frac{x \ g \ salt}{100 \ mL \ of \ solution}$$

Because the unknown, or *x*, is set to 100 mL, it will give you the percentage strength. Before solving, however, convert the 1 L to 1,000 mL so that the units in the denominators are the same.

$$\frac{5 \ g \ salt}{1000 \ mL \ of \ solution} = \frac{x \ g \ salt}{100 \ mL \ of \ solution}$$
$$\frac{5}{1000} = \frac{x}{100}$$

Cross-multiply

$$500 = 1000x$$
$$x = 0.5$$

Therefore, if 5 g of salt are mixed with 1 L of water, a 0.5% solution results.

Ratio Solutions

Another means of expressing the strength of a solution is a ratio. In review, the ratio represents the parts of the solute related to the parts of the solution. For example, a 1:200 solution of isoproterenol ($\frac{V}{V}$) contains 1 mL of isoproterenol (liquid solute) in 200 mL of a sterile-water solution.

We can solve word problems involving ratios by way of the same system used for solving word problems involving percent solutions. You should first write down what is given; then, relate this to the unknown; next, make sure all units in the numerators and denominators are the same; and, finally, solve for *x* by cross-multiplying the proportion.

Example:

How many milliliters of isoproterenol are in 1 mL of a 1:100 solution?

Write down what is given

$$1{:}100 \ solution = \frac{1 \ mL \ isoproterenol}{100 \ mL \ sterile \ water}$$

Relate the given to the unknown with a proportion

$$\frac{1 \ mL \ isoproterenol}{100 \ mL \ sterile \ water} = \frac{x \ mL \ isoproterenol}{1 \ mL \ sterile \ water}$$
$$\frac{1}{100} = \frac{x}{1}$$

Cross-multiply

$1 = 100x$

$x = 0.01$

There are .01 mL of isoproterenol in 1 mL of a 1:100 solution.

Now consider a problem involving a $(\frac{W}{V})$ solution in milligrams; use the same steps.

Example:

How many milligrams of epinephrine are in 1 mL of a 1:200 solution?

Write down what is given

$$1:200 \; solution = \frac{1 \; g \; epinephrine}{200 \; mL \; solution}$$

Relate the given to the unknown with a proportion

$$\frac{1 \; g \; epinephrine}{200 \; mL \; solution} = \frac{x \; mg \; epinephrine}{1 \; mL \; solution}$$

Before solving, convert grams to milligrams in the numerator so that the units are the same

$$\frac{1000 \; mg \; epinephrine}{200 \; mL \; solution} = \frac{x \; mg \; epinephrine}{1 \; mL \; solution}$$

$$\frac{1000}{200} = \frac{x}{1}$$

Cross-multiply

$1000 = 200x$

$x = 5 \; mg$

Therefore, 5 mg of epinephrine is found in 1 mL of a 1:200 solution of epinephrine.

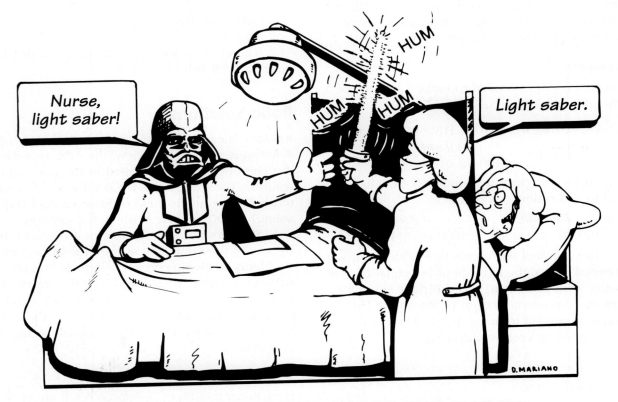

Nurse, light saber!

Light saber.

HUM

HUM

D. MARIANO

APPLIED LASER SURGERY OF THE FUTURE

Source: Delmar/Cengage Learning

Professional Profile
Surgical Technology

If you follow any of the soap operas on television, chances are you have seen at least one scene in an operating room, where the hero or heroine is saved from a terminal illness. (Of course, you had to wait until Monday to find that out!) You may have thought that the people in masks and gowns were either doctors or nurses. (*Reality check*: They were only actors!) In the real world, however, a variety of allied health professions are represented in any given operating room. One of these professions is surgical technology. Surgical technologists, who are usually supervised by either surgeons or registered nurses, help to provide the best care possible for surgical patients.

Surgical technologists have a wide range of responsibilities, which may include setting up the operating room for surgery by preparing the instruments and equipment; preparing fluids, such as saline and glucose, for intravenous administration; and transporting and preparing patients for surgery. A surgical technologist may also pass instruments to the surgeon during the actual procedure, as well as adjust lighting and operate suctioning or diagnostic devices. Surgical technologists may prepare specimens for laboratory analysis and apply dressings to wound areas. And a relatively new area opening up to surgical technologists is assisting in the use of lasers for surgery.

The need for a thorough understanding of math in this profession is pretty obvious. For instance, math is used for tasks such as tallying the number of sponges and instruments before and after a surgical procedure. While this may seem to be a very simple task, it is also a very important one. Counting these items before and after a procedure ensures that no equipment was left in the patient! And what about laser surgery? Intensity and distances for this procedure must be exact or a patient could be seriously injured. Finally, drawing up and administering special drugs or solutions require not only dexterity but also math skills. There is little margin for error in the operating room environment.

Job opportunities in this field are expected to grow faster than average. In addition to operating rooms, surgical technologists may also work in delivery rooms and emergency departments.

Most surgical technology programs take from 9 to 10 months to complete and are usually hospital based. However, there are also 2-year associate degree programs available at the college level.

For more information concerning this exciting field, visit the Association of Surgical Technologists website at www.ast.org.

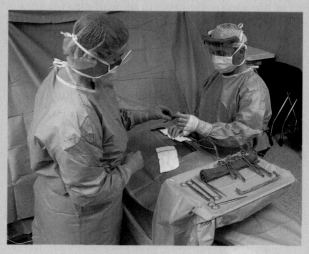

Source: Delmar/Cengage Learning

■ CHAPTER REVIEW

Exercises

1. The distance around a rectangular garden is given by $d = 2l + 2w$ where l is the length and w is the width. If the distance around the garden is 140 meters, and the width is 20 meters, what is the length?

2. In physics, the formula $V = IR + Ir$ might describe an electrical circuit. What is R if $V = 16$, $I = 2$, and $r = 3$?

3. Write each of the following as an equation and then solve for the variable.

   a. Ten fewer than x equals 3.

   b. The number represented by t divided by 2 is 9.

   c. Twice m equals 32.

   d. The quotient of F and 4 is 12.

   e. Three fourths of a number, n, is 24.

   f. An amount, a, divided by 20 is 1.5.

   g. A quantity, q, doubled and then increased by 7 is 29.

4. A doctor uses 10 needles from a box. There are now 14 needles remaining in the box. How many needles were originally in the box?

5. A patient is allowed 14,000 mg of salt over a 7-day period. How much salt can the patient have each day if the patient is to have the same amount each day?

6. A vial contains 1,800 mg of a drug that is to be used for 5 equal doses. How much of the drug should be given at each dose?

7. How much albuterol, a medication used to treat asthma, was originally in a bottle if 30% of the original amount was 600 mL?

8. At the end of the year, the receipts in a gift shop were $100,000. Of this, 90% went toward expenses, and the remainder was profit. How much profit did the gift shop make?

9. A man weighing 300 pounds joined a weight loss program and lost 72 pounds. What percent of his original weight did he lose?

10. A technician mixed 40 mL of alcohol with 160 mL of water to make a solution. What percent of the solution is alcohol?

11. A nursing student answered 80% of the questions on an exam correctly. If she answered 40 questions correctly, how many questions were on the exam?

12. This year a pharmacy school received 823 applications for admission which was 125 more than last year. How many did it receive last year?

13. Normal body temperature is $37°$ Celsius. A patient has a fever and has a temperature of $40.3°$ Celsius. The temperature is how many degrees above normal?

14. A fitness club has a membership of $100 to join plus an additional fee of $25 per month. In how many months will a member pay a total of $600 to belong to the club?

15. Solve for the variable in each of the following.

   a. $\dfrac{2}{x} = \dfrac{6}{18}$

   b. $\dfrac{2}{5} = \dfrac{x}{15}$

   c. $\dfrac{t}{9} = \dfrac{2}{3}$

16. A certain solution must be mixed 6 parts concentrate to 5 parts water. How much water is needed if 3 gallons of concentrate are to be used?

17. If a baseball player hits 23 home runs in 54 games, how many home runs would he be expected to hit in 162 games?

18. A medication is to be made in capsule form. It consists of two substances in a ratio of 8 parts medication to 3 parts filler. If the total amount of medicine available is 120 grams, how much filler material is needed?

19. The scale on a map is one-fourth centimeter to 40 kilometers. What is the actual distance between two towns that are 6 centimeters apart on the map?

20. A homeowner is preparing a solution of lawn fertilizer. The directions are to mix 3 parts fertilizer to 32 ounces of water. How much fertilizer is needed to mix with 160 ounces of water?

21. If the daily recommended allowance of protein for adults is 0.8 grams for every 1 pound of body weight, how many grams of protein should a man weighing 200 pounds consume per day?

22. For every water molecule, 2 atoms of hydrogen combine with 1 atom of oxygen. How many hydrogen atoms would be needed to combine with 80 oxygen atoms to form water molecules?

23. Fifty liters of fluid flow through a tube in 15 hours. At this rate, how long will it take 130 liters to flow though the tube?

24. A woman takes a 24-mg zinc tablet each day. If this amount represents 300% of the recommended daily allowance, how many milligrams are recommended?

25. Twenty kilograms of sodium hydroxide is needed to neutralize 45 kg of sulfuric acid. At this rate, how many kg of sodium hydroxide are needed to neutralize 180 kg of sulfuric acid?

26. A jogger weighing 140 pounds burns 4 calories per minute. How many calories would she burn in 2 hours?

27. Each cubic foot of water weighs 62.4 pounds. How much would the water in a bathtub containing 25 cubic feet weigh?

Drug Dosage Problems

28. How would you make 500 mL of a 10% salt water solution?

29. How much salt and water are present in 300 mL of a 4% solution?

30. How would you make 100 mL of a 10% solution of isoproterenol? (Remember, this is now a $\frac{V}{V}$ solution.)

31. How much liquid isoproterenol and saline are present in a 5% solution of isoproterenol?

32. How many milliliters of isoproterenol are in 10 mL of a 1:1,000 solution?

33. How many milligrams of epinephrine are in 5 mL of a 1:100 solution?

Real Life Issues and Applications

Ethics of Miscalculation

You are responsible for giving patient John his medication. The physician's order specifies that a low dosage of a very safe medicine should be given once in the morning and once in the evening. Through a calculation mistake, however, you give patient John twice the amount of medication ordered for the A.M. Because the drug is very safe, your drug dosage calculation error luckily caused no side effects and no harm was done to the patient. What should you do?

Additional Activity

Arrange to take a tour of the operating and recovery rooms of a local hospital. Note the vast array of equipment. Investigate the variety of health care professions involved with the surgery and recovery of patients. Investigate how math relates to surgery and recovery. Discuss your findings with the class.

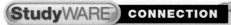

StudyWARE CONNECTION

Go to your StudyWARE™ DVD and have fun learning as you play interactive games, view animations and videos, and take practice tests to help reinforce key concepts you learned in this chapter.

Workbook Practice | *Go to your Workbook for more practice questions and activities.*

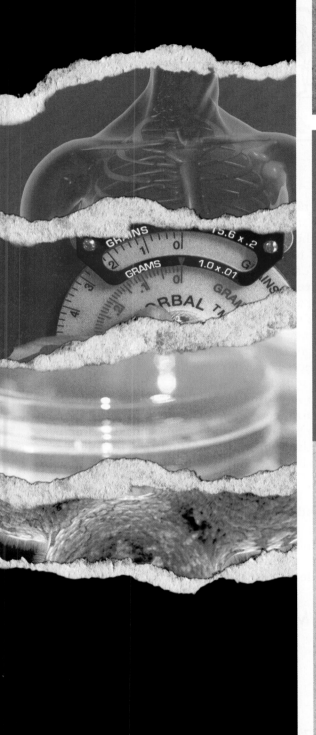

CHAPTER 20

STATISTICS AND GRAPHS

Objectives

Upon completion of this chapter, you should be able to

- Find the mean, median, and mode for a group of values

- Determine which measure best describes the center of a distribution

- Use various types of graphs to interpret and analyze information

- Relate the construction of a dosage response curve

- Interpret and analyze data from dosage response curves

Key Terms

average
bar graph
circle graph
data
graphs
line graph
mean

measures of central tendency
median
mode
picture graph
slope
statistics

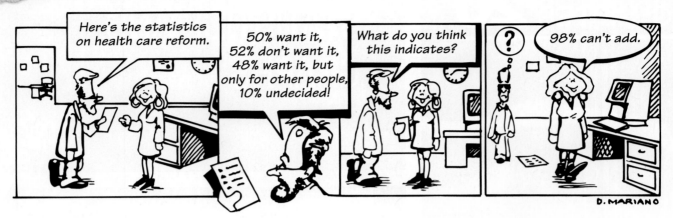

Source: Delmar/Cengage Learning

■ INTRODUCTION

Statistics is the branch of mathematics concerned with the collection, organization, and display of information. This information is commonly referred to as **data**. Hardly a day goes by that statistics is not used by everyone. Phrases such as "for sale 20% off"; "his batting average is 0.300"; and "she is just an average basketball player" all involve statistics.

The focus of this chapter is to introduce some often-used terminology for the word **average**, and to help you understand how to interpret graphical information.

Types of Statistics

This section will present the most basic statistics, those used to find averages.

Average

The word *average* means "in between" or "in the middle." For example, an average student is neither the best nor the worst student, and an average raise is between the highest raise and the lowest raise. So the "average" is some measure of the center of data. Three statistical terms are used to describe the center of a distribution of data. Usually referred to as the **measures of central tendency**, these terms are the **mean**, the **median**, and the **mode**.

The *mean* is the most commonly used statistical average and is sometimes called the *arithmetic average*. To find the mean, you simply add all the numbers in a group and divide by the number of items added.

The *median* is the middle value when values are arranged from highest to lowest or from lowest to highest. To find the median, you simply arrange the values in order and find the middle value; half the values will be above the median and half will be below. If there are an even number of values, you simply add the middle two values and divide by 2.

The *mode* is the value that occurs most often. There may not even be a mode for a given set of data, or there may be more than one mode.

SOMEWHAT INTERESTING MATH FACTS

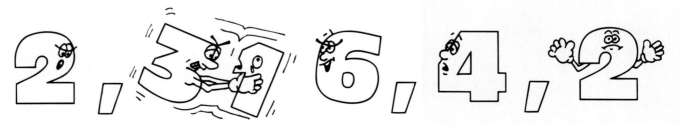

You don't always need math to determine the MEAN number.

Source: Delmar/Cengage Learning

Example:

Find the mean, median, and mode for the following set of data:

0, 1, 2, 2, 5, 5, 7, 7, 7

The mean is

$$\frac{0 + 1 + 2 + 2 + 5 + 5 + 7 + 7 + 7}{9} = \frac{36}{9} = 4$$

The median is 5 because when the numbers are arranged in order, the middle value is 5. The mode is 7 because it is the number that occurs most often.

To emphasize the importance of understanding the average, and particularly the differences between the measures of central tendency, consider the following story.

GREAT MOMENTS IN MATH HISTORY

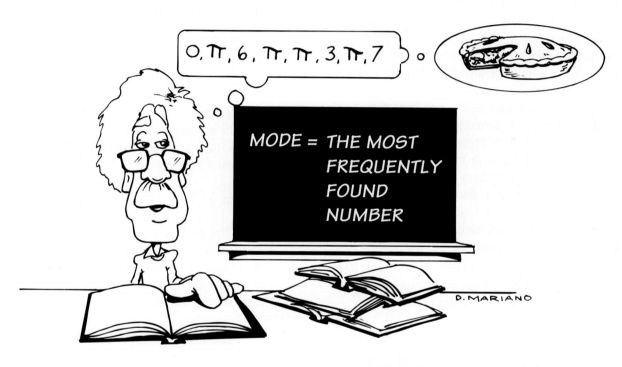

Mathematicians discover PI A LA MODE

Source: Delmar/Cengage Learning

Clinical Relevancy

Cholesterol

Another medical term with which nearly everyone is familiar is *cholesterol*. But do you know what cholesterol is? Cholesterol is a substance found in the fats and oils of animals, as well as in egg yolks and milk. It is also found in human brain tissue, parts of human nerve fibers, and in the human liver and kidneys.

Cholesterol plays an important role in good health. Specifically, cholesterol is used to form cholic acid in the liver. This acid forms bile salts, which are needed in order for us to digest fat. Our bodies require large amounts of cholesterol to prevent our skin from absorbing water-soluble substances. Smaller amounts of

(continues)

(*continued*)

cholesterol are used by the ovaries, testes, and adrenal glands in the formation of hormones.

Although a certain amount of cholesterol is good, as is the case with other good things, you can have too much cholesterol. High levels of cholesterol appear to be a major factor in the development of coronary artery disease. High levels of cholesterol in the blood (known as *hypercholesterolemia*) can be caused by liver disease, pancreatic disease (including diabetes mellitus), and hypothyroidism.

The normal serum (or blood) level for cholesterol is 150 to 200 mg/dL. This value varies depending on diet and age and, oddly enough, from country to country. A serum level of greater than 200 mg/dL would indicate *hypercholesterolemia*.

Individuals can also suffer from *hypocholesterolemia*. In such cases, serum levels of cholesterol are below 150 mg/dL. Low cholesterol levels can result from poor dietary habits or malnutrition, severe liver disease, and hyperthyroidism.

From the preceding discussion, the importance of monitoring cholesterol level should be clear. Now, let's apply what we have learned so far in this chapter. Consider the following scenario:

> One of your patients had cholesterol levels taken each month for 10 months. Those results were as follows (all in mg/dL units of measure):

140, 160, 180, 120, 200,

160, 240, 160, 200, 220

Given this information, how would you find the mean, median, and mode?
The mean cholesterol value would be:

$$\frac{the\ sum\ of\ the\ values}{number\ of\ values} = \frac{1780}{10} = 178$$

So the mean is 178 mg/dL.

To find the median, place the values in order:

120, 140, 160, 160, 160,

180, 200 , 200, 220, 240

Because there are an even number of values (10), the median lies between the fifth and sixth values, that is, between 160 and 180. This is expressed as follows:

$$median = \frac{160 + 180}{2} = 170$$

Thus, the median is 170 mg/dL, even though there is no actual value of 170 mg/dL.
Given all of the patient's cholesterol values, what is the mode? Remember, the value repeated most often is the mode.

Stop and Review 20-1

The heights, measured to the nearest centimeter, for 10 students in a class were: 120, 130, 125, 120, 129, 140, 120, 139, 132, 145. Find the mean, median, and mode.

Sally interviewed for a job as an occupational therapist at a small private medical care company. The company consists of a president, two vice presidents, three managers, and five medical specialists. At the interview, the president told Sally that the average weekly salary was $800, that she would earn $250 per week while in training, and that her salary would increase after training. She was pleased with this description and accepted the position.

After one week on the job, Sally discovered that the medical specialists each earned only $300 per week. She was angry, and asked to see the president.

"Mr. Twister, you misled me!" she complained after telling him what she had learned.

He responded that he had been quite accurate in his statements, and to prove his point, he showed her the following salary-scale chart:

Position	Salary	Number Employed
President	$3,800	1
Vice President	$1,000	2
Manager	$ 500	3
Medical Specialist	$ 300	5
Total	$8,800	11
Average Salary	$8,800/11 = $800	

Source: Delmar/Cengage Learning

"The average salary can also be called the mean salary," Mr. Twister said. "The middle salary, or the median, is also a way to state average." He showed her the following list:

$300, $300, $300, $300, $300, $500,

$500, $500, $1,000, $1,000, $3,800

Sally studied the set of figures. "But what about all of us who earn $300 a week! There are more of us than anyone else!" she protested.

"Ah! Well, that's another matter. That's called a mode. It is also a type of average."

"I see," said Sally, "and I quit."

As can be seen from the preceding story, the concept of average is extremely important. Furthermore, the mean is not always the best measure of central tendency. In fact, the mean is affected by extreme values more than is either the median or the mode; that is, the mean is the most sensitive measure of central tendency. As an illustration, consider the following 10 cholesterol levels, each in milligrams:

120, 140, 140, 150, 160,

160, 160, 180, 190, 350

The median and mode are both 160, while the mean is 175. But notice that the value of 350 is extremely high relative to the other values. Because of the relatively extreme nature of this value, this may be an invalid reading and, therefore, should be rechecked. Furthermore, if the extreme value of 350 were discarded, the mean would be approximately 155; the median and mode, however, would both remain at 160. The value of 350, therefore, had much more of an effect on the mean than it did on either the median or the mode.

Stop and Review 20-2

The number of pills given daily to five patients are 2, 3, 4, 4, 12, respectively. Which value best describes the average number of pills taken daily by these patients?

Special Focus

Statistical Concepts in the Health Care Field

Do you remember the formula used to find mean arterial pressure (MAP)? The answer to the formula represents the "average" pressure exerted upon the arterial walls. This pressure varies depending on the phase of the cardiac cycle. During contraction, or the systolic phase, the pressure is very high as compared to when the heart is not pumping during relaxation, or the diastolic phase.

Another important factor is that the relaxation phase is normally two times longer than the contraction phase. In essence, your heart spends one part of its cycle in contraction and two parts in relaxation. To find the arithmetic mean, you would therefore add the one part systolic pressure and two parts diastolic pressure and divide the total by 3. Hence the following formula:

$$MAP = \frac{(2 \times diasolic) + systolic}{3}$$

An increase in MAP represents more stress placed on the walls of the arterial system. Factors that can increase MAP include arteriosclerotic heart disease and disease states that increase the rate and force of heart contraction.

A decrease in MAP may indicate a lack of blood flow (perfusion) to the brain or kidneys. Lack of blood flow to the brain can prevent the body from receiving signals from the central nervous system (CNS) that are needed in order to sustain life. Lack of blood flow to the renal system or kidneys can result in the body's inability to filter and rid itself of toxic waste products. Both situations can lead quickly to death. A classic example would be a patient in "shock," where low blood pressure would lead to poor renal perfusion.

Cost of goods	$ $ $ $ $ $ $ $ $ $ $ $	(12 needed)
Marketing	$ $ $ $ $ $ $ $ $	(9 needed)
Research	$ $ $ $ $ $ ^	($6^2/_5$ needed)
Profits	$ $ $ $ $ ^	($5^1/_5$ needed)
Administration	$ $ $ $	(4 needed)
Taxes	$ $ $ ^	(approx. $3^1/_3$ needed)

Source: Delmar/Cengage Learning

Graphing

A **graph** is used to give a visual representation of numbers. Just as it is said that a picture is worth a thousand words, it might be said that a graph is worth a thousand numbers. The focus of this section is on interpreting the information given in picture graphs, circle graphs, bar graphs, and line graphs.

Picture Graphs

To understand the concept of a **picture graph**, or pictograph, consider a hypothetical manufacturer and seller of medicinal drugs. Suppose that the total yearly cost to manufacture and sell these drugs is $1,000,000. Following is a list showing the revenue breakdown for the manufacture and sale of these drugs.

Cost of goods	$300,000	(30%)
Marketing	$225,000	(22.5%)
Research	$160,000	(16%)
Profits	$130,000	(13%)
Administration	$100,000	(10%)
Taxes	$ 85,000	(8.5%)

Source: Delmar/Cengage Learning

A picture graph uses pictures to represent numerical facts. Each picture should be appropriate and represent a predetermined number of items. For this example, a dollar bill symbol, $, might be chosen to represent $25,000. The following graph would result.

$ = $25,000

The reason for choosing $25,000 to represent each picture is so that the number of pictures

necessary will neither be so large as to be cumbersome nor so small as to be fruitless.

Because $25,000 was chosen to represent each picture, simply divide by $25,000 to find the number of pictures necessary. For example, the $225,000 marketing figure divided by $25,000 is 9; therefore, 9 dollar bill symbols would be needed to represent marketing costs in this picture graph. Had $10,000 been chosen to represent each picture, then 22.5 pictures would be needed to represent the costs of marketing.

The advantage of this graph is that you can quickly see that the cost of goods accounts for the largest portion of the total manufacturing cost, while the taxes account for the smallest portion.

Circle Graphs

For this same hypothetical example, a **circle graph**, or pie graph, may be a more appropriate type of graph. A circle graph is usually used to represent a whole when divided into parts. Given that 100% represents the whole, by changing each value into a percent, the circle, or pie, can be used to represent the whole (see Figure 20-1).

Again, observe how quickly you can see that taxes account for the smallest portion of the manufacturing costs, while cost of goods accounts for the largest portion.

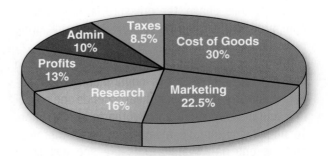

Figure 20-1   *Circle graph illustrating the costs and profits of a hypothetical drug manufacturer.*

Source: Delmar/Cengage Learning

Bar Graphs

A third type of graph often used for comparisons is the **bar graph**. In a bar graph, the length of each bar indicates the number of items represented (see Figure 20-2). The bars may be drawn horizontally or vertically. Notice from Figure 20-2 that in a horizontal bar graph, a scale is drawn at the bottom for easy reference. In a vertical bar graph, the scale is usually drawn on the left side.

Example:

Suppose that for our hypothetical company, profits each year of a 6-year period beginning in 2005 were as follows:

2005	$ 90,000
2006	$ 95,000
2007	$ 98,000
2008	$110,000
2009	$120,000
2010	$130,000

Source: Delmar/Cengage Learning

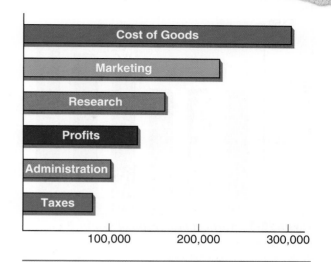

Figure 20-2 *Horizontal bar graph illustrating the costs and profits of a hypothetical drug manufacturer.*

Source: Delmar/Cengage Learning

This information can be illustrated using a bar graph, as shown in Figure 20-3.

Again, note the ease with which the information can be read in Figure 20-3. Furthermore, it can easily be seen that profits have increased over this 6-year period. It is, thus, evident that graphs

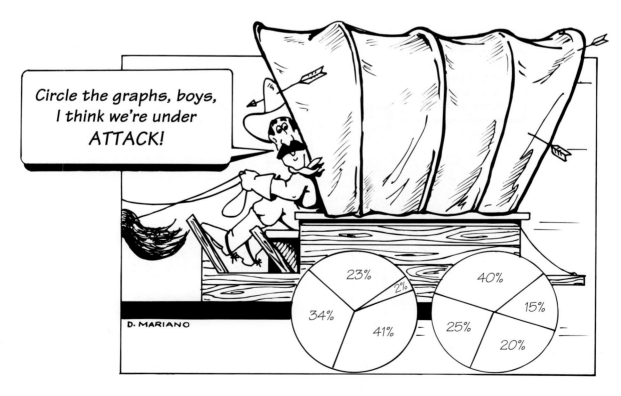

A MATHEMATICIAN'S VIEW OF THE OLD WEST

Source: Delmar/Cengage Learning

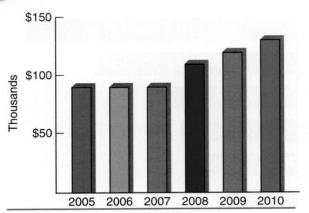

Figure 20-3   *Vertical bar graph of profits for a 6-year period.*

Source: Delmar/Cengage Learning

can represent trends that may not be as apparent when looking at a "sea of numbers."

Line Graphs

The type of graph with which you may be most familiar is the **line graph**. A line graph is usually used to show trends or changes over a period of time. A line graph uses two scales at right angles to one another. The vertical scale usually indicates a measured quantity such as temperature, dollars, or population. The horizontal scale usually indicates a uniform change such as time or distance.

A line graph is constructed by drawing a dot on the graph at the appropriate point for each given value and connecting the dots.

Example:

Using the profits noted in the previous example about the manufacture of drugs, construct a line graph.

A line graph is constructed much like a bar graph, where the height of the bar represents a given amount. In a line graph, the amount is represented as a point at that same height.

In this example, profits in 2005 were $90,000. Therefore, draw a point directly above 2005 and directly across from $90,000; next, draw a point directly above 2006 and directly across from $95,000; and so on. After you have done this for all six points, connect the points (see Figure 20-5).

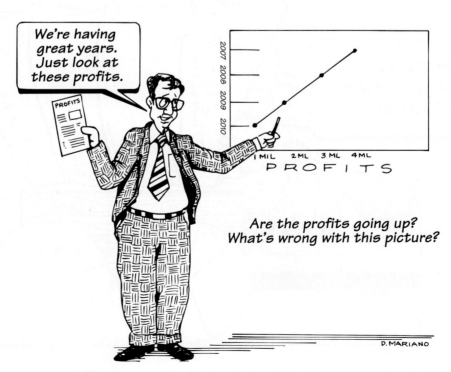

Source: Delmar/Cengage Learning

Clinical Relevancy

Graphing in the Health Care Field

Each year in the United States, approximately 500,000 people suffer strokes. Of these people, more than 150,000 die. Many stroke survivors require special rehabilitation and extended care. This costs millions of dollars annually and often places tremendous burdens on family members. It is sad to note that while stroke is one of the leading causes of death in the United States, many of the risk factors for stroke are potentially treatable.

One such risk factor is high blood pressure. A person with moderately high blood pressure may have twice the risk of stroke as a person with normal blood pressure. People having very high blood pressure may be at a *four times* greater risk for stroke than individuals having normal blood pressure. This is why it is so important to have blood pressure checked on a regular basis. If there is a problem, most often it can and should be treated.

The bar graph in Figure 20-4 clearly shows the relationship between increased blood pressure and the incidence of stroke. In looking at Figure 20-4, what can you conclude about age and its effects on blood pressure and the incidences of stroke?

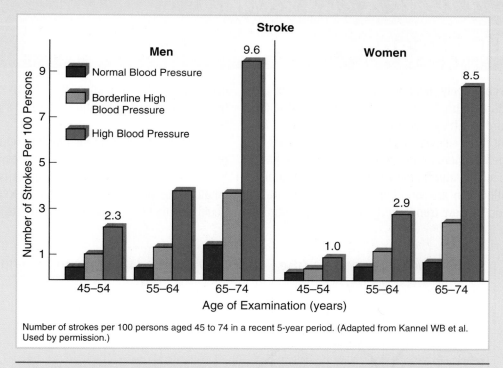

Number of strokes per 100 persons aged 45 to 74 in a recent 5-year period. (Adapted from Kannel WB et al. Used by permission.)

Figure 20-4 *Bar graph showing the relationship between blood pressure and incidence of stroke.*

Source: Delmar/Cengage Learning

Again, it can easily be seen from Figure 20-5 that profits are increasing. In fact, when the line rises from left to right, the quantity increases. When the line falls from left to right, the quantity decreases. When the line is horizontal, the quantity remains the same.

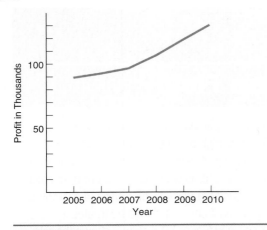

Figure 20-5 *Line graph illustrating the profits of a hypothetical drug manufacturer over a 6-year period.*

Source: Delmar/Cengage Learning

Line Graphing in the Sciences

A concept important in chemistry that will be discussed is "change of states." Line graphing can be used, for example, to illustrate the change of the state of ice to a liquid (water) and then to steam. Suppose we wanted to change 1 g of ice, which has a temperature of -50° Celsius, to steam. The ice would first need to be heated and changed to water, and then be heated further and changed to steam.

Clinical Relevancy

Line Graphs in the Health Care Field

A graph commonly included in patient charts is the temperature graph. The patient's temperature is taken and recorded at various times throughout the day and night. This allows health care professionals to determine whether patients are developing fevers and may also aid in determining whether certain therapies (e.g., antibiotics) are working. A temperature graph allows you to view trends in a patient's temperature over time and at a glance. It is much quicker than going page by page through a patient's chart to find temperatures.

Look, for instance, at the graph in Figure 20-6. This graph shows a pneumonia patient's increasing temperature over time. Note the change in the patient's temperature after an antibiotic was administered on 9/09/10. Could it be that the antibiotic was doing its job?

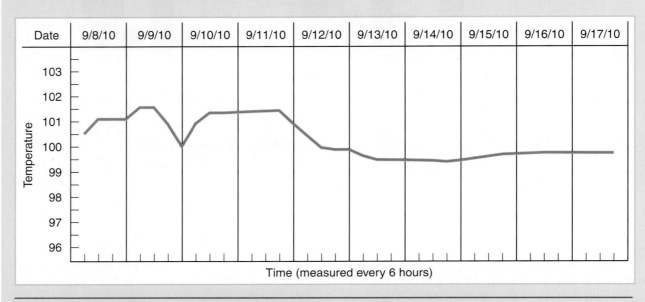

Figure 20-6 *Graph of patient's temperature over a 10-day period.*

Source: Delmar/Cengage Learning

Increasing the temperature of ice 2° Celsius requires 1 calorie of heat. Using proportions as discussed in previous chapters, given that 1 calorie of heat will raise the temperature of ice 2° C, x calories will raise the temperature 50° C:

$$\frac{1 \ calorie}{2 \ degrees} = \frac{x \ calories}{50 \ degrees}$$

Cross-multiply

$2x = 50$

$x = 25$

It, therefore, takes 25 calories of heat to raise the temperature of the ice to 0° Celsius, the temperature at which ice begins to change to water. This is represented graphically in Figure 20-7. Notice that as heat is added and the temperature rises, the graph rises from left to right.

At this point in time, the ice will need to be melted. The temperature will not change until the last bit of ice has melted. Most substances possess this quality. The amount of heat required to change a solid to a liquid is called the *latent heat of fusion*, illustrated graphically in Figure 20-8. Notice that 80 calories were added to change the ice to water. The horizontal line indicates that the temperature does not change even though heat is being added.

Water begins changing to steam at 100° C. After the ice has been changed to water at 0° Celsius, it will take 1 calorie of heat to raise the temperature 1° Celsius. Therefore, adding 100 calories will change the temperature of water to 100° C, the temperature at which water begins to change to steam. This is represented graphically in Figure 20-9.

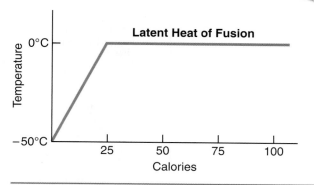

Figure 20-8 *Graphic representation of the concept of latent heat of fusion.*
Source: Delmar/Cengage Learning

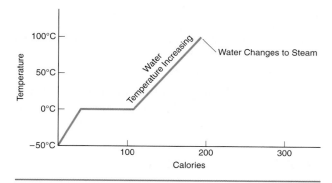

Figure 20-9 *Graphic representation of changing water to steam.*
Source: Delmar/Cengage Learning

If more heat is added after the water reaches 100° C, the water will begin changing to steam. It will take another 539 calories to change this 1 g of water to steam. This is called the *latent heat of vaporization* and is represented graphically in Figure 20-10.

Although an additional 539 calories of heat has been added, the temperature remains at 100° C. The water has vaporized and changed to steam, but the temperature of the steam is still 100° C. Additional heat must be added to raise the temperature of the steam. It will take 1 calorie of heat to raise the temperature of steam 2° Celsius, just as with ice. For example, adding another 56 calories of heat will raise the temperature of the steam by 112° C.

In Figure 20-10, look at the steepness of the lines between 0 calories and 25 calories and 744 calories and 800 calories, respectively. The steepness looks the same. The graph between 105 calories and 205 calories is not as steep, however. This is because 1 calorie of heat will raise the temperature of ice or steam 2° Celsius, whereas 1 calorie of heat will raise the temperature of water only 1° Celsius. This concept of the steepness of a

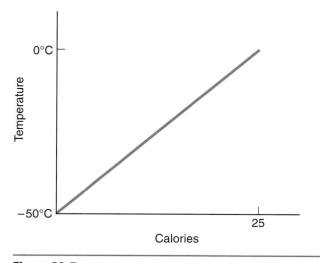

Figure 20-7 *Graph of temperature versus calories.*
Source: Delmar/Cengage Learning

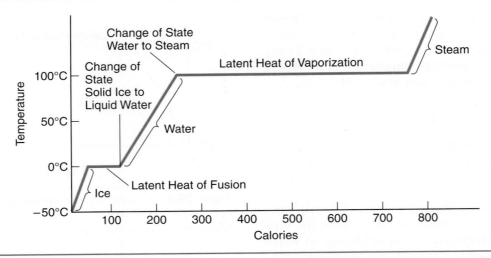

Figure 20-10   *Putting it all together: This graph shows the changes of states and the latent heat of fusion and vaporization. Notice how calories are added during the latent periods (flat lines), but there is no change in temperature.*

Source: Delmar/Cengage Learning

graph, called **slope**, is an important one. If units are consistent between graphs, the steeper the line, the faster the quantity is increasing.

Drug Dosage Response Graphs

Much of the health sciences is concerned with the proper dispensing of medications to treat illness. These medications must undergo testing to determine potency, safety, and maximal effect. A simple dose-effect relationship is illustrated in Figure 20-11. The shape of the curve in this figure tells a lot about this drug. For instance, the desired physiologic response is not attained until 20 g of the drug has been administered. After

that, there is a rise (slope), which reaches a peak, or maximal effect. Beyond the maximal effect, not only are little or even no additional positive effects seen, but the patient may in fact be placed in danger of toxicity or death. The general rule is to give the lowest dosage possible to produce the desired physiologic effects.

This type of graph can take on different shapes depending on how the given drug affects the body. For instance, if a drug reaches its maximal effects very rapidly, the slope of the graph would be steep, as in Figure 20-12, graph line A. The range of dosages that would give the desired response would be relatively narrow for this drug.

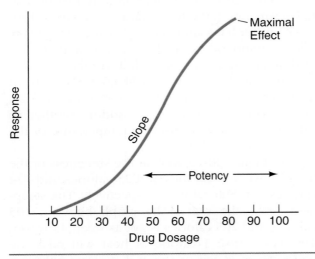

Figure 20-11   *Drug dosage response graph showing the dose-effect relationship.*

Source: Delmar/Cengage Learning

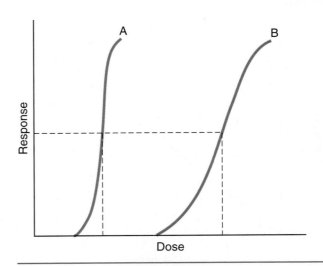

Figure 20-12   *Graph comparing two drugs and their effects.*

Source: Delmar/Cengage Learning

Now consider a graph that combines several concepts (Figure 20-13). In an earlier chapter, the concepts of ED_{50}, LD_{50}, and therapeutic index were discussed in relationship to fractions. The ED_{50} is the dose required to produce a desired effect in 50% of the individuals tested; this is by definition a median value. The LD_{50} is the median lethal dose. Both the ED_{50} and LD_{50} can be graphed to show the therapeutic index for a given population, as illustrated in Figure 20-13. (Of course, human subjects are not used.)

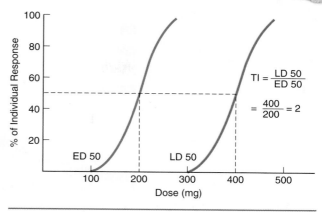

Figure 20-13   *Graph of the therapeutic index.*
Source: Delmar/Cengage Learning

CHAPTER REVIEW

Exercises

1. Find the mean, median, and mode for each of the following.

   a. 2, 3, 3, 4, 7, 9, 1, 0, 3

   b. 2, 9, 10, 15, 21, 20, 11, 12

   c. 2.1, 3.2, 5.7, 1.1, 2.6, 7.9, 2.0

2. The lengths of stay in days for 10 patients at a particular hospital were as follows:

   $$3, 7, 2, 12, 22, 2, 5, 2, 103, 12$$

   Find the mean, median, and mode for this data. Which of these measures of central tendency is the best indicator of the average length of stay?

3. The birth weights in ounces for the first 9 babies born in 2010 at a given hospital were as follows:

   $$80, 59, 84, 112, 100, 95, 59, 120, 24$$

   Find the mean, median, and mode for this data. Which of these measures of central tendency is the best indicator of the average birth weight?

4. Answer each of the following questions regarding the graph in Figure 20-14.

   a. Which of the four age groups is rising most rapidly?

   b. During what decades was the 85-and-older age group not significantly represented?

   c. What is happening to the 55–64 age group from 1900 to 2040?

   d. Write several paragraphs concerning the information provided by this graph. Cite possible health science–related explanations for these trends. In addition, discuss the potential impact of these trends on the health care system of the years 2000–2040.

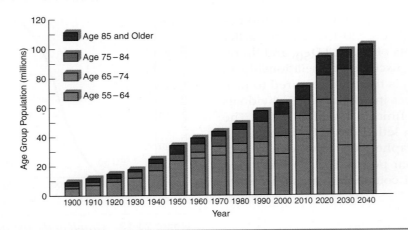

Figure 20-14   *The actual and projected populations of persons 55 years or older for four different age groups between the years 1900 and 2040.*

Source: Delmar/Cengage Learning

5. As we age, our bodies react to different stimuli in different ways. One way the body reacts to stress is by increasing heart rate. Maximum heart rate (measured in beats per minute, or bpm) is estimated by using the following formula:

maximum heart rate = 220 − age

Thus, the maximum heart rate for a 55-year-old individual is:

220 − 55 = 165 bpm

Maximum heart rate per age can be represented by a line graph, as in Figure 20-15. Answer each of the following questions regarding this figure.

a. Looking at the graph, what is the maximum heart rate for a 60-year-old?

b. In general, what does this graph lead you to conclude? You may draw a number of conclusions, including:

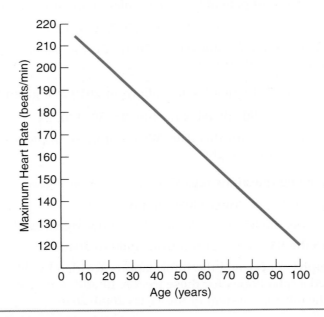

Figure 20-15   *Graph of maximum heart rate per age.*

Source: Delmar/Cengage Learning

- As we age, the supply of oxygen for heart tissue may decrease. Remember: oxygen is our fuel.
- As we age, the flexibility of the heart muscle decreases.
- As we age, the electrical pathways of the heart may become less effective.

Can you think of any more possible explanations?

It is important to note that as we age, it takes a longer time for the heart to both accelerate and return to a normal rate after a stressful situation. Thus, an elderly patient may not demonstrate the expected cardiac response to a variety of clinical stimulations, including pain and anxiety.

6. Answer each of the following questions regarding the graph in Figure 20-16, which illustrates the effects of aging on cardiac output (CO).

a. What general conclusion can you draw from this graph?

b. What is the cardiac output at ages 20, 30, 40, and 50, respectively?

c. What do you think the cardiac output would be at age 10?

d. What do you think the cardiac output would be at age 90?

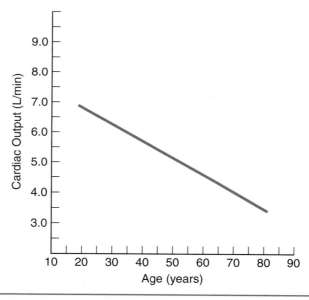

Figure 20-16 *Graph of the effects of aging on cardiac output.*
Source: Delmar/Cengage Learning

7. Answer each of the following questions regarding the therapeutic index graph in Figure 20-17 on the next page.

a. How many milligrams of this drug are needed to produce an effective dose in 50% of the subjects tested? How many milligrams are needed to produce a lethal dose in 50% of the subjects?

b. How many milligrams of the drug are needed to be effective in 100% of the subjects? How many milligrams are needed to be lethal in 100% of the subjects?

c. In order for the therapeutic index to increase, what would need to happen to the distance between the two lines in the graph? Would this result in a safer or more toxic medication?

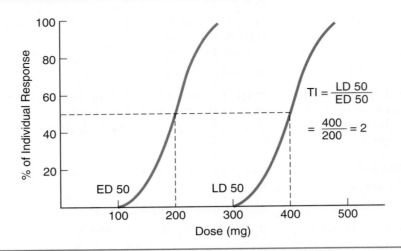

Figure 20-17 *Graph of therapeutic index.*
Source: Delmar/Cengage Learning

Real Life Issues and Applications

Statistics at Home

A growing body of evidence suggests that a parent who smokes cigarettes in the home may increase his or her child's risk of developing respiratory diseases such as bronchitis. Furthermore, the parent's smoking may increase the incidence of asthmatic attacks in an asthmatic child. Knowing this, if a parent continues smoking in an area of the home that is shared with a child, and that child develops bronchitis, should that parent be arrested and tried for child endangerment?

As a class project, determine the number of smokers and nonsmokers in each student's household. Use this information to develop a bar graph. Next determine the amount of cigarettes smoked in each household on a daily basis, and use this information to make another bar graph. Finally, determine the approximate number of colds that occur in each household over a period of 1 year, and use this information to create a third bar graph. Using these three bar graphs, determine the relationship between the number of people who smoke, the amount of cigarettes smoked, and the number of colds that occur annually in a given household.

Additional Activity

Contact your local chapter of the American Lung Association or American Cancer Society and ask for information regarding smoking. Areas on which to focus can include the median age of smokers, the average number of cigarettes smoked by smokers, the types of diseases caused by smoking, and the average increase in life expectancy after quitting smoking. Share this information with your class.

StudyWARE   **CONNECTION**

Go to your StudyWARE™ DVD and have fun learning as you play interactive games, view animations and videos, and take practice tests to help reinforce key concepts you learned in this chapter.

Workbook Practice | *Go to your Workbook for more practice questions and activities.*

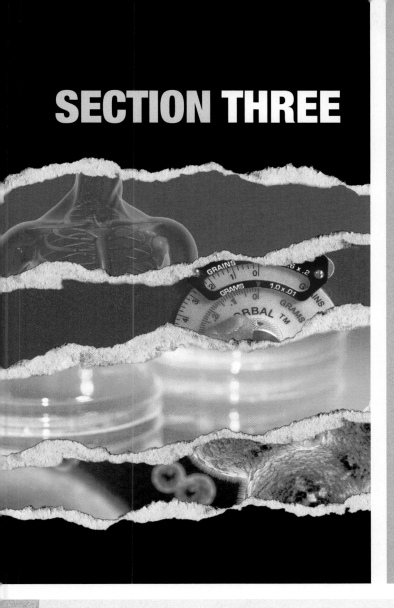

SECTION THREE

Chemistry in the Health Sciences

SECTION OVERVIEW

Chemistry plays an extremely important role in all aspects of health care. A basic understanding of chemistry is necessary to understand human physiology and the pathologic activities that occur in the human body. In addition, some relevant physics topics are discussed. The concepts learned here relate strongly to the anatomy, physiology, and microbiology sections. In the first chemistry chapter, one of the topics we will discuss is the physics and chemistry concept of states of matter. Why is this important, you may ask? This is the cornerstone of X-ray interpretation. The three main states—solid, liquid, and gas—can be found in the body as bone, blood, and air. These substances vary in density and, as you will later discover, affect how X-rays travel through your body and show up as variations of light and dark on an X-ray image. The other chemistry chapters will then focus on a more atomic and molecular level and provide additional concepts with clinical examples that have relevancy to a variety of health care professionals.

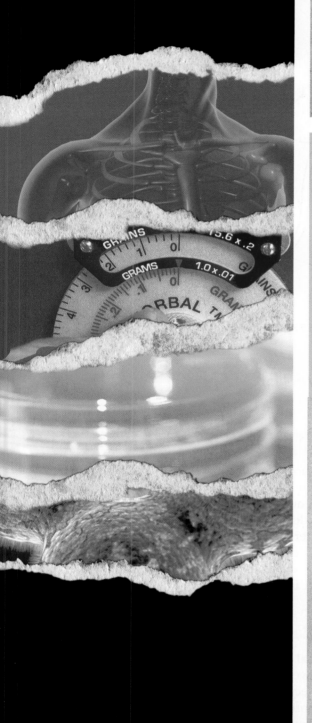

CHAPTER 21

ENERGY AND STATES OF MATTER

Objectives

Upon completion of this chapter, you should be able to

- Define the terms *potential energy* and *kinetic energy*
- List and describe the various states of matter
- Solve basic energy problems
- Solve basic problems relating to density and pressure
- Describe the various temperature scales

Key Terms

absolute zero
adhesive force
capillarity
capillary action
cohesive force
density

heat
kinetic energy
potential energy
pressure
temperature
thermal energy

SUPER HERO TRADING CARDS

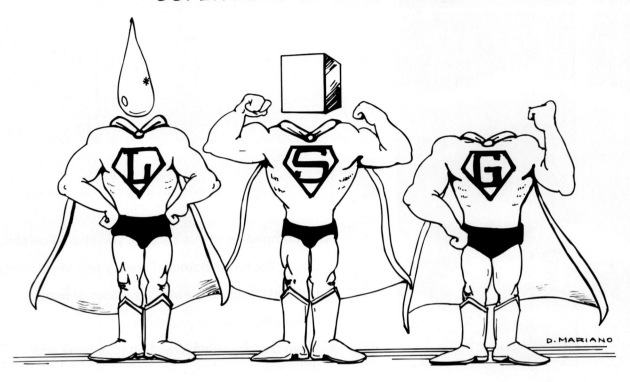

THE MANY FACES OF WATERMAN

Source: Delmar/Cengage Learning

■ INTRODUCTION

The sciences of chemistry and physics are often interrelated. Physics is the study of the laws of matter and their interactions with energy. The purpose of this chapter is to examine the concepts of energy and states of matter which have implications in both chemistry and physics.

For example, one of the abstract concepts in physics is that of energy. When you rise from bed in the morning you are full of energy—or, at least, you should be full of energy. Electricity, coal, and heat are all considered forms of energy. What do all of these energy forms have in common? The answer is that they all are capable of doing work. Energy has the capacity to do work. Work is defined as the product of the force (f) exerted on a body and the distance (d) the body moves in the direction of the force ($W = fd$). Energy is expressed in units of work such as foot-pounds or joules. The state or form of matter is very much related to the molecular energies. Therefore, we will begin with a discussion of the concept of energy.

Energy

This section contains a discussion of energy. The understanding of the concepts of kinetic energy and potential energy will be useful in later chapters. Understanding potential energy will help you better understand the concept of chemical potential energy discussed later. Kinetic energy will be used to explain the concept of temperature later in the chapter.

Potential Energy

Potential energy is stored energy. A hammer held above a nail has the capacity to drive the nail into a piece of wood. The hammer, therefore, has the potential to do work. Likewise, a drawn bow has the capacity to fire an arrow into a target, and a flexed spring has the capacity to do work.

Potential energy can be thought of as the *energy of position*. If an object has potential energy because of its height above the ground, it is called *gravitational potential energy*. In the case of the hammer held above the nail, the potential energy depends on the hammer's weight and the height to which the hammer is raised. This would yield an equation of:

$$PE = (W)(h)$$

Because weight is mass times the acceleration due to gravity (g); however, the equation for potential energy can become:

$$PE = (m)(g)(h)$$

Example:

A rock weighing 150 pounds is at the top of a cliff 100 feet high. What is the potential energy of the rock?

$$PE = (W)(h)$$

$$PE = (150 \text{ lb}) \times (100 \text{ ft}) = 15,000 \text{ ft-lb}$$

Kinetic Energy

Kinetic energy is the *energy of motion*. Many objects can do work because of their motions. A hammer drives a nail into a board because of its motion. Kinetic energy depends on the mass of the object and how fast the object is moving (i.e., its velocity):

$$KE = \tfrac{1}{2}(mv^2)$$

Example:

How much kinetic energy does a car weighing 3,500 pounds have if it is moving at a velocity of 40 feet per second?

$$KE = \tfrac{1}{2}(3,500)(40)^2$$

$$= \tfrac{1}{2}(3,500)(1,600)$$

$$= 2,800,000 \text{ (ft-lb/sec)}$$

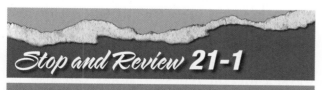

Stop and Review **21-1**

If the velocity of the car in the preceding example were increased to 80 feet per second, what would happen to the kinetic energy?

Conservation of Energy

In our discussion of gravitational potential energy, we determined that a rock weighing 150 pounds on top of a cliff 100 feet high has 15,000 foot-pounds of potential energy. Because the rock is not moving, however, its kinetic energy is zero. When the rock hits the ground, its potential energy is zero because its height (h) is zero. What has happened is that its potential energy was transformed into kinetic energy. In fact, the instant the rock hits the ground, the rock's kinetic energy is 15,000 foot-pounds, which is the same as its initial amount of potential energy (see Figure 21-1). This demonstrates the important principle of the conservation of energy that states *energy cannot be created or destroyed*. There may be

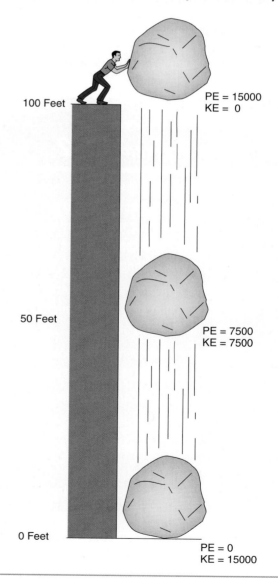

Figure 21-1 *The relationship between potential energy and kinetic energy.*

Source: Delmar/Cengage Learning

a transformation from one form of energy to another or a transfer of energy from one object to another, but the *total* energy is always conserved.

In the example of the falling rock, the kinetic energy is actually slightly less than 15,000 foot-pounds because air resistance causes a slight temperature change in the rock. As a result, some of the energy is transformed into **heat** energy. This is similar to how friction produces heat when we rub our hands together. The air "rubbing" the falling rock causes heat energy and warms the rock. Because this is so slight, we will ignore it for our purposes. With regard to a space shuttle's reentry into the Earth's atmosphere, however, the effects of this type of energy transformation could not be neglected. The heat energy transformed is so great, in fact, that special tiles had to be designed and adhered to the exterior of the shuttle to absorb the tremendous heat. Typically, though, we will use "ideal" models, wherein energy is either potential or kinetic in nature.

Stop and Review 21-2

a. A ball with a mass of 2 kilograms is dropped from the top of a building. If the ball's kinetic energy when it hits the ground is 200 kilogram-meters per square second, how high is the building?

b. Explain the changes in kinetic energy and potential of a child sled riding from the top of a hill to the bottom of the hill.

c. Choose either kinetic energy or potential energy for each of the following statements:

1. the energy in a gallon of gasoline

2. the energy in sugar

3. the energy in a football as it travels to a receiver

4. a race car speeding around a track

Matter and Its Interactions

In the following section, we will discuss the concept of states of matter. This is a fundamental concept to the study of science. We will also discuss the concept of density.

States of Matter

Ordinarily, matter exists in one of three physical states: *solid*, *liquid*, or *gas*. Another state is encountered only under extremely high temperatures; it is called the *plasma state*.

Temperature is an important factor related to states of matter. In fact, temperature is one of the main determining factors for the state of matter. For example, water, which is a liquid state, can be frozen to form ice, which is a solid state, or heated to form steam, which is a gaseous state.

All matter is composed of atoms. In most substances, these atoms are joined to form molecules. For example, one molecule of water is composed of two hydrogen atoms and one oxygen atom. These atoms are held together by electrical forces generated by the particles of the atoms themselves. Whether the water molecule is frozen, liquid, or gaseous, it is always composed of two hydrogen atoms and one oxygen atom. Change of state does not chemically alter the makeup of the molecule.

The states of matter can generally be described as follows. Solids have definite shapes. Liquids have definite volumes but not definite shapes. A liquid takes on the shape of the container within which it is held. A gas spreads out and fills the entire container within which it is held. Gases have no definite volumes, or shapes (see Figure 21-2). If enough heat is added to a gas, the molecules and then the atoms themselves will separate, and a plasma state will result. (Note: Although it is pronounced and spelled the same, this plasma is completely different from blood plasma.)

Solids

As mentioned previously, solids have definite shapes and volumes. The atoms and molecules, however, are not fixed but, instead, vibrate within a fixed position. The molecules are in a constant state of motion but are confined to a very small space. You could think of atoms as being connected by "springs", which are the forces that hold the atoms together. Although the atoms vibrate, they are held together by these forces.

Atoms can be combined in different ways. Different types of atoms can also be combined. The different kinds of atoms combined in different ways determine the type of matter formed by the molecules. Again the molecular form does not change from one state of matter to another.

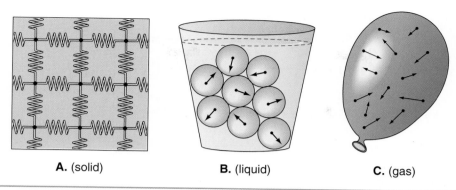

A. (solid)   **B.** (liquid)   **C.** (gas)

Figure 21-2 *The states of matter.*
Source: Delmar/Cengage Learning

QUOTES & NOTES

The planet Saturn is large but not very dense. If there were an enormous ocean in space, Saturn would float in it!

A black hole occurs when a star collapses to such a small diameter and becomes so dense that not even light can escape its gravitational pull.

Density

One of the obvious differences between objects is the compactness of the objects. For example, equal volumes of Styrofoam and lead do not weigh the same. This is because the lead is much more compact. The masses of the particles in relation to the spaces between the particles will determine the **density** of a material. Density, then, is a measure of the compactness of the particles in a material. Density is defined as mass divided by volume.

$$\text{density} = \text{mass/volume}$$

$$d = m/v$$

Units for density are units of mass/units of volume. For example:

$$\text{gram/cm}^3 \text{ or kg/m}^3$$

Example:

What is the density of a block of wood with a mass of 700 grams and a volume of 1,000 cubic centimeters?

$$\text{density} = \text{mass/volume}$$

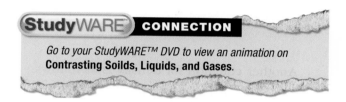

There are two important things to keep in mind regarding density. The first is that for equal volumes of material, the more dense the material the more it weighs. A block of iron measuring 1 cubic foot and having a density of about 7.9 grams per cubic centimeter will weigh approximately three times as much as a block of aluminum measuring 1 cubic foot and having a density of 2.7 grams per cubic centimeter. Thus, it would take approximately three times a given volume of aluminum to obtain the same weight as the same given volume of lead.

The second important thing to keep in mind regarding density is that an object immersed in a liquid or gas will float if it is less dense than the liquid or gas. If it is denser it will sink. Figure 21-3 shows objects of various densities in water. The objects that are less dense than water (cork and ice) float while the objects with a larger density than water (aluminum and lead) sink. Water has a density of 1 gram per cubic centimeter, whereas ice has a density of approximately 0.92 gram per cubic centimeter. Ice is, therefore, less dense than water; this is why ice cubes float in water. The density of a typical human body is slightly less than 1 gram per cubic centimeter. Thus, most humans float in water. People whose bodies are denser will, of course, sink.

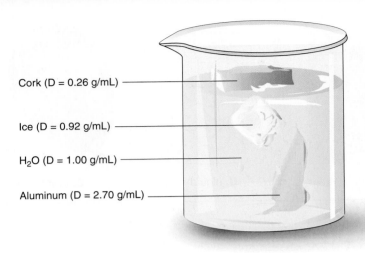

Cork (D = 0.26 g/mL)

Ice (D = 0.92 g/mL)

H_2O (D = 1.00 g/mL)

Aluminum (D = 2.70 g/mL)

Figure 21-3   *Objects of varying densities in water.*

Source: Delmar/Cengage Learning

Another equation for density is as follows:

$$\text{density} = \text{weight}/\text{volume}$$

This equation is sometimes used to yield easier calculations. Fresh water has a density of 62.4 pounds per cubic foot. Thus, 1 cubic foot of fresh water weighs 62.4 pounds. Salt water is slightly denser, at 64 pounds per cubic foot.

Special Focus

Density and Measuring Body Fat

This idea can be applied to the health sciences. It is more important to know a person's percent of body fat than his or her weight. There are different ways to measure body fat. One way involves the concept of density. If you have ever seen Italian dressing, you should remember that the oil floats on top of the vinegar. Fats and oils are less dense than water and hence float on water. Therefore, a person who has a higher percent of body fat will float in water more readily than a person with a low percent of body fat.

To determine a person's percent of body fat, you must first determine the person's mass on land. The second step is to determine his or her mass while submerged in water. This is done by lowering the person into water on a large platform that is part of an apparatus to measure mass. The difference between the mass on land and the mass in water can be used to calculate the buoyant force. The buoyant force is used to determine the body volume. The person's density (M/V) can be found by dividing the mass on land by the body volume. The person's body density can then be used to determine the percent of body fat from a chart. The higher a person's percent of body fat, the lower the person's density. The lower the person's percent of body fat, the higher his or her density.

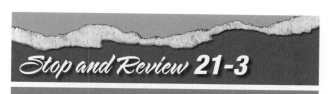

Stop and Review 21-3

a. A(n) _____ spreads out and fills the entire container within which it is held.

b. A(n) _____ takes on the shape of the container within which it is held.

c. You could think of atoms as being connected by springs in a(n) _____.

d. Explain how a life jacket decreases a person's density, thus enabling the person to float in water.

So, an object with a density of 63 pounds per cubic foot will float in salt water but sink in fresh water.

Pressure

Another very important concept is that of **pressure**. As will be further discussed in Chapter 24, a force is a push or a pull. Pressure, likewise, is the push or pull per area of the surface acted on. Thus, pressure takes into account not only the force but also the area of application.

$$\text{pressure} = \text{force/area}$$
$$p = f/a$$

Some units for pressure are pounds/square inch and newtons/square meter.

Clinical Relevancy

The Specific Gravity of Urine

Much can be learned by measuring the density of an individual's urine. The density of this fluid is related to its specific gravity. Determining the specific gravity is a normal part of routine urinalysis in the hospital setting. The specific gravity of urine can be measured using a hydrometer, which is a glass bulb that floats in the liquid of interest. The urinometer has a scale that is used to determine the specific gravity. See Figure 21-4.

When measuring specific gravity, we are actually measuring the concentration of particles in the urine. These particles include waste and electrolytes from the body. Specific gravity of urine, then, is a good indicator of how well the kidneys are functioning and is also an indicator of the body's hydration level. This lets us know whether a patient's fluid intake should be restricted or increased.

The normal range of specific gravity for urine is 1.010 to 1.030. If a urine sample has a high specific gravity, it is considered concentrated. Diluted urine has a low specific gravity. Higher-than-normal specific gravities can be caused by dehydration, a decrease in blood flow to the kidneys (resulting from heart failure or hypotension), fever, vomiting, excessive sweating, or diarrhea. Lower-than-normal specific gravities can

be caused by overhydration, diabetes insipidus, renal failure (wherein the kidneys cannot reabsorb water), diuretics, or hypothermia.

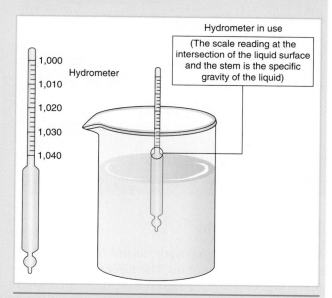

Figure 21-4   *A hydrometer designed to serve as a urinometer.*

Source: Delmar/Cengage Learning

Examples:

A man weighing 200 pounds stands on both feet. If the area of the bottom of each shoe is 40 square inches, how much pressure is exerted on the floor?

$$p = f/a$$
$$p = 200 \text{ lb}/80 \text{ sq in.}$$
$$p = 2.5 \text{ lb/sq in.}$$

Does a woman weighing 100 pounds and standing on heels each having an area of 5 square inches exert more or less pressure on the floor than does the man in the preceding example?

$$p = f/a$$
$$p = 100 \text{ lb}/10 \text{ sq in.}$$
$$p = 10 \text{ lb/sq in. } 10 \text{ lb/in}^2, \text{ or four times the}$$
pressure exerted by the man in the preceding example.

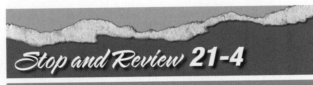

Stop and Review 21-4

a. Using the equation for pressure, explain why a sharp hypodermic needle does not require as much pressure to puncture the skin as does a dull one.

b. What units are used to measure gas pressure?

c. A woman weighs 100 lb and wears high heels with a heel area of 1/16 sq in. (¼ in. x ¼ in.). Calculate the force of the heel on the floor when the woman takes a step. Assume all her weight is exerted on the heel.

Change of State

As mentioned previously, the atoms in solids are in a constant state of motion. The forces that hold the atoms together are analogous to springs. In a solid substance, the atoms vibrate about fixed positions. As the temperature of the substance increases, the activity of the atoms also increases. The atoms begin to vibrate more rapidly. The molecules then begin to flow and take on the shape of the container within which they are held. The substance,

thus, forms a liquid. The molecules, however, stay approximately the same distance apart. This means that, for the most part, liquids cannot be compressed. Thus, a liquid will, generally speaking, keep its same volume under pressure.

As the temperature of the substance again increases, the molecules begin to vibrate even more rapidly—so rapidly, in fact, that they begin to break apart and form a gas. The molecules of the gas are now free to move apart and fill the container within which they are held. Unlike the liquid, however, the gas is compressible. (This is discussed further in Chapter 24.)

Because both liquids and gases flow, they are often referred to collectively as *fluids*. Many of the principles of physics apply equally to both liquids and gases. Some principles, such as compressibility, however, apply to liquids in a manner different from gases.

Liquid Pressure

Under the surface of any liquid, there exists pressure resulting from the weight of the liquid. Water in a swimming pool, for instance, exerts a force on the bottom of the pool because of the weight of the water above it. It is analogous to piling books one on top of another. The more books on the pile, the greater the pressure on the bottom book. The deeper the water, the greater the weight of water exerting force on the bottom of the pool. The pressure caused by any liquid can be determined using the following equation:

$$\text{pressure} = \text{weight density} \times \text{depth}$$
$$p = (D)(d)$$

Liquid pressure does not depend on the size or shape of the container. Liquid pressure depends only on the density of the liquid and the depth. Therefore, the pressure at the bottom of a swimming pool 10 feet deep is the same as the pressure at the bottom of a reservoir 10 feet deep,

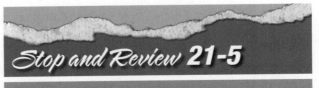

Stop and Review 21-5

If salt water has a density of 64 pounds per cubic foot, what is the pressure exerted on a swimmer 10 feet below the surface of the ocean?

which is the same as the pressure 10 feet below the surface of the water behind the Hoover Dam.

Capillary Action

The force of attraction between molecules of like substances is called **cohesive force**. The force of attraction between molecules of unlike substances is called **adhesive force**.

If you look at a glass filled halfway with water (or a half-empty glass if you are a pessimist), you will see that the water appears to climb up the sides of the glass ever so slightly. This is because the adhesive forces between the glass and the water are stronger than the cohesive forces within the water itself. If the glass were filled halfway with mercury, however, the surface of the mercury would bow upward toward the center. This is because the cohesive forces within the mercury are stronger than the adhesive forces between mercury and the glass. Don't try this at home, as mercury is a poisonous substance.

When a tube having a very small diameter (called a capillary tube) is inserted in a liquid, the liquid will rise in the tube. This is called **capillary action**, or **capillarity**. The adhesive forces cause the liquid to climb up the walls of the tube, while the cohesive forces cause the center of the liquid to rise. The combination of these forces causes the center of the liquid to rise until the upward force is balanced by the weight of the liquid in the tube. In other words, the adhesive force, which pulls the water up, equals the weight of the column of water, which pulls the water down, causing the liquid to stop rising (see Figure 21-5).

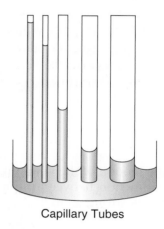

Capillary Tubes

Figure 21-5 *Capillary tubes: notice that the volume of liquid in each tube is the same.*

Source: Delmar/Cengage Learning

Clinical Relevancy

Baby Blood Gases (Capillary Sticks)

Premature newborns often have breathing mechanisms that have not yet matured enough to sustain life on their own. In other situations, a baby may be born healthy but something may happen subsequent to birth to make breathing difficult.

A sample of blood taken from an infant's artery (known as an *arterial blood gas*, or *ABG*) enables us to determine how well the child is breathing. By examining the level of carbon dioxide in the infant's blood, we can determine how well air is moving in and out of the infant's lungs (ventilation); by looking at the oxygen levels, we can determine whether we need to supply more oxygen to the infant; and the bicarbonate levels help us determine the metabolic status of our little patient.

The most common site for obtaining a blood gas is the radial artery located in the wrist. The radial artery of a newborn is extremely tiny, however. In addition, arteries are located deeper in the body in comparison to veins; because you cannot see arteries, it is necessary to, instead, feel for the artery before inserting the needle to obtain the sample. Locating an infant's radial artery can be made somewhat easier by placing the infant's wrist over a bright, *cool* light. Because the infant's wrist is relatively thin, enough light can pass through to provide a view of the internal anatomy of the wrist. This makes arterial identification and needle insertion much easier.

Historically, an alternative to ABGs has been the *capillary blood sample* (known as the *capillary stick*, or *heel stick*). In this procedure, the infant's heel is warmed, usually by wrapping the foot with a clean

(continues)

(continued)

diaper soaked in warm, not hot, water. This warming process "arterializes" the capillary blood in the tissue of the heel so that it closely reflects the carbon dioxide and oxygen levels of the arteries.

When the infant's heel has been sufficiently heated, it is wiped with an alcohol-saturated pad. The heel is then pricked with a lancet (a small razor blade) and gently squeezed to cause bleeding. The first drop of blood is wiped away, and a capillary tube with heparin (an anticoagulant) coating the lumen (to prevent clotting of the blood in the tube) is placed at the incision site. Because of capillary action, the blood travels right up the inside of the tube. Two tubes are usually filled. A bandage is then placed on the heel and the blood sample is taken to a blood gas analyzing machine to be "run" (a term used with regard to blood samples that means "analyzed").

The advantage of the capillary stick method is that it requires small amounts of blood; this is particularly important if many samples are needed over a period of time, such as when an infant is severely ill. If larger samples were used, there would be a possibility of severely depleting the infant's blood supply.

Perhaps now you can see how the concept of capillarity applies to practical situations in the health care field.

Surface Tension

Because of the motion of the vibrating molecules, the force of attraction between the molecules in a liquid is not as strong as that of the molecules in a solid. The molecules in a liquid are still attracted to one another, however. The molecules below the surface of the liquid are attracted to the molecules on all sides, which results in a net force of zero. See Figure 21-6. The molecules at the surface of a liquid, however, are attracted in all directions except upward. These molecular attractions tend to pull the surface molecules into a liquid film where the water meets the gaseous atmosphere. Surface tension allows the water level to be increased beyond the rim of a glass. The surface of the water becomes stretched almost like an elastic film (see Figure 21-7).

The effects of surface tension can be demonstrated by carefully placing a razor blade on the surface of a glass of calm water. Placing a few drops of detergent into the water will cause the razor blade to sink. This is because detergent reduces the surface tension and makes water "wetter." In fact, that is the purpose of detergent: to reduce surface tension and stop water from beading up. Using soap while washing your hands, therefore, allows the water to penetrate the pores of your hands, thus facilitating cleaning.

Because hand washing is one of the best ways to stop the spread of germs, perhaps you can understand why it is so important to use soap instead of just rinsing your hands with water before and after working with patients.

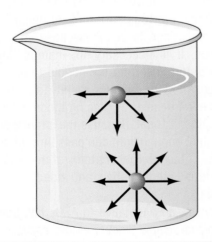

Figure 21-6 *A surface molecule is pulled only sideways and downward by neighboring molecules. A subsurface molecule is pulled equally in all directions.*

Source: Delmar/Cengage Learning

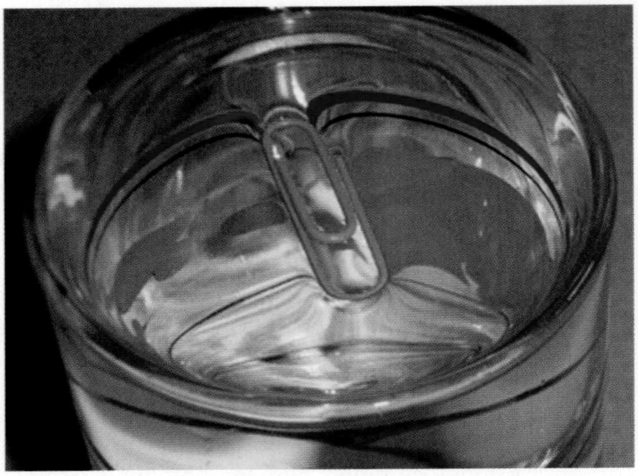

Figure 21-7 *A paper clip can float on water due to surface tension.*

Source: Delmar/Cengage Learning

Clinical Relevancy

Surfactant in the Lungs

Surfactant is a liquid produced in the lungs by type-II cells. This liquid forms a continuous layer around the alveoli (the small microscopic structures where gas exchange takes place) and has the ability to alter surface tension. As the radius of an alveolar unit decreases, a greater pressure is required to keep the sphere-like structures from collapsing. This decrease of radius coincides with end exhalation when the alveoli are smallest. Surfactant lessens the pressure needed to keep the alveoli and small airways open at end exhalation. It also lessens pressure needed to inflate the lungs. This concept is very important because reduced or insufficient amounts of surfactant can lead to alveolar instability and eventual collapse (atelectasis). This means that less air will be used in the gas exchange between the lungs and the blood, thus decreasing oxygen levels while increasing carbon dioxide levels.

Decreased surfactant can result from near drowning (where water washes it away); exposure to high levels of oxygen; air pollution; neonatal and adult respiratory distress syndromes; and pulmonary edema. There also appears to be a relationship between monotonous breathing and low breathing volumes leading to decreased surfactant levels, and atelectasis.

Ground-up cow and sheep lungs possessing surfactant have been successfully instilled into human lungs to increase surfactant levels. Synthetic surfactants also have brought remarkable improvement in many patients, especially premature infants. In many cases, instillation of surfactant into human lungs has prevented the need for mechanical ventilation and the complications that potentially accompany this serious medical intervention.

Temperature and Heat

As discussed earlier, changing the temperature of a substance is one way of changing its form. An increase in temperature causes an increase in the motion of the molecules; they vibrate more rapidly. All the molecules within the substance do not necessarily move with the same speed, however. Some move more rapidly than others. Temperature is a measure of the average energy per molecule of a substance; it is a measure of the hotness or coldness of a substance.

The temperature of a body is the condition that determines the direction of energy flow between that body and other bodies. **Thermal energy** always moves from a substance having a higher temperature to one having a lower temperature.

How does the temperature of a substance change? Obviously, there must be some kind of energy transfer. Because energy can be neither created nor destroyed, the increase in molecular motion (i.e., energy) must come from some other source. This energy transfer is called *heat*.

Heat is the thermal energy added to, or removed from, a substance.

The distinction between temperature, thermal energy, and heat is an important one, especially to chemists and physicists. Temperature is a measure of the average molecular energy of a substance; thermal energy is a measure of the total energy of a substance; and heat is the energy transferred from one substance to another.

QUOTES & NOTES

The heart of a star reaches nearly 30 million° F. A grain of sand that hot would kill a person up to 100 miles away!

Measuring Temperature

Certainly, human beings have the ability, through the sense of touch, to determine whether a substance is hotter or colder than their own body temperatures. But how can we measure that hotness or coldness and fix some number to it?

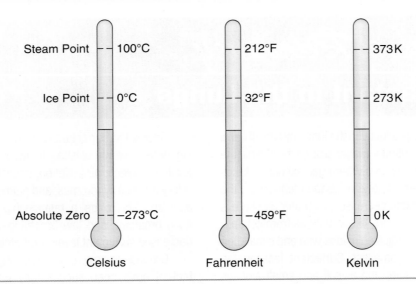

Figure 21-8 *Comparison of the Celsius, Fahrenheit, and Kelvin temperature scales.*
Source: Delmar/Cengage Learning

A thermometer is the most common device used to measure temperature. A thermometer operates on the principle that most substances expand when their temperatures rise and contract when their temperatures fall.

The most common type of thermometer is constructed of a small glass capillary tube containing a liquid (usually mercury or colored alcohol). A bulb (or reservoir) at the base of the thermometer holds the liquid; as the temperature rises, the liquid expands and flows into the tube. This provides a means of measuring temperature.

For example, if you were to first place a thermometer in ice water and calibrate it to read 0, then place it in boiling water at standard pressure and calibrate it to read 100, and, finally, separate the difference between these points into 100 sections (degrees), the resulting thermometer would reflect the Celsius temperature scale. Had the freezing and boiling points been labeled 32 and 212, respectively, with 180 sections (degrees) in between, the thermometer would reflect the Fahrenheit temperature scale.

Another temperature scale often used in science and research is the Kelvin scale. Similar to the Celsius scale, the Kelvin temperature scale also has 100 sections between the freezing and boiling points of water. In the Kelvin scale, however, water freezes at 273 Kelvin (*not* degrees) and boils at 373 Kelvin. A

measurement of 0 Kelvin, which corresponds to −273 degrees Celsius, is called **absolute zero**. Absolute zero is, theoretically, the lowest limit of temperature. (This concept is discussed further in Chapter 24 on gas laws.) Figure 21-8 compares the Celsius, Fahrenheit, and Kelvin temperature scales.

QUOTES & NOTES

*T*hought to ponder: Why are you unable to determine whether you are running a temperature by touching your own head?

Measuring Heat

As previously discussed, heat is the transfer of thermal energy from one body to another. This transfer usually causes a change in temperature, and the amount of heat transferred is related to the change in temperature. The units most often used to measure heat are the *calorie* and the *BTU* (British thermal unit). A calorie is the amount of heat required to change the temperature of 1 gram of water 1 degree Celsius. A BTU is the amount of heat required to change the temperature of 1 pound of water 1 degree Fahrenheit. One BTU equals 252 calories. Figure 21-9 shows the amount of calories needed to change the state of water.

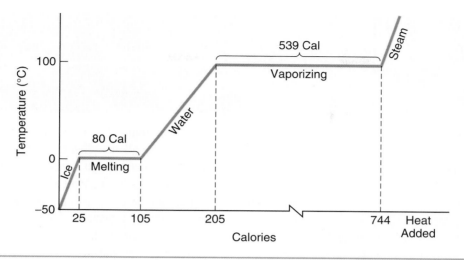

Figure 21-9   *Graph showing the changes in temperature of one gram of water as heat is added to it. Notice the changes of state.*

Source: Delmar/Cengage Learning

Special Focus

Calories, Calories, Calories!

The United States is a nation of dieters. No matter where you go, you are constantly bombarded with commercials telling you how to lose weight via dieting, exercise, pills, or even hypnosis. There are some definite disadvantages to being truly overweight. In an obese individual, the heart must work harder. In fact, for every pound of fat in the body, the heart must pump blood through approximately an additional 2/3 mile of blood vessels!

True obesity is a condition wherein a person weighs 20% more than that person's ideal body weight (IBW). Ideal body weight (in pounds) is determined by the following formulas:

male IBW = 106 + [(ht. in inches − 60) × 6]
female IBW = 105 + [(ht. in inches − 60) × 5]

Calculate your ideal body weight and see where you are!

You have, no doubt, heard the word *calorie*. A calorie is a measurement of the energy value of food. The higher the number of calories, the more energy the food has to offer.

As we work or, even, as we breathe, we utilize energy. Certain disease states can alter the rate at which we use, or "burn up," calories. Patients with lung disease, for instance, use ten times the calories to breathe as do healthy individuals.

Normally, we lose or gain weight based on two things: the amount of calories we take in and the amount of calories we burn up. If you were to maintain your current intake of calories and decrease your activity level, you would gain weight. If you were to increase your activity level and maintain your current intake of calories, you would lose weight. If you were to maintain your current activity level and increase your caloric intake, you would gain weight. If you were to maintain your current activity level, and decrease your caloric intake, you would lose weight. Other factors may, of course, affect weight; but this is how it generally works.

Why does dieting often seem to fail? It is most likely because many people who diet fail to undertake other necessary lifestyle changes. A balanced diet (i.e., one utilizing all of the food groups) and a realistic regular exercise program are necessary in order to take weight off and keep it off. These two things should not be abandoned when weight is lost but, rather, should become an integral part of a healthier lifestyle.

Professional Profile
Occupational Therapy

As a rule, we have provided information on health professions whenever those professions have related to particular chapters. As in life, however, there are always exceptions to rules. Although occupational therapy does not exactly "fit in" with this chapter, we felt that it was too important a profession to not include it.

Occupational therapists work with patients who are disabled as a result of mental, physical, developmental, or emotional disorders. These health professionals help patients deal with both activities of daily living and the physical and emotional stress that can accompany disability.

If you watch an occupational therapist at work, you will see that these professionals use a variety of activities in working with patients. Many of these activities appear to be fun or recreational, but they each serve a specific purpose. Some things that many of us take for granted, such as baking a cake or cleaning house, are activities that aid in the development of memory, sequencing of events, coordination, and dexterity. Other similar everyday activities may be used to help patients develop perceptual skills in areas as simple as recognizing colors or shapes.

Because of their disabilities, some patients require special equipment in order to aid their independence. For instance, special eating utensils may be necessary for those patients who do not have full use of their hands. Occupational therapists help patients learn to use this specialized equipment.

Occupational therapists work not only in the hospital setting, but also are employed in public schools, nursing homes, rehabilitation centers, and patients' homes. The minimal educational requirement for this field is a bachelor's degree.

An alternative to an occupational therapy degree is an occupational therapy assistant certificate. Individuals having high school diplomas and 1- or 2-year degrees from accredited colleges or universities can work as occupational therapy assistants under the supervision of occupational therapists.

For more information on this diverse field, contact the American Occupational Therapy Association by visiting their website at www.aota.org.

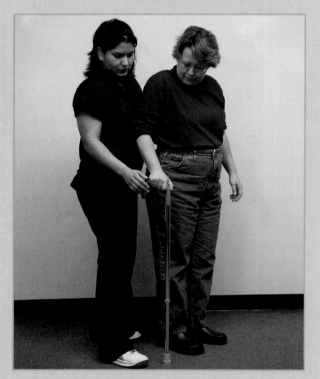

Source: Delmar/Cengage Learning

■ CHAPTER REVIEW

Exercises

1. You want to smash an egg; therefore, you hold a 600-pound anvil 2 feet above a large, grade A chicken egg. That anvil suspended above the egg is an example of what type of energy? (*Hint*: It is the energy of position.)

2. If a 400-pound can of banana pudding were on a shelf 6 feet above the ground, what would be the potential energy of that can of pudding?

3. If you were to roll a 600-pound can of pudding down the isle of the grocery store at a rate of 60 feet per second, what would be the kinetic energy of that can of pudding?

4. Why are special tiles needed on the space shuttle so that it can reenter the Earth's atmosphere?

5. List the four physical states of matter.

6. What is the basic difference between atoms and molecules?

7. What is the density of a sponge having a mass of 100 grams and a volume of 2,000 cubic centimeters?

8. A 600-pound man is standing on one foot. If the bottom of his shoe is 3 square inches, how much pressure is he exerting on the floor?

9. Why does a can of Diet Coke float while regular Coke sinks?

10. Explain why a liquid will travel up a capillary tube.

11. Two scientists approach a container holding some fluid. The first scientist sticks a thermometer into the fluid, and the thermometer reads 275. The second scientist also sticks a thermometer into the fluid. This thermometer reads 2. If the thermometers are not broken, what is going on?

12. A teacher place two beakers on a desk. The one beaker contains 50 mL of water at 25°C and the other contains 150 mL at 25°C. They are both at the same temperature, but do they contain the same amount of heat energy? Explain.

Real Life Issues and Applications

Extra Weight and Its Strain on the Heart

A male patient presents with heart failure (HF). After the acute episode is treated, he is told that he should lose weight to lessen the work of his heart. He is 5 feet 6 inches tall and weighs 200 pounds. Ideally, how much weight should he lose? What suggestions would you give him?

Additional Activity

In this chapter, we learned about temperature. Oral, rectal, axillary, and otic temperatures are taken in health care settings. Research these routes of obtaining body temperature, such as the advantages and disadvantages, and share your findings with the class.

StudyWARE　**CONNECTION**

Go to your StudyWARE™ DVD and have fun learning as you play interactive games, view animations and videos, and take practice tests to help reinforce key concepts you learned in this chapter.

Workbook Practice　*Go to your Workbook for more practice questions and activities.*

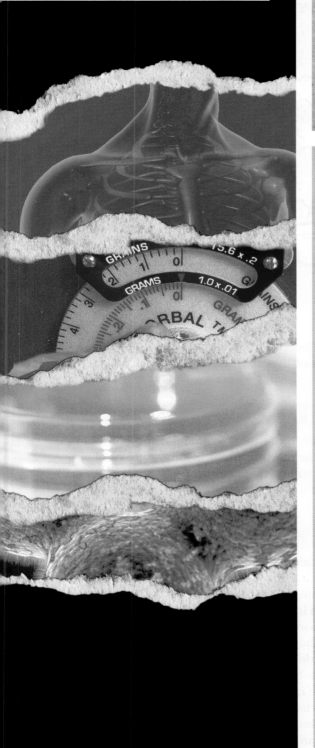

CHAPTER 22

BASIC CONCEPTS OF CHEMISTRY

Objectives

Upon completion of this chapter, you should be able to

- ■ Relate the importance of chemistry to students studying the health professions and to various body processes

- ■ Define and differentiate between atoms, elements, and isotopes

- ■ Explain and illustrate atomic structure, including the major particles that make up the atom

- ■ Explain the importance of and the information that can be obtained from the periodic table

- ■ Draw the Bohr model and the electron dot structure for any of the first 20 elements of the periodic table

- ■ Distinguish between alpha radiation, beta radiation, and gamma radiation

- ■ Relate radioisotopes to the treatment and diagnosis of disease

- ■ State the advantages and disadvantages of MRI, PET scan, X-rays, and CT scan

Key Terms

alpha radiation
atom
atomic number
beta radiation
compounds
computer tomography (**CT**) scan

electron dot structure
electrons
element
energy levels
gamma radiation
isotopes

(continues)

magnetic resonance imaging (**MRI**)   neutrons   protons
mass number   nucleus   **X**-rays
metastasized   positron emission tomography (**PET**)

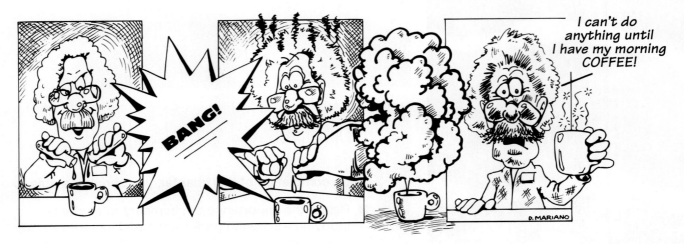

I can't do anything until I have my morning COFFEE!

BANG!

D. MARIANO

Source: Delmar/Cengage Learning

■ INTRODUCTION

People entering the health professions sometimes feel that they do not need to study chemistry. Nothing could be further from the truth. The body is a complex chemical factory within which a variety of reactions take place that are integral to good health. For example, the energy required in playing sports or any physical activity comes from chemical reactions that break down glucose (a type of sugar) to carbon dioxide and water. When the body is not functioning properly, different chemical reactions occur that upset the delicate balance and result in the symptoms associated with various maladies. An understanding of the chemical processes that occur in the body can help in making diagnoses, giving proper therapies, and responding appropriately in emergency situations.

Chemistry has a wide variety of applications to the health professions. Before we can discuss these applications, however, you must first learn the basics of chemistry, including vocabulary. This chapter introduces you to these basics. All of the chapters in this section build on each other; therefore, it is necessary for you to understand the introductory material before proceeding. For this reason, we include the periodic table here (see Figure 22-1)—because this table is like an owner's manual for chemistry. During your study of chemistry you will need to reference this table many times. The periodic table is further explained throughout this chapter.

What Makes Up Our World?

A discussion of atoms, elements, and compounds will be the starting point in our study of chemistry. This will be the basis for the study of chemical bonds in a later chapter.

Atoms

The ancient Greeks were among the first to develop a theory about atoms. Given the lack of equipment in ancient times, their theory was based on logic rather than experimental evidence. They reasoned that if you were to cut a bar of gold in half, then cut the half in half, and continue to do so, you would eventually end up with a particle that, if cut in half, would no longer be a particle of gold. They labeled this smallest complete particle an **atom**. See Figure 22-2.

Today, we still use this concept to define the atom of an **element**. By definition, then, an atom is the smallest particle of an element that still retains the properties of that element. An *element* is a pure substance that cannot be broken down into a simpler substance by ordinary chemical means. Thus, gold is an element, and the actual particles that make up gold are gold atoms.

Periodic Table of the Elementsᵃ

Atomic Number

Noble
Gases
0

Periods	IA																	

1 1 **H** 1.00794

Atomic weight

IIA

2 3 **Li** 6.941 / 4 **Be** 9.01218

3 11 **Na** 22.98977 / 12 **Mg** 24.3050

IIIB IVB VB VIB VIIB   VIII   IB IIB

4 19 **K** 39.0983 / 20 **Ca** 40.078 / 21 **Sc** 44.95591 / 22 **Ti** 47.88 / 23 **V** 50.9415 / 24 **Cr** 51.9961 / 25 **Mn** 54.9380 / 26 **Fe** 55.847 / 27 **Co** 58.93320 / 28 **Ni** 58.69 / 29 **Cu** 63.546 / 30 **Zn** 65.39 / 31 **Ga** 69.723 / 32 **Ge** 72.61 / 33 **As** 74.92159 / 34 **Se** 78.96 / 35 **Br** 79.904 / 36 **Kr** 83.80

5 37 **Rb** 85.4678 / 38 **Sr** 87.62 / 39 **Y** 88.90585 / 40 **Zr** 91.224 / 41 **Nb** 92.90638 / 42 **Mo** 94.94 / 43 **Tc** 98.9072 / 44 **Ru** 101.07 / 45 **Rh** 102.90550 / 46 **Pd** 106.42 / 47 **Ag** 107.8682 / 48 **Cd** 112.411 / 49 **In** 114.82 / 50 **Sn** 118.710 / 51 **Sb** 121.75 / 52 **Te** 127.60 / 53 **I** 126.90447 / 54 **Xe** 131.29

6 55 **Cs** 132.90543 / 56 **Ba** 137.327 / 57 *****La** 138.9055 / 72 **Hf** 178.49 / 73 **Ta** 180.9479 / 74 **W** 183.85 / 75 **Re** 186.207 / 76 **Os** 190.2 / 77 **Ir** 192.22 / 78 **Pt** 195.08 / 79 **Au** 196.96654 / 80 **Hg** 200.59 / 81 **Tl** 204.3833 / 82 **Pb** 207.2 / 83 **Bi** 208.98037 / 84 **Po** 208.9824 / 85 **At** 209.9871 / 86 **Rn** 222.0176

7 87 **Fr** 223.0197 / 88 **Ra** 226.0254 / **89 †Ac** 227.0278 / 104 **Unq** 261.11 / 105 **Unp** 262.114 / 106 **Unh** 263.118 / 107 **Uns** 262.12 / 108 **Uno** 265 / 109 **Une** 273

IIIA IVA VA VIA VIIA

2 **He** 4.00260

5 **B** 10.811 / 6 **C** 12.011 / 7 **N** 14.00674 / 8 **O** 15.9994 / 9 **F** 18.99840 / 10 **Ne** 20.1797

13 **Al** 26.98154 / 14 **Si** 28.0855 / 15 **P** 30.97376 / 16 **S** 32.066 / 17 **Cl** 35.4527 / 18 **Ar** 39.948

* *58 **Ce** 140.115 / 59 **Pr** 140.90765 / 60 **Nd** 144.24 / 61 **Pm** 144.9127 / 62 **Sm** 150.36 / 63 **Eu** 151.965 / 64 **Gd** 157.25 / 65 **Tb** 158.92534 / 66 **Dy** 162.50 / 67 **Ho** 164.93032 / 68 **Er** 167.26 / 69 **Tm** 168.93421 / 70 **Yb** 173.04 / 71 **Lu** 174.967

† **90 **Th** 232.0381 / 91 **Pa** 231.0359 / 92 **U** 238.0289 / 93 **Np** 237.0482 / 94 **Pu** 244.0642 / 95 **Am** 243.0614 / 96 **Cm** 247.07003 / 97 **Bk** 247.0703 / 98 **Cf** 251.0796 / 99 **Es** 252.083 / 100 **Fm** 257.0951 / 101 **Md** 258.10 / 102 **No** 259.1009 / 103 **Lr** 260.150

Figure 22-1 *The periodic table of elements.*

Source: Delmar/Cengage Learning

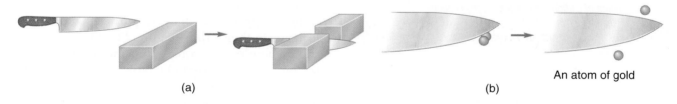

(a)   (b)

An atom of gold

Figure 22-2 *Cutting a piece of gold until all that is left is an atom of gold.*

Source: Armold, Melvin T., *Essentials of General, Organic, and Biochemistry*, 1e, Brooks/Cole, Cengage Learning

Elements and Compounds

There are 109 known elements. Each element has its own symbol, usually consisting of one or two letters. Table 22-1 lists some of the more common elements.

Of the common elements in Table 22-1, oxygen, carbon, hydrogen, and nitrogen make up 96% of the mass of the human body. As can be seen in Table 22-1, 99.3% of the body's mass is made up of elements that are found within the first 20 elements of the periodic table. Because of this we will focus our attention to this part of the periodic table.

Elements that are necessary to maintain a healthy body are called *minerals.* Mineral elements are interrelated to each other in their functions within the body. For example, sodium, potassium, calcium, phosphorous, and chlorine are important ingredients of body fluids. The

TABLE 22-1
Chemical Elements in the Human Body

ELEMENT	SYMBOL	PERCENT BY MASS IN HUMAN BODY
Oxygen	O	65
Carbon	C	18
Hydrogen	H	10
Nitrogen	N	3
Calcium	Ca	1.5
Phosphorous	P	1.0
Potassium	K	0.35
Sulfur	S	0.25
Sodium	Na	0.15
Magnesium	Mg	0.05

response of the muscles in our body depends on these minerals being present in the correct concentrations. Calcium, magnesium, phosphorous, and others are used to make bone tissue. A deficiency of one element will affect the functioning of the others. The main source of these minerals is our diet. It is important to eat foods that contain adequate amounts of these nutritionally important minerals. The recommended daily allowance of a few of these minerals is shown in Table 22-2.

QUOTES & NOTES

The amount of carbon in the human body is enough to fill 9,000 "lead" pencils.
—From: http://www.sciensational.com/chemistry-facts-pg3.html

TABLE 22-2
Recommended Dietary Allowance (RDA) for Some Minerals

ELEMENT	AMOUNT PER DAY	
	YOUNG FEMALE ADULTS	YOUNG MALE ADULTS
Calcium	1.2 g	1.2 g
Copper	1.5–3.0 mg	1.5–3.0 mg
Iodine	150 mcg	150 mcg
Iron	15 mg	10 mg
Magnesium	280 mg	350 mg
Phosphorous	1.2 g	1.2 g
Zinc	12 mg	15 mg

(Arnold, Melvin T., *Essentials of General, Organic, and Biochemistry*, 1e, Brooks/Cole, Cengage Learning)

Some elements such as gold and silver are found uncombined in nature. Some other elements, however, are found bonded together. The common substance water, for example, consists of two hydrogen atoms and one oxygen atom bonded together. These types of substances are called **compounds**. A compound, then, is two or more elements joined together by a chemical bond. (Bonding is discussed in detail in Chapter 23.)

Atomic Structure

Many particles compose an atom. To simplify things, we will discuss the three most important particles: **protons**, **neutrons**, and **electrons**. A *proton* (symbol p) is positively charged and has approximately the same mass as a neutron. A *neutron* (symbol n) is neutral—that is, it has no electrical charge. An *electron* (symbol e) is negatively charged, and its mass is extremely small as compared to that of a proton or neutron. Because the mass of an electron is so small, the mass of an atom is concentrated in the **nucleus**, which houses the protons and neutrons.

As described by the *Bohr model*, the protons and neutrons of an atom are located in a dense, central core called the nucleus; the electrons orbit the nucleus much like the planets orbit the sun. The electrons' orbits are called **energy levels**, because the electrons must maintain certain energy levels to remain in their pathways, or orbits. As mentioned previously, electrons are negatively charged and protons are positively charged; the attraction of these oppositely charged particles holds the electrons in their orbits. Figure 22-3 illustrates the arrangement of electrons in the shells for the first 20 elements of the periodic table.

It is important to remember that all elements, and therefore matter in general, is composed of protons, neutrons, and electrons. The arrangement and number of protons, neutrons, and electrons are what determine the various elements and their respective characteristics. This is similar to the DNA molecules that comprise our genes. While we are all human and composed of the same basic genetic material, it is the arrangement of the genetic material that determines our characteristics.

QUOTES & NOTES

If an atom was expanded to the size of the Astrodome, the nucleus would be approximately the size of a fly.

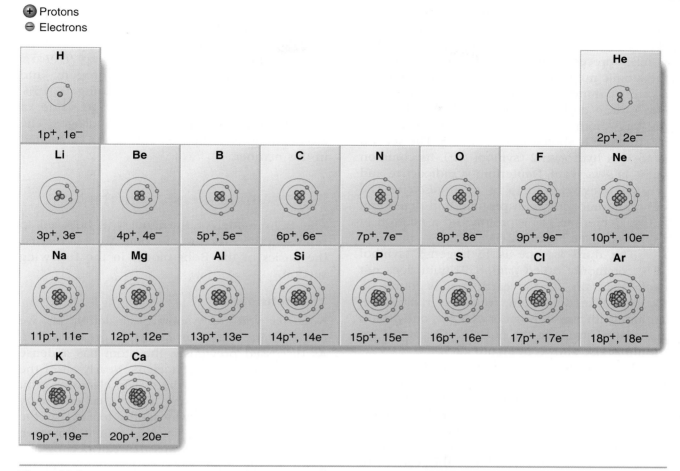

Figure 22-3 *The arrangement of the electrons in shells for the first 20 elements.*

Source: Armold, Melvin T., *Essentials of General, Organic, and Biochemistry*, 1e, Brooks/Cole, Cengage Learning

Isotopes

To better understand the structure of the atom, it is necessary to first learn several more definitions. The **atomic number** of an atom is the number of protons in the nucleus of the atom. Atoms of the same element always have the same number of protons in their nuclei. This number, therefore, determines the element. Atoms are electrically neutral. Therefore, the number of protons must equal the number of electrons. That is, the number of positively charged particles must be equal to the number of negatively charged particles.

The **mass number** of an atom is the sum of the protons and neutrons in the nucleus. (As mentioned previously, the protons and neutrons are the only particles that have any appreciable mass.) While atoms of the same element must have the same number of protons, they can have varying numbers of neutrons. Atoms of the same element that have different numbers of neutrons

in their nuclei are called **isotopes**. The mass number and atomic number of an element are sometimes written with the symbol for that element, as shown in Figure 22-4 (where *a* represents the atomic number, *m* represents the mass number, and *X* represents any element).

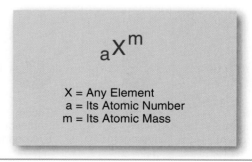

Figure 22-4 *Mass number and atomic number written with the symbol of an element.*

Source: Delmar/Cengage Learning

To illustrate what we have discussed thus far, consider the three isotopes of hydrogen. The simplest of these is hydrogen-1 (symbol $_1H^1$). The number preceding the symbol of the element is the atomic number of that element. $_1H$, then, has an atomic number of 1; its nucleus, therefore, has one proton and one electron which orbits the nucleus. Another name for this isotope is *protium*; its structure is shown in Figure 22-5. The second isotope is hydrogen-2 (symbol $_1H^2$). Its common name is *deuterium*. Deuterium is radioactive and is sometimes referred to as a *radioisotope*. The only difference between protium and deuterium is that deuterium has a proton and a neutron in its nucleus (see Figure 22-5).

The third isotope is hydrogen-3 (symbol $_1H^3$), commonly called *tritium*. Tritium does not occur naturally on the earth, but is found on the sun. Like deuterium, tritium is radioactive. Tritium, with a mass number of 3, has one proton and two neutrons in the nucleus. The model for tritium is also shown in Figure 22-5.

We now have enough information to see how the atomic weights on the periodic table (Figure 22-1) are determined. The atomic weights given on the periodic table are not the actual masses of the elements in grams. The actual masses of the atoms are extremely small, so a relative mass scale was established. To do this, carbon-12 was assigned a value of 12.00. The actual masses of the other elements were then compared to this value and assigned values accordingly. For example, the hydrogen-1 isotope has an actual mass approximately 1/12 that of the carbon atom; its relative mass, therefore, is 1/12 that of carbon-12's assigned value of 12, giving it a relative mass of approximately 1. Its actual relative mass is 1.008. But we give it a 1 to simplify matters. Likewise, an isotope of magnesium has an actual mass approximately two times that of the actual mass of carbon; its relative mass is, therefore, 24.

The atomic weight values given on such tables are weighted averages based on percent abundances of the isotopes as found in nature. For example, hydrogen-1 makes up 99.985% of the naturally occurring hydrogen, and hydrogen-2 makes up the remaining 0.015%. These abundances yield an average value of 1.00797 for the atomic weight of hydrogen. The atomic weights of the elements are all calculated in this manner.

Representing Atomic Structure

The Bohr model of the atom will be used to represent the structure of atoms. We will discuss the basics of the Bohr model in the following section.

The Bohr Model

Now that you know some basic definitions, we can examine the Bohr model in greater detail. As discussed previously, the atom has a dense central part called the nucleus. Nearly all of the atom's mass is located here. The electrons orbit the nucleus in orbits, or pathways, called energy levels, or shells, in a way similar to the way the planets orbit the sun. There is a limit, however, to the number of electrons that can occupy any given energy level. Because it is sufficient for our purposes, we will examine only the first 20 elements on the periodic table. The maximum number of electrons per energy level for these elements is listed in Table 22-3.

Keep in mind that the numbers in Table 22-3 are valid only for the first 20 elements and that the fourth energy level is not completely full. We now have all the necessary information to build specific Bohr models for each atom. Let's build the model for the nitrogen-13 atom. From the periodic table, we know that the atomic number of nitrogen is 7. From the definition of atomic number, we know that this is the number of protons in the nucleus. We can determine the number of neutrons in a nitrogen atom by subtracting the atomic number, that is, 7, from the mass number,

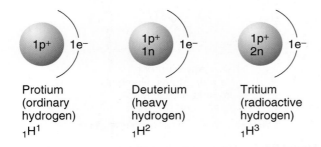

Figure 22-5   *The isotopes of hydrogen.*

Source: Delmar/Cengage Learning

TABLE 22-3				
Maximum Number of Electrons per Energy Level for the First 20 Elements				
Energy level	1	2	3	4
Maximum number of electrons	2	8	8	2

that is, 13. This gives 6 as the number of neutrons in the nucleus. This gives us all that we need to know about the nucleus.

The next step in completing the Bohr model is to determine the electron configuration. Atoms are neutral; that is, they have no net electrical charge. This means that they have the same number of electrons (negatively charged particles) as they do protons (positively charged particles). Thus, because nitrogen-13 has 7 protons, it must also have 7 electrons. The electrons are distributed throughout the various energy levels, filling up each energy level until all the electrons are distributed. In the nitrogen-13 atom, then, 2 electrons would be distributed to the first energy level, and because 2 is the maximum number of electrons that can occupy the first energy level, the remaining 5 electrons must be distributed to the second energy level. How we determined the Bohr model for the nitrogen-13 atom is illustrated in Figure 22-6.

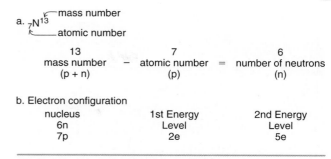

a. $_7N^{13}$ mass number / atomic number

| 13 mass number (p + n) | − | 7 atomic number (p) | = | 6 number of neutrons (n) |

b. Electron configuration

| nucleus 6n 7p | 1st Energy Level 2e | 2nd Energy Level 5e |

Figure 22-6   *The Bohr model for the nitrogen-13 atom.*

Source: Delmar/Cengage Learning

Electron Dot Structure

It is possible to simplify the Bohr model when discussing bonding. We can reconfigure our model of the atom to what is called an **electron dot structure**. In an electron dot structure, we use the symbol of the element to represent the

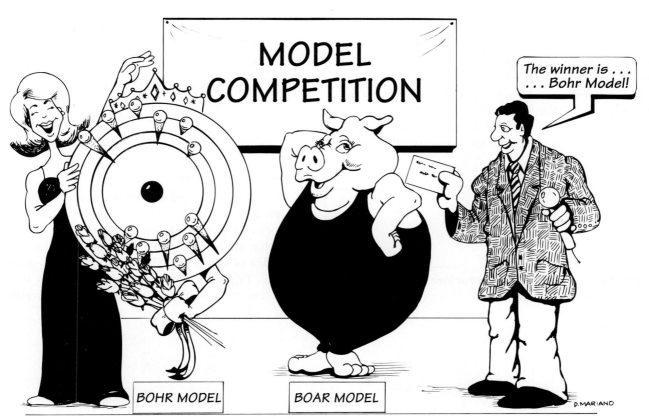

KNOW YOUR ATOM.

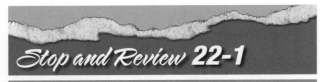

Stop and Review 22-1

a. Draw the specific Bohr model for the aluminum-27 atom.

b. How are elements different from compounds?

c. What are the three subatomic particles that make up an atom and where are they located in the atom?

QUOTES & NOTES

*H*ydrogen, oxygen, carbon, and nitrogen account for 99% of the atoms in the human body. Amazing Fact: Approximately 99% of the calcium present in the body is found in the bones and teeth.

nucleus of the atom and dots to represent the number of electrons in the outermost energy level of the atom. This outermost shell is crucial. Because each element will attempt to completely fill its outermost shell, this is where the majority of element reactivity takes place. When atoms react chemically with one another, they do so by sharing or transferring electrons in the outer energy level. Relate this to a human who has a great desire to feel like a complete person. If only it were as simple as having a completely filled outermost shell!

The electron dot structure of nitrogen is illustrated in Figure 22-7. As we know from our previous discussion, the nitrogen atom has an atomic number of 7, which puts 2 electrons in its first energy level and 5 electrons in its outermost energy level. Note that, rather than being randomly placed around the symbol, the dots

are placed in a particular pattern. The reason for this is beyond the scope of this text, but Figure 22-8 shows the general pattern for dot placement.

Let's look at another example. This time, we will draw the Bohr model and electron dot structure for neon-20. The atomic number of neon-20 is 10. Neon-20, then, has 10 protons in its nucleus. We can find the number of neutrons by subtracting the atomic number, 10, from the mass number, 20. The number of neutrons, then, is 10. The number of electrons is equal to the number of protons, that is, 10. Thus, there are 2 electrons in the first energy level and 8 in the second energy level. The Bohr model and electron dot structure for neon-20 are illustrated in Figure 22-9.

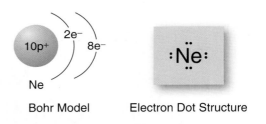

Bohr Model   Electron Dot Structure

Figure 22-9 *The Bohr model and electron dot structure for neon-20.*

Source: Delmar/Cengage Learning

Octets of Electrons

The electron configuration of an atom is important because it is the electrons, and particularly the electrons in the outermost energy level of an atom, that determine the chemical and physical properties of the atom. The neon atom is a good example. Eight electrons completely fill its outermost energy level. This produces a very stable

Figure 22-7 *The electron dot structure of nitrogen.*

Source: Delmar/Cengage Learning

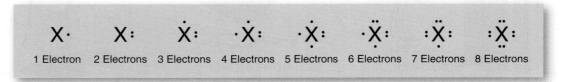

1 Electron   2 Electrons   3 Electrons   4 Electrons   5 Electrons   6 Electrons   7 Electrons   8 Electrons

Figure 22-8 *The general pattern of dot placement in an electron dot structure.*

Source: Delmar/Cengage Learning

electron configuration, which, in turn results in a chemically inert, or nonreactive, atom. This atom is said to have an *octet* of electrons, that is, 8 electrons in its outermost energy level. The outermost energy level is the one farthest from the nucleus. Atoms having less than 8 electrons try to complete their outer energy levels by losing, gaining, or sharing electrons in the process of forming a chemical bond. An exception to the rule is helium which only requires two electrons to fill its outermost energy level.

Stop and Review 22-2

a. Draw the Bohr model and electron dot structure for oxygen-16.

b. What are the mass number, atomic number, and electron configuration for an atom with 6 protons and 5 neutrons?

The Periodic Table

We can organize and simplify much of the preceding information by using the periodic table introduced at the beginning of this chapter. The periodic table arranges the elements in order of increasing atomic number, from left to right. See Figure 22-10. This done, it becomes apparent that certain elements are similar in their chemical properties. These elements are arranged in vertical columns called *families*, which are numbered with Roman numerals followed by the letter "A" at the top of the columns. We call a vertical column on the periodic table a family because the elements within the columns labeled with an A have similar chemical properties. The atoms in these element families have the same electron configuration. The number at the top of each column, called the *group number*, reveals the number of electrons in the outermost energy levels of these atoms. For example, the atoms in group IIA all have 2 electrons in their outer energy levels. This means that, in general, "X:" would be the electron dot structure for the atoms of each element in this family (with "X" being any one of Be, Mg, Ca, Ba, Sr, or Ra).

Periodic Table of the Elements

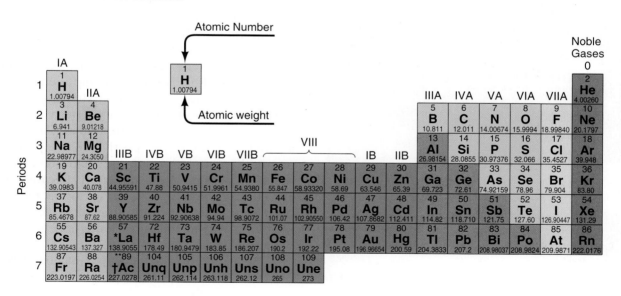

Figure 22-10 *The periodic table of elements.*

Source: Delmar/Cengage Learning

Stop and Review 22-3

a. Using the periodic table, determine the electron dot structure for each of the following elements.
  1. potassium (K)
  2. magnesium (Mg)
  3. boron (B)
  4. silicon (Si)
  5. phosphorus (P)
  6. oxygen (O)
  7. chlorine (Cl)
  8. neon (Ne)

b. Give the group number (Roman numeral A groups) for the following elements. Write the symbol and electron dot structure for each also.
  1. lithium
  2. nitrogen
  3. magnesium
  4. sulfur

Nuclear Chemistry

Nuclear chemistry is a useful tool in the diagnosis and treatment of various medical conditions. The following section will introduce you to some of the basics of nuclear chemistry.

Types of Radiation

Thus far, we have made only passing mention of the nucleus of the atom. The reactions that occur within the nucleus are important to the health field, however. Many health problems are diagnosed and treated via the use of radiation formed in nuclear reactions. Before discussing these types of reactions, it is necessary to briefly review our earlier discussion regarding atomic structure.

As you recall from our earlier discussion of isotopes, we said that it is possible for atoms of the same element to have different mass numbers. These atoms have a different number of neutrons in their nuclei. Whenever the ratio of protons to neutrons deviates from a one-to-one ratio, the nucleus of an atom can become unstable. When this happens, the atom emits various forms of radiation and continues to do so until the nucleus again becomes stable.

Although there are many forms of radiation, we will concentrate on three of the more common types of ionizing radiations: **alpha radiation**, **beta radiation**, and **gamma radiation**. We will examine the properties of these radiation forms to help you better understand how they are used in the health field.

Alpha radiation consists of particles called *helium nuclei*, which consist of two protons and two neutrons. Alpha particles are represented by the Greek letter alpha (α) and the chemical symbol $_2He^4$. Relative to the components of the other forms of radiation, these particles are slow moving. The most important property of radiation, from a diagnosis and treatment perspective as well as a safety perspective, is the penetrating ability. It is important to shield ourselves as much as possible from radiation. Because they are so large and slow moving, alpha particles have very little penetrating power. A few centimeters of dry air will sufficiently shield against alpha particles.

Beta radiation (β), consists of fast-moving electrons. The chemical symbol for beta particles is $_{-1}e^0$. Being small and fast, they have more penetrating power than alpha particles. The outer layer of skin or a thin piece of aluminum metal is sufficient to shield against beta particles.

Gamma radiation (γ) is a form of electromagnetic energy similar to X-rays. In fact, gamma rays can be thought of as high-energy X-rays.

Special Focus

The Periodic Table as It Relates to the Health Professions

Let's look at a few elements from the periodic table that are of interest to health professionals. One of these is calcium (Ca), from group IIA. Calcium not found in the skeletal structure must be present in the correct concentration to allow for both contraction of muscles and proper clotting of blood. Phosphorus (P), from group VA, is also found in the teeth and bones. Magnesium (Mg), another group IIA element, is required for muscle contraction and proper transmission of nerve signals.

The roles of the elements potassium (K), sodium (Na), and chlorine (Cl) are closely related; thus, we will discuss them together. These elements control the balance of the positive and negative charges in the cells, tissues, and blood. This balance is necessary to maintain the normal flow of fluids

and to control the amounts of acids and bases in the blood.

Iodine and iron are two elements found in the body in tiny amounts. Iodine is necessary for maintaining a healthy thyroid gland. Lack of iodine in the diet can cause the thyroid to become enlarged, a condition referred to as a *goiter*. Iron is an important constituent in the hemoglobin of blood that carries the vital oxygen needed for cellular respiration. A reduction of iron in the blood results in anemia, or a decrease in red blood cells.

The preceding are just a few of the many elements that are found in the body and are necessary for maintaining good health. We will discuss the roles of these elements further in later chapters, as your knowledge of chemistry increases.

They have the most penetrating power of the three radiations discussed and are, therefore, very useful in the diagnosis and treatment of disease. These three types of radiation are summarized in Table 22-4.

TABLE 22-4
Common Types of Radiation

	SYMBOL	MASS NUMBER	CHARGE
Alpha	α	4	+2
Beta	β	0	–1
Gamma	γ	0	0

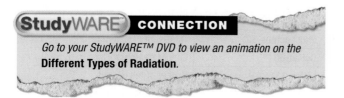

StudyWARE CONNECTION

Go to your StudyWARE™ DVD to view an animation on the **Different Types of Radiation**.

Stop and Review 22-4

a. What type of radiation consists of fast-moving electrons?

b. What type of radiation is like high-energy X-rays?

c. What type of radiation consists of helium nuclei?

d. Write the names and symbols of the three common forms of ionizing radiations.

Dangers of Radiation

Radiation exposure is dangerous because of the ions produced when radiation passes through the human body. If this ionization occurs on a cell membrane, the cell can die. More importantly, if the ionization takes place in the molecules that carry genetic information, a mutation can occur. Mutations of this nature can result in cells becoming cancerous. Cancer and radiation were first linked in the 1920s. Women who painted luminous dials (radioactive radium) on watches and who removed loose bristles from their paint brushes using their teeth developed oral and bone cancer after several years. These cases of cancer were later linked to radium exposure.

Danger from exposure to radon is related to our study of the nucleus. Radon is formed in the environment by the radioactive decay of uranium found in certain rock formations. Being a gas, radon can move through the ground and become concentrated in the basements of homes. It can also be breathed into the lungs, where it can undergo decay, as shown in the following equation:

$$_{86}Rn^{222} \text{ radon (gas)} \rightarrow _{2}He^{4} \text{ (a particle)} \\ + _{84}Po^{218} \text{ polonium (solid)}$$

When the element radon decays, it gives off an alpha particle and then changes into polonium, a solid. This polonium can remain in the lungs. Polonium is also an alpha emitter. Although it is easy to shield against alpha particles, they can be very dangerous once inside the body. Being heavy particles, they can produce large numbers of ions as they pass through human tissue. Exposure over long periods of time can lead to cancer.

Clinical Relevancy

Beneficial Uses of Radiation in the Health Sciences Field

Despite some of the dangers linked to radioisotopes, radiation can be safely used in the diagnosis and treatment of disease. Technetium-99m, for example, is used in the diagnosis of cancer. It is a gamma emitter and can be easily detected. In combination with phosphate, technetium-99m can be used to determine whether cancer cells have metastasized (i.e., spread) to the bones. Cancerous bone cells will absorb the compound faster than will other cells. Areas of high radioactivity, thus, would indicate the presence of cancer cells. Technetium-99m can also be used in diagnosing heart damage resulting from a heart attack.

Iodine-123 is used in the diagnosis of thyroid problems. A drink containing iodine-123 is given to the patient, and detectors are placed near the patient's thyroid gland. The alpha particles emitted by the iodine can be detected. From the rate at which the iodine is absorbed, the diagnosis of an overactive or underactive thyroid can be made.

Iodine-131 is a radioisotope used in the treatment of thyroid cancer. Iodine-131 is both a gamma and beta emitter. The beta particles are helpful in treating certain types of thyroid cancer. Radiation affects cells that reproduce more rapidly and, hence, is useful in the treatment of cancer.

The radioisotope cobalt-60 is also used in the treatment of cancer. In some cases, the cobalt is placed in a small metal container the size of a needle. This, in turn, is placed near the tumor, with shielding being used to minimize exposure of healthy cells.

Tables 22-5 and 22-6 list some isotopes used in diagnosis and treatment of disease.

TABLE 22-5
Radioisotopes in Diagnosis of Disease

ISOTOPE	DIAGNOSTIC USE
Iodine-123	Thyroid function
Sodium-24	Blood flow and volume
Technetium-99m	Bone and bone marrow and many other tissues
Fluorine-18	PET scans
Strontium-85	Bone scans

TABLE 22-6
Radioisotopes in Treatment of Disease

ISOTOPE	USE
Phosphorous-32	Treatment of leukemia
Cobalt-60	Cancer treatment
Iodine-131	Cancer of the thyroid
Radium-226	Implantation cancer therapy

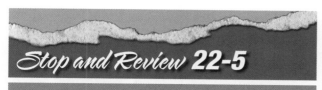

Stop and Review 22-5

a. Define the term *ionizing radiation*.

b. What is the danger from exposure to radon gas?

c. What ionizing radiation is formed from the decay of polonium?

d. Why is exposure to radiation harmful?

Medical Imaging

It is sometimes necessary for a doctor to see inside a patient to make a proper diagnosis. A variety of noninvasive medical imaging techniques are available to doctors. Each technique has its own advantages and disadvantages. We will look at four different imaging techniques, X-rays, CT scans, MRIs, and PET scans, and discuss some of the advantages and disadvantages of each.

X-rays

X-rays are a common type of imaging technique familiar to most people. The first X-ray image of the human body was taken in 1895. X-rays are produced when high-energy electrons bombard a metal. X-rays are high-energy electromagnetic radiation and are classified as ionizing radiation. Because of their high energy, they easily pass though the soft tissues of the body but are absorbed by the denser areas such as bone tissue. A film similar to photographic film is used to detect the X-rays. The dark areas represent the area detecting X-rays and the light areas represent the areas where the X-rays were absorbed. See Figure 22-11. The primary use of X-rays is in the imaging of bones.

CT scans

Computerized tomography (CT) scans are a more recent development in imaging techniques. The word *tomography* is derived from the Greek words *tomos* meaning "slice" and *graphien* meaning "to write." The image produced in a CT scan is many cross-sectional slices of the body put together by the computer to make a three-dimensional picture.

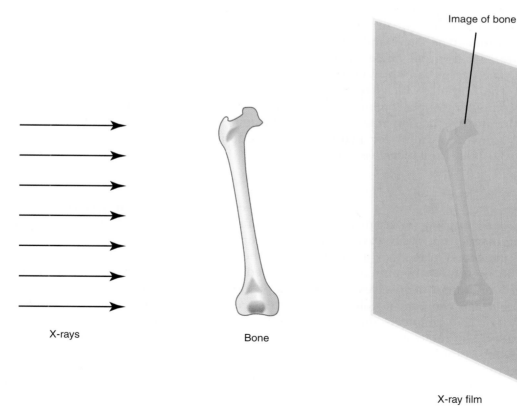

Figure 22-11   *X-ray images are formed when the X-rays are absorbed by dense tissue such as bone.*

Source: Delmar/Cengage Learning

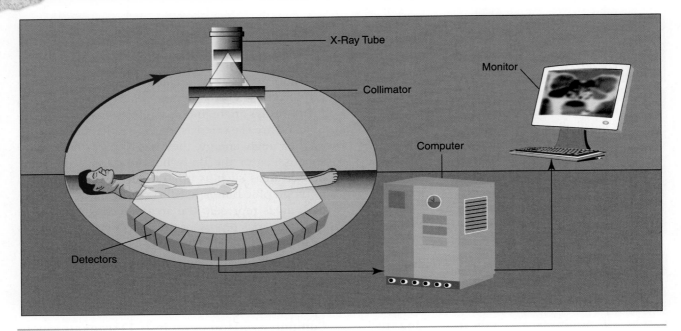

Figure 22-12   *A CT scan produces an image of a cross-sectional slice of the body.*

Source: Delmar/Cengage Learning

A CT scan uses X-rays to produce the image. An X-ray generator and detectors are arranged in a circle. The array is rotated as a unit and a brief pulse of X-rays are sent from all angles across one cross section. The person is moved and the process repeated. The output of the detector is analyzed by the computer which combines the information together to produce an image. See Figure 22-12. CT scans are useful for making images of bones, soft tissue, and blood vessels.

MRI

Magnetic resonance imaging (MRI) produces an image by using magnetism, radio waves, and a computer. The patient is placed in a strong magnetic field. The protons in hydrogen atoms act as little magnets and align themselves to the strong magnetic field like compass needles. See Figure 22-13A and B. The sample is then subjected to radio waves. The radio wave energy is absorbed by some of the protons and causes them to flip opposite to the direction of the magnetic field. See Figure 22-13C. This causes some of the radio frequency energy to be absorbed. The amount of absorption depends on the concentration of protons in the path of the radio waves. A detector measures the amount of absorption

of the energy, and a computer then produces an image based on the absorption.

Unlike the CT scan and PET scan, MRI imaging does not require the use of ionizing radiation. Since hydrogen atoms are found in many places in the body, such as fats, proteins, and water, images of soft tissue can be easily made. The MRI image of soft tissue is much clearer than the image formed by a CT scan.

PET Scans

Positron emission tomography (PET) is a scanning technique used in the diagnosis of cancer, brain disorders, and heart disease. Some synthetic radioactive isotopes emit a particle called a *positron.* A positron is an electron with a positive charge. When a positron and an electron come into contact, they annihilate each other and form gamma radiation. That is, they change from matter into electromagnetic radiation (gamma rays) g. See Figure 22-14.

Certain radioactive substances are positron emitters. Positron emitters of interest in the medical field are oxygen-15, nitrogen-13, and carbon-11. For example, an oxygen-15 atom can replace an oxygen atom in glucose. The glucose can then be traced by the gamma radiation

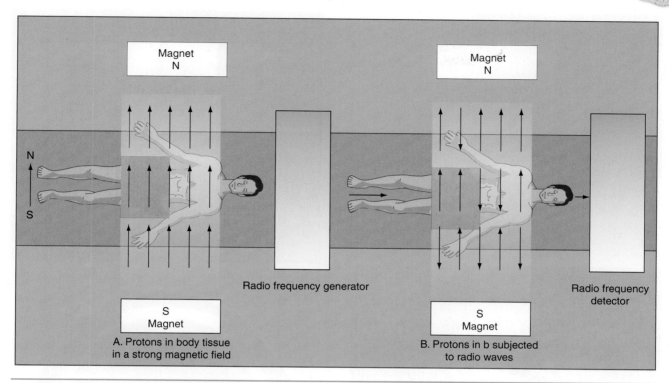

Figure 22-13   *(A) Protons in body tissue will align in a strong magnetic field. (B) Some protons will absorb energy from radio waves and align against the magnetic field.*
Source: Delmar/Cengage Learning

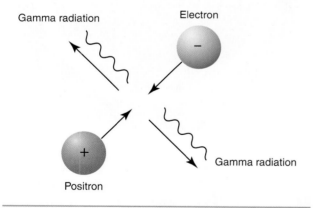

Figure 22-14   *When a proton and positron annihilate each other, gamma rays are produced. The gamma rays can then be detected and used to produce an image.*
Source: Delmar/Cengage Learning

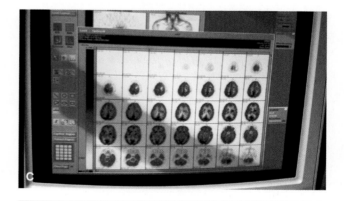

Figure 22-15   *PET scan output images.*
Source: Delmar/Cengage Learning

produced. Since glucose can enter the brain, the activity of the brain in certain areas can be measured using this technique. Figure 22-15 shows PET scan output images.

To contrast some of the imaging that has been discussed, see Figure 22-16 for a comparison of images from an X-ray, a CT scan, a PET scan, and an MRI.

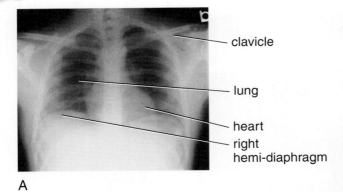

clavicle

lung

heart

right hemi-diaphragm

A

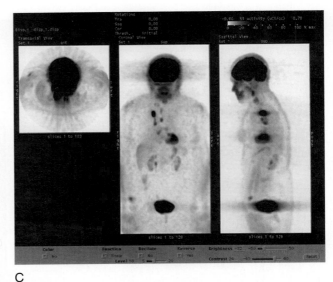

C

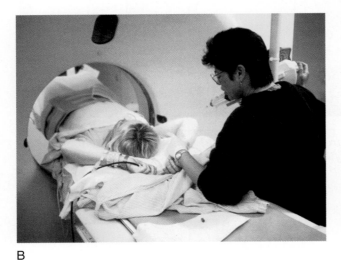

B

Figure 22-16 *(A) An X-ray view of the chest. (B) A patient preparing for a computerized tomography (CT) scan. (C) A PET body scan showing a tumor in the right lung. (D) An MRI of the brain with a "bleed" visual at the lower right region.*

Source: Delmar/Cengage Learning

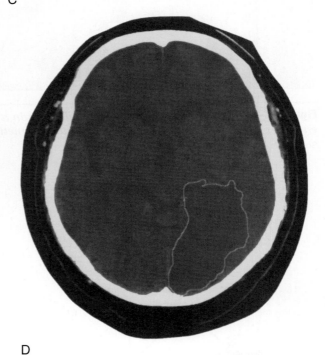

D

Stop and Review 22-6

a. What medical imaging technique(s) use(s) ionizing radiations?

b. Define the term *tomography*.

c. Which imaging technique(s) use(s) radio waves?

d. How can we get positron emitters into various parts of the body?

■ CHAPTER REVIEW

Exercises

1. Write the symbol for the following elements.
   a. iodine
   b. sulfur
   c. iron
   d. potassium
   e. sodium

2. Name each of the following elements.
   a. C
   b. I
   c. Cl
   d. Pb

3. Which of the following substances are elements and which are compounds?
   a. sodium chloride
   b. water
   c. iron
   d. carbon dioxide
   e. sugar

4. A sample of table salt contains sodium and chlorine. Is salt an element or a compound? Explain your answer.

5. Given the symbol $_{11}Na^{23}$, answer each of the following questions.
   a. How many protons are in the nucleus of an atom of this element?
   b. How many neutrons are in the nucleus of an atom of this element?
   c. How many electrons orbit the nucleus of an atom of this element?
   d. What is the Bohr model for an atom of this element?

6. Which pairs of the following elements are isotopes?
   a. element A: atomic number 10, mass number 11
   b. element B: atomic number 11, mass number 11
   c. element C: atomic number 10, mass number 10
   d. element D: atomic number 11, mass number 10

7. Using the periodic table, draw the electron dot structure for each of the following.
   a. calcium
   b. nitrogen
   c. sulfur
   d. magnesium
   e. argon

8. Which of the elements in exercise number 6 has an octet of electrons?

9. Why is potassium iodide added to table salt?

10. What condition results from inadequate amounts of iron in the diet?

11. What role does each of the following elements play in the body?
   a. calcium
   b. phosphorus
   c. potassium, sodium, and chlorine

12. Answer each of the following questions regarding nuclear chemistry.
   a. Which type of radiation consists of fast-moving electrons?
   b. Which type of radiation has the greatest penetrating power?
   c. What are some ways of shielding yourself from radiation?

13. How are each of the following isotopes used in the health field?

    a. technetium-99m

    b. iodine-123

    c. iodine-131

    d. cobalt-60

14. In general terms, how is an X-ray image formed?

15. What is the difference between a positron and an electron?

16. Why are X-rays, CT scans, and PET scans more harmful than an MRI?

17. *Directions*: Match each of the following to the element having the atomic number provided in parentheses. (*Warning:* Some of the answers are more than a little corny, and some are far-fetched.)

    a. What did the Greek warrior say when he got out of the wooden horse? (atomic number 1)

    b. The word meaning "to keep drilling" (atomic number 5)

    c. What Mr. and Mrs. Claus call their male offspring? (atomic number 33)

    d. When President Calvin Coolidge had visitors who were requesting an audience, he asked his aide what to do. His aide said, "(atomic number 20)."

    e. When asked if they departed, the reply was "Yes, they (atomic number 18)."

    f. Two equally hairless men (atomic number 27)

    g. A word meaning "to fix the dike" (atomic number 101)

    h. When asked how he did on the exam, the student replied, "I didn't get all of them, but I got (atomic number 72)."

    i. What I bought my girlfriend for her birthday (atomic number 32)

    j. When you kneel down, what do you put on the floor? (atomic number 10)

    k. The divorced man paid his ex-wife (atomic number 51).

    l. Where you drive your car (atomic number 45)

    m. The man was buried in a (atomic number 36) the hill.

    n. The church couldn't ring its bell, because it had (atomic number 102).

    o. He is a good (atomic number 62).

    p. What one cowboy said to the other on the cattle drive: "I'll ride (atomic number 63)!"

    q. We have roaches, so I'll spray (radon number 86) them.

18. *Directions*: Fill in the numbered blanks with the name of the element having the atomic number as shown in the table following the paragraph below.

    The a._____ and jewels b._____ That c._____ must have stolen them. Call the d._____ before he has a chance to e._____ or f._____. There should be a g._____ his place before he has gotten h._____. When they break i._____ the j._____ will k._____ and l._____ to give them back. If he doesn't, I wouldn't give a plugged m._____ for his chances. He will be behind n._____ bars in no time. Maybe that will o._____.

Blank Number	Atomic Number	Blank Number	Atomic Number
a.	79	i.	49
b.	18	j.	29
c.	14	k.	55
d.	29	l.	52
e.	56	m.	28
f.	66	n.	26
g.	86	o.	96
h.	77		

Real Life Issues and Applications

Patient Education

You are assigned to instruct a group of patients on the importance of elemental minerals in the diet. You will need to list the various elements from the periodic table that have nutritional value, tell where they are found, and explain why they are important for optimal body functioning. Visiting a nutritional store and reading supplement labels may be a very good place to start. Develop a sample chart that shows this information.

Radon Gas

A patient with a family medical history of lung cancer is highly concerned about radon gas in his home. How would you educate this patient regarding identifying and correcting any radon problems in his home? First, of course, you must educate yourself. *Hint*: The American Lung Association and the American Cancer Society may be good places to start.

Additional Activities

1. Invite a nutritionist or hospital dietician to come to class and discuss the importance of minerals and trace elements in the diet.

2. Beginning chemistry students sometimes wonder how scientists can know so much about atoms when they cannot even see them. Ask your instructor to place an object in a box and seal the box. Try to determine what is in the box by manipulating it. Also, list some things that you might be able to do using equipment that is not available in school to determine the contents of the box.

3. Go to the library and research how radioisotopes are used in the health professions. Discuss your findings, including the advantages and disadvantages of using radioisotopes, with the class.

4. Check the newspaper daily for articles related to chemistry. Share your findings with the class and, in particular, discuss the importance of chemistry in our daily lives.

5. Ask your teacher to invite a geologist to class to discuss the prevalence of radon in your area.

6. Contact the nuclear medicine department of a nearby hospital. Ask a representative how isotopes are used in diagnosis and treatment of disease. Share your findings with the class.

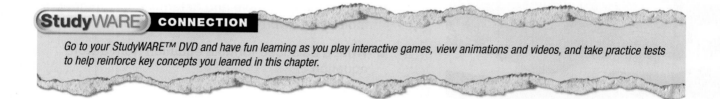

StudyWARE CONNECTION

Go to your StudyWARE™ DVD and have fun learning as you play interactive games, view animations and videos, and take practice tests to help reinforce key concepts you learned in this chapter.

Workbook Practice *Go to your Workbook for more practice questions and activities.*

CHAPTER 23

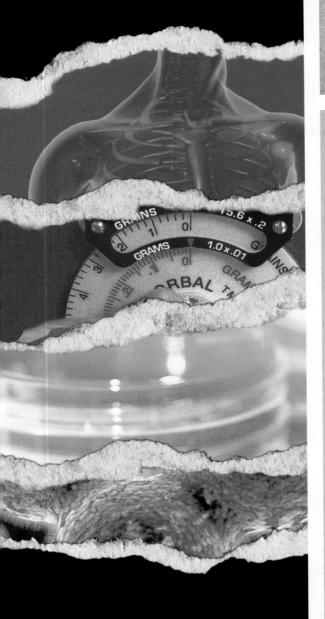

BONDING AND CHEMICAL FORMULAS

Objectives

Upon completion of this chapter, you should be able to

- Define and differentiate between the various types of chemical bonding, including ionic, pure covalent, polar covalent, and hydrogen

- Explain the concept of *osmosis* and what happens to a blood cell in an isotonic solution, a hypotonic solution, and a hypertonic solution

- Distinguish between molecules and ions

- Determine the number of atoms in a compound, given the formula

- Name a compound, given the formula, and write the formula for a compound, given the name

- Use the periodic table to determine the charge on a monatomic ion

- Define the term *mole* and determine the number of moles of a given element in a compound

- Write a balanced formula equation from a word equation

Key Terms

anemia (uh-**NEE**-me-uh)
anion
antitussive
astringent
Avogadro's number (av-oh-**GAH**-droe)

cation
compound
covalent bonding
crenation (cree-**NAY**-shun)
electrolytes (ee-**LEC**-trow-lites)
empirical formula

(continues)

expectorant
hemoglobin (hee-ma-**GLOW**-bin)
hypertonic solution
hypotonic solution
ionic bond

ions
isotonic solution
metabolic acidosis
mole
osmosis

polar covalent bond
pure covalent bond
quantitative terms
structural formula

LITTLE KNOWN CHEMISTRY FACTS

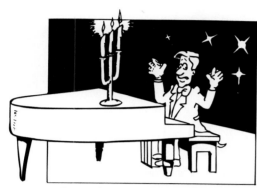

*The discoverer of super glue
was originally going to be
a great concert pianist.*

Source: Delmar/Cengage Learning

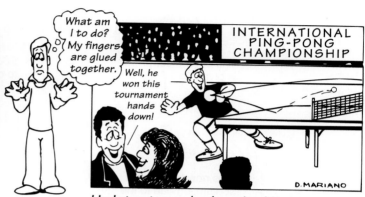

*He later turned adversity into success
as a world class ping-pong player.
You certainly have to "hand" it to him!*

■ INTRODUCTION

You now have an understanding of atoms, elements, and isotopes. These are analogous to the cellular building blocks of your body. Cells are put together in specific ways to form tissues; tissues to form organs; organs to form systems, and systems to form the human organism. Likewise, the various arrangements of protons, neutrons, and electrons form the atom, which determines the element. The element can then be put together or joined with other elements to form compounds and molecules.

We come into contact with many *compounds* every day. Examples include sugar (sucrose) we put into our coffee or tea in the morning to other compounds we use in cooking such as baking soda (sodium bicarbonate). Vinegar that is used in salad dressing is a solution of acetic acid. When we have an upset stomach we can use a mixture of magnesium hydroxide and aluminum hydroxide to neutralize any excess stomach acid (hydrochloric acid). These are just a few of the types of substances that we will discuss in this chapter.

This chapter will address how atoms can be joined together, or bonded. Also discussed are atoms having positive or negative charges. These atoms, called **ions**, are very important to the chemistry of the human body. Many ions are found dissolved in the bloodstream; these are referred to as the body's **electrolytes**. Finally, this chapter introduces the basics of naming compounds and writing formulas.

Bonding

There are two basic types of chemical bonding. We will look at ionic bonding first. Ionic compounds are important in the body. They make up the compounds called electrolytes that are found in the blood and cells of the body.

Ions and Electrolytes

Many compounds are found in the body, including carbohydrates (sugars), lipids (fats), and proteins. To better understand the roles of compounds in the body, it is necessary to also understand how atoms chemically bond to form compounds. We introduced the basis for this in Chapter 22 when we mentioned that atoms like to complete their outer shells by losing or gaining electrons. This process is called *ionization*.

Figure 23-1 illustrates the process of losing and gaining electrons. As you can see, the sodium-23 atom (atomic number 11) has a single

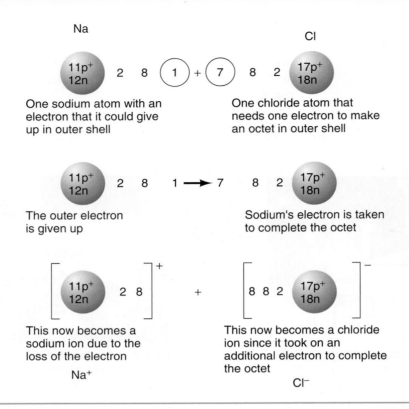

Figure 23-1 *The process of losing and gaining electrons: the ionization of sodium and chloride. Now with opposite charges, they can combine to form the compound NaCl.*

Source: Delmar/Cengage Learning

electron in its outer shell. This electron is weakly held by the nucleus because it is so far away from the nucleus. As shown in Figure 23-1, it is relatively easy to remove this electron, which results in the formation of a sodium ion. An ion can be thought of as a particle having either a positive or negative charge.

When you compare the sodium atom to its ion, you see that the electrical charge in the ion is no longer balanced. Whereas the atom has 11 protons and 11 electrons, the ion has 11 protons and only 10 electrons, because the outermost electron was removed. The ion, therefore, has one more positive charge than negative charge. This ion, then, is said to have a $+1$ charge. The symbol for this ion is Na^{1+}. Another name for a positive ion is **cation**. It is important to note that this sodium

ion now has 8 electrons, or an octet, in its outer shell. This is a stable electron configuration.

Chlorine can also ionize (form ions), but it does so in a different manner. Chlorine-35 has an atomic number of 17. The atom is electrically neutral and has 7 electrons in its outer shell. The easiest way for it to obtain an octet is to add an electron to its outer shell. When it does so, the ion formed has 18 electrons and only 17 protons and, therefore, has a charge of 21. The symbol for the ion is Cl^-. A negative ion is called an **anion**.

In the ionization process, then, electrons move from one atom to another. Because electrons are negatively charged, when an atom loses an electron, the resulting ion is positively charged, and when an atom gains an electron, the resulting ion is negatively charged.

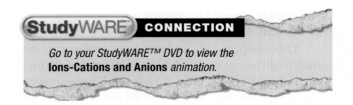

StudyWARE CONNECTION

Go to your StudyWARE™ DVD to view the **Ions-Cations and Anions** *animation.*

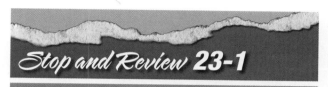

Stop and Review 23-1

a. Define the term *ion*.

b. When an electrically neutral potassium atom loses an electron, the resulting ion will have what type of charge?

c. When an electrically neutral oxygen atom gains two electrons, the resulting ion will have what type of charge?

d. What is meant by an octet of electrons?

QUOTES & NOTES

An average adult body contains around 250 g (1/2 lb) of salt.

Special Focus

Electrolytes: The Ions in Your Body

When salt is dissolved in water, the sodium (Na^+) and chloride (Cl^-) break apart and are surrounded by water molecules. Salt is also dissolved in our bloodstream in a concentration of 0.9%. If the salt did not break down into ions and, instead, remained combined in its crystallized form, we would be in serious trouble! Our arteries, veins, and capillaries would clog, which would eventually lead to death.

Sodium, chloride, calcium, magnesium, potassium, and phosphorus are all found dissolved in their ionic forms and in specific concentrations within the bloodstream. Because they are charged ions in solution, they are referred to as *electrolytes*. This is similar to the electrolyte solutions found in sport drinks that allow you to "recharge yourself." Table 23-1 lists some of the more important electrolytes that are found in the blood and cells and their concentrations.

As we can see from Table 23-1, the concentrations of the positive ions and negative ions are equal. We must always have the same concentrations of positive and negative ions in a solution. Also, the sodium ion (Na^+) and chloride ion (Cl^-) are found in the largest concentration in the blood while the potassium ion (K^+)

and other negative ions are found in the largest concentration in the intracellular fluids.

TABLE 23-1
Electrolytes Found in the Blood and Cells

ELECTROLYTE	BLOOD PLASMA (mEQ/L)	INTRACELLULAR FLUID (mEQ/L)
Positive Ions (Cations)		
Ca^{2+}	5	1
K^+	4	159
Mg^{2+}	2	40
Na^+	142	10
Total number of positive ions	153	210
Negative Ions (Anions)		
Cl^-	103	3
HCO_3^-	25	7
Protein	17	45
Other	8	155
Total number of negative ions	153	210

(Adapted from Armold, Melvin T., *Essentials of General, Organic, and Biochemistry*, 1e, Brooks/Cole, Cengage Learning)

Clinical Relevancy

Clinical Significance of Electrolytes in the Body

We have used the term *homeostasis* to describe the smooth operation of the body. Ideally, everything is in balance or can be brought back into balance, or homeostasis. What happens when electrolytes become out of balance as a result of either too little or too much of a given element? Following is a discussion of conditions that can result from electrolyte imbalances within the body.

As stated earlier in this text, calcium (Ca) is needed for strong bones and teeth; in fact, 98 to 99% of the calcium present in the body is stored in the bones and teeth. Calcium is also needed for proper muscle contraction and relaxation, heart action, the transmission of nerve impulses, and proper blood clotting. The condition known as *hypercalcemia* (meaning higher-than-normal levels of calcium in the blood) can cause confusion, abdominal pain, and muscle pain and weakness. If calcium levels are high enough, shock and death can occur. While hypercalcemia is often associated with cancer, high levels of calcium can also result from prolonged immobilization, excessive intake of vitamin D, prolonged use of diuretics, or acidosis caused by breathing problems. If the calcium levels are too low (a condition known as *hypocalcemia*), cardiac arrhythmia, muscle twitching, tetany, and hyperparesthesia (an intense feeling of "pins and needles") of the lips, tongue, hands, and feet can occur. Hypocalcemia can be caused by the excessive use of IV fluids, an inability to absorb nutrients, acute pancreatitis, and diarrhea.

Because magnesium (Mg^{2+}) is commonly found in food, deficiencies of this element are relatively rare in individuals who maintain normal diets. Magnesium is needed for carbohydrate utilization, protein synthesis, muscle contraction, nerve impulse conduction, and proper blood clotting. Magnesium levels are related to calcium levels in the sense that magnesium is needed in order for the body to absorb calcium from nutrients in the intestines and to metabolize this calcium after it is absorbed. Low levels of magnesium hamper this process, causing the body to take calcium from the bones. Because magnesium is filtered through the kidneys, a decrease in renal function will result in increased magnesium levels in the blood.

Increased levels of magnesium can also be caused by diabetes, dehydration, and the use of antacids containing magnesium. Increased levels of magnesium can cause lethargy, weak deep tendon reflexes, drowsiness (so if you fall asleep in this class, blame it on high magnesium levels!), slurred speech, and even respiratory depression. Lower-than-normal levels of magnesium can be caused by chronic diarrhea, hemodialysis, cirrhosis, alcoholism, the use of diuretics, and chronic pancreatitis. Low levels of magnesium can lead to muscle tremors, twitching, and even tetany. The individual may also exhibit nausea, vomiting, anorexia, and lethargy.

Chloride (Cl^-) is an important blood electrolyte responsible for helping to maintain fluid balance within the cells of the body. Lower-than-normal levels of chloride (called *hypochloremia*) can be caused by severe vomiting, diarrhea, or severe burns; heat exhaustion; diabetic acidosis; the use of diuretics; fever; and acute infection. Higher-than-normal levels of chloride (called *hyperchloremia*) can be caused by anemia, dehydration, hyperventilation, and some kidney disorders. A variety of drugs can also cause changes in chloride levels.

Potassium (K^+) is the main electrolyte of the intracellular fluid in the body. In fact, approximately 90% of the potassium present in the body is found in the cells; the remainder is spread throughout the bones and blood. Note that the kidneys do not save potassium in reserve; thus, a potassium-poor diet can result in a severe deficiency of this element. Potassium is needed for proper nerve impulse conduction, proper muscle function (including the rate and force of heart contraction), and maintenance of proper acid-base and fluid balances. Lower-than-normal levels of potassium (called *hypokalemia*) can result from diarrhea, starvation, severe vomiting, severe burns, excessive consumption of licorice, chronic stress or fever, liver disease, the use of diuretics, or the use of steroids. The most common cases of hypokalemia that you will encounter will likely involve patients on IV therapy who do not receive adequate daily potassium supplements. Increased potassium levels (known as *hyperkalemia*)

(continues)

(continued)

can be caused by renal failure (wherein the kidneys are unable to excrete potassium), cell damage or injury, internal bleeding, uncontrolled diabetes, or acidosis.

Sodium (Na^+) is the most abundant electrolyte found in the blood. Sodium is needed for the maintenance of osmotic pressure (fluid balance) and acid-base balance as well as for the transmission of nerve impulses. Lower-than-normal levels of sodium (called *hyponatremia*) can be caused by water retention, which dilutes the overall concentration of sodium in the blood. Other potential causes include severe burns, severe diarrhea, vomiting, and the use of diuretics. *Hypernatremia* (high levels of sodium) can be caused by dehydration (resulting from insufficient intake of water), coma, diabetes insipidus, or tracheobronchitis.

Finally, phosphorus in the form of phosphate (PO_4^{3+}) is needed for the building of bony tissue, the metabolism of fats and sugars, and maintenance of the acid-base balance. Interestingly, as phosphorus levels increase, calcium levels decrease, and vice versa. As the level of one of these electrolytes increases, the kidneys excrete the other. A rapid rise in phosphorus will cause calcium levels to drop rapidly. This can result in cardiac arrhythmia and twitching muscles. Increased levels of phosphorus (called *hyperphosphatemia*) can be caused by hypocalcemia, excessive vitamin D intake, bone tumors, healing bone fractures, and renal insufficiency. Lower-than-normal levels of phosphorus (called *hypophosphatemia*) can result from rickets and continuous IV administration of glucose.

We hope that this brief discussion highlights the importance of maintaining proper electrolyte balances in the body.

QUOTES & NOTES

Chlorine is a poisonous gas. The chloride ion, however, is not poisonous. In fact, it is found in all body fluids.

Ionic Bonding

Figure 23-1 illustrated how sodium and chlorine atoms interact when ionized. Electrons are transferred from the sodium atom to the chlorine atom. To indicate the formation of a negative ion, the name is changed from chlor*ine* to chlor*ide*. The ions resulting from this ionization are attracted to each other because they are oppositely charged. In this way, they form the compound *sodium chloride*, or ordinary table salt. This attraction between oppositely charged particles that results in the formation of a compound is called an **ionic bond**.

A **compound** is two or more atoms joined by a chemical bond. A chemical change occurs when two elements join to form a compound. This is evident in the formation of sodium chloride. Sodium is a metal that reacts violently with water. Chlorine is a poisonous gas. When they react, however, they form a substance having none of the properties associated with the elements from which it was derived—and one integral to human life.

Sodium chloride is represented by NaCl. This formula tells us, by the lack of subscripts (which is understood as 1), that there is an ion of sodium for every ion of chloride. They combine in a one-to-one ratio because of their respective charges. The total charge of a compound must add up to zero, as is the case with sodium chloride. The formulas for ionic compounds are called **empirical formulas**. An empirical formula gives the whole number ratio of the ions that combine to form an ionic compound.

For example, consider the ionic compound that forms when magnesium and chlorine react. Magnesium is in group IIA of the periodic table; thus, we know each magnesium atom has 2 electrons in its outer shell. The electron dot structure for magnesium is "Mg:". Chlorine is in group VIIA, and thus each chlorine atom has 7 electrons in its outer shell. The magnesium atom, then, must lose 2 electrons to form an octet, and the chlorine atom can accept only 1 electron to form an octet. That means 2 chlorine atoms are needed for every magnesium atom. This is illustrated by the following equation:

$$Mg: + \ 2\ Cl \rightarrow Mg^{2+} + \ 2\ Cl^-$$

In this reaction, the magnesium atom loses 1 electron to each of the 2 chlorine atoms. In doing so, the magnesium ion gains a charge of +2, while the chlorine ions each gain a charge of −1. The empirical formula for magnesium chloride, then, is $MgCl_2$.

Osmosis

Elsewhere in this text, we discuss the roles of sodium and chloride ions in the body. These roles become more apparent when we consider the movement of water into and out of cells. This movement is determined by the concentrations of dissolved substances in the water and cells. If you were to place a stalk of celery in a concentrated saltwater solution, the celery would shrink because of the movement of water from the cells of the celery into the saltwater solution. The movement of water through a cell membrane from a lower concentration of dissolved substances (more water and less dissolved salt in the celery) to a higher concentration of dissolved substances (more dissolved salt in the saltwater solution) is called **osmosis**. Osmosis represents an attempt to dilute the solution with the higher concentration so that there are equal concentrations on both sides of the membrane. The flow of water under these conditions is always in the same direction, that is, from the lower concentration to the higher concentration of dissolved substances.

The significance of osmosis becomes evident when considering the cells in the body. The cells in the body have a certain concentration of dissolved substances. If a solution is injected into the body, it is important that the concentration of the solution being injected match the concentration of dissolved substances in the cells. If the solution being injected possesses a lower concentration of NaCl than the concentration of NaCl in the cells, for example, water will flow into the cell (see Figure 23-2B, and note that Figure 23-2A

represents an isotonic solution with no flow). It is possible that enough water will flow into the cell to burst the cell.

Solutions having lower concentrations of dissolved substances than are present in the body's cells are called **hypotonic solutions** (*hypo* meaning "less than"); they are said to be hypotonic relative to the solution in the cell. Solutions having higher concentrations of dissolved substances than are present in the body's cells are called **hypertonic solutions** (*hyper* meaning "greater than"); they are said to be hypertonic relative to the solution in the cell. If a hypertonic solution is injected into the body, fluid will flow out of the cell, and the cell will shrink (see Figure 23-2C). **Crenation** is the term that describes the shrinking of the cells.

Ideally, solutions injected into the body should be of the same concentration as the solution in the cells. Solutions of this kind are called **isotonic solutions** (*iso* meaning "same"); they are said to be isotonic with respect to the solution in the cell (see Figure 23-2A). A 0.9% NaCl solution, then, is isotonic with respect to the fluid inside a red blood cell (RBC). This solution is called a *physiological saline solution*.

QUOTES & NOTES

Osmotic pressure is one of the factors responsible for sap rising in trees, and by tapping a maple tree the sap can be boiled down to make maple syrup.

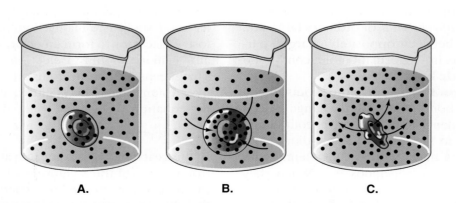

A. **B.** **C.**

Figure 23-2 *(A) Cell in an isotonic solution; (B) Cell in hypotonic solution; (C) Cell in a hypertonic solution.*
Source: Delmar/Cengage Learning

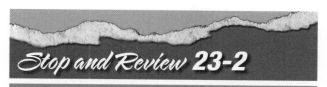

Covalent Bonding

Another type of bonding is exhibited in the formation of a chlorine molecule (Cl_2). In this type of bonding, called **covalent bonding**, the atoms share electrons to gain an octet rather than transferring them from one atom to another, as is done in ionic bonding. Chlorine, from group VIIA, has 7 electrons in its outer energy level and needs 1 electron to form an octet. In the case of a chlorine molecule, two chlorine atoms share a pair of electrons to form an octet. This is illustrated by the electron dot structure in Figure 23-3.

A molecule, then, is a structure held together by the attraction of the nuclei of a pair of atoms that are sharing electrons. Counting shared and unshared electrons, then, both chlorine atoms have an octet of electrons. We can simplify the electron dot structure by drawing a **structural formula**. In a structural formula, the nonbonding electrons are removed and a single line is used to represent the pair of electrons being shared. The

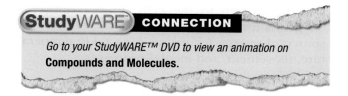

Figure 23-4 *Structural formula for the chlorine molecule.*

Source: Delmar/Cengage Learning

structural formula for the chlorine molecule is illustrated in Figure 23-4.

Another way of expressing molecular structure is via a *molecular formula*. The molecular formula for the chlorine molecule is Cl_2. The subscript 2 means that 2 chlorine atoms are bonded together. In future chapters, we will be using both structural and molecular formulas; therefore, you should be familiar with both representations.

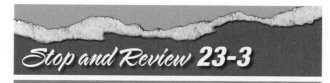

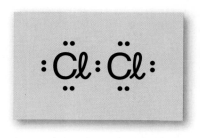

Figure 23-3 *Electron dot structure for the chlorine molecule.*

Source: Delmar/Cengage Learning

The oxygen found in the air we breathe is another example of a molecule. The oxygen atom has 6 electrons in its outer shell and needs 2 electrons to complete its outer energy level. It achieves this by sharing 2 pairs of electrons with another oxygen atom. The three structures for the resulting molecule are shown in Figure 23-5.

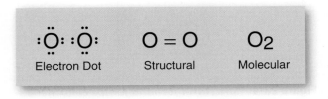

Figure 23-5   *Electron dot structure, structural formula, and molecular formula for the oxygen molecule.*

Source: Delmar/Cengage Learning

A covalent bond wherein 2 pairs of electrons are shared is called a *double covalent bond*. This is the structure of the oxygen found in the air. Oxygen composes approximately 21% of the air. Nitrogen makes up about 78%. The remainder of the air is composed of some inert gases, carbon dioxide, and water vapor. The oxygen in the air is taken into our lungs. From the lungs, it passes into the bloodstream. The bloodstream then carries the oxygen to the cells. In the cells, the oxygen is used along with other substances as a source of energy for maintaining body temperature, movement, and mental processes.

Chemical Formulas

Being able to write and read chemical formulas will be essential in this and following chapters. Chemical formulas are a shorthand way of writing chemical compounds.

Empirical Formulas

As noted earlier, empirical formulas are useful in expressing the composition of ionic compounds. As previously discussed, ionic compounds are composed of ions. The ratio of ions in an ionic compound is determined by the charge of the bonding ions. For example, in sodium chloride (NaCl), the sodium (Na) ion has a charge of +1 and the chlorine (Cl) ion has a charge of −1. The sum of the charges in a compound must add up to zero. As illustrated in Figure 23-6, a crystal of NaCl is an aggregate of Na and Cl ions (Figure 23-6C). These ions are always found in a one-to-one ratio, as shown in Figure 23-6A and B. Thus, when considering the empirical formula of an ionic compound, you must remember that the formula represents the ratio in which the ions are found and that crystal formations of the compound contain large numbers of ions in this one-to-one ratio.

Table 23-2 lists the symbols and charges of some common ions. When examining the table, you will see that the metal ions all have positive charges equal to their group numbers on the periodic table. Thus, if you have a periodic table, you need not memorize these charges.

Likewise, the charges of negative ions can be determined using knowledge you gained from our discussion of bonding earlier. We told you that atoms always try to complete their outer shells and obtain an octet of electrons. Accordingly, atoms of the group VI elements, for example, all have 6 electrons, and therefore

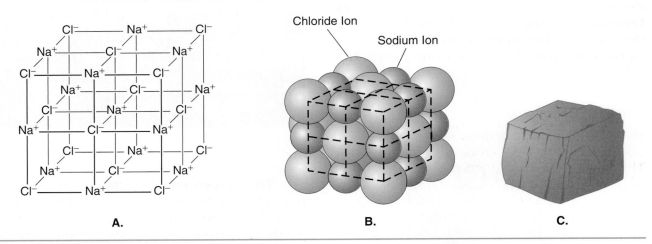

A.   **B.**   **C.**

Figure 23-6   *(A) Schematic showing how the ions are distributed in a sodium chloride crystal. (B) Sodium ions are smaller than chloride ions and these ions are arranged in the crystal as shown. (C) The actual crystal of sodium chloride.*

Source: Delmar/Cengage Learning

TABLE 23-2
Symbols and Charges for Various Ions

GROUP	ELEMENT	SYMBOL FOR THE NEUTRAL ATOM	SYMBOL FOR ITS COMMON ION	NAME OF ION
IA	Lithium	Li	Li^+	Lithium ion
	Sodium	Na	Na^+	Sodium ion
	Potassium	K	K^+	Potassium ion
IIA	Magnesium	Mg	Mg^{2+}	Magnesium ion
	Calcium	Ca	Ca^{2+}	Calcium ion
	Barium	Ba	Ba^{2+}	Barium ion
IIIA	Aluminum	Al	Al^{3+}	Aluminum ion
VIA	Oxygen	O	O^{2-}	Oxide ion
	Sulfur	S	S^{2-}	Sulfide ion
VIIA	Fluorine	F	F^-	Fluoride ion
	Chlorine	Cl	Cl^-	Chloride ion
	Bromine	Br	Br^-	Bromide ion
	Iodine	I	I^-	Iodide ion
Transition elements				
	Silver	Ag	Ag^+	Silver ion
	Zinc	Zn	Zn^{2+}	Zinc ion
	Copper	Cu	Cu^+	Copper (I) ion (cuprous ion)
			Cu^{2+}	Copper (II) ion (cupric ion)
	Iron	Fe	Fe^{2+}	Iron (II) ion (ferrous ion)
			Fe^{3+}	Iron (III) ion (ferric ion)

must gain 2 electrons to create an octet of electrons in their outer shell. Gaining 2 electrons results in a charge of −2, as is the case for oxygen and sulfur (Table 23-2). The same reasoning yields a charge of −1 for the ions of the group VII elements. Although there are exceptions to this rule, it does apply to the ions listed in Table 23-2.

The only ions for which you will need to memorize charges are those of the four transition elements listed at the bottom of Table 23-2. This is easy to do with the elements having ions of various charges because the charge is implied in the name. For example, Iron (Fe) has ions with +2 and +3 charges, and these ions are named Iron (II) and Iron (III), respectively. However, because the older names of *ferrous* (Fe^{2+}) and *ferric* (Fe^{3+}) are still used in some circles, you should be familiar with these names also.

Molecular Formulas

The particles formed in covalent bonding are called *molecules*. The formulas of these substances are referred to as *molecular formulas* because they represent the makeup of the actual molecules. The molecular formula of water, for example, is H_2O. This shows that the water molecule is made up of 2 hydrogen atoms and 1 oxygen atom. The gaseous elements hydrogen, nitrogen, oxygen, fluorine, chlorine, and bromine and the solid element iodine are all diatomic (*di* meaning "two"). Their molecular formulas are H_2, N_2, O_2, F_2, Cl_2, Br_2, and I_2, respectively.

In summary, then, ions make up ionic compounds. The crystals of ionic compounds consist of ions in the ratio given by the empirical formula of the ionic compound. Covalently bonded substances consist of molecules. The molecular formula gives the ratio of atoms in the molecular compound.

Stop and Review 23-4

a. Without referring to Table 23-2, write the symbol and charge for each of the following ions using the periodic table.

 1. sodium

 2. calcium

 3. chloride

 4. iron (III)

b. Without referring to Table 23-2, name each of the following ions.

 1. K^+

 2. Mg^{2+}

 3. O^{2-}

 4. Zn^{2+}

c. Use the periodic table to determine the charge of the following ions.

 1. sulfide

 2. strontium

 3. lithium

 4. aluminum

 5. fluoride

TABLE 23-3
Common Polyatomic Ions

NAME	FORMULA
Ammonium ion	NH_4^+
Hydronium ion	H_3O^+
Hydroxide ion	OH^-
Acetate ion	$C_2H_3O_2^-$
Carbonate ion	CO_3^{2-}
Bicarbonate ion (Hydrogen carbonate)	HCO_3^-
Sulfate ion	SO_4^{2-}
Hydrogen sulfate ion	HSO_4^-
Phosphate ion	PO_4^{3-}
Monohydrogen phosphate ion	HPO_4^{2-}
Dihydrogen phosphate ion	$H_2PO_4^-$
Nitrate ion	NO_3^-
Nitrite ion	NO_2^-
*Aerosmith	$HVYMTL^+$
Cyanide ion	CN^-

*Not a true "heavy" metal ion but rather a "light" attempt at humor by the authors.

In some cases, molecules become ionized. The resulting covalently bonded ions are called *polyatomic ions*. Table 23-3 lists some common polyatomic ions.

Naming Compounds

The preceding information can be useful in naming compounds. For example, the name for ZnO is zinc oxide, a compound sometimes found in skin ointments. In ionic compounds, the first ion is always the positive ion, and we just use its name. The second ion is the negative ion. Negative ions other than polyatomic ions end in *ide*. Thus, the negative ion of oxygen is called *oxide*. As another example, consider MgO, a substance used as a mineral supplement in vitamin pills. The name of the compound is magnesium oxide.

Many compounds are used in the health field either alone or in combination with other substances. Furthermore, most compounds have more than one use. Sodium fluoride (NaF) is used either alone or in children's vitamin tablets to prevent tooth decay. Calcium chloride ($CaCl_2$), along with other substances, is used as an oral electrolyte rehydration solution for people who have become dehydrated. Sodium chloride or table salt (NaCl) is one of the substances used with $CaCl_2$ for this purpose. Sodium chloride is also used in solution for saline nose drops and contact lens solution. Calcium iodide is used along with codeine for symptomatic relief of coughs. Together they act as an **expectorant** and **antitussive**. An expectorant helps clear the lungs, and an antitussive helps reduce coughing.

When naming compounds composed of polyatomic ions, the name of the polyatomic ion is all that is needed. For example, the compound $NaHCO_3$ is called *sodium bicarbonate*. Sodium bicarbonate is injected into the blood to treat **metabolic acidosis**. Metabolic acidosis is a condition characterized by too much acid in the blood resulting from a metabolism problem, such as diabetes. The name of Li_2CO_3 is *lithium carbonate*, a compound used to treat manic depression. As you can probably see, it is extremely difficult to name the compounds if you do not know the polyatomic ions. It is therefore important to memorize these and any other polyatomic ions that your instructor feels are necessary.

Magnesium hydroxide $(Mg(OH)_2)$ is used in antacids such as Maalox. Disodium hydrogen phosphate (Na_2HPO_4) is used as a urinary acidifier. Iron supplements, with iron (II) sulfate $(FeSO_4)$ as an ingredient, are used to treat **anemia**, a condition characterized by an insufficient number of red blood cells (RBCs) in the blood. Calcium acetate $(Ca(C_2H_3O_2)_2)$ is used to prepare an **astringent** wet dressing. Astringents have the power to draw together, or contract, organic tissue. A styptic pencil containing potassium aluminum sulfate $KAl(SO_4)_2$ (alum) is another example of an astringent.

Writing Chemical Formulas

Now that you know how to name compounds, we will learn how to write the formula for a compound given the compound's name. It is necessary to know the symbols and charges to be able to do this. In writing the formula for a compound, it is often easiest to write the symbol and charge for each ion, and then determine how many of each ion are necessary to make the total charge of the compound equal to zero. Writing the symbol and charges for the compound sodium sulfate, for example, gives the following:

$$Na^+SO_4^{2-}$$

Two sodium ions for every sulfate ion, then, are needed to balance the charges. This gives the following formula:

$$Na_2SO_4$$

An easy way to determine the subscripts for the ions in a formula is to use the numerical value of the charge of one ion as the subscript for the other ion. Thus, for the sodium sulfate example, we would get the following:

Remember Na^{1+} and SO_4^{2-}

$$Na_2SO_4$$

This gives the formula Na_2SO_4, as before.

Note that a subscript of 1 is understood and never written. Also, if the charges are equal and opposite, the ions always combine in a one-to-one ratio. As an example, consider the formula

for zinc oxide. The symbols and charges for zinc and oxide are Zn^{2+} and oxide O^{2-}, respectively. Because the charges are equal and opposite, the formula is written as ZnO.

You have to be particularly careful when writing formulas involving polyatomic ions. When more than one of these ions is present in the formula, it must be enclosed within parentheses. This means that the formula for barium hydroxide, for example, is $Ba(OH)_2$, and not $BaOH_2$.

Stop and Review 23-5

a. Write the formula for each of the following compounds.
   1. sodium chloride
   2. sodium hydrogen carbonate

b. List 10 chemicals that you come into contact with on a daily basis. Hint: Read some of the lists of ingredients on food labels.

The Mole

In our daily lives, we use terms that represent a certain number of items. When we talk about a *pair* of socks, for example, everyone knows that we mean two socks. Similarly, the terms *dozen*, *case*, and *gross* represent the numbers 12, 24, and 144, respectively. We call terms such as these **quantitative terms**, that is, names for a number of objects.

The quantitative term **mole** is used by chemists to describe that amount of a substance that contains an Avogadro number of particles. **Avogadro's number** is 6.02×10^{23}, an extremely large number. Because atoms are extremely small, you can easily hold an Avogadro number of atoms in your hand. But to give you an even better idea of the size of Avogadro's number, consider this: If an Avogadro number of M&Ms were spread uniformly over the 48 contiguous states, the blanket of M&Ms would be more than 50 miles deep.* Thus, the term *mole* means 6.02×10^{23} particles. These particles can be atoms, molecules, ions, or even M&Ms!

---

*This calculation was performed by Merlo, C., & Turner, K. E., *Journal of Chemical Education*, 1993, volume 70, p. 453.

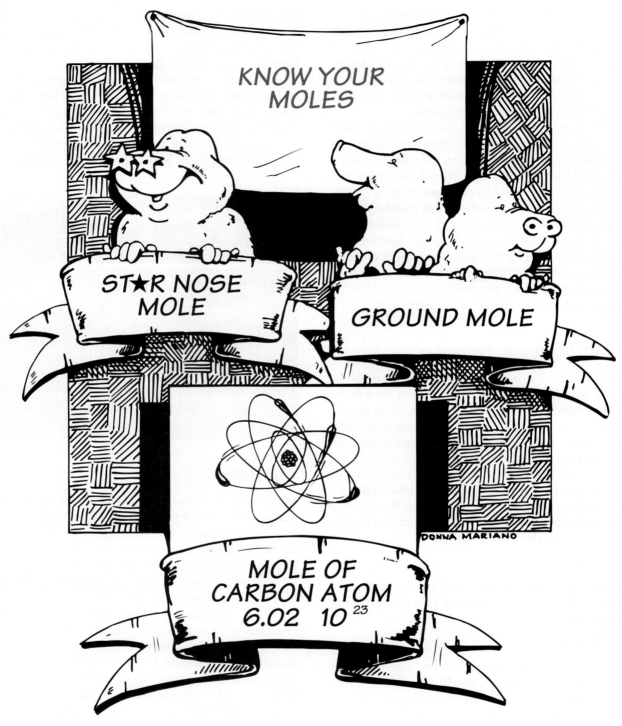

KNOW YOUR MOLES

ST★R NOSE MOLE

GROUND MOLE

MOLE OF CARBON ATOM 6.02 10²³

DONNA MARIANO

Source: Delmar/Cengage Learning

In our discussion of compound formulas, we implied that the subscripts represent the number of atoms of each element present in the compound. It also can be said that subscripts represent the number of moles of each atom. Consider, for example, the molecular formula for methane (natural gas): CH_4. As this formula indicates, a single molecule of methane is composed of 1 carbon

Clinical Relevancy

Oxygen Toxicity: Too Much of a Good Thing

By now, you undoubtedly realize that oxygen is essential to life. Patients suffering from certain diseases require additional oxygen. For example, additional oxygen decreases myocardial work in heart attack victims and increases blood oxygen levels in patients having lung disease, thus allowing them to be more active.

But you can actually get too much of a good thing when it comes to oxygen. If oxygen is given in excessive amounts, the results can be life threatening. Excessive amounts of oxygen affect the integrity of cell membranes in the body. This occurs as a result of *free radicals*. A free radical is an extremely reactive atom or molecule possessing at least one unpaired electron. These atoms normally remain in a free form for only a brief moment before combining with other atoms. Free radicals result from oxygen's participation in biochemical actions at the

cellular level, where oxygen takes on electrons, becoming reduced, while the electron donors (in this case the cell membrane) become oxidized. Cell membranes are affected as electrons are removed from the cells; the cells then begin to disintegrate.

Free radicals can stop the growth of tissue and, even, inactivate certain enzymes needed for cellular metabolism. It is a proven fact that the growth of tissue can be inhibited in an environment of 100% oxygen at 1 atmosphere of pressure. Furthermore, if a laboratory rat is suddenly placed in an environment of 100% oxygen, the rat could die within 72 hours. While there is some evidence showing that oxygen is safe up to a concentration of 50%, some studies point to oxygen toxicity in patients who have received low levels of supplemental oxygen in their homes.

atom and 4 hydrogen atoms. Likewise, 1 mole of methane consists of 1 mole of carbon and 4 moles of hydrogen, or 6.02×10^{23} molecules of methane (1 mole) consists of 6.02×10^{23} carbon atoms (1 mole) and 24.08×10^{23} hydrogen atoms (4 moles).

Other Types of Bonds

Thus far in our discussion of covalent bonding we have focused on bonding between two atoms of the same element. Under these circumstances, the shared pairs of electrons are equally shared, and a **pure covalent bond** results because the charge on the nuclei of the atoms is the same.

If the atoms sharing the electrons are of different elements, it is possible for the electrons to be shared unequally; this results in a **polar covalent bond**. An example of this type of bonding is the hydrogen chloride molecule. The electron dot structure for hydrogen chloride is "H:Cl". The hydrogen atom has only 1 proton attracting the shared pair of electrons, while the chlorine atom has 17 protons attracting the shared pair. It is only reasonable, then, that the electrons would be more closely attracted to the chlorine atom than to the hydrogen atom. For this reason, we attribute a slight negative charge to the chlorine

and a slight positive charge to the hydrogen, as shown in Figure 23-7A.

This type of bonding is also found in water. The structural formula of water is illustrated in Figure 23-7B. As you can see, the hydrogen atoms are slightly positive, and the oxygen atoms are slightly negative. If water molecules are placed together in a container, the atoms will arrange themselves so that the opposite charges are attracted. This means that the hydrogen of one atom will be attracted to the oxygen of another atom. This force of attraction between the hydrogen and oxygen is called a *hydrogen bond*. Hydrogen bonding, illustrated in Figure 23-7C, is somewhat of a misnomer, however, because the process does not result in the formation of a true bond; rather, it is an attraction between opposite charges that occurs.

In summary, then, ionic bonding results from the formation of oppositely charged ions. These ions are attracted to each other because of their opposite charges. In covalent bonding, molecules are formed by the attraction of the atoms that share electrons. The polar covalent bond is a bond somewhere between equal sharing of electrons and a complete transfer of electrons, that is, somewhere between a neutral molecule and an ionic compound. The resulting molecules have partial charges attributed to them.

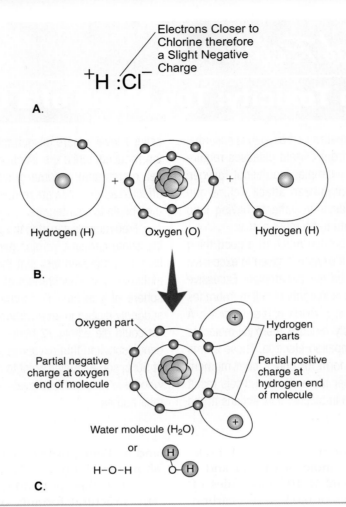

Figure 23-7   *Forms of polar covalent bonding (A and B) and hydrogen bonding (C).*
Source: Delmar/Cengage Learning

Translating Reactions into Equations

Chemical equations are a way of expressing complex chemical reactions in a more efficient way. We will start our discussion of chemical equations using word equations and move on to balancing formula equations.

Chemical Word Equations

The easiest way to express chemical reactions is via word equations. In the simplest terms, a reaction is expressed as follows:

reactants → products

This is read "reactants yield products." The reactants are those substances that combine together and change, or react. The products are the outcome of this combining process. For instance, when oxygen reacts with hydrogen, they combine to form water. The word equation for this reaction is as follows:

hydrogen + oxygen → water

This word equation is read "hydrogen plus oxygen yields water."

Clinical Relevancy

The Hemoglobin-Oxygen Word Equation

After oxygen crosses the barriers of the lung, it enters the blood. Oxygen is transported by the blood in two ways. It can either be dissolved in the plasma (liquid portion) of the blood, in which case it is free to move about the plasma in its usual gaseous state, or as happens with most of the oxygen, it can quickly attach to the **hemoglobin** (Hb) in the red blood cells (RBCs). Each RBC in your body contains 280 million hemoglobin molecules, and each hemoglobin molecule possesses four heme groups to which oxygen can attach. Thus, each hemoglobin molecule can transport four molecules of oxygen. If all four sites of attachment are utilized, it is said that the hemoglobin is 100% saturated; if three sites hold oxygen, the hemoglobin molecule is 75% saturated. When oxygen is attached to hemoglobin, it is referred to as *oxyhemoglobin*. If there is less than 75% saturation (oxygen attached to the hemoglobin molecule), hemoglobin is considered to be *reduced hemoglobin*, or *deoxyhemoglobin*.

This phenomenon of hemoglobin attracting oxygen is represented by the following equation:

$$Hb + O_2 \rightleftharpoons HbO_2$$

The arrows in this equation indicate that hemoglobin can both combine with and readily release oxygen. This can be compared to a bus (Hb) that picks up passengers (O_2, from the lungs), drives them to work (through the circulatory system), and drops them off (at the tissues of the body, which need oxygen to survive).

Formula Equations

As you can see, the only information provided by word equations is the reactants and their products. A more useful type of equation, therefore, is the formula equation, which gives information regarding the amounts of the substances reacting. Using the example of water again, the formula equation is as follows:

$$H_2 + O_2 \rightarrow H_2O$$

As discussed earlier, hydrogen and oxygen are diatomic elements. For this reason, their symbols are written with the subscript 2. The preceding equation is incorrect as written, however. As you can see, there are two oxygen atoms on the left side of the equation and only one on the right side. This violates the law of the conservation of atoms, which states that there must be the same number of atoms on both sides of the equation. You cannot do this by changing the formulas of the reactants or products.

If we were to change the formula to H_2O_2, we would satisfy the law of conservation of atoms, but the compound indicated would be hydrogen peroxide rather than water. Because water and not hydrogen peroxide is formed when oxygen and hydrogen react, this formula cannot be correct. To obtain the same number of atoms on each side of the equation, then, we must change the coefficients rather than the subscripts. To obtain two oxygen atoms on the right side, we must therefore use a coefficient in front of the water:

$$H_2 + O_2 \rightarrow 2H_2O$$

While this yields the correct number of oxygen atoms, there are now four hydrogen atoms on the right side and only two on the left. Putting a coefficient of 2 for the hydrogen on the left yields an equal number of hydrogen atoms on both sides of the equation. Thus, the correct formula equation for water is as follows:

$$2H_2 + O_2 \rightarrow 2H_2O$$

This process is called *balancing an equation*. The purpose of balancing an equation is to get the same number of atoms of each element on opposite sides of the equation. This is similar to the process of balancing mathematical equations, as discussed in Section Two. When an equation is balanced, it is more useful to us because it shows the numbers of substances reacting. The preceding equation, for example, tells us that 2 molecules of hydrogen react with 1 molecule of oxygen to produce 2 molecules of water.

Example:

We know that potassium chlorate decomposes to yield potassium chloride and oxygen. The word equation for this reaction is as follows:

potassium chlorate → potassium chloride + oxygen

The formula equation is as follows:

$$KClO_3 \rightarrow KCl + O_2$$

To balance this equation, three molecules of oxygen are needed on the right side. If we use a coefficient of 1.5 for the oxygen we will have the correct number of oxygen atoms, as shown in the following equation:

$$KClO_3 \rightarrow KCl + 1.5O_2$$

While this balances the equation, we cannot in actuality have 1.5 molecules of oxygen. Therefore, we must change 1.5 to a whole number. To do so, we would multiply both sides of the equation by 2, which yields the following equation:

$$2KClO_3 \rightarrow 2KCl + 3O_2$$

There are now (2)K, (2)Cl, and (6)O on both sides of the equation; the equation is, therefore, balanced.

Note: As is the case with subscripts, coefficients represent both the number of molecules and the number of moles of a given substance in a reaction.

To summarize, then, the steps for writing a balanced formula equation are as follows:

1. Write the correct formula equation from the word equation, being especially careful when working with formulas including diatomic elements.

2. Adjust coefficients to get the same number of atoms of each element on opposite sides of the equation; do not change subscripts.

3. Check your results by adding the number of atoms on each side of the equation.

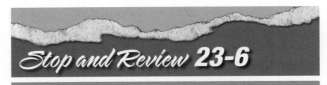

Stop and Review 23-6

Write a balanced formula equation for the following reactions.

a. calcium + oxygen yields calcium oxide

b. sodium + sulfur yields sodium sulfide

■ CHAPTER REVIEW

Exercises

1. An ion has 9 protons in its nucleus and 10 electrons orbiting its nucleus. What is the charge on this ion?

2. An ion has 20 protons in its nucleus and 18 electrons orbiting its nucleus. What is the charge on this ion?

3. Distinguish between ionic bonding and covalent bonding. What particles are formed in each type of bonding?

4. Why would you not want to inject pure water into a person's body?

5. Is a solution having a concentration of 0.8% isotonic, hypotonic, or hypertonic with respect to a physiological saline solution?

6. How many atom(s) are present in each of the following compounds?

   a. $CaCl_2$

   b. Al_2O_3

   c. $C_6H_{12}O_6$

7. Name the following compounds.

   a. NaF

   b. $CaCl_2$

   c. NaCl

   d. CaI_2

8. Name each of the following compounds.

   a. $Mg(OH)_2$

   b. Na_2HPO_4

   c. $FeSO_4$

   d. $Ca(C_2H_3O_2)_2$

9. Write the formula for each of the following compounds:

   a. calcium oxide

   b. lithium nitrate

   c. aluminum oxide

   d. sodium sulfate

   e. calcium hydroxide

10. How many atoms of each element are in each of the following compounds?

    a. $BaCl_2$

    b. Al_2O_3

    c. $K_2Cr_2O_7$

    d. $Ca(C_2H_3O_2)_2$

11. What is an ion? How are ions formed?

12. What is the charge on a neutral atom if it gains 3 electrons?

13. What is the charge on a neutral atom if it loses 2 electrons?

14. Write the symbol and charge for each of the following ions.

    a. sodium ion

    b. iron (III)

    c. barium ion

    d. potassium ion

    e. bicarbonate ion

    f. monohydrogen phosphate ion

    g. hydroxide ion

    h. ammonium ion

15. Name each of the following ions.

    a. I^-

    b. K^+

    c. Cl^-

    d. Fe^{2+}

    e. H_3O^+

    f. CO_3^{2-}

    g. $C_2H_3O_2^-$

    h. $H_2PO_4^-$

16. The formula for an ozone molecule is O_3. What does the subscript 3 tell us?

17. Name each of the following compounds.

    a. NaF

    b. $FeBr_2$

    c. NH_4CN

    d. KOH

18. Write the formula for each of the following compounds.

    a. aluminum sulfide

    b. iron (II) bromide

    c. iron (III) nitrate

    d. silver nitrate

19. What is the amount of a substance containing an Avogadro number of particles called?

20. How many moles of each atom are present in each of the following compounds?

    a. NaF

    b. $CaSO_4$

    c. $Mg(H_2PO_4)_2$

21. Write a balanced formula equation for each of the following reactions.

    a. zinc + hydrogen chloride → zinc chloride + hydrogen

    b. iron + sulfur → iron (II) sulfide

    c. nitrogen + hydrogen → ammonia (NH_3)

22. Balance each of the following equations.

    a. $Mg + O_2 \rightarrow MgO$

    b. $Zn + H_2SO_4 \rightarrow ZnSO_4 + H_2$

    c. $NaI + Br_2 \rightarrow NaBr + I_2$

Additional Activities

1. Refer to a book on nutrition in the library and determine the percentage of the U.S. recommended daily allowances for the various minerals discussed in this chapter. Read the nutritional information on the labels of your favorite foods. Discuss with your classmates why it is necessary to eat a well-balanced diet. Also, are there any minerals that should be limited in the diet? Look up Wilson's disease in an encyclopedia. Did any foods list copper? Do you see why?

2. Invite a dietician, nurse, or physician in to discuss the importance of electrolytes in the human body.

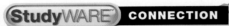 **CONNECTION**

Go to your StudyWARE™ DVD and have fun learning as you play interactive games, view animations and videos, and take practice tests to help reinforce key concepts you learned in this chapter.

Workbook Practice | *Go to your Workbook for more practice questions and activities.*

CHAPTER 24

THE GAS LAWS

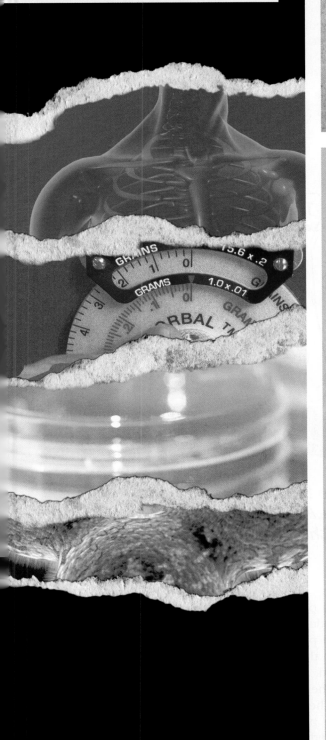

Objectives

Upon completion of this chapter, you should be able to

- Explain the kinetic theory in relationship to gases

- Relate the concepts of volume, temperature, and pressure to gases

- Define Boyle's law, Charles' law, and Gay-Lussac's law and solve gas law problems according to each of these gas laws

- Solve problems according to both the combined gas law and Dalton's law of partial pressure

- Define and differentiate between the terms *STPD*, *ATPS*, and *BTPS*

- Convert between equivalent expressions of gas pressure

- Define both Henry's law and gas diffusion and relate each to physiologic processes

- Explain how barometers measure barometric pressure

- Explain what is meant by the temperature of a substance in terms of molecular motion

- Explain conditions necessary for chemical reactions and factors that affect reaction rates in terms of the collision theory

Key Terms

absolute humidity
absolute temperature

absolute zero
activation energy

(continues)

antipyretics
ATPS
Avogadro's law
barometer
barometric pressure
Boyle's law
BTPS
Charles' law
combined gas law

Dalton's law
diffusion
enzymes
external respiration
fractional distillation of liquid air
Gay-Lussac's law
gram molecular weight
Henry's law
hyperpyrexia

hypothermia
internal respiration
Kelvin scale
kinetic theory
relative humidity
STPD
vasodilator
water vapor

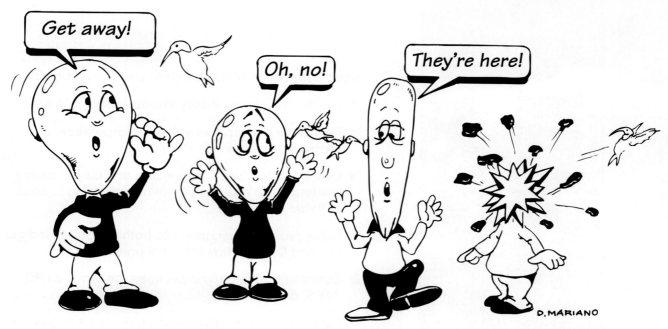

While taking a stroll through the park, the balloon head family unwittingly demonstrate BOYLE'S LAW when four nearsighted hummingbirds mistake them for flowers.

Source: Delmar/Cengage Learning

■ INTRODUCTION

Medical gases are used extensively in the health professions. Oxygen is a therapeutic gas used in many situations. Anesthetic gases are used in surgery, and several other gas mixtures are used in diagnostics and research. In addition, many of the machines utilized in the health care setting are pneumatically powered, which is another way of saying they run on pressurized gas.

In Chapter 21, we discovered that matter exists in one of four states depending on the arrangement of particles and the forces that act on these particles. In a gaseous state, the particles of matter are widely scattered and act independently of each other. Unlike a solid, a gas does not possess a definite shape. Instead, a gas takes on the form of the container within which it is held, and the gaseous particles evenly distribute themselves throughout the container. The kinetic theory will help us to better understand why the physical condition or state of any gas is affected by four quantities: the temperature, pressure, volume, and mass of the gas. Note that a change in any one of these four quantities will result in a change or alteration in the other three. The kinetic theory will also help us to understand the various factors that affect the rate of a chemical reaction.

How Gas Behaves

The characteristics of gases can be explained using the kinetic theory. Initially, we will discuss the kinetic theory and the properties of gases, and then we will tie them all together in the gas laws sections.

The Kinetic Theory

Before discussing how the previously mentioned four quantities affect matter in a gaseous state, it is necessary to develop an understanding of the **kinetic theory**. The main points of this theory were developed over a period of time to describe the characteristics of gases on a molecular level. Simply stated, these points assume that:

1. All matter is composed of extremely small particles.

2. These tiny particles generate their own energy and are in constant, rapid, and random motion.

3. Because of this motion, these particles collide with each other and with the wall of the container within which they are held. When they collide with each other, the particles appear to be "perfectly elastic"; in other words, they neither gain nor lose energy on impact. This is not the case, however, when the particles collide with the nonelastic sides of the container within which they are held.

Pressure and Gases

If a gas is placed in a closed container, the gas particles will collide with the container's walls. Each time a particle collides with a wall, it exerts a force on the wall, even if for only the briefest moment. This may seem trivial until you realize the mind-boggling number of gas particles in a given container and the fact that these collisions occur equally against *all* walls of the container. It stands to reason, then, that as the number of gas particle "hits" within the container increases, so does the pressure.

If you were to throw a ball at a bathroom scale glued to a wall, you would see a temporary increase in pressure, as evidenced by the deflection of the scale when the ball hit the scale. The scale would then quickly return to zero. If you were to continuously throw many balls at the scale, however, the scale would never get a chance to reset to zero, and the "pressure" (i.e., how high the scale climbed) would depend on the number of hits.

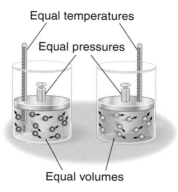

Figure 24-1 *At a given temperature and pressure, equal volumes of all gases contain the same number of molecules.*

Source: Arnold, Melvin T., *Essentials of General, Organic, and Biochemistry*, 1e, Brooks/Cole, Cengage Learning

To visualize the magnitude of the number of molecules involved in a gaseous state, it is important to understand **Avogadro's law**, which states that at any given temperature and pressure, equal volumes of *all* gases contain equal numbers of molecules (i.e., 6.02×10^{23}, known as Avogadro's number). Thus, the **gram molecular weight** of any gas contains the same number of molecules (6.02×10^{23}), and the gram molecular weight of any gas occupies 22.4 liters at standard temperature and pressure. See Figure 24-1. The importance of the concept of standard temperature and pressure will become clearer as we perform some gas law problems.

Temperature and Gases

Now that you have an appreciation for the number of molecules present in any given gas, we will focus on how temperature affects the activity of these molecules. The average kinetic energy of a gas is directly proportional to its **absolute temperature** (to be discussed further in a moment). This means that as you increase the temperature of a gas, you increase the kinetic energy of that gas. As a result, you increase the velocity of the gas particles, which in turn increases the frequency of gas particle collisions. As stated earlier, an increase in the number of "hits" leads to increased pressure in the container. Absolute temperature, then, is directly proportional to the pressure of a gas.

The absolute temperature scale was developed in 1848 by Lord Kelvin, based on his belief that the lowest obtainable temperature is –273 degrees Celsius and that this is the temperature at which the kinetic activity of a substance is theoretically zero. Kelvin referred to this temperature as **absolute zero**, and it is the starting point for the absolute scale, or

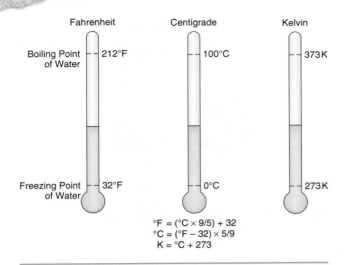

Fahrenheit   Centigrade   Kelvin

Boiling Point — 212°F   — 100°C   — 373K
of Water

Freezing Point — 32°F   — 0°C   — 273K
of Water

$$°F = (°C \times 9/5) + 32$$
$$°C = (°F - 32) \times 5/9$$
$$K = °C + 273$$

Figure 24-2 *Comparison of the three temperature scales along with conversion formulas.*

Source: Delmar/Cengage Learning

The Specific Gas Laws

Understanding Boyle's law is essential to understanding how we breathe and cough, which are discussed in the section following Boyle's law.

Boyle's Law

In the 1600s, a British chemist and physicist named Robert Boyle developed a gas law that demonstrates the relationship between the volume and the pressure of a gas. **Boyle's law** states that, assuming that the temperature of a given sample of gas remains constant, the volume of that sample of gas will vary inversely with the pressure of the gas. Thus, as the volume of a container holding a given sample of gas increases, the pressure exerted by the gas decreases. So, if you want to increase the pressure exerted by a given amount of a gas, simply decrease the volume of the container holding the gas (see Figure 24-3).

what we now call the **Kelvin scale**. Increments in the Kelvin scale are the same as those in the Celsius scale. Thus, to convert from Celsius to Kelvin all you need to do is add 273 to any Celsius temperature:

Kelvin = Celsius temperature + 273

When referring to absolute temperatures, we use the word "Kelvin" rather than "degrees"; so 285 K (which we all know is 12 degrees Celsius) is called "285 Kelvin." Remember that you must use the Kelvin temperature scale when considering temperature's relationship to gases. Figure 24-2 compares the three different temperature scales.

To illustrate how Boyle's law works mathematically, we will begin with the following equation:

$$P = 1/V$$

In this equation, P = pressure, V = volume, and 1 = a mathematical constant. If we juggle this

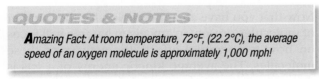

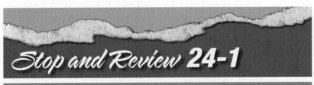

Stop and Review 24-1

a. What is 352 Kelvin equivalent to on the Celsius temperature scale?

b. What is −5 degrees Celsius equivalent to on the Kelvin temperature scale?

c. What property of a gas describes the force of the gas particles hitting the walls of its container?

d. What property of a gas is related to the kinetic energy of its particles?

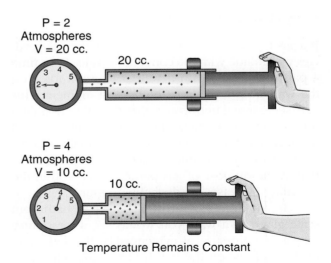

P = 2
Atmospheres
V = 20 cc.

20 cc.

P = 4
Atmospheres
V = 10 cc.

10 cc.

Temperature Remains Constant

Figure 24-3 *An application of Boyle's law: hand-applied pressure compresses an equal number of molecules into a smaller space, resulting in increased pressure.*

Source: Delmar/Cengage Learning

equation around, we arrive at the following equation:

$$P \times V = 1$$

Thus, if 1 (sometimes represented by the letter "K") is to remain constant, when we want to increase pressure, we must decrease volume. Conversely, if we want to decrease pressure, we must increase volume in order to maintain the constant.

Although we have mathematically represented the statement of Boyle's law, this alone does not allow us to fully apply this law. It would be useful to be able to use this law to predict change. With this in mind, we can develop a second equation that will allow us to compare a gas before and after a change occurs. This equation is written as follows:

$$P_1 V_1 = P_2 V_2$$

In this equation, P_1 = initial pressure, P_2 = final pressure, V_1 = initial volume, and V_2 = final volume.

This formula can be manipulated in a number of ways to solve for volume or pressure. For example:

$$P_2 = P_1 V_1 / V_2$$

or

$$V_2 = P_1 V_1 / P_2$$

Example:

A given amount of oxygen occupies 250 mL on a day when the barometric pressure is 720 mm Hg. What will be the volume of that same gas the next day, when the barometric pressure is 750 mm Hg?

What we know:

P_1 = 720 mm Hg

P_2 = 750 mm Hg

V_1 = 250 mL

The unknown is V_2, the changed volume resulting from the change in pressure.

If we rearrange our original formula $(P_1 V_1 = P_2 V_2)$ to solve for the unknown volume, we get the following formula:

$$V_2 = P_1 V_1 / P_2$$

Now, insert the known values:

$$V_2 = (720 \text{ mm Hg})(250 \text{ mL})/750 \text{ mm Hg}$$

So V_2 = 240 mL. Because this amount is less than the original volume, this example proves that gas is compressible.

Another illustration of Boyle's law is provided in Figure 24-4.

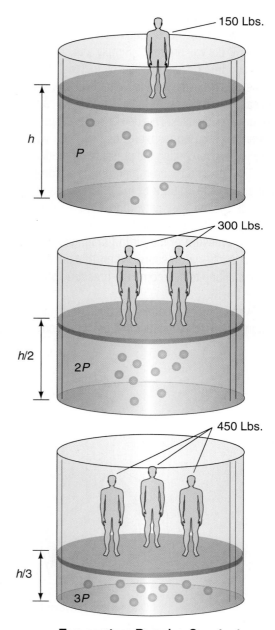

Temperature Remains Constant

Figure 24-4 *An illustration of Boyle's law: if the temperature of a gas remains constant, the volume of the gas will vary inversely with the pressure.*

Source: Delmar/Cengage Learning

Special Focus

Boyle's Law as It Relates to Breathing and Coughing

Breathing: Each of us begins and ends our respective lives with a breath. And all the breaths in between usually occur with no conscious efforts on our parts.

How do we breathe? Simply put, inspiration (i.e., breathing in) is accomplished by increasing the volume of the chest cavity. As the volume of the chest cavity increases, the pressure inside the chest cavity (and in the lungs) decreases. This decreased pressure allows the higher-pressure atmosphere to "push" its way into the lungs, thus overcoming the pressure difference.

Exhalation (i.e., breathing out) is accomplished by decreasing the volume of the chest cavity. As the volume of the chest cavity (and lungs) decreases, the pressure of the air in the lungs increases to the point that the pressure of the air in the lungs is greater than the atmospheric pressure. When this occurs, air flows out of the lung to overcome the pressure difference (see Figure 24-5).

A variation on breathing is coughing. A good, effective cough is necessary in order to protect the body's airways; coughing helps to prevent accumulation of secretions and foreign bodies in the airways, thus decreasing the chance of lung infections. In coughing, inhalation is performed as usual, with an inspiratory pause that allows for an even distribution of gases in the lung. Instead of passively exhaling, however, the glottis is closed and rapid exhalation against the closure is attempted, thus temporarily closing the container (the lungs). This resistance increases intrathoracic pressure.

With a sudden opening of the glottis, the air inside the lungs is then rapidly expelled, along with any foreign bodies or secretions that happen to be in the way. Coughing, like breathing, represents a physiologic application of Boyle's law. With coughing, a rapid decrease in the volume of the lungs causes a rapid increase in the pressure within the lungs, which greatly enhances both the flow of gases and the expulsion of foreign material from the lungs (see Figure 24-6). Gas traveling through the airways during a cough can easily reach speeds of over 100 miles per hour!

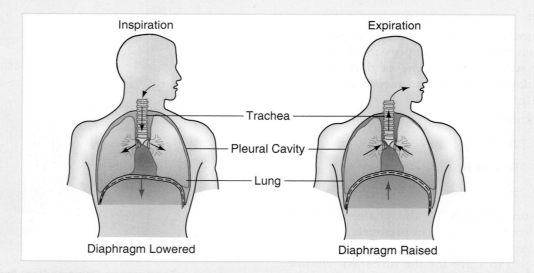

Figure 24-5   *Boyle's law and breathing: as the diaphragm lowers, the volume of the chest cavity increases, thereby decreasing the intrathoracic pressure.*

Source: Delmar/Cengage Learning

(continues)

(continued)

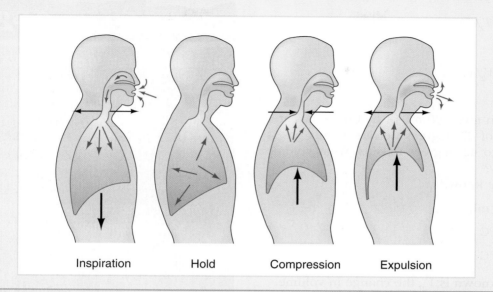

Inspiration   Hold   Compression   Expulsion

Figure 24-6 *Boyle's law and coughing: the body uses rapid changes in volume to increase the pressure and, therefore, the effectiveness of the cough.*
Source: Delmar/Cengage Learning

Charles' Law

Whereas Boyle's law addresses the relationship between the volume and the pressure of a gas, **Charles' law** addresses the relationship between the volume and temperature of a gas. Developed by Jacques Charles (1746–1823), this law states that if the mass and pressure of a gas remain constant, volume and temperature of the gas are directly related. Thus, if you increase the temperature of a fixed amount of gas, its volume will also increase (see Figure 24-7). The formula we will use to initially represent Charles' law is as follows:

$$V/T = K$$

As with Boyle's law, the constant is constant—it cannot change. So whatever affects the volume will also affect the temperature, and vice versa.

Again as with Boyle's law, we can develop a second equation that will allow us to compare a

gas before and after it is acted on. This equation is written as follows:

$$V_1/T_1 = V_2/T_2$$

In this equation, V_1 = initial volume, V_2 = final volume, T_1 = initial temperature, and T_2 = final

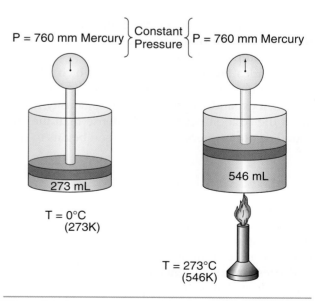

P = 760 mm Mercury ⎱ Constant ⎰ P = 760 mm Mercury
               ⎰ Pressure ⎱

273 mL

546 mL

T = 0°C
(273K)

T = 273°C
(546K)

Figure 24-7 *An illustration of Charles' law: as the temperature of the gas increases, so does the volume.*
Source: Delmar/Cengage Learning

temperature. We can solve for new volume or new temperature by rearranging our formula as follows:

$$V_2 = V_1 \, T_2/T_1$$

and

$$T_2 = T_1 \, V_2/V_1$$

Example:

We have been given 90 mL of hydrogen gas at a temperature of 27 degrees Celsius. If this gas is warmed up to 42 degrees Celsius, what volume will it occupy?

What we know:

$$V_1 = 90 \text{ mL}$$

$$T_1 = 27°C$$

$$T_2 = 42°C$$

The unknown is V_2, the change in volume. As is the case in all gas law problems involving temperature, we must first convert Celsius degrees to Kelvin.

$$K = T(C) + 273$$

$$T_1 = 27 + 273 = 300 \text{ K}$$

$$T_2 = 42 + 273 = 315 \text{ K}$$

Now using the formula to solve for new volume, insert the known values:

$$V_2 = V_1 \, T_2/T_1$$

$$V_2 = (90 \text{ mL})(315 \text{ K})/300 \text{ K}$$

So, V_2 is 94.5 mL, proving that an increase in the temperature of a gas will lead to an increase in the volume of the gas.

Charles' law is the principle on which a hot air balloon functions. As the air entering the balloon is heated, it expands, thus decreasing its density. As the air in the balloon becomes less dense than the surrounding atmospheric air, the balloon begins to rise.

Gay-Lussac's Law

Gay-Lussac's law addresses the relationship between the temperature and pressure of a gas. According to Joseph Gay-Lussac, if the volume and mass of a gas remain constant, the temperature and pressure of the gas are directly related (see Figure 24-8). Thus, if you increase the pressure of a gas, you will also increase its temperature, and vice versa. The equation we will use initially to represent Gay-Lussac's law is as follows:

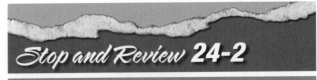

Stop and Review 24-2

a. A container held 40 cc of gas at 20 degrees Celsius. The volume later changed to 60 cc. What was the temperature of the gas at this later point in time?

b. A person placed a sandwich in a sealed plastic bag and drove to the top of a high mountain. Why did the bag expand?

c. If we increase the pressure exerted on a gas in a sealed container, what will happen to the gas volume?

d. A balloon at room temperature is placed in a freezer. What will happen to its volume?

$$P/T = K$$

As with the other gas laws, to maintain the constant (that is, K), if we increase one variable, we must also increase the other variable.

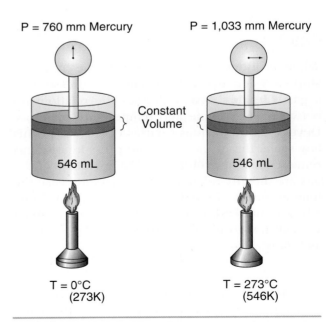

P = 760 mm Mercury   P = 1,033 mm Mercury

} Constant Volume {

546 mL   546 mL

T = 0°C (273K)   T = 273°C (546K)

Figure 24-8 *An illustration of Gay-Lussac's law: if the volume of a gas remains constant, the temperature and pressure of the gas will vary directly.*

Source: Delmar/Cengage Learning

Likewise, if we decrease one variable, we must also decrease the other variable. So, if we increase P, we must also increase T, and if we decrease P, we must also decrease T.

Again as with the other gas laws, we can develop a second equation that will show the relationship between the initial and the final states of a given gas. This equation is written as follows:

$$P_1/T_1 = P_2/T_2$$

We can solve for the new temperature or new pressure by rearranging this formula as follows:

$$T_2 = T_1 P_2/P_1$$

and

$$P_2 = P_2 T_2/T_1$$

Example:

A car tire is filled to a pressure of 24 pounds per square inch (psi) when the temperature is 20 degrees Celsius. After running at high speed, the tire temperature rises to 60 degrees Celsius. What is the new pressure within the tire, assuming that the tire's volume did not change?

What we know:

$$P_1 = 24 \text{ psi}$$

$$T_1 = 20°C = 293 \text{ K}$$

$$T_2 = 60°C = 333 \text{ K}$$

The unknown is P_2, the change in pressure. Now, using the formula to solve for new pressure, insert the known values:

$$P_2 = P_1 T_2/T_1$$

$$P_2 = (24 \text{ psi})(333 \text{ K})/293 \text{ K}$$

The new pressure, then, would be 27.3 psi.

For the sake of consistency, this is why tire manufacturers suggest that you always inflate your tires at a "cold" temperature.

Historically, one of the favorite pastimes of youth has been to throw aerosol cans into a fire. This mindless act leads to explosive results that probably explain why this is a pastime of youth— those who practice it may not live to adulthood! A rapid increase in temperature combined with an inflexible container leads to a tremendous increase in pressure. This pressure causes a violent rupturing of the can, spewing shrapnel in all directions.

Happily, the effects of temperature on pressure can be demonstrated on a far less violent level. Medical gas cylinders stored in outside tank cages during the winter exhibit relatively low gauge pressure readings when first brought into a hospital. As the cylinders slowly warm to room temperature, however, the gauge pressure readings increase. Does someone sneak extra gas into these tanks when no one is looking? No: this is just Gay-Lussac's law in action!

The Combined Gas Law

The three previously discussed gas laws can be "put together" to form the **combined gas law**. This law shows the relationship between the pressure, temperature, and volume of a given gas. The combined gas law is written mathematically as follows:

$$P_1 V_1/T_1 = P_2 V_2/T_2$$

If we cross-multiply, the equation becomes:

$$T_2 \times V_1 \times P_1 = T_1 \times V_2 \times P_2$$

Example:

If a given gas measures 400 mL at a temperature of 25 degrees Celsius while under a pressure of 800 mm Hg, to what temperature would you need to cool this gas in order to reduce its volume to 350 mL and its pressure to 740 mm Hg?

What we know:

$$V_1 = 400 \text{ mL}$$

$$V_2 = 350 \text{ mL}$$

$$P_1 = 800 \text{ mm Hg}$$

$$P_2 = 740 \text{ mm Hg}$$

$$T_1 = 25°C$$

The unknown is T_2, the new temperature. As in previous examples involving temperature, don't forget to convert to Kelvin.

Rewrite the formula to solve for T_2:

$$T_2 = (T_1)(P_2)(V_2) / (P_1)(V_1)$$

Now, simply insert the known values:

$$T_2 = (298 \text{ K})(740 \text{ mm Hg})(350 \text{ mL})/(800 \text{ mm Hg})(400 \text{ mL})$$

Thus, you would need to cool the temperature to 241.19 K, or −31.81°C.

Special Focus

Fractional Distillation of Liquid Air

Let's take a close look at how the gas laws apply to a process that saves millions of lives. This process is the manufacturing of medical oxygen used to treat critically ill patients.

If you have ever walked around the outside of a hospital building, you may have noticed structures that resemble enormous white thermos bottles. This is where liquid oxygen is stored until needed by patients. Oxygen is utilized in liquid form because the costs required to ship bulk oxygen in liquid form are much less than those required to ship an equivalent amount of oxygen in gas-filled cylinders. Furthermore, storage space requirements for liquid oxygen are much less than those for an equivalent volume of gaseous oxygen. In fact, when liquid oxygen changes to a gaseous state at room temperature, it expands to almost 862 times its original volume!

The process of creating liquid oxygen, called **fractional distillation of liquid air,** was developed in 1907 by Dr. Carl von Linde. The following is how the process is accomplished:

1. A given amount of air is cleaned to remove all impurities (such as dust). The temperature of the purified air is then reduced to nearly freezing, thus removing all of the air's moisture.
2. The clean, dry air is then compressed to a pressure of 200 atmospheres (atm). Per Gay-Lussac's law, as we pressurize (i.e., increase the pressure of) a given volume of gas, we increase the temperature of that gas.
3. The compressed air is then cooled to room temperature.
4. When the air is cooled, it is expanded from 200 atm to only 5 atm of pressure. This rapid drop in pressure greatly reduces the air's temperature in a very efficient manner.
5. The air has now cooled to the point that it becomes a liquid!
6. The liquid air is poured into a distilling column and allowed to warm. In this case, "warm" means approximately −320.4 to −297.3 degrees Fahrenheit! Each gas in the warming liquid air will boil off at a known temperature. (Nitrogen, for example, boils off at −196 degrees Celsius, while oxygen boils off at −183 degrees Celsius.) The trick to obtaining liquid oxygen is to stop warming the liquid air when its temperature reaches just below the boiling point of oxygen. At that point in the process, only liquid oxygen remains.
7. The distillation process is performed again to remove any remaining impurities and ensure that the oxygen is at least 99% pure, as required by the Food and Drug Administration (FDA). Most medical oxygen is actually more than 99% pure.
8. When the desired level of purity is reached, the liquid oxygen is drawn off to cold converters for delivery to hospitals or medical equipment suppliers.

Figure 24-9 shows the relationship of all three variables (pressure, temperature, and volume) in a combined schematic.

Dalton's Law

The final gas law we will discuss concerns the actions of gases when they are mixed together. Because oxygen is vital to our survival, we often assume that the bulk of our atmosphere is oxygen. In actuality, however, oxygen makes up approximately one-fifth (20.9%) of our atmosphere, with nitrogen making up nearly all the rest (79%). This means that less than 1% of our atmosphere is composed of such gases as carbon dioxide (which is exhaled as a waste product of the body's metabolism), carbon monoxide, and methane (see Table 24-1).

TABLE 24-1 Atmospheric Gases		
ELEMENT	**PROPORTION OF THE ATMOSPHERE (%)**	**TRACE AMOUNTS**
Nitrogen (N_2)	78.08	Helium (He)
Oxygen (O_2)	20.95	Hydrogen (H_2)
Argon (Ar)	0.93	Krypton (Kr)
Carbon dioxide (CO_2)	0.03	Neon (Ne)
		Ozone (O_3)
		Radon (Rn)

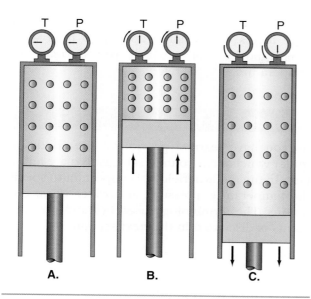

Figure 24-9 *Relationship of the variables of pressure, temperature, and volume in a gas. As shown in part B, when volume decreases, temperature and pressure increase. As shown in part C, when volume increases, temperature and pressure decrease.*

Source: Delmar/Cengage Learning

Simply put, **Dalton's law** states that each gas in a gas mixture exerts a partial pressure equal to its fractional concentration. This law also states that the sum of the partial pressures in a gas mixture will always equal 100%. The mathematical formula representing Dalton's law is as follows:

fractional concentration of a specific gas × total pressure = partial pressure of that gas

As a real-life example, let's assume that a hospital patient is receiving 28% oxygen from a mask when the barometric pressure is 600 mm Hg. Substituting these values into our formula gives us the following:

$$0.28 \times 600 \text{ mm Hg} = 168 \text{ mm Hg}$$

We therefore know that the oxygen is exerting a partial pressure of 168 mm Hg within the mask.

There is one other variable that we must consider, however: the effect of **water vapor**. Water molecules in water vapor are so small that they behave like a gas. Because water vapor behaves like a gas, it also exerts a pressure. The partial pressure exerted by water vapor depends on temperature and the amount of water available. Whenever we calculate the partial pressure of a gas where water vapor is present (such as in our airways or in the surrounding air), we must subtract the water vapor pressure from the barometric pressure before we can solve for the partial pressures of any other gases. Thus, Dalton's law can be modified as follows:

$$P_{partial} = (P_{barometric} - P_{H_2O})(\text{fractional concentration})$$

Example:

The partial pressure of water vapor (P_{H_2O}) is maximally 47 mm Hg at body temperature (37 degrees Celsius). If the barometric pressure is 747 mm Hg, what is the partial pressure of oxygen in the lungs of a patient inspiring a gas mixture containing 50% oxygen?

Clinical Relevancy

Hyperbaric Therapy

An interesting application of Dalton's law is the use of hyperbaric chambers to treat people with burns or suffering from carbon monoxide (CO) poisoning. In a hyperbaric (*hyper* meaning "above") chamber, the pressure can be raised to two or thee times atmospheric pressure. This will increase the partial pressure of oxygen, resulting in more oxygen being dissolved into the blood. High levels of oxygen in the blood can be toxic to bacteria and help treat infections. In the case of carbon monoxide poisoning, the carbon monoxide binds with hemoglobin and blocks the oxygen from combining with hemoglobin. The high concentration of oxygen can force out the carbon monoxide that was attached to the hemoglobin, allowing oxygen to take its place.

$$P_p = (747 \text{ mm Hg} - 47 \text{ mm Hg})(0.50)$$

$$P_p = (700 \text{ mm Hg})(0.50)$$

$$P_p = 350 \text{ mm Hg}$$

The partial pressure of the oxygen in the lungs of this patient is, therefore, 350 mm Hg.

Stop and Review 24-3

a. How much pressure is exerted by nitrogen if the barometric pressure is 760 mm Hg and the water vapor pressure is 20 mm Hg?

b. Why would an aerosol paint can explode if placed in a fire?

c. What is meant by the partial pressure of a gas?

Humidity

Since we have just gotten our feet wet concerning water vapor, let's look at some other ways of expressing water vapor content. **Absolute humidity** is the actual weight of the water vapor contained in a given amount of gas. This is usually expressed either as grams per cubic meter (g/m^3) or milligrams per liter (mg/L). At 37 degrees Celsius (body temperature), the most humidity that air can hold is 43.8 grams per cubic meter, or 43.8 milligrams per liter. **Relative humidity**, on the other hand, is a comparison of the actual amount of water vapor to the amount of water vapor that a given gas can hold at a given temperature. Relative humidity is expressed as a percentage and is determined using the following equation:

$$RH = \text{content/capacity} \times 100$$

So, if water vapor content is 25 milligrams per liter at 37 degrees Celsius, what is the relative humidity?

$$RH = 25 \text{ mg/L} / 43.8 \text{ mg/L} \times 100$$

$$RH = 57\%$$

If you can keep the water content of a given gas constant while increasing the gas's temperature,

the relative humidity will decrease because you have increased the air's capacity to hold water. The opposite will occur if you decrease the temperature.

Other Gas Topics

As you have learned previously, the conditions under which a gas volume is measured are important. In the medical field, it is important to specify the temperature, pressure, and water vapor conditions. The terminology used in these measurements is discussed in the next section.

STPD, ATPS, and BTPS

(What does it all spell?)

By now it should be apparent that gas laws are necessary in the study of respiratory physiology. In time, you will learn that many important measurements are made using various instruments for specific circumstances. Three such measurements are represented by the acronyms **STPD**, **ATPS**, and **BTPS**. STPD stands for a *standard temperature* (0 degree Celsius) *pressure* (760 mm Hg) and *dry* (0 mm Hg water vapor pressure.) ATPS stands for *ambient temperature*, *pressure*, and *saturated* with water vapor, which basically means room temperature, barometric pressure, and saturated water vapor pressure at that particular room temperature. BTPS means *body temperature* (37 degrees Celsius), *pressure* (barometric), and *saturated* with water vapor at that particular temperature. Keep these terms in the back of your mind for now; they will be important in upcoming chapters.

QUOTES & NOTES

Helium is the lightest medical gas. For this reason, it is also the most expensive gas to package (compress) into cylinders. The lightness, or low density, of helium is what causes a helium balloon to rise rapidly in our atmosphere.

Equivalent Expressions of Normal Atmospheric Pressure

While we are on the subject of remembering things for the future, there are several equivalent units for standard atmospheric pressure (each of these values equals one atmosphere) that you will need to understand to be able to convert between units. These are as follows:

> 760 mm Hg (millimeters of mercury)
>
> 14.7 psi (pounds per square inch)
>
> 1,034 cm H_2O (centimeters of water)
>
> 33 ft of salt H_2O (feet of salt water)
>
> 33.9 ft of fresh H_2O (feet of fresh water)
>
> 29.9 in. mm Hg (inches of mercury)

You can use the factor label method covered in the math section to easily convert between these units. A quick example to refresh your memory follows.

Example:

How many mm Hg are there in 10 psi?
First write down what is given, placing the unit you have in the denominator and the unit for which you want to solve in the numerator:

$$\frac{10 \text{ psi}}{1} \times \frac{\text{mm Hg}}{\text{psi}}$$

Now, insert the equivalent numbers and solve:

$$\frac{10 \text{ psi}}{1} \times \frac{760 \text{ mm Hg}}{14.7 \text{ psi}} = 517 \text{ mm Hg}$$

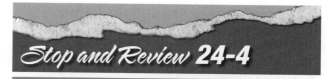

Stop and Review 24-4

a. What is the difference between ATPS and STPD?

b. List the different units used to measure air pressure.

Special Focus

Mercury Barometers

The Earth is surrounded by a blanket of gases we call the atmosphere. This blanket exerts a force on everything on our planet. **Barometric pressure** is the term used to describe this force, or pressure. We can measure this pressure using a device called a **barometer**. The principle by which a barometer works is that the atmosphere exerts a pressure on a reservoir of mercury, which causes the mercury to be pushed up into an evacuated (i.e., depressurized) glass tube (see Figure 24-10). This tube is calibrated in either millimeters or inches. Barometric pressure is thus measured by how high the column of mercury is pushed up the calibrated tube. The pressure reading is given in millimeters of mercury (mm Hg). Some scientists refer to 1 mm Hg as 1 torr, in memory of the Italian scientist Evangelista Torricelli (1608–1647), who developed the mercury manometer.

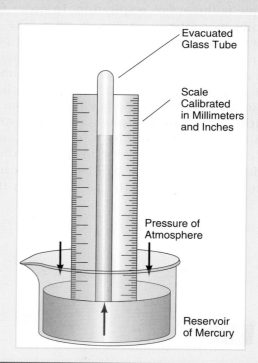

Figure 24-10   *A mercury barometer.*
Source: Delmar/Cengage Learning

Diffusion

Diffusion is the movement of gas from an area of high concentration of that gas to an area of low concentration of that gas (see Figure 24-11). In the opening paragraph of this chapter, we touched on the process of diffusion when we learned that a gas will distribute itself equally throughout a container if given sufficient time. This is how perfume works: it diffuses away from the wearer and permeates the room.

The diffusion rate of a gas is directly related to the concentration gradient, the temperature, and the cross-sectional area for diffusion. Thus, if any of these increases, so will the rate of diffusion. The rate of diffusion is indirectly related to the molecular weight of the gas (a heavier gas is slower to distribute) and the distance that the gas has to diffuse.

A good physiologic illustration of this principle is the act of respiration. In order for the body to continue to live, it must take in nutrients and expel waste products. The primary purpose of our lungs and blood vessels is to take in oxygen from the external atmosphere and get rid of carbon dioxide, which is a waste product of the body's metabolism. If too little oxygen were brought in, our tissues would starve and be unable to function. Coma and death would follow. If too much carbon dioxide were allowed to build up as a result of insufficient expulsion of this gas from the

lungs, the body's pH would become very acidic and, again, we could die.

How do we exchange these gases with the external environment and within our bodies? Several processes are at work, the most important one being diffusion and the factors related to it. Our lungs simply ventilate, or bring in, a bulk flow of fresh gas from the atmosphere. This gas is relatively high in oxygen and low in carbon dioxide. This gas mixture flows to the functional unit of gas exchange in the lung, known as the alveolar capillary membrane (see Figure 24-12).

The alveolus and the capillaries surrounding it possess very thin walls and, therefore, allow for the diffusion of gas across their surfaces. As you can see from Figure 24-13, the blood in the capillary is relatively low in oxygen because it has just come from the tissues, where it has given off its oxygen for cellular metabolism. Conversely, it has taken on carbon dioxide, the waste by-product of metabolism, which it now transports to the alveoli. A pressure gradient is established wherein the oxygen will flow from an area of higher concentration of oxygen (the alveolus) to an area of lower concentration of oxygen (the capillary) and will attach to the hemoglobin molecule, which will then carry the much-needed oxygen to the tissues. Likewise, carbon dioxide will flow from an area of higher concentration of carbon dioxide (the capillary) to an area of lower concentration of carbon dioxide (the lungs) where it will be exhaled on the next breath. This explains why, although we inhale virtually no carbon dioxide, we exhale a substantial amount of this gas.

The process of exchanging gases with the external environment (atmosphere) is called **external respiration**. Basically the reverse process of gas exchange occurs at the tissue level. This process, termed **internal respiration**, has been explained in more depth in the Anatomy and Physiology section.

Henry's Law

Just when you thought you were done learning about gas laws, here is yet one more. **Henry's law** (1803) helps to describe the physiologic process of respiration, where gas molecules move from a gaseous state in the alveoli to a liquid state in the blood.

Henry's law states that the amount of gas that enters a physical solution in a liquid is directly

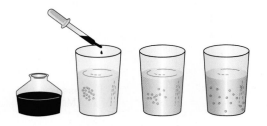

Figure 24-11 *The process of diffusion: the dye molecules go from an area of high concentration to one of low concentration.*

Source: Delmar/Cengage Learning

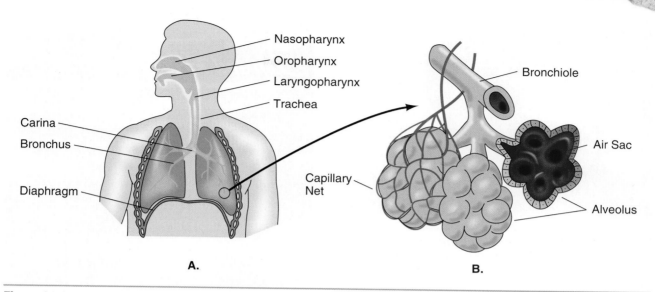

Figure 24-12 *(A) The conducting airways that ventilate, or bring atmospheric gases into contact with, the functional alveolar capillary unit. (B) An expanded view of one of the millions of alveolar capillary units.*
Source: Delmar/Cengage Learning

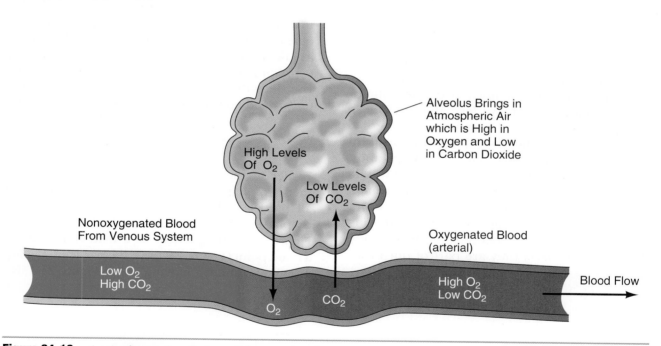

Figure 24-13 *A one-dimensional view of the process of external respiration, or gas exchange with the atmosphere: the pressure gradient causes diffusion from areas of high concentration to areas of low concentration.*
Source: Delmar/Cengage Learning

proportional to the partial pressure of the gas above the surface of the liquid. Therefore, placing a person on a high concentration of oxygen would not only increase the pressure gradient and facilitate diffusion, but would also increase the driving pressure above the liquid blood, thus allowing oxygen to saturate the hemoglobin molecules. This is why hospital patients are given

supplemental oxygen by either cannula or mask when sufficient blood oxygen levels cannot be maintained via breathing atmospheric air (see Figure 24-14).

A nonphysiologic example of Henry's law is the carbonation of beverages. In this process, carbon dioxide is compressed above a liquid mixture of water, sweeteners, artificial

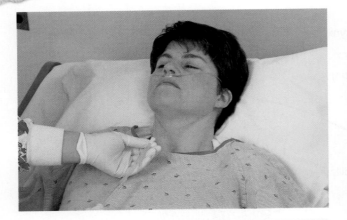

Figure 24-14   *A patient receiving additional oxygen in order to increase the pressure gradient and, thus, cause more oxygen to be loaded into the bloodstream (Henry's law).*

Source: Delmar/Cengage Learning

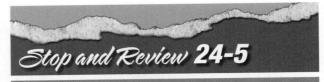

Stop and Review 24-5

a. State the law that addresses the relationship between the following variables. Also, write the formula for the law.

   1. pressure-volume
   2. temperature-volume
   3. temperature-pressure

b. State the law of partial pressures and write the formula for this law.

coloring, and artificial flavors. The high driving pressure of carbon dioxide forces the gas molecules into solution, thus giving the mixture its effervescence. The resulting mixture is, of course, capped so that the carbon dioxide cannot escape and is maintained in the liquid by vapor pressure. When uncapped, the solution will eventually go flat and lose almost all of its carbon dioxide to the atmosphere.

How many other examples can you think of where gas laws come into play? What about pressurized airplane cabins or the need to take supplemental oxygen on high-altitude climbs? What about scuba diving and space exploration? As you can see, the gas laws are not just some lofty scientific theories or meaningless academic exercises; they are part of our everyday lives.

Rates of Reaction

Initially, one would not think that the study of rates of reaction would have anything to do with the medical field. One application of reaction rates involves explaining why a moderate fever is beneficial. After you study the following sections, you should better understand how a moderate fever can be beneficial.

The Kinetic Theory

Earlier in the chapter we discussed the kinetic theory of matter. In review, this theory states that all particles of matter, regardless of their state or phase, are in constant motion. As shown in Figure 24-15, the particles of a solid vibrate about a fixed point (Figure 24-15A); the particles of a liquid vibrate about a moving point (Figure 24-15B);

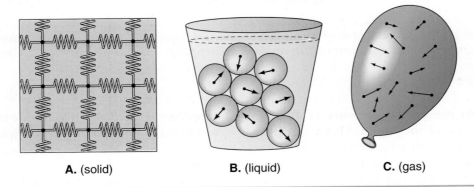

A. (solid)   **B.** (liquid)   **C.** (gas)

Figure 24-15   *(A) The particles of a solid vibrate about a fixed point. (B) The particles of a liquid vibrate about a moving point. (C) The particles of a gas move independently of one another.*

Source: Delmar/Cengage Learning

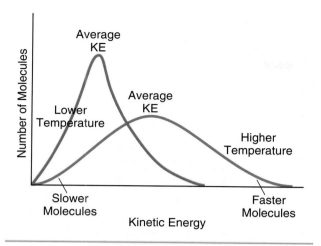

Figure 24-16 *The average kinetic energy of a gas is directly proportional to its Kelvin temperature.*
Source: Delmar/Cengage Learning

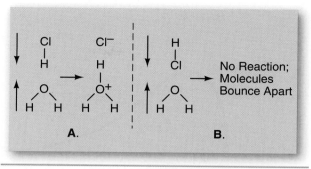

Figure 24-17 *(A) Effective collision, with proper orientation of the molecules. (B) Ineffective collision, with no reaction taking place.*
Source: Delmar/Cengage Learning

and the particles of a gas are in constant random motion, traveling in straight lines until they collide with either one another or the walls of their container (Figure 24-15C).

We learned earlier that the average kinetic energy of a solid, liquid, or gas is proportional to the Kelvin temperature. If, for example, you were to increase the temperature of gas, the gas molecules, on average, would move faster. It is important to realize, however, that not *all* of the molecules in a gas at a given temperature move at the same speed. Some move more slowly; some move more quickly. Most of the molecules, however, move at the same average speed, as shown in Figure 24-16.

The Collision Theory

The kinetic theory can be helpful in explaining the rates of chemical reactions. Before discussing rate of reaction and its applications to the health sciences, however, we must first examine how chemical reactions take place. The collision theory helps explain chemical reactions. As the name implies, the collision theory describes chemical reactions in terms of collisions between the reacting particles. Per this theory, the particles must be oriented properly and possess sufficient energy to break the bonds of the old molecules so that new molecules can be formed. Figure 24-17 illustrates both effective collision and ineffective collision for the following reaction:

$$H_2O + HCl \rightarrow H_3O^+ + Cl^-$$

In an effective collision as shown in Figure 24-17A, the H$_2$O molecule collides with the HCl

molecule, the old bonds break, and new bonds form to yield H$_3$O$^+$ + Cl$^-$. Without proper orientation, the molecules just bounce off each other and no reaction takes place (Figure 24-17B). Keep in mind that an efficient collision is not enough for a reaction to take place. For a chemical reaction to take place, sufficient energy is needed to break the bonds of the reacting molecules. Once the bonds of the reacting molecules are broken, the reactant molecules can form. The minimum energy required for a reaction to occur is called **activation energy**. If the H$_2$O molecules and HCl do not possess at least this amount of energy, they will just bounce off each other, and no reaction will take place.

In summary, then, chemicals react by colliding with each other. For a new substance to be formed, the colliding molecules must be properly oriented and possess sufficient energy.

Factors Affecting Rate of Reaction

Figure 24-18 shows the effect of increasing the temperature of a reacting substance. In Figure 24-18A, the molecules in the shaded portion have energy greater than the activation energy. If we increase the temperature, the distribution of molecular speeds changes. As you can see from Figure 24-18B, the number of molecules with energy greater than the activation energy increases. Thus, higher temperatures result in a higher number of collisions that have sufficient energy to react, which in turn result in a faster reaction rate. The general rule of thumb is that for every 10°C increase in temperature, the rate of reaction will approximately double.

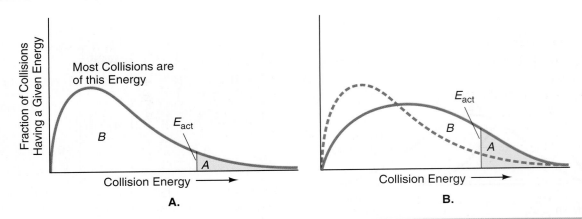

Figure 24-18   *(A) Distribution of energies at a given temperature. (B) Distribution of energies at a higher temperature.*

Source: Delmar/Cengage Learning

Another factor that may affect the rate of reaction is concentration. This is due to the fact that we have more molecules that will bump into each other and increase the possibility of them having the proper orientation. It only makes sense that an increase in the number of molecules will increase the incidence of effective collisions. The increase in reaction rate depends on the type of reaction taking place. Thus, while it does not hold true for *every* reaction, it is generally true that increasing concentration will increase rate of reaction.

The last factor that affects the rate of a reaction is the presence of catalysts. A *catalyst* is a substance that increases the rate of a reaction without being consumed. The effects of catalysts can be very dramatic. In some cases, catalysts increase rates of reactions by as much as 1 million times. Catalysts work by lowering the activation energy. As a result, more molecules possess energy greater than the activation energy and the rate of reaction thereby increases.

In summary, then, the three factors that affect the rate of reaction are temperature, concentration, and catalysts. These factors affect the reaction rate by affecting the energy of the reacting molecules, by increasing the number of effective collisions, and by lowering the activation energy, respectively.

At the other extreme is a condition called **hypothermia**, meaning lower-than-normal body temperature. Exposure to cold is the usual cause of hypothermia. This does not necessarily mean extremely low temperatures, however. For instance, a person who falls into a river or stream on a

Stop and Review 24-6

a. Why does increasing the temperature increase the rate of a reaction?

b. What is the rule of thumb for rates of reactions when the temperature is raised 10°C ?

cool spring day and neglects to change from the resulting wet clothing can develop hypothermia. Likewise, a person who drinks alcoholic beverages outdoors on a cold day can develop hypothermia because the alcohol acts as a **vasodilator**. In other words, the alcohol dilates the blood vessels of the vascular system, resulting in excessive heat loss from the body. Symptoms of hypothermia are weakness, confusion, lack of coordination, and irregular heartbeat. These symptoms are understandable when you apply your knowledge of reaction rate. Each of these symptoms is related to conduction of nerve signals. The conduction of nerve signals involves chemical reactions. At lower temperatures, the rates of these reactions will be slower. Thus, we would expect the person's strength, coordination, and heartbeat to be affected. Treatment for hypothermia centers on preventing further heat loss. This is accomplished by wrapping the person in blankets and allowing a spontaneous, slow rewarming to occur.

Clinical Relevancy

Body Temperature and Rate of Reaction

What does rate of reaction have to do with the human body? Reaction rates are linked to numerous body processes. For example, without the increase in reaction rate caused by the catalysts known as our digestive enzymes, it would take each of us 50 years to digest a single meal!

As another example, consider body temperature. Most people think of fever as being a bad thing. Some researchers, however, believe that a person with a moderate fever (lower than 101°F, or 38.3°C) should not be given antipyretics. Antipyretics are substances that reduce fevers (such as acetaminophen and aspirin). The reasoning behind this belief is that fighting disease involves chemical reactions and that increased temperature increases the rate of these reactions. It is important to note, however, that a high fever can be fatal and should be treated.

Normal body temperature is considered to be 37.0°C (98.6°F). Variations of only a few degrees Celsius from the normal can have serious consequences. **Hyperpyrexia** is the term used to define a condition of higher-than-normal body temperature, as in the case of heatstroke. Heatstroke can result from a combination of prolonged exposure to high temperatures and strenuous exercise. A decrease or cessation of sweating may precede an attack of heatstroke by several hours. Body temperature rises rapidly to between 40.6°C (105°F) and 41.1°C (106°F). A body temperature this high requires immediate attention. Treatment for this condition may include lukewarm baths to help lower body temperature. Rectal temperature should not be allowed to fall below 38.3°C (101°F), however.

■ CHAPTER REVIEW

Exercises

1. What is the movement of a gas from an area of high concentration of that gas to an area of low concentration of that gas called?

2. Why is the air pressure at the top of Pike's Peak lower than at sea level?

3. Define each of the following abbreviations.

   a. STPD   c. ATPS

   b. BTPS

4. What is the difference between relative humidity and absolute humidity?

5. How much pressure is exerted in your lungs by the oxygen that you are breathing in now (assuming that the barometric pressure is 747 mm Hg)?

6. If water vapor pressure is 47 mm Hg at 37 degrees Celsius, what is the relative humidity?

7. Which gas law states that each gas in a gas mixture exerts a pressure equal to its fractional concentration?

8. A sealed container holds a gas that exerts a pressure of 20 pounds per square inch at 20 degrees Celsius. If we heat this container to 40 degrees Celsius, what pressure will this gas exert?

9. If 100 mL of helium gas is collected at 20 degrees Celsius, what will the volume of that gas be if the gas is warmed to 40 degrees Celsius?

10. Write a formula representing Charles' law.

11. If a set volume of a gas occupies 250 mL on a day when the barometric pressure is 720 mm Hg, what volume will that same gas occupy when the barometric pressure rises to 750 mm Hg?

12. What is the measure of the average kinetic energy of a substance called?

13. According to the collision theory, what two criteria must be met in order for a reaction to occur?

14. What is the minimum energy needed for a reaction to occur called?

15. What effect will a 10°C increase in temperature have on the rate of reaction?

16. What is a substance that increases the rate of reaction without being consumed called?

17. What are catalysts that are found in the body called?

18. What is the general name for substances that reduce fever?

19. Does hyperpyrexia describe a body temperature that is above or below normal?

20. What is the name of the condition characterized by lower-than-normal body temperature?

21. Why shouldn't you give alcohol to a victim of hypothermia?

Real Life Issues and Applications

Temperature and Medical Gas Cylinders

Your department is in charge of maintaining the inventory of oxygen tanks used in patient transport. These oxygen cylinders are stored outside in a protective cage. During a severe cold spell this past winter, several of these tanks were brought inside for patient use. When the pressure gauges were put on the tanks, the gauges showed that the tanks were only one-half full. As a result, the oxygen company was called and told to bring a new supply of tanks because the shipment they had previously sent had, apparently, been incorrectly filled. One tank left over from the "defective" shipment sat in your department for 3 hours. At the end of this 3-hour period, you looked at the pressure gauge, and it showed that the tank was full. A somewhat agitated employee from the oxygen company subsequently called to tell you that when the "defective" tanks were tested, they were at maximum service pressure. What happened?

Additional Activities

1. Give each member of your class five balloons. Working either in teams or as individuals, use the balloons to explain three of the gas laws discussed in this chapter.

2. Invite a respiratory therapist to class to discuss the relevancy of gas laws to his or her professional practice.

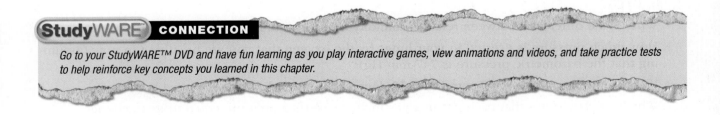

StudyWARE CONNECTION

Go to your StudyWARE™ DVD and have fun learning as you play interactive games, view animations and videos, and take practice tests to help reinforce key concepts you learned in this chapter.

Workbook Practice   *Go to your Workbook for more practice questions and activities.*

CHAPTER 25

ACIDS AND BASES

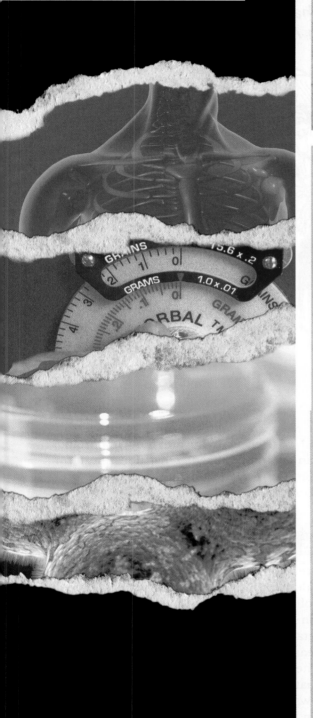

Objectives

Upon completion of this chapter, you should be able to

- List common properties of acids and bases

- Define the terms *acid*, *base*, *neutralization*, *buffer*, and *pH*

- Determine whether a solution is acidic or basic, given its pH

- Explain how the lungs and kidneys help maintain constant and proper blood pH

- Distinguish between acidosis and alkalosis

Key Terms

acid
acid-base indicators
acidosis
alkalosis
base
buffer solution

caustic
hydronium ion (H_3O^+)
neutralization
pH
salt

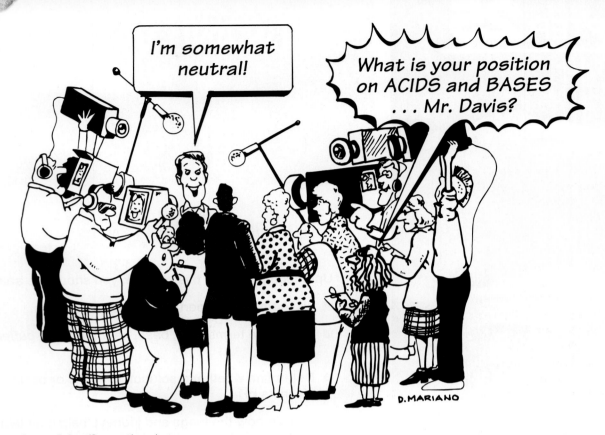

Source: Delmar/Cengage Learning

■ INTRODUCTION

We come into contact with many different **acids** and **bases** during our lifetimes. The gastric juice in our stomach contains hydrochloric acid. Lactic acid is produced when milk sours. Lactic acid is also produced in our bodies when we exercise vigorously. The orange juice we drink contains citric acid; vinegar contains acetic acid; car batteries contain a sulfuric acid electrolyte solution; and our bodies contain several acids that assist in body functioning—assuming, that is, that the acids remain in the proper range of concentration.

Bases are substances that combat acidity. Antacids (*ante* meaning "against") contain basic substances, such as calcium carbonate or sodium bicarbonate, that help reduce the acidity of (i.e., neutralize) a solution. Over-the-counter antacids are used quite heavily in our society to combat oversecretion of stomach acid, which can lead to a breakdown of the stomach lining, commonly known as ulcers. Much of this oversecretion is due to stress, which makes you wonder why we don't concentrate more of our efforts on discovering methods to cope with and alleviate excessive stress—but that is another story.

Just what are these substances that we call acids and bases, and why are they important? How is an acid neutralized? What does the term **pH** mean? The answers to these questions will soon become clear.

Acids, Bases, and Neutralization

The process of the oxygenation of hemoglobin is dependent on the acid concentration in blood. Uncontrolled diabetes can lead to an increase of acid in the blood. Respiratory problems and some metabolic problems can lead to an increase or decrease in the acid concentration in the blood. These are just a few of the health-related issues that involve acids and bases. Hopefully, this shows how important studying acids and bases can be.

Acids

By definition, an *acid* is a proton donor, the symbol for a proton being the hydrogen ion, H^+. Hydrogen has an atomic number of 1, meaning that each hydrogen atom has one proton and one electron. If the electron is removed, the atom changes to an ion with a net charge of +1. Thus, when a citric acid molecule (found in citrus juice) or an acetic acid molecule (found in vinegar) is present in water, the molecules of the acid give off protons to the water molecules and form **hydronium ions, H_3O^+**.

When hydrogen chloride gas dissolves in water, it acts as an acid. The equation for hydrogen chloride gas dissolving in water, for example, is as follows:

$$\textbf{H}Cl + H_2O \Leftrightarrow \textbf{H}_3O^+ + Cl^- \text{ hydronium ion}$$

In this equation, the hydrogen chloride acts as an acid by giving up a proton (H^+) to the water, thereby forming the hydronium ion. The bold symbol for hydrogen (**H**) shows the pathway the proton takes from the hydrogen chloride to the hydronium ion. An older definition of acids defines them as substances that produce hydronium ions in solution. In essence, then, the more hydrogen ions floating free in a solution, the more acidic the substance.

> **QUOTES & NOTES**
>
> **H**ydrochloric acid is the acid present in the stomach. The term acid *is derived from the Latin word meaning "sour."*

Properties of Acids

If you have ever tasted vinegar, a lemon, or a lime, you are aware of one of the properties of acids. Dilute solutions of acids taste sour. This is one reason that carbonic acid (H_2CO_3) and sometimes phosphoric acid is added to soda. There is a large amount of sugar in soda, and to counteract this sweet taste, manufacturers add acids. The next time you drink a can of soda, read the list of ingredients and see what acids are present in your soda. You will probably not find carbonic acid listed as such because carbonic acid is made by dissolving carbon dioxide (CO_2) in water. Another name manufacturers typically use for carbonic acid is carbonated water.

Another important property of acids is that they affect indicators. **Acid-base indicators** are chemicals that change colors in the presence of acids and bases. One such indicator is litmus. The chemical litmus is dissolved in a water solution and paper is soaked in the solution. The resulting litmus paper can be used to distinguish

acids and bases by placing a drop of the solution on the paper. If the solution is acid, the paper will turn red, and if it is basic, the solution will turn blue.

Figure 25-1 shows another property of acids. Certain metals in an acid solution will dissolve. This is a photo of magnesium dissolving in an acid solution. The equation for this reaction is

$$Mg + 2HCl \rightarrow MgCl_2 + H_2$$

Bases

In order to regulate a solution to the desired homeostatic level, there must be a counterpart mechanism to balance the production of acid. Alkalinity is the opposite of acidity and is measured by how basic the solution becomes.

Bases act as proton acceptors. The most common base is the hydroxide ion, OH^-. Bases can be defined as substances that produce hydroxide ions in solution. In a neutral solution such as pure water, you will find both hydrogen ions and hydroxide ions in very small but equal amounts (see Figure 25-2). In an acid solution, the hydrogen ion concentration is greater than the hydroxide ion concentration. In a basic solution, there are more hydroxide ions than hydrogen ions (see Figure 25-3). As illustrated in Figure 25-3, the balance of these two ions determines the level of acidity or alkalinity. The body must have some way of bringing a solution that is too acidic or too basic back to the desired homeostatic state—of neutralizing the effects of a solution that is out of balance.

Properties of Bases

Dilute solutions of bases are bitter tasting. This taste can sometimes be noticed when taking antacids, although sometimes the bitter taste is counteracted by the presence of sugar and flavoring such as mint.

Solutions of strong bases are **caustic**. Caustic compounds are substances that will dissolve human tissue. They will dissolve things such as wool, flesh, and hair. Bases such as sodium hydroxide (NaOH) are used as drain cleaners because of this property. Two substances that will generally cause a drain to become blocked are hair and fats from cooking. Using sodium hydroxide will clear both substances from the drain. First, sodium hydroxide reacts with fats to make soap, which will dissolve in water. We will discuss this reaction in more detail later. This reaction leads to another property of bases.

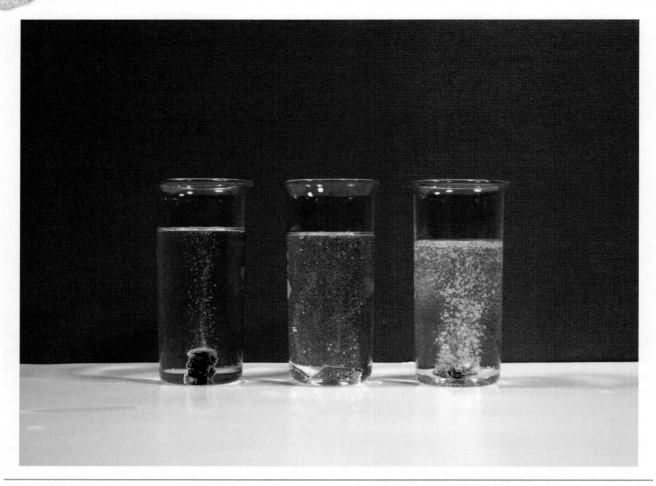

Figure 25-1   *When magnesium metal dissolves in an acid, hydrogen gas (H_2) is produced.*
Source: Spencer, L., & Slabaugh, Michael R., *Chemistry for Today,* GOB, 6e, Brooks/Cole, Cengage Learning

Neutral Solution

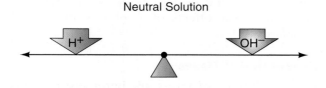

Figure 25-2   *In a neutral solution, the number of hydrogen ions and the number of hydroxide ions are equal.*
Source: Delmar/Cengage Learning

When we place a basic solution on our fingers, the bases react with the fats on our skin to form soap, and this makes the solution feel slippery. Second, the sodium hydroxide dissolves any hair that may be clogging the drain.

Neutralization

Neutralization is a property common to both acids and bases. In **neutralization**, the hydronium ion gives up its proton to a hydroxide ion and forms water. As mentioned earlier, pure water is a neutral substance; that is, it contains equal numbers of hydronium ions and hydroxide ions. An example of neutralization is the reaction of hydrochloric acid (a strong acid), HCl, and sodium hydroxide (a strong base), NaOH. The equation for this reaction is as follows:

$$HCl + NaOH \rightarrow NaCl + H_2O$$

To get the proper results, exact amounts of acid and base must be mixed—that is, one molecule of acid for every molecule of base. When these conditions are met, a **salt** (NaCl) and water are formed. A *salt* is an ionic substance formed from the positive ion of a base and the negative ion of an acid. Because sodium chloride is neither acidic nor basic and water contributes equal amounts of hydronium ions and hydroxide ions, a neutral solution results from mixing equal amounts of a strong acid and a strong base.

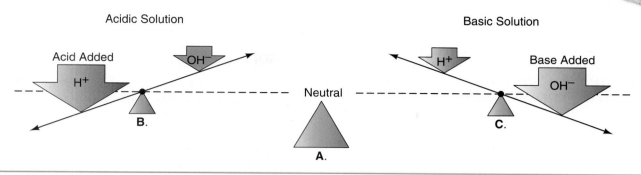

Acidic Solution

Basic Solution

Acid Added

OH⁻

H⁺

Neutral

H⁺

Base Added

OH⁻

B.

C.

A.

Figure 25-3 *The relationship between hydrogen ions and hydroxide ions in (A) a neutral solution, (B) an acid solution, and (C) a basic solution.*
Source: Delmar/Cengage Learning

Hydrochloric acid is found in the stomach. Under certain conditions, this acid is overproduced, resulting in heartburn or, in severe cases, an ulcer. Antacids neutralize excess acid in the stomach. Table 25-1 lists the bases present in some common antacids.

The neutralization reaction for an antacid that uses calcium carbonate is as follows:

$$CaCO_3 + 2HCl \rightarrow CaCl_2 + H_2CO_3$$

The calcium carbonate reacts with the acid and forms calcium chloride. The hydrogen ions (in boldface) from the acid combine with the carbonate to form carbonic acid (H_2CO_3). The carbonic acid is unstable and breaks down to water and carbon dioxide gas, as shown in the following equation:

$$H_2CO_3 \rightarrow H_2O + CO_2$$

Thus, the hydrogen ions from the acid become part of the water molecule. Given that water is a neutral solution, the calcium carbonate has effectively neutralized the hydrochloric acid.

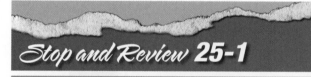

Stop and Review **25-1**

a. A solution is tested with litmus paper and the paper turns red. Is the solution an acid or a base?

b. What is a base? List three properties of a base and write the names of two common bases.

c. What is an acid? List three properties of acids and write the names of two common acids.

Expressing Acid-Base Concentration

When chemists talk about acid-base concentration, they refer to the pH of the solution. In the following section, we will discuss the strengths of acids and the concept of pH.

TABLE 25-1 Bases Present in Common Antacids	
ANTACID	**BASE(s)**
Amphojel	$Al(OH)_3$
Milk of Magnesia	$Mg(OH)_2$
Mylanta-II	$Mg(OH)_2$, $Al(OH)_3$
Maalox	$Mg(OH)_2$, $Al(OH)_3$
Di Gel	$Mg(OH)_2$, $Al(OH)_3$
Gelusil M	$Mg(OH)_2$, $Al(OH)_3$
Riopan	$Mg(OH)_2$, $Al(OH)_3$
Bisodol	$CaCO_3$, $Mg(OH)_2$
Titralac	$CaCO_3$
Pepto-Bismol	$CaCO_3$
Tums	$CaCO_3$
Alka-Seltzer	$NaHCO_3$, $KHCO_3$

Strengths of Acids

The strength of an acid is related to the degree of ionization; the more free-floating hydrogen ions (H^+) in a solution, the more hydronium ions (H_3O^+) that will be formed. Strong acids are nearly 100% ionized. Examples of strong acids include hydrochloric acid and sulfuric acid. In a solution of hydrochloric acid, nearly all the HCl molecules will ionize—that is, they will eventually take the form of H_3O^+ and Cl^-.

In a solution of a weak acid such as acetic acid, however, only about 0.5% of the molecules will produce hydrogen ions. Thus, of 1,000 acetic acid molecules in solution, 995 would be in molecular form and only 5 would be in ionic form, as shown in the following equation:

$$HC_2H_3O_2 + H_2O \rightarrow H_3O^+ + C_2H_3O_2^-$$

995 molecules   5 ions   5 ions

The Measure of pH

You have likely heard the term *pH* used with respect to shampoos and soaps. The pH, which stands for the "potential of Hydrogen," is an expression of a solution's hydronium ion (H_3O^+) concentration. The pH therefore tells us the degree to which a solution is acidic (many hydronium ions) or basic (few hydronium ions).

The actual formula for determining pH is as follows:

$$pH = -\log[H_3O^+]$$

Although we will not calculate pH, it is important that you understand this equation. Because of the negative sign, as the hydronium ion concentration increases, the pH decreases. This can be confusing initially, but it is important to keep in mind. By substituting any numerical value for the $[H_3O^+]$, you prove that as the concentration goes up, the numerical value goes down. For example, an arbitrarily chosen initial value of 3 becomes −3 (disregarding the log function) in the equation to determine pH. If more hydronium ions were added and the value increased to 9, this would become −9, which is clearly less than −3. As mathematically illustrated by this example, then, as the concentration of hydronium ions goes up, the pH goes down, and vice versa. This is illustrated in Figure 25-4.

Earlier, we stated that a neutral solution has equal concentrations of hydronium and hydroxide ions. Pure water would be a neutral solution. The pH of a neutral solution such as pure water is 7; this solution is neither acidic nor basic. Solutions with a pH of less than 7 are considered acidic. In an acidic solution, there are more hydronium ions than hydroxide ions. Basic solutions have a pH greater than 7. In a basic solution, there are more hydroxide ions than hydronium ions. Table 25-2 lists the pHs of some common substances.

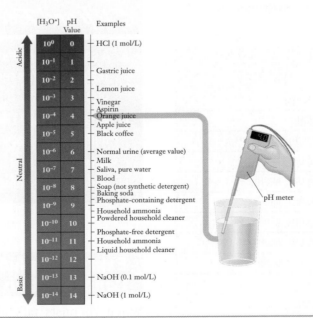

Figure 25-4   *The relationship between hydronium ion concentration, hydroxide ion concentration, and pH.*

Source: Armold, Melvin T., *Essentials of General, Organic, and Biochemistry*, 1e, Brooks/Cole, Cengage Learning

TABLE 25-2
pHs of Some Common Substances

SOLUTION	pH
1.0 M HCl	0
Gastric juice	1.6
Lemon juice	2.2
Vinegar	2.8
Carbonated beverages	3.0
Coffee	5.0
Urine	6.0
Rainwater	6.2
Water (pure)	7.0
Blood	7.4
Bile	8.0
Detergents	8.0–9.0
Milk of magnesia	10.5
Ammonia	11.0
Bleach	12.0
1.0 M NaOH	14.0

Stop and Review 25-2

a. Examine each of the following solution pHs and determine whether each solution is acidic, basic, or neutral.

   1. pH = 7.00

   2. pH = 8.65

   3. pH = 2.91

b In a solution of pure water, the concentrations of hydronium ions and hydroxide ions are

   _____.

c. A solution contains a higher concentration of hydroxide ions than hydronium ions. This solution is _____.

d. A solution contains a higher concentration of hydronium ions than hydroxide ions. This solution is _____.

Maintaining Constant and Proper Blood pH

As we mentioned earlier, the process of oxygenation of hemoglobin is pH dependent. It is important that the blood pH be maintained at the proper level for this process to occur. One way the body maintains the proper pH of the blood is by the use of buffers. This is discussed in the following sections.

The pH of Blood

The pH level of the body must be maintained within a very narrow range. A pH level outside of this range would cause cellular and tissue disruption that would lead to death. Acceptable pH ranges vary throughout the body. Stomach pH, for example, is normally low (i.e., very acidic) to facilitate proper digestion of food. The average pH value of blood, on the other hand, is 7.4, which is slightly alkaline, or basic. As noted in the math section, however, it is important to remember that *average* means there are some values above and below the given point. There exists, then, a clinically acceptable range of values for blood pH; even patients who have normal acid-base levels may have blood pH values slightly above or below the average value of 7.4.

The normal range of acceptability for blood pH is 7.35–7.45. If blood pH falls below 6.8 or rises above 7.8, life is normally not possible. Variations outside of the acceptable range but not life threatening require prompt attention, nonetheless. When blood pH falls below 7.35, the condition is labeled **acidosis** (osis meaning "condition of"). Although the condition is called acidosis, you should note that the pH is greater than 7; hence, the solution is basic. The term *acidosis* in this case means that the solution is more acid than is normal. A blood pH above 7.45 is referred to as **alkalosis**. The ways whereby the body maintains proper blood pH are described in the following discussion.

QUOTES & NOTES

Small changes in the concentration of acids can turn enzymes either on or off.

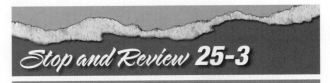

Stop and Review 25-3

a. What is acidosis?

b. What is alkalosis?

Buffer Solutions

It should now be evident that it is important to maintain blood pH within narrow limits. How does the body do this? Substances in the blood act as buffers to help maintain the pH within a narrow range. **Buffer solutions** have the ability to neutralize acids and bases within certain limits, thereby maintaining a constant pH. Another way to think of buffers is that they attempt to prevent extreme changes in pH.

The main buffer in the blood is the *carbonate buffer system* which consists of H_2CO_3 (carbonic acid) and HCO_3^- (bicarbonate). These two substances arise from the presence of carbon dioxide (CO_2) in the body. The following equation illustrates how CO_2 and H_2O react:

$$CO_2 + H_2O \Leftrightarrow H_2CO_3 \Leftrightarrow H^+ + HCO_3^-$$

The double arrow, $\Leftrightarrow$, means that the reactions can go in either direction. They are reversible. The direction is determined by the concentrations of the substances in the equation. The body is constantly producing CO_2 via metabolism. This

CO_2 dissolves in the blood. As shown in the preceding equation, this produces more hydrogen ions, which can then combine to form hydronium ions (H_3O^+). These hydronium ions cause excess acidity.

When there is an excess of H_3O^+, it will react with the HCO_3^-, as shown in the following equation:

$$HCO_3^- + H_3O^+ \rightarrow H_2CO_3 + H_2O$$

Thus, any excess hydrogen ions are removed by the bicarbonate ion. An excess of hydroxide ions will react with carbonic acid in the following manner:

$$H_2CO_3 + OH^- \rightarrow H_2O + HCO_3^-$$

Thus, HCO_3^- and H_2CO_3 in the blood will react with small amounts of either hydronium or hydroxide ions to help keep blood pH within normal range.

It is important to note that carbonic acid is unstable, and when its concentration increases, it decomposes, as shown in the following equation where (aq) stands for aqueous or watery solution:

$$H_2CO_{3(aq)} \rightarrow H_2O + CO_{2(aq)}$$

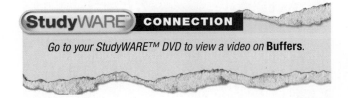

StudyWARE CONNECTION

*Go to your StudyWARE™ DVD to view a video on **Buffers**.*

Special Focus

The pH of Soaps and Shampoos

Elsewhere in this chapter we made reference to the pH of soaps and shampoos. Some of these products are labeled "pH balanced." But what does this mean, and is it significant?

The pH of the skin is approximately 5, which is, of course, acidic. The acidic nature of the skin lends the skin antibacterial (*anti* meaning "against") properties, which help the skin ward off infection.

This is very important because the skin is the first line of defense of the body.

Most commercially prepared soaps are alkaline; these soaps, therefore, will neutralize the acid on the skin. A pH-balanced soap, on the other hand, has a pH closer to that of the skin. Using these soaps will therefore help maintain the acidic nature of the skin and, thus, help inhibit the growth of bacteria.

The Role of the Lungs in Maintaining Blood pH

When blood passes through the lungs, the pCO_2 (concentration of CO_2) in the blood is greater than the pCO_2 in the alveoli; thus, the CO_2 passes from the blood, into the alveoli, and out of the body (see Figure 25-5). This process causes the following reaction:

$$CO_{2(aq)} \rightarrow CO_{2(g)}$$

in blood   in lungs

The "(g)" in this equation indicates that the CO_2 is in the gaseous state. Remember that the "(aq)" symbol indicates that these substances are in aqueous solution—that is, they are dissolved in water. These two things show that the lungs are an important part of the system to maintain a constant blood pH. The following equation puts these concepts together.

$$\mathbf{H^+}_{(aq)} + HCO_{3\ (aq)}^- \Leftrightarrow \mathbf{H}-HCO_{3(aq)} \Leftrightarrow CO_{2(aq)} + \mathbf{H}-OH$$

Lungs move equation in this direction →

← kidneys move equation in this direction

The double arrows in this equation represent reversible reactions. The single arrows represent the favored direction of the reaction in the lungs and in the kidneys. The hydrogen ion is indicated by boldface. Hydrogen ions in the blood react with the bicarbonate (buffer) to form carbonic acid. As noted earlier, when the carbonic acid concentration becomes high, the carbonic acid decomposes to yield CO_2 and H_2O.

In the lungs, the reaction unfolds from left to right as indicated in the preceding equation. Here, the volatile (changeable from dissolved form in the blood to gaseous form) CO_2 leaves the blood to be exhaled from the body. The lungs can therefore remove excess H^+ from the body by reacting with the bicarbonate ion to form carbonic acid, which then dissociates into H_2O and CO_2. The volatile CO_2 is blown off by the lungs.

The Role of the Brain in Maintaining Blood pH

As noted previously, each reaction is reversible. This enables the body to use these reactions to keep the hydrogen ion concentration constant. If the hydrogen ion concentration becomes too high, the amount of CO_2 builds up in the blood. This is detected by the brain, which tells the lungs to increase the breathing rate or depth to get rid of the excess CO_2. For every CO_2 molecule expelled, one H^+ is removed from the blood. In the opposite case, if the hydrogen ion concentration is too low, the CO_2 concentration will also be low. The body then decreases either the rate or depth of breathing to

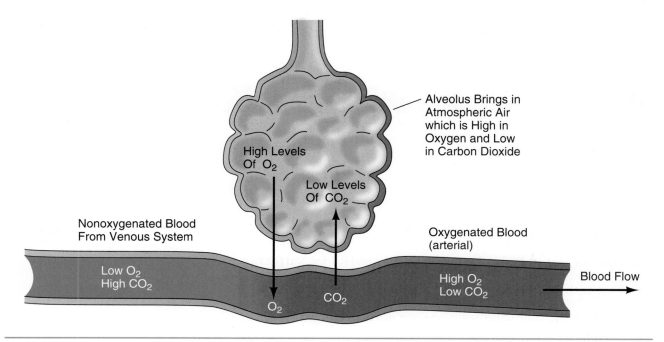

Figure 25-5 *Illustration of O_2 and CO_2 exchange across the alveolar capillary membrane.*
Source: Delmar/Cengage Learning

Clinical Relevancy

Lactic Acidosis

The limits of physical endurance are imposed on us by the chemistry of the body. A person who is physically fit has an efficient oxygen distribution system, meaning that the heart and lungs do a good job of getting oxygen to the cells. A person who is not very physically fit does not have as good a distribution system, however. When people of this description exert themselves, their muscle cells soon run out of oxygen and must break down glucose without oxygen. This is called *anaerobic metabolism.*

While this process supplies needed fuel, it does so in an inefficient manner that results in a buildup of lactic acid. The muscle pain and cramping associated with overexertion is caused by lactic acid. If exercise is continued, the amount of lactic acid in the blood will increase to the point of exceeding the buffer capacity. This will result in *lactic acid acidosis.* If the acidosis becomes severe enough, it can cause a person to collapse. This is the body's way of saying, "Stop! The supply of oxygen is not meeting the demand!"

retain CO_2. This reverses the previously mentioned reactions, resulting in an increase in H^+. Thus, the brain regulates H^+ concentration by increasing or decreasing breathing rate and depth.

The Role of the Kidneys in Maintaining Blood pH

The kidneys also have a role in maintaining acid-base balance in the blood. Their main purpose is to maintain the proper amounts of base, HCO_3^-, in the blood. The kidneys accomplish this task by making or excreting HCO_3^-. From the previous equation (now going in the reverse direction to the way it was written), you can see that as CO_2 levels increase in the blood, the kidneys turn more of the carbonic acid into hydrogen ions (H^+) and bicarbonate ions (HCO_3^-). The kidneys then secrete more H^+ ions via the urine to rid the body of the excess acid and at the same time retain (by reabsorbing back into the bloodstream) the bicarbonate ions to help buffer the excess acid in the blood.

■ CHAPTER REVIEW

Exercises

1. What is a proton donor called?

2. List three common acids.

3. Define the term *neutralization.*

4. Write the equation for the neutralization of HCl by $NaHCO_3$.

5. What is the difference between a strong acid and a weak acid?

6. Which of the following solutions are acidic? Which are basic?

   a. baking soda, pH = 8.8

   b. gastric juice, pH = 1.9

   c. soda, pH = 3.5

   d. blood, pH = 7.4

7. Blood work is performed on a blood sample taken from a patient in the emergency room. If the pH of the sample is 7.21, is the person suffering from alkalosis or acidosis?

8. A person who took an overdose of bicarbonate is found to have a blood pH of 7.68. Is this person suffering from acidosis or alkalosis?

9. What is a solution that maintains a constant pH called?

10. What is the name of the main buffer system in the blood?

11. What does carbonic acid yield when it decomposes?

12. How many hydrogen ions are removed from the blood for every CO_2 molecule exhaled?

13. The body can adjust blood pH by exhaling or retaining what substance?

Real Life Issues and Applications

Patients with Acidic Conditions

A patient has a high acid level in the metabolic system (i.e., kidneys). How will the respiratory system attempt to neutralize the acid? What type of medication can be given intravenously to this patient to help combat this situation? If this same patient also has very low levels of oxygen in the blood, how will this contribute to the acidosis? What treatment would you recommend?

Additional Activities

1. The muscle pain associated with exercising is caused by lactic acid in the muscles. The lactic acid is eventually chemically broken down by the body. Think back to the discussion of reaction rates. Why is applying a warm compress or taking a hot bath a good way to relieve pain? Investigate some ways to prevent lactic acid from accumulating in the body.

2. As a class, break down into teams. Research one of the following topics, as assigned by your instructor. Report your findings to the class. Good sources of information include the *Merck Manual*, *The Physicians' Desk Reference*, and *The Physicians' Desk Reference for Nonprescription Drugs*.

   a. How do some antacids inhibit the antibiotic tetracycline?

   b. What are some advantages, disadvantages, and cautions that should be followed when using the following antacids?

   - Amphojel
   - Maalox tablets
   - Tums
   - Alka Seltzer

   c. What are some common basic (alkali) compounds found around the home? Which of these substances could be used by a trained individual to neutralize a caustic alkali?

StudyWARE™ **CONNECTION**

Go to your StudyWARE™ DVD and have fun learning as you play interactive games, view animations and videos, and take practice tests to help reinforce key concepts you learned in this chapter.

Workbook Practice   *Go to your Workbook for more practice questions and activities.*

CHAPTER 26

BIOCHEMISTRY

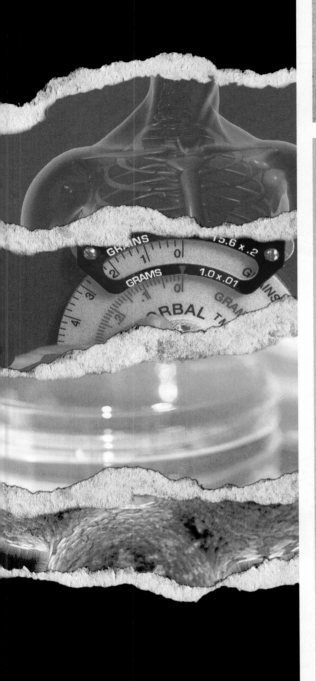

Objectives

Upon completion of this chapter, you should be able to

- Define the term *isomer*

- Discuss the differences between organic compounds and inorganic compounds

- Explain the difference between saturated hydrocarbons and unsaturated hydrocarbons

- State the differences in structure between glucose, galactose, and fructose

- Define the terms *monosaccharide*, *disaccharide*, and *polysaccharide*

- Explain how excess glucose is stored in the body

- Distinguish between saturated fats and unsaturated fats

- Explain the difference between saponifiable lipids and nonsaponifiable lipids

- Name two ways that the body uses cholesterol

Key Terms

alkane
alkene
alkynes
amylopectin
amylose (**AM**-eh-lace)
cellulose
disaccharide (dye-**SACK**-eh-ride)

fats
glucosuria (GLOO-koh-SEW-ree-uh)
glycogen
hydrocarbons
hyperglycemia
hypoglycemia

(continues)

isomers
lipids
monosaccharide

oils
polysaccharide
renal threshold

saturated fatty acids
unsaturated fatty acids

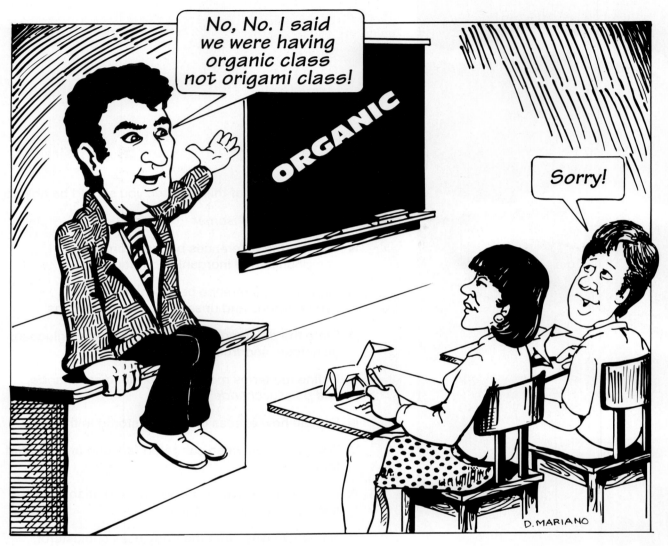

Source: Delmar/Cengage Learning

■ INTRODUCTION

While chemistry and chemical reactions are constantly occurring in our world, the special chemistry that occurs in the human body is called *biochemistry*. Before beginning our discussion of biochemistry, it is important that you first understand the basics of organic chemistry, or the study of the compounds of carbon. All life is based on carbon and its special properties. Carbon is unique among the elements in that carbon atoms can form covalent bonds between themselves to a greater extent than can the atoms of any other element. This yields a wide variety of

organic compounds. In addition, long chains of carbon atoms can be arranged in a variety of configurations, making it possible for organic compounds to have the same molecular formulas or components but different structures. The structure determines the properties of the compound.

Biochemistry is an application of organic chemistry to living systems. In this Biochemistry section, we are going to study the major compounds of living systems, carbohydrates (sugars) and lipids (fats and oils). Carbohydrates and lipids are used for energy in the body. In the next chapter we will devote the entire chapter to a discussion of proteins.

The Chemistry of Life

The structure of organic compounds determines the physical and chemical properties of these compounds. Therefore, it is important to be able to express the formulas of organic compounds. An important concept in organic structure is isomers, which are discussed in the next section.

Isomers

Compounds having the same molecular formulas but different structural formulas are called **isomers**. An example of isomerism can be seen in the organic compounds ethyl alcohol and dimethyl ether (see Figure 26-1). While both substances share the same molecular formula, C_2H_6O, you need only consider the properties of these substances to realize the effects of their different structures. For instance, whereas ethyl alcohol is a liquid at room temperature, dimethyl ether is a gas; and whereas ethyl alcohol is soluble in water, dimethyl ether is only slightly soluble in water. This represents only a sampling of the different properties exhibited by these two substances. But this sampling shows that molecular formula is not very useful in organic chemistry. To distinguish between different organic compounds, you must examine the structure of the molecules that compose the compounds.

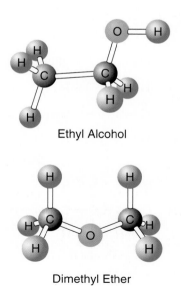

Ethyl Alcohol

Dimethyl Ether

Figure 26-1 *The isomers ethyl alcohol and dimethyl ether.*

Source: Delmar/Cengage Learning

QUOTES & NOTES

The term isomer *is derived from two Greek words:* iso *meaning "equal" and* meros *meaning "parts."*

Properties of Organic Compounds

The chemical and physical properties of organic compounds are very different from those of inorganic compounds. For one thing, most organic compounds are nonpolar and therefore do not dissolve in water, a polar substance. Thus, nonpolar solvents must be used when making solutions of organic compounds. In terms of chemical properties, organic compounds are more easily decomposed by heat than are inorganic compounds. For example, were you to heat sugar, it would decompose to carbon; were you to instead heat table salt, however, it would vaporize before having the chance to decompose. Finally, whereas most inorganic reactions occur instantaneously upon mixing, organic compounds react at a much slower rate. Some reactions involving organic compounds take many hours or even days to complete.

Hydrocarbons

The simplest of the organic compounds are the **hydrocarbons**. The molecules of hydrocarbons are composed of only carbon and hydrogen. Because hydrocarbons are the basic structures of all organic and biochemical compounds, we will begin with them.

Hydrocarbons can be classified into three basic groups: **alkanes**, **alkenes**, and **alkynes**. *Alkanes* are straight or branched-chain hydrocarbons wherein the carbon atoms are joined by single covalent bonds. Alkanes are sometimes referred to as *saturated hydrocarbons*, because they are saturated with respect to hydrogen atoms. The first five members of the alkane family and their structural formulas are shown in Figure 26-2. These structures are important foundations for some of the compounds we will be discussing later in this chapter.

You should note that it is sometimes easier to represent alkane molecules via their condensed structural formulas. For example, the condensed structural formula for ethane is CH_3CH_3, while the condensed structural formula for propane is $CH_3CH_2CH_3$ (see Figure 26-2). Comparing the condensed structural formula for propane to the

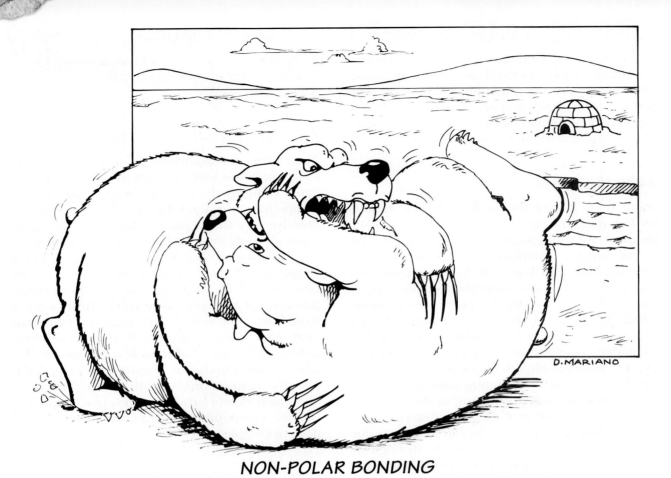

NON-POLAR BONDING

Source: Delmar/Cengage Learning

structural formula for propane in Figure 26-2, we can see that the number of hydrogen atoms that are attached to a carbon atom in the structural formula is written following that carbon, and written with an H H H subscript. For example, the structural formula for propane is

$$\begin{array}{ccc} H & H & H \\ | & | & | \\ H - C - C - C - H \\ | & | & | \\ H & H & H \end{array}$$

The first carbon has 3 hydrogen atoms attached. In the condensed structural formula, we write this as CH_3. The middle carbon has two hydrogen atoms attached and we write it as CH_2. The third carbon has three hydrogen atoms attached, like the first, and we write it as CH_3. Putting the three together gives the condensed structural formula of $CH_3CH_2CH_3$.

Alkenes are straight or branched-chain hydrocarbons wherein at least two of the carbon

Figure 26-2   *The first five members of the alkane family, with corresponding structural formulas. Each line in the structural formulas represents a pair of shared electrons.*

Source: Delmar/Cengage Learning

Name	Structure
Ethene	$CH_2\!=\!CH_2$
Propene	$CH_2\!=\!CHCH_3$
1-Butene	$CH_2\!=\!CHCH_2CH_3$
1-Pentene	$CH_2\!=\!CHCH_2CH_2CH_3$

Figure 26-3   *Some members of the alkene family, with corresponding structural formulas.*
Source: Delmar/Cengage Learning

atoms are joined by a double covalent bond. The alkenes are sometimes called *unsaturated hydrocarbons* because they have room for more hydrogen atoms in their molecules. Several members of the alkene family are shown in Figure 26-3.

Double lines in the structural formulas represent double covalent bonds. Hydrogen can be added to these molecules across the double bond. Doing so changes the alkene to an alkane—that is, it changes an unsaturated hydrocarbon into a saturated hydrocarbon. An equation for this reaction is as follows:

$$CH_2 = CH_2 + H_2 \rightarrow CH_3CH_3$$

This is how corn oil can be converted into solid shortening. We will further examine other organic reactions in our discussion of lipids.

Alkynes are straight or branched-chain hydrocarbons wherein at least two of the carbon atoms are joined by a triple covalent bond. Because alkynes are generally not found in living systems, we will not discuss them any further.

QUOTES & NOTES

*T*he fragrances of lemons, oranges, cloves, and peppermint are generated by unsaturated hydrocarbons.

Carbohydrates and Lipids

The body uses three types of food: carbohydrates, lipids, and proteins. The remainder of this chapter is devoted to examining the properties of carbohydrates and lipids.

Stop and Review 26-1

a. Classify each of the following compounds as being alkane or alkene.
   1. $CH_3CH_2CH_3$
   2. $CH_2 = CH_2$
   3. CH_3CHCH_2
      |
      CH_3
   4. $CH_3CH_2CH_2CH = CH_2$

b. How many carbon atoms are present in butane? Ethane?

c. Are the following formulas of organic or inorganic compounds?
   1. $CH_3CH_2CH_3$
   2. NaCl
   3. CH_4
   4. NaOH

d. What is meant by *saturated organic compound*?

e. Define the term *hydrocarbon* and list the three types of hydrocarbons.

Carbohydrates

While many people may not know them by their chemical names, nearly everyone is familiar with carbohydrates. Sugar, including table sugar (sucrose), glucose, and milk sugar (lactose), are a type of carbohydrate, as is starch, a **polysaccharide** found in potatoes and pasta.

The name *carbohydrate* is derived from the fact that the general formula for carbohydrates is $(CH_2O)n$. The carbohydrates are made up of carbon, hydrogen, and oxygen. The hydrogen and oxygen are found in the same ratio as in water. For example, glucose has the molecular formula $C_6H_{12}O_6$. This could be rewritten as $(CH_2O)_6$ where $n = 6$ in our general formula above. The presence of carbon in sugar can be shown using sulfuric acid. Sulfuric acid has a strong affinity for water and will pull the hydrogen atoms and oxygen atoms from the sugar to make water. The equation for the reaction is

$$H_2SO_4 + (CH_2O)n \rightarrow nC(s) + n(H_2O)g$$

Heat is produced in the reaction and the water is given off in the gaseous state (steam).

There are three broad classifications of carbohydrates: **monosaccharides**, **disaccharides**, and **polysaccharides**. Monosaccharides, the simplest of the sugars, consist of a single sugar molecule. Disaccharides consist of two sugar molecules bonded together. Polysaccharides consist of long chains of monosaccharide molecules, such as those of glucose, bonded together.

Monosaccharides

The most common and most important monosaccharide is *glucose*. The structure of the glucose molecule is shown in Figure 26-4. The presence of the polar —OH group in the molecule renders glucose very soluble in water. In nature, glucose is found in grapes and other fruits.

Because it is the most common carbohydrate in the blood, glucose is sometimes referred to as blood sugar. Glucose is the major source of energy in the cells of the body. Normal glucose concentration in the blood ranges from 70–100 mg/100 mL of blood. In the case of diabetes, the level is higher than normal. A higher-than-normal blood sugar level is called **hyperglycemia**. **Hypoglycemia** is the term used to describe a lower-than-normal blood sugar level. If blood sugar level becomes too high, the excess sugar is excreted by the kidneys via the urine. The presence of glucose in the urine is called **glucosuria**. The **renal threshold** for glucose is 140–160 mg/100 mL blood. Glucosuria will occur within this range or higher.

As shown in Figure 26-4, *galactose* is a monosaccharide similar to glucose. The only difference between glucose and galactose is the position of the —OH group on the fourth carbon. Although galactose does not frequently occur in nature as a monosaccharide, it is found in the disaccharide lactose.

The sweetest of all the sugars is *fructose*. As shown in Figure 26-4, fructose is similar in structure to glucose. The only difference between glucose and fructose is the position of the C = O (on the first carbon in glucose and on the second carbon in fructose). Fructose is found in many fruits and in honey.

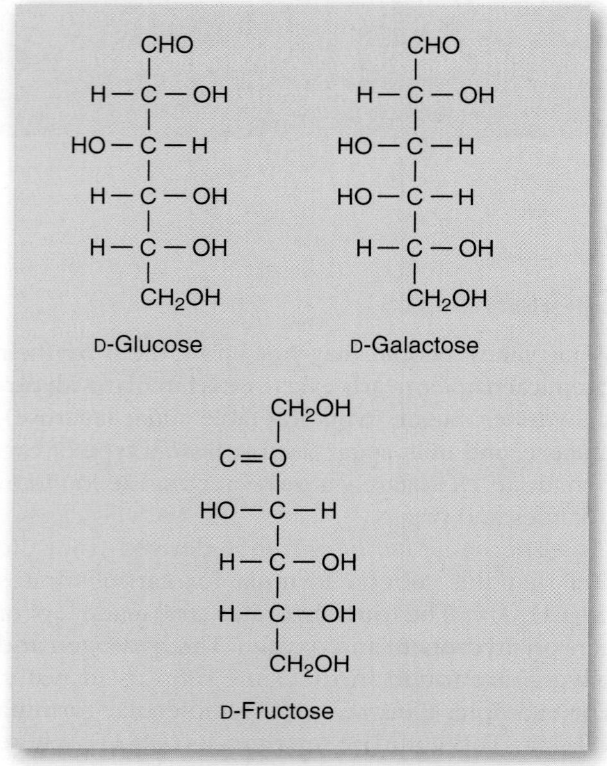

Figure 26-4 *Glucose, galactose, and fructose molecules.*
Source: Delmar/Cengage Learning

Disaccharides

Monosaccharides combine in various ways to create disaccharides. *Sucrose*, *lactose*, and *maltose* are the three nutritionally important disaccharides. The following word equations show the monosaccharides that create these disaccharides:

sucrose + water → glucose + fructose

lactose + water → glucose + galactose

maltose + water → 2 glucose

The reactions represented by these word equations in general are referred to as *hydrolysis reactions* (*hydro* meaning "water," *lysis* meaning "to break down"). Reactions of this type use water, as indicated in the preceding equations, to split a larger molecule into smaller molecules. Digestion of disaccharides in the body is an example of a hydrolysis reaction.

QUOTES & NOTES

The term saccharide is derived from the Latin word saccharum, *meaning "sugar."*
Honey does not spoil and is also antibacterial.
—From www.sciensational.com/chemistry-facts-pg3.htm

Clinical Relevancy

Donating Blood

Have you ever donated blood for a blood drive? Those of you who answered yes realize an important factor in this process is to determine your blood type. There are four different blood types designated by the letters A, B, AB, and O. The percentages of these blood types in the general population are approximately 43% O, 40% A, 12% B, and 5% AB. Whenever a person is given a transfusion, it is necessary to know the type of blood he or she is receiving because certain blood types are incompatible. This can be seen on Table 26-1 below.

Looking at Table 26-1, we can see that Type O blood is the universal donor. That is, Type O blood can be given to a person with any other blood type. On the other hand, Type AB is the universal recipient. That is, a person with Type AB can obtain blood from a person in any of the other blood groups.

The relevance of this topic to carbohydrates, monosaccharides in particular, is that one of the distinguishing features in the structures of the various blood types is the monosaccharide galactose. The different blood types have certain chemical compounds attached to the red blood cells. Some of the structures are complex, so we will just look at a block diagram of the different blood types. The diagram in Figure 26-5 shows the differences between the different structures attached to the red blood cells.

As can be seen in Figure 26-5, Type O contains a single galactose molecule attached indirectly to the red blood cell. Type A has a different structure attached to the galactose molecule. Type B contains two galactose molecules. There is no structure for Type AB blood because Type AB contains both A and B blood types.

TABLE 26-1
Compatibility of Blood Groups

	RECIPIENT BLOOD TYPES		
DONOR BLOOD TYPE	A	B	AB
A	+	−	+
B	−	+	+
AB	−	−	+
O	+	+	+

+ = compatible; − = incompatible

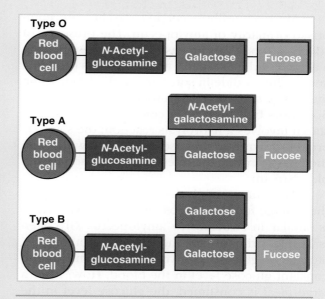

Figure 26-5 *Block diagrams for the structures of the different blood types.*

Source: Delmar/Cengage Learning

Polysaccharides

A polysaccharide is a large molecule composed of the same monosaccharide molecules linked together. Three polysaccharides are relevant to our discussion: *starch*, **glycogen**, and **cellulose**. These polysaccharides all contain glucose molecules as the building blocks. The only difference between starch, glycogen, and cellulose is the manner whereby the glucose molecules are linked together.

Plants use starch to store the excess glucose produced by photosynthesis. As shown in Figure 26-6, there are two kinds of starch found in nature: **amylose**, which has a linear structure, and **amylopectin**, which has a branched structure.

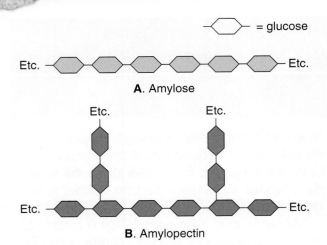

Figure 26-6 *Structures of (A) amylose and (B) amylopectin, the two types of starch found in nature.*
Source: Delmar/Cengage Learning

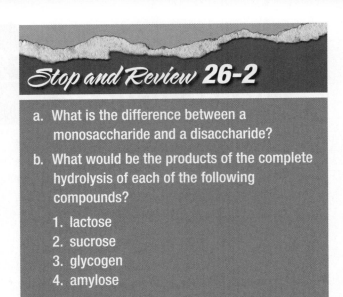

Stop and Review 26-2

a. What is the difference between a monosaccharide and a disaccharide?

b. What would be the products of the complete hydrolysis of each of the following compounds?

 1. lactose
 2. sucrose
 3. glycogen
 4. amylose

c. What is meant by the term *polysaccharide*?

Most naturally occurring starches are composed primarily of amylopectin. The presence of starch in foods can be easily detected by placing a drop of iodine reagent, which consists of iodine and sodium iodide in solution, on the food. When the iodine solution encounters a starch, the solution turns bluish-black in color. The digestion of starch involves a hydrolysis reaction; the starch is broken down into glucose molecules, which can then pass through the intestinal walls and into the bloodstream.

The human equivalent of starch is *glycogen*, the storage form of glucose in animals. Glycogen is similar in structure to amylopectin. Glycogen is stored primarily in the liver and in muscle. Storage of glucose as glycogen helps maintain a constant glucose level in the blood. How? After a large meal is consumed, the glucose level in the blood increases. Glucose not needed for energy is stored as glycogen, thus lowering the glucose level. After a period of fasting, the glucose level decreases. Glycogen is then broken down to glucose, which is released into the bloodstream.

Cellulose is the most abundant of the polysaccharides. The glucose molecules in cellulose are linked in a manner different from those in starch. This subtle difference renders cellulose undigestible by humans. Whereas cows, horses, and other such animals can break down the cellulose in plant fibers and, thus, use the cellulose as a source of energy, humans cannot. Despite its indigestibility, cellulose is nonetheless important for proper digestion. Cellulose is a major component of dietary fiber, which provides the bulk necessary to keep food moving through the digestive tract. Fiber can be thought of as "nature's broom."

Lipids

Lipids have a variety of functions in the body. They can be used to store energy or as a source of energy, and some lipids are used to make various hormones. The following discussion will introduce you to the basics of lipids.

Lipid Classification

Thus far in our discussion of biochemistry, we have used structure to identify compounds. Lipids, however, are classified according to solubility rather than structure. **Lipids** are plant or animal substances that are soluble in nonpolar solvents. Thus, if you were to place any plant or animal tissue in a nonpolar solvent, the lipid portion of the tissue would dissolve. Lipids can be subdivided into two classes of compounds: *saponifiable lipids* and *nonsaponifiable lipids*. Saponifiable lipids are *esters*, while nonsaponifiable are not. The term *ester* will be defined later in this chapter.

To understand saponifiable lipids, you must first understand the organic compounds called *carboxylic acids*. A very common carboxylic acid is the acid found in vinegar: acetic acid. The structure of acetic acid is as follows:

$$CH_3\overset{\displaystyle O}{\overset{\displaystyle \|}{C}}OH$$

Special Focus

Disaccharides

Sucrose is the substance we refer to as sugar, or table sugar. It is found naturally in sugar cane, sugar beets, and honey. Jams and jellies contain sucrose that is partially hydrolyzed to yield glucose and fructose. The presence of glucose and fructose makes jams and jellies sweeter than they would be if they contained only unhydrolyzed sucrose.

Maltose, also called *malt sugar*, is produced by germinating grain. Maltose is hydrolyzed by the enzyme *maltase* into two glucose molecules.

Lactose is found in cow's milk and human milk. In fact, it is sometimes referred to as *milk sugar*. Lactose is an important ingredient in commercially prepared infant formula. The souring of milk occurs when lactose is oxidized by bacteria to form lactic acid. People who lack the enzyme *lactase*, which breaks down lactose into glucose and galactose, are labeled as *lactose intolerant*. In these individuals, the undigested lactose molecules absorb water and cause a sensation of fullness in the intestine. Bacteria then act on the lactose, producing gas. This results in severe cramping and diarrhea. Milk treated with an enzyme that breaks down lactose can remedy the symptoms of lactose intolerance.

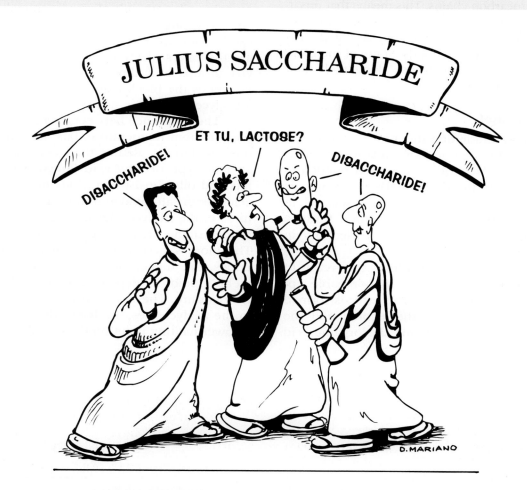

ET TU, LACTOSE?

Source: Delmar/Cengage Learning

The characteristic feature of all organic acids is the structure:

$$\begin{array}{c} O \\ \| \\ CH_3COH \end{array}$$

This is sometimes written as —COOH or —CO$_2$H.

The carboxylic acids present in lipids are called *fatty acids*. Fatty acids have four or more carbons in their hydrocarbon chains. The most common fatty acids have 16 or 18 carbons in their hydrocarbon chains. Earlier in the chapter we stated that hydrocarbons are not soluble in water. The long hydrocarbon chains on the fatty acids are what make these acids insoluble in water. Acids with shorter hydrocarbon chains, such as acetic acid, are water soluble, however.

Saturated fatty acids contain alkane hydrocarbon chains; **unsaturated fatty acids** contain alkene hydrocarbon chains. This means that unsaturated fatty acids contain one or more carbon-to-carbon double bonds, while the saturated fatty acids contain no double bonds. Some of the more common fatty acids are listed, along with their structures, in Table 26-2.

Organic Alcohol

Before further examining the structure of lipids, we must first discuss one more organic structure: *organic alcohol*. Alcohol has an —OH bonded to a hydrocarbon chain. (The —OH should not be confused with the hydroxide ion discussed in Chapter 25.) The condensed structural formula for a simple alcohol is CH$_3$CH$_2$OH. Alcohols do not ionize in water solution.

Organic acids and alcohols can react to form compounds called *esters*. Saponifiable lipids contain ester structures. The ester is formed by removing the H from the alcohol and the OH from the acid and linking the organic acid and alcohol together, as shown in the following equation:

$$\begin{array}{ccc} O & & O \\ \| & \rightarrow & \| \\ CH_3COH + HOCH_2CH_3 & & CH_3COCH_3 \end{array}$$

The ester structure is the basis of the saponifiable lipids. The simplest saponifiable lipids are the waxes that occur in nature. Beeswax, lanolin (a wax from wool), and the waxy coating on fruits are some examples of natural waxes. Because fatty acids do not dissolve in water, beeswax and lanolin can be used as water repellents. They contain a fatty acid linked to a long-chained alcohol having from 16 to 30 carbons. Figure 26-7 includes a diagram of a wax and lists some common waxes along with their corresponding structures, sources, and uses.

Fats and Oils

The substances that we call **fats** and **oils**, such as palm oil, corn oil, olive oil, animal fats, and lard, have slightly more complex structures than esters; they are referred to as *triglycerides*. They are the esters of glycerol, an alcohol with three OH groups and three fatty acids. Figure 26-8 illustrates the block diagram for the structure of a triglyceride.

The difference between fats and oils is simple. At room temperature, fats are solids, while oils are liquids. Rather than consisting of one specific type of fatty acid linked with glycerol, fats and oils consist of various mixtures of fatty acids, both saturated and unsaturated. The structures of the triglycerides that make up the fat or oil determine the melting point of the fat or oil. The more saturated fats present in the triglycerides, the higher the melting point. A higher melting point renders a substance solid at room temperature. The more unsaturated fats present in the triglycerides, the lower the melting point. A lower melting point renders a substance liquid

TABLE 26-2
Some Common Fatty Acids and Their Structures

NAME	NUMBER OF DOUBLE BONDS	TOTAL NUMBER OF CARBONS	STRUCTURE
Palmitoleic acid	1	16	$CH_3(CH_2)CH_5 = CH(CH_2)_7CO_2H$
Oleic acid	1	18	$CH_3(CH_2)_7CH = CH(CH_2)_7CO_2H$
Linoleic acid	2	18	$CH_3(CH_2)_4CH = CHCH_2CH = CH(CH_2)_7CO_2H$
Linolenic acid	3	18	$CH_3CH_2CH = CHCH_2CH = CHCH_2CH = CH(CH_2)_7CO_2H$

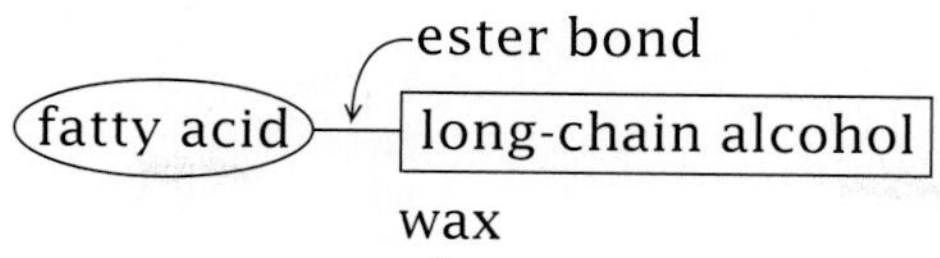

ester bond

(fatty acid) — [long-chain alcohol]

wax

A.

Type	Structural formula	Source	Uses
Beeswax	$CH_3(CH_2)_{14}$—$\overset{\overset{\displaystyle O}{\|}}{C}$—$O$—$(CH_2)_{29}CH_3$	Honeycomb	Candles, shoe polish, wax paper
Carnauba wax	$CH_3(CH_2)_{24}$—$\overset{\overset{\displaystyle O}{\|}}{C}$—$O$—$(CH_2)_{29}CH_3$	Brazilian palm tree	Waxes for furniture, cars, floors, shoes
Spermaceti wax	$CH_3(CH_2)_{14}$—$\overset{\overset{\displaystyle O}{\|}}{C}$—$O$—$(CH_2)_{15}CH_3$	Sperm whale	Candles, soaps, cosmetics, ointments

B.

Figure 26-7 *(A) The core structure of a wax. (B) The structures, sources, and uses of some common waxes.*
Source: Delmar/Cengage Learning

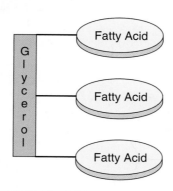

Figure 26-8 *The block diagram of a triglyceride.*
Source: Delmar/Cengage Learning

at room temperature. Table 26-3 shows the types of fats and oils and their corresponding fatty-acid constituents.

Steroids

All of the lipids discussed thus far have been saponifiable lipids. Steroids are classified as non-saponifiable lipids. Steroids can be identified by the presence of the steroid nucleus, shown in Figure 26-9. In this figure, which represents a condensed structure of the actual molecule, each of the vertices of the geometric figures represents a carbon atom with the appropriate number of hydrogen atoms. Cholesterol is a steroid familiar to most people. Its structure is shown in Figure 26-10. Cholesterol, the most common steroid in animal tissue, is an important constituent of cell membranes and is used to make steroid hormones. Cholesterol does not have an ester group and therefore is a nonsaponifiable lipid.

TABLE 26-3
Fats and Oils and Their Corresponding Fatty Acid Constituents

TYPE	FAT OR OIL	AVERAGE COMPOSITION OF FATTY ACIDS (%)				
		MYRISTIC ACID	PALMITIC ACID	STEARIC ACID	OLEIC ACID	LINOLEIC ACID
Animal Fats	Butter	8–15	25–29	9–12	18–33	2–4
	Lard	1–2	25–30	12–18	48–60	6–12
	Beef tallow	2–5	24–34	15–30	35–45	1–3
Vegetable Oils	Olive	0–1	5–15	1–4	67–84	8–12
	Peanut	–	7–12	2–6	30–60	20–38
	Corn	1–2	7–11	3–4	25–35	50–60
	Cottonseed	1–2	18–25	1–2	17–38	45–55
	Soybean	1–2	6–10	2–4	20–30	50–58
	Linseed	–	4–7	2–4	14–30	14–25
Marine Oils	Whale	5–10	10–20	2–5	33–40	–
	Fish	6–8	10–25	1–3	–	–

Steroid Nucleus

Figure 26-9 *The steroid nucleus.*

Source: Delmar/Cengage Learning

Stop and Review **26-3**

How do we determine if a substance is a lipid?

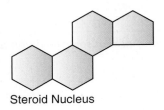

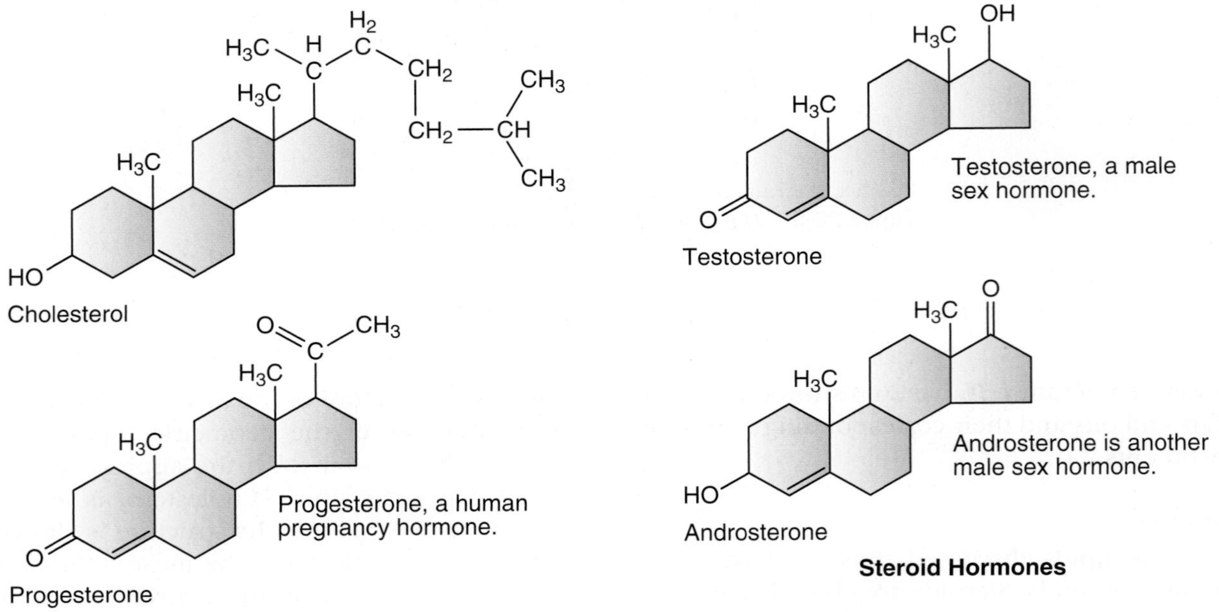

Cholesterol

Progesterone, a human
pregnancy hormone.

Progesterone

Testosterone, a male
sex hormone.

Testosterone

Androsterone is another
male sex hormone.

Androsterone

Steroid Hormones

Figure 26-10 *The structures of cholesterol and some common steroid hormones.*

Source: Delmar/Cengage Learning

Professional Profile
Nutritional Therapy

What is the one thing that all hospital patients have in common? For this profile, the correct answer is that they all need to be fed. Not all patients have the same nutritional requirements, however. For example, some patients require low-salt diets; some require salt-free diets. Some patients need low-fat diets; some need diets higher in fat. And the nutritional needs of an infant are certainly different from those of an 80-year-old diabetic.

Food form can also be important. For instance, it would be very difficult for a patient who has just had major reconstructive surgery of the jaw to chew a piece of steak. In this situation, it would be desirable to provide food in a more liquid yet still appetizing form. In other cases, nutritional formulas must be created and administered to the patient via an intravenous route.

This chapter has focused on the breakdown of carbohydrates and fats in our diets into usable energy sources. The upcoming chapter will focus on the protein we ingest and how it is used in our bodies. See Figure 26-11 which shows the phases in digestion of carbohydrates (starches), fats, and proteins and their usable end products.

What member of the hospital staff is responsible for determining the nutritional needs of and developing nutritional plans for patients? These professionals are known as *dieticians*, or *nutritionists*. Dieticians also evaluate the success of the patient's nutritional program, report results to physicians, ensure that food consumed by the patient does not conflict with medications given to the patient, and promote good eating habits. Dieticians

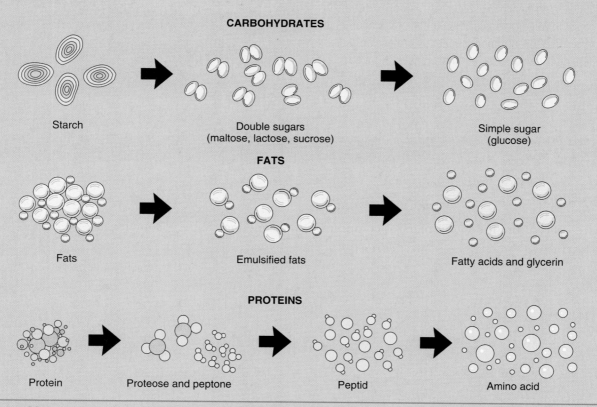

Figure 26-11 *The phases in the digestion of carbohydrates (starch), fats, and proteins with their usable end products.*

Source: Delmar/Cengage Learning

(continues)

(continued)

often are in charge of the food service departments of institutions. Here, responsibilities can include not only meal and nutritional planning, but also managerial and administrative tasks. Nutritionists work in a variety of places including hospitals, schools, nursing homes, home health agencies that produce home-delivered meals, food manufacturing companies, grocery store chains, and prisons.

    The minimal educational requirement to become a dietician is a bachelor's degree with a concentration in foods, nutrition, or institutional management. Courses of study include biology, chemistry, physiology, behavioral science, food science, food service systems management, math, computer science, statistics, business, and communications. A master's degree allows for further specialization within the field.

    As a result of an increased understanding of both the connection between nutrition and health and the nutritional needs of a varied population, the future outlook for dieticians is very bright. With the national trend of developing healthier lifestyles, it is believed that this profession will grow faster than the average nonmedical professions. To learn more about this profession, visit the American Dietetic Association at www.eatright.org/.

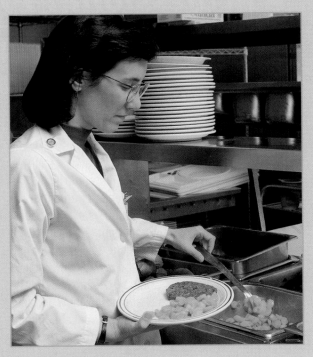

Source: Delmar/Cengage Learning

■ CHAPTER REVIEW

Exercises

1. Are each of the following pairs of compounds the same, or are they isomers?

   a. CH_3CHCH_3 CH_3CH_2CHOH
         |
         O
         |
         H

   b. CH_3CHCH_3 CH_2
        | |
        CH_3 $CH_2CH_2CH_3$

   c. CH_3COOH $HOOCCH_3$

2. Which of the following compounds are saturated, and which are unsaturated?

   a. $CH_2 = CH_2$

   b. $CH_3CH_2CH_3$

   c. $CH_3CH = CH_2$

3. A carbohydrate consisting of a single sugar molecule is called a:

   a. monosaccharide

   b. disaccharide

   c. polysaccharide

   d. starch

4. A diabetic has a higher-than-normal blood sugar level. This condition is called:

   a. hypoglycemia

   b. hyperglycemia

   c. glucosuria

   d. hyperdiabetes

5. What is the name for the condition wherein glucose is found in the urine? Within what range of blood sugar levels does this condition occur?

6. What monosaccharides are present in each of the following disaccharides?

   a. sucrose

   b. lactose

   c. maltose

7. What is the difference between the structures of the polysaccharides amylose and amylopectin?

8. The storage form of glucose in animals is called:

   a. amylose

   b. amylopectin

   c. glycogen

   d. starch

9. Plant or animal products that are soluble in nonpolar solvents are called:

   a. carbohydrates

   b. lipids

   c. proteins

   d. starches

10. Draw a generalized diagram for a triglyceride.

11. What is the difference between a fat and an oil?

12. List two ways that the body uses cholesterol.

Real Life Issues and Applications

Dietary Concerns of Glucose

A patient presents with a blood glucose level of 150 mg/100 mL of blood. The patient is disoriented. What is a possible treatment? What dietary modifications would you recommend?

Additional Activities

1. Contact an exercise physiologist, sports trainer, or other related health professional. Ask this professional to speak to the class regarding the benefits of aerobic exercise and how it can be used for weight control.

2. The recommended daily amount of fat in the diet should not exceed 60 g for men and 45 g for women. Record the foods you eat on a given day. Using label information and other sources as suggested by your instructor, determine how many grams of fat you ingested. How did your intake of fat compare to the daily recommended amounts? How did your intake compare to the intakes of other students in the class?

3. Determine the grams of fat per one serving for as many different foods as possible, being sure to note what one serving represents (e.g., a 1.5-oz bag of pretzels equals one serving). If possible, obtain information from fast-food restaurants. Combining your information with that of your classmates, list the foods in descending order according to fat content (i.e., place the food having the highest fat content at the top of the list, and the food having the lowest fat content at the bottom of the list). Does a single serving of any one food contain the recommended daily amount of fat? In general, what types of foods have the highest fat content?

StudyWARE CONNECTION

Go to your StudyWARE™ DVD and have fun learning as you play interactive games, view animations and videos, and take practice tests to help reinforce key concepts you learned in this chapter.

Workbook Practice   *Go to your Workbook for more practice questions and activities.*

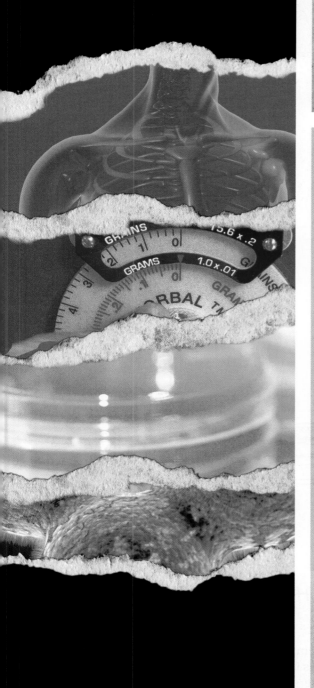

CHAPTER 27

THE AMAZING PROTEINS

Objectives

Upon completion of this chapter, you should be able to

- Define the term *amino acid* and differentiate between a complete protein and an incomplete protein

- Write the word equation for the hydrolysis of proteins

- Give an example of each of the four classes of proteins and their respective functions in the body

- Explain the term *specificity*

- Define the terms *apoenzyme*, *cofactor*, *coenzyme*, and *activator*

- Write the equation describing enzyme action and explain the process of enzyme action

- Distinguish between lock-and-key theory and induced-fit theory

- Give two examples of how enzymes can be used in the diagnosis of disease

Key Terms

activator
active site
amino acid
apoenzyme
catalyst
coenzyme
cofactor
complete protein
denaturation

essential amino acid
fibrous protein
globular protein
incomplete protein
primary structural feature
protein
substrate
zymogen

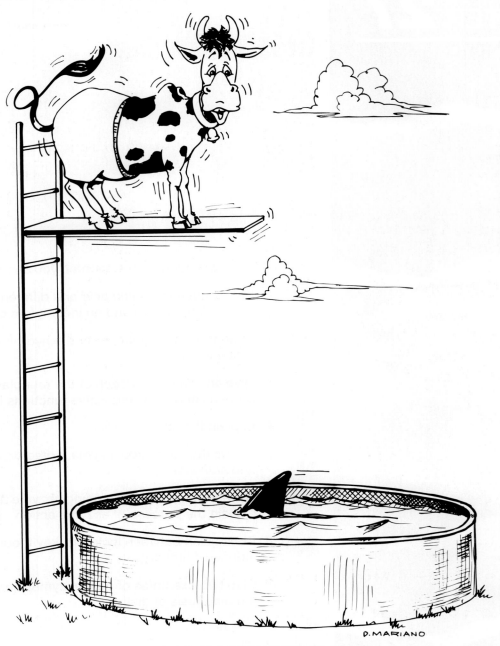

A HIGH PROTEIN SHAKE

Source: Delmar/Cengage Learning

■ INTRODUCTION

The word **protein** is derived from the Greek word *proteios*, meaning "of first rank." Proteins are very diverse substances that provide for a variety of functions within the body. Structural proteins compose in part the skin, hair, and cartilage; the muscles in our bodies consist of proteins; and enzymes, which act as catalysts in the body, also consist primarily of proteins. In addition, the antibodies in the blood, which protect our bodies from foreign substances,

are proteins; and various proteins transport oxygen and lipids in the bloodstream. As you can see, without these substances, our bodies could not function. Proteins, thus, deserve the title of "first rank."

Proteins

We will start our discussion of proteins by looking at the foundation of proteins—amino acids. This will be followed by the topics of protein structure and the properties of proteins.

Amino Acids

The building blocks of proteins are the **amino acids**. The general structure of amino acids is as follows:

NH$_2$CHCOOH
|
G

The symbol *G* represents a side chain group attached to this structure. The various side chains are listed in Table 27-1.

It is interesting to note that the same set of 20 amino acids is used by all plants and animals. These amino acids are bonded together in various combinations and in long chains to form proteins. **Essential amino acids** are amino acids that cannot be synthesized from the carbohydrates and lipids in the body. Because they cannot be made by the

TABLE 27-1
Amino Acid Side Chains

TYPE	SIDE CHAIN, *G*	NAME	SYMBOL
Nonpolar Side Chain	—H	Glycine	Gly
	—CH$_3$	Alanine	Ala
	—CH(CH$_3$)$_2$	Valine	Val
	—CH$_2$CH(CH$_3$)$_2$	Leucine	Leu
	—CHCH$_2$CH$_3$ | CH$_3$	Isoleucine	Ile
	—CH$_2$— (phenyl ring)	Phenylalanine	Phe
	—CH$_2$— (indole ring)	Tryptophan	Trp
	(complete structure, proline ring)	Proline	Pro
Side Chain having a Hydroxyl Group	—CH$_2$OH	Serine	Ser
	—CHOH | CH$_3$	Threonine	Thr
	—CH$_2$—(ring)—OH	Tyrosine	Tyr
Side Chain having a Carboxyl Group (or an amide)	—CH$_2$CO$_2$H	Aspartic Acid	Asp
	—CH$_2$CH$_2$CO$_2$H	Glutamic Acid	Glu
	—CH$_2$CONH$_2$	Asparagine	Asn
	—CH$_2$CH$_2$CONH$_2$	Glutamine	Gln
Side Chain having a Basic Amino Group	—CH$_2$CH$_2$CH$_2$CH$_2$NH$_2$	Lysine	Lys
	—CH$_2$CH$_2$CH$_2$NH—C(=NH)—NH$_2$	Arginine	Arg
	—CH$_2$— (imidazole ring)	Histidine	His
Side Chain Containing Sulfur	—CH$_2$SH$_2$	Cysteine	Cys
	—CH$_2$CH$_2$SCH$_2$	Methionine	Met

TABLE 27-2
The Essential Amino Acids

Lysine	Tryptophan
Leucine	Valine
Isoleucine	Phenylalanine
Methionine	Histidine
Threonine	Arginine

body, the essential amino acids must be part of the diet. Table 27-2 lists the essential amino acids.

A **complete protein** contains all of the essential amino acids in the proper amounts. An **incomplete protein** is low in one or more of the essential amino acids. Animal protein from eggs, milk, meat, fish, and poultry is complete. All vegetable protein is incomplete. In order to obtain all of the essential amino acids, vegetarians, therefore, must eat a wide variety of grains and legumes.

As stated earlier, proteins are composed of long chains of amino acids covalently bonded to one another. The sequence of amino acids in the chain is called the **primary structural feature** of the protein. Hydrogen bonding and interactions between the side chain groups cause a twisting and folding of the primary structure into a three-dimensional shape, as shown in the myoglobin structure in Figure 27-1.

Protein Reactions

Two chemical reactions of proteins are of interest to us: hydrolysis and **denaturation**. The hydrolysis process is involved in the digestion of proteins in the

body. In this process, the covalent bonds that hold the amino acids together in the protein are broken apart, thus yielding the individual amino acids. In equation form, this is represented as follows:

$$\text{protein} + H_2O \rightarrow \text{amino acids}$$

The amino acids formed by this process can then be absorbed into the bloodstream through the intestinal wall.

As stated previously, the three-dimensional shape of proteins is caused and maintained by hydrogen bonding and the interactions between the side chain groups. Rather than being covalent bonds, these interactions are weaker, electrostatic (i.e., between positive and negative charges) forces of attraction. The shape of a protein is critical to its function. Any change in shape can result in the protein being unable to perform its function. *Denaturation* is the disorganization of the protein structure in such a manner as to render the protein incapable of performing its function (see Figure 27-2). Some poisonous substances cause problems by denaturing proteins. Because our bodies contain many proteins that

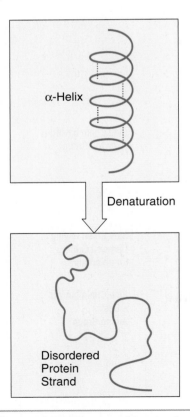

Figure 27-2   *Denaturation resulting in the breakdown of protein structure.*

Source: Delmar/Cengage Learning

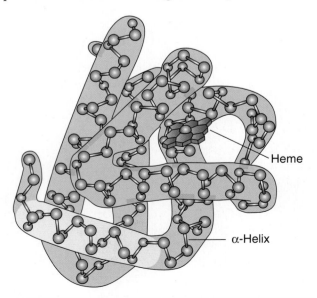

Figure 27-1   *The myoglobin structure.*

Source: Delmar/Cengage Learning

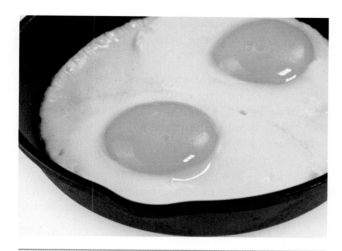

Figure 27-3 *When an egg is heated in a frying pan, the protein in the egg white is denatured.*

Source: Stoker, Stephen H., *General, Organic, and Biological Chemistry*, 5e, Brooks/Cole, Cengage Learning

are essential to life, this type of breakdown of protein structure could easily result in death.

Denaturing agents are not necessarily chemicals. Some physical processes can cause denaturation of protein. For example, when you fry an egg, the egg white solidifies as a result of protein denaturation as shown in Figure 27-3. As illustrated by this example, a denatured protein is not very soluble, and thus will solidify. Heat, therefore, can be considered a denaturing agent. We make use of this fact whenever we heat something to sterilize it. The heat denatures the protein of various bacteria. Alcohol solutions such as ethyl alcohol and isopropyl also act as disinfectants by denaturing the protein of bacteria. Table 27-3 shows some examples of denaturing agents and their effect on proteins.

TABLE 27-3
Denaturing Agents and Their Effects

DENATURING AGENT	EFFECT OF AGENT/APPLICATIONS
Heat	Causes the protein molecules to vibrate violently
	Examples: Heating an egg white (e.g., by frying an egg), causing it to coagulate; autoclaving surgical instruments to kill bacteria
Microwave radiation	Causes violent vibrations and thus heating of protein molecules
Ultraviolet radiation	Similar to the action of heat
	Example: Damage to proteins in the skin from sunlight (sunburn)
Violent whipping or shaking	Mechanical action of whipping disrupts the protein structure
	Example: Beating egg white into meringue
Soaps/detergents	Disrupt hydrogen bonding of the protein structure
	Example: Killing bacteria by washing hands with soap
Organic solvents (e.g., ethyl alcohol)	Interfere with the hydrogen bonds of the protein
	Example: Using ethyl alcohol or isopropyl alcohol to denature proteins in bacteria, killing them
Strong acids and bases	Disrupt hydrogen bonds initially; prolonged exposure results in hydrolysis of the protein
	Example: Lactic acid from bacteria, which denatures milk proteins causing them to coagulate
Salts of heavy metals (e.g., mercury, lead)	The positive ions of the metals disrupt neurotransmission
	Example: Brain damage due to mercury exposure (Mad Hatters)

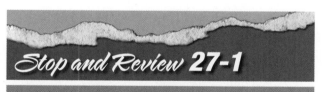

Stop and Review 27-1

a. What element is present in an amino acid that isn't present in carbohydrates and lipids?

b. What are the building blocks of proteins?

c. What is an essential amino acid? How does this relate to a complete protein?

d. How does autoclaving (heat and pressure) surgical instruments kill bacteria?

Protein Classification

Studying substances having a wide variety of functions and structures can be confusing. Such is the case with proteins. One way to simplify the study of proteins is to classify them. Note, however, that because of the different methods of classification and the diversity of proteins, there is some overlap in the classification of these substances; that is, the same protein may be classified in multiple ways. This is analogous to a classification system for houses. Classification could be done by color, number of stories, or presence of a garage. Thus, if you live in a blue, one-story house without a garage, your house would appear under two of the three possible classes. The same holds true for proteins. Classification of proteins is done by solubility, composition, and biological function; and the same protein may be found in more than one class.

Protein Classification According to Solubility

There are two major subclasses of proteins based on solubility: **fibrous proteins** and **globular proteins**. Fibrous proteins tend to have long, string-like structures that can intertwine to form fibers. These proteins are insoluble in water. Globular proteins consist of spherically shaped molecules and are water soluble.

Following are four classes of fibrous proteins:

- *collagens*—found in the various connective tissues
- *elastins*—found in the elastic tissue of ligaments and arteries
- *keratins*—found in hair, wool, skin, and hooves
- *myosins*—found in muscles (*myo* meaning "muscle"); responsible for the contraction and extension of muscles

Following are two classes of globular proteins:

- *albumins*—found in the blood; carriers of molecules that are not soluble in the blood
- *globulins*—include enzymes and blood proteins involved in the immune system

QUOTES & NOTES

The protein in the cornea of the eye is a member of the collagen class of proteins. A collagen fibril measuring 1 mm in diameter can hold a suspended mass as heavy as 22 pounds.

Protein Classification According to Composition

Some complex proteins contain nonprotein structures. These proteins can be classified according to the groups to which they are attached. Following are several examples of protein classes based on composition:

- *phosphoroproteins*—contain a phosphate group; an example is casein, which is found in milk
- *glycoproteins*—contain a carbohydrate group; an example is gamma globulin, which helps protect the body against disease and is also classified as a globular protein
- *hemoproteins*—contain a heme group; an example is hemoglobin, which transports oxygen

Protein Classification According to Biological Function

A newer method of classifying proteins is according to function. This classification method best shows the diversity of proteins. Following are several examples of protein classes based on biological functions:

- *enzymes*—act as **catalysts** within the body; without enzymes, our bodies could not function because the chemical reactions in the body would take place too slowly
- *hormones/neurotransmitters*—act as chemical messengers within the body; hormones such as insulin tell the cells to absorb glucose, while neurotransmitters such as acetylcholine carry nerve impulses across the synapses between neurons
- *protection proteins*—defend the body against disease by combining with and destroying viruses, bacteria, and other foreign substances within the body
- *structural proteins*—serve as the major components of connective tissue, bones, skin, hair, and ligaments; compose the largest percentage of proteins in the human body
- *transport proteins*—carry other molecules in cells and blood; examples include hemoglobin, which carries oxygen from the lungs to the cells, and lipoproteins, which carry lipids in the blood

Stop and Review 27-2

a. What type of experiment could you perform to distinguish between globular and fibrous proteins?

b. Describe the function of the following proteins.

   1. lipoproteins

   2. hemoproteins

   3. albumins

   4. globulins

c. Classify the following proteins.

   1. hemoglobin, used to carry oxygen in the blood

   2. protease, an enzyme that hydrolyzes proteins

   3. gamma globulin, a protein that protects the body from disease

Enzymes

Enzymes are essential to life, and their properties are important to people in the medical field. As we will see later, enzymes can be used in the diagnosis and treatment of disease.

Properties of Enzymes

Enzymes are organic catalysts. As discussed earlier, a catalyst is a substance that increases the rate of a reaction without being consumed. Life would be impossible without enzymes. They play vital roles in controlling the various reactions within the body.

Those properties of enzymes that are relevant to our discussion are the ability to enhance rate of reaction and specificity. By "enhance rate of reaction," we mean increase the rate of a reaction. It is mind-boggling how much faster reactions take place in the presence of catalysts. Some reaction rates increase by more than 10 million times in the presence of catalysts.

Specificity means the extent to which an enzyme is "choosy." Some enzymes will react with only one type of compound. For example, urease will catalyze only those reactions involving urea. Other enzymes are not as specific and will, instead, react with a certain class of compounds, such as esters. It is important to note, however, that all enzymes possess a certain degree of specificity ranging between the extremes.

Enzyme Structure

Before continuing our discussion of enzymes, we need to define several terms relating to the structure of enzymes. Most enzymes are not pure proteins—that is, there is usually a nonprotein part attached to the protein. The purely protein part of the enzyme is called the **apoenzyme**; the nonprotein part of the enzyme is called the **cofactor**. Cofactors can be organic compounds, in which case they are called **coenzymes**. Some cofactors are metal ions called **activators**.

Coenzymes are the substances we call *vitamins*. The apoenzymes and cofactors must be joined together in order for the enzyme to function.

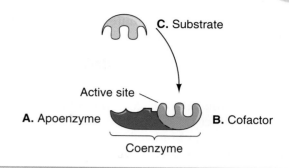

Figure 27-4 *An enzyme: (A) the apoenzyme, (B) the cofactor, and (C) the substrate. The enzyme is formed by the joining of the apoenzyme and the cofactor.*
Source: Delmar/Cengage Learning

Enzyme action typically takes place in coenzymes; specifically, catalytic action occurs in an area of the enzyme called the **active site**. Figure 27-4 illustrates an enzyme and enzyme action. The substance acted on by the enzyme is called the **substrate**.

It is sometimes necessary to control enzyme action. Such is the case with the enzymes involved in digestion. These enzymes are produced in one place and then are moved to the stomach, where they catalyze reactions. Naturally, it is undesirable for these enzymes to exhibit enzyme activity in the areas where they are produced. These enzymes, therefore, are produced in inactive forms called **zymogens**, which are activated only when they enter the stomach.

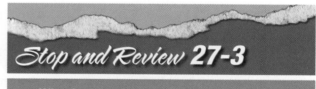

Stop and Review **27-3**

a. Why does our body need enzymes?

b. Define each of the following terms:

  1. apoenzyme
  2. activator
  3. cofactor
  4. coenzyme
  5. active site
  6. zymogen

Enzyme Specificity

The specificity of enzymes can best be understood by examining the way these substances act. Basically, the enzyme and substrate bind, a chemical reaction occurs, a product forms, and the enzyme and substrate separate. This is illustrated in the following equation:

$$E + S \rightarrow ES \rightarrow EP \rightarrow E + P$$

where E = the enzyme, S = the substrate, and P = the product.

Enzymes can bind only with particular substrates because of the need for complementary binding sites on the enzymes and substrates. The binding takes place via hydrogen bonding or some form of electrostatic attraction (i.e., attraction between opposite charges). Figure 27-5 is a simplified representation of enzyme and substrate binding.

It is important to remember that only a substrate having a structure complementary to the structure of a given enzyme can bind with that enzyme. This is analogous to a lock and key: In order for a key to work a particular lock, the key must have a shape complementary to that of the lock. This theory of enzymes is sometimes referred to as the *lock-and-key theory* (see Figure 27-6).

According to the *induced-fit theory*, an enzyme will change its shape slightly to accommodate a substrate (see Figure 27-7).

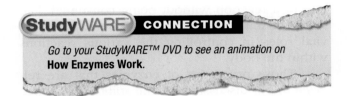

Go to your StudyWARE™ DVD to see an animation on **How Enzymes Work**.

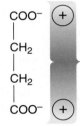

Figure 27-5   *The binding of an enzyme to a substrate occurs via electrostatic forces of attraction.*

Source: Delmar/Cengage Learning

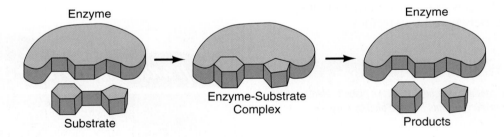

Figure 27-6   *The substrate must have a shape complementary to that of the enzyme in order for the substrate to bind with the enzyme. This is termed the* **lock-and-key theory**.

Source: Delmar/Cengage Learning

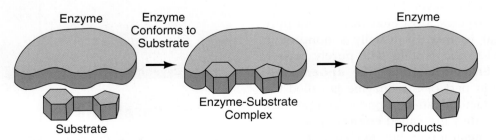

Figure 27-7   *According to the* induced-fit theory, *an enzyme will alter its shape slightly to facilitate substrate binding.*

Source: Delmar/Cengage Learning

Clinical Relevancy

Enzymes in the Health Science Field

Enzymes are useful in the health science field for both the treatment and diagnosis of disease. Enzymes are not usually found in the blood. When the tissue of a particular organ is damaged by disease, however, the enzymes specific to that organ can be released into the bloodstream. Thus, a disease affecting a particular organ can be diagnosed by determining the presence of enzymes in the blood. For instance, while several body tissues contain the enzyme glutamate pyruvate transferase, abbreviated GPT, the liver contains approximately three times as much GPT as does any other tissue. Thus, the appearance of GPT in the blood may indicate liver damage or a viral infection such as hepatitis.

A heart attack can be diagnosed in a similar manner. A person who has suffered a heart attack will have higher-than-normal levels of the enzymes creatine kinase (CK), glutamate oxaloacetate aminotransferase (GOT), and lactate dehydrogenase (LDH) within a few hours or days after suffering the heart attack. The diagnosis of a heart attack can be made by measuring the concentrations of these enzymes at various times after a suspected heart attack. Figure 27-8 shows the change in concentration of these isoenzymes in the days following a myocardial infarction.

Heart attacks can be caused by blood clots blocking coronary arteries. Enzymes capable of dissolving blood clots can be used to treat heart attacks. The three enzymes currently used to dissolve blood clots are tissue plasminogen activator (TPA), streptokinase, and a modified form of streptokinase called acylated plasminogen-streptokinase activator complex (APSAC). These enzymes must be administered shortly after the first symptoms of a heart attack for effective treatment.

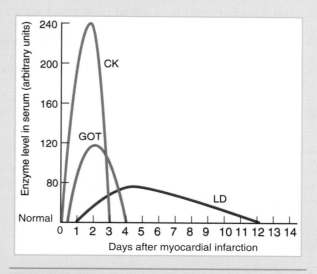

Figure 27-8   *Changes in isoenzyme concentrations.*
Source: Delmar/Cengage Learning

■ CHAPTER REVIEW

Exercises

1. What is the general formula for an amino acid?

2. What do we mean when we say that amino acids are the building blocks of proteins?

3. What do we mean when we say that a piece of roast beef is a complete protein?

4. The disorganization of a protein's structure in such a manner as to render the protein incapable of performing its function is called:

   a. killing the protein   c. precipitating the protein

   b. debugging the protein   d. denaturing the protein

5. Prior to giving a patient an injection, a nurse will rub the injection site with isopropyl alcohol to kill any bacteria. How does alcohol kill bacteria?

6. What are two major subclasses of proteins classified by solubility? Give two examples of each subclass.

7. What are three classes of proteins classified by biological function?

8. What does the term *specificity* mean in relation to proteins?

9. Draw the diagram of a complete enzyme. Include and identify the apoenzyme, coenzyme, activator, and substrate.

10. What is the difference between the lock-and-key theory and the induced-fit theory?

11. Give two examples of how enzymes can be used to diagnose disease.

12. How can enzymes be used to treat heart attacks?

13. The presence of GPT in the blood could indicate the presence of what viral infection?

14. After a myocardial infarction, the concentration of what three enzymes increases?

Real Life Issues and Applications

Cardiac Enzymes

After being admitted for chest pain and shortness of breath, a patient's cardiac enzyme levels are determined to be elevated. What do you predict the diagnosis to be? What would be some possible treatments, both during the acute phase and for the long-term?

Additional Activities

1. Research the warning signs of a myocardial infarction and preventive measures that can be taken to minimize the risk of heart attack. (*Hint:* The American Heart Association may be a good place to start.)

2. Many people believe erroneously that the only type of pain associated with a heart attack is chest pain. How would you educate a group of patients regarding the possible signs and symptoms of a heart attack? Which teaching method would be most effective: straight lecture, demonstration, or role play?

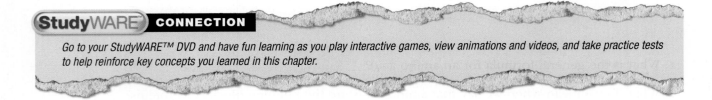

StudyWARE CONNECTION

Go to your StudyWARE™ DVD and have fun learning as you play interactive games, view animations and videos, and take practice tests to help reinforce key concepts you learned in this chapter.

Workbook Practice | *Go to your Workbook for more practice questions and activities.*

SECTION FOUR

Medical Microbiology

SECTION OVERVIEW

While cells were discussed in the Anatomy and Physiology section, this section will give a more in-depth discussion of microorganisms that can cause disease. This section will contrast the different types of organisms, discuss identification and classification systems, and focus on clinical applications such as specimen collection and infection control.

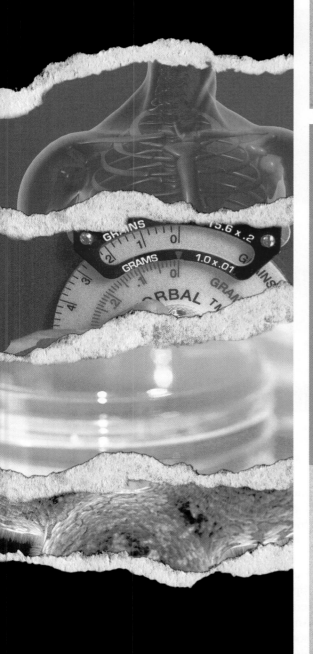

CHAPTER 28

INTRODUCTION TO MICROBIOLOGY

Objectives

Upon completion of this chapter, you should be able to

- List various areas of medical microbiology specialization and study

- Describe bacterial structure and morphology

- Discuss the process and importance of bacterial staining

- Describe the technique and importance of bacterial culture and sensitivity

- List parasites, fungi, and viruses and their causative diseases

- List medical treatments for microbial infections

Key Terms

acid-fast (Zeil-Neelsen) stain
aerobic (er-**OH**-bick)
anaerobic (**AN**-er-**OH**-bick)
antibiotic
asexual reproduction
bacilli (bah-**SILL**-eye)
bactericidal
bacteriology
bacteriostatic
binary fission
broad-spectrum drug
broth dilution
capsid
capsule

cocci (**COCK**-sye)
culture and sensitivity (C&S)
    test
disk diffusion
flagella (flah-**GELL**-eh)
flora
Gram stain
microbiology
mycology
narrow-spectrum drug
nosocomial infections
    (**NO**-soh-**KOME**-ee-al)
opportunistic infections
parasitolgy

(continues)

pathogen   *spirilla (spur-**ILL**-ah)*   *virology*
resistant   *spores*   *virulence*

GREAT MOMENTS IN MEDICAL HISTORY

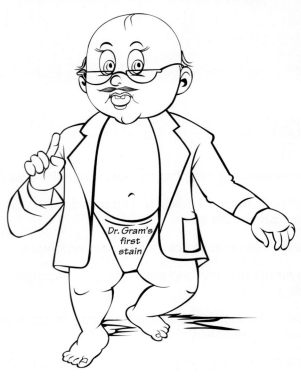

Source: Delmar/Cengage Learning

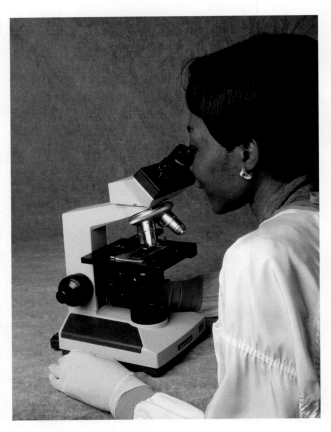

Source: Delmar/Cengage Learning

■ INTRODUCTION

Microbiology is the study of microscopic organisms. You learned about normal microscopic cells of the human body in the Anatomy and Physiology section of this textbook, and now we will focus on other microorganisms that can exist in the body, and especially on those that can cause disease. Keep in mind that the majority of these microorganisms are beneficial to the body and are known as *normal flora*. However, a small percentage can cause disease or be classified as **pathogenic**. **Virulence** is the increased ability for an organism to produce an infection.

Classification of Microorganisms

Microorganisms are classified according to their cell type, and some of the classification systems do vary. Historically, living organisms were broadly divided into two "kingdoms" called plants and

animals. With the invention of the microscope, a whole new kingdom was discovered that was neither plant nor animal. This new kingdom was classified as *protista,* and the one-celled organisms of this kingdom were known as *protists*.

Two groups of protists are important in health care. The first group of protists is called prokaryotes and consists of bacteria, blue-green algae, rickettsiae, and mycoplasmas. The second group of protists is classified as eukaryotic cells and includes algae (other than blue-green), protozoa, fungi, and slime molds. Another separate category of microorganisms was also discovered called *viruses*; this category has huge implications in the field of medicine.

Medical Microbiology

How do all of these microorganisms relate to health care? Organisms from each of these groups have the potential to cause disease, but how can you systematically study and test for the multitude of organisms found in each of these categories?

Medial microbiology is dedicated to collecting and identifying disease-producing (pathogenic) organisms and suggesting effective medical treatments.

Medical microbiology laboratories are usually divided into departments or sections that specialize in the following areas:

- **Bacteriology**: This is usually the largest department and is responsible for the growth, isolation, identification, and suggestions for optimal treatment of bacterial infections.
- **Virology**: This department specializes in identification, study, and treatment of viral infections.
- **Mycology**: This area focuses on the identification of fungi, including yeasts and molds which can cause infection.
- **Parasitology**: This area is responsible for identifying specific parasites that may be inhabiting the host's body and adversely affecting physiologic functions.

Microbiology departments, however, have responsibilities that go beyond the isolation and identification of potential pathogens and the suggestion of possible treatments. These departments also work closely with infection control departments in monitoring hospital-acquired infections, which are termed **nosocomial infections**. Such infections must be closely monitored to determine their origin and to prevent further spread, especially in an environment where patients may have compromised immune systems. Patients whose immune systems and normal protective **flora** are compromised are very susceptible to **opportunistic infections**.

Let's take a more in-depth look at the four specialties of medical microbiology, beginning with the largest, bacteriology.

Bacteriology

As mentioned earlier, bacteria are prokaryotic cells and are single-cell organisms that have no nucleus. See Figure 28-1 which shows an example of a bacterial cell. Bacteria reproduce rather easily by a process called **binary fission**. During this process a bacterial cell copies its DNA and divides up the cytoplasm and splits in half. When cells

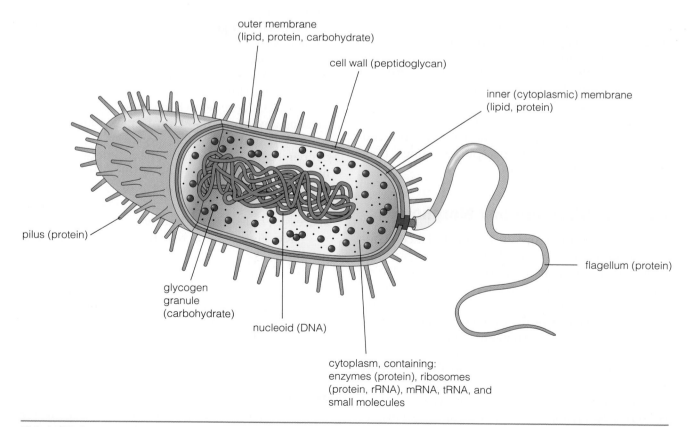

Figure 28-1   *Structures of a bacterial cell.*

source: Ingraham, John L., & Ingraham, Catherine A., *Introduction to Microbiology: A Case-History Study Approach*, 3e, Brooks/Cole, Cengage Learning

make identical copies of themselves without the involvement of another cell, this is called **asexual reproduction**. In essence, two identical daughter cells result from a single parent cell.

Many bacteria live within the human body and are either harmless or serve a vital function that is essential for life. For example, normal intestinal bacterial flora helps to digest your food and synthesize vitamin K, which is vital to the blood-clotting process.

> **QUOTES & NOTES**
>
> **B**acteria can reproduce so rapidly that under certain conditions, their population can double every 30 minutes. It's no wonder a bacterial infection can rapidly spread.

Naming Bacteria

A binomial nomenclature (two-name) system is used to give names to various types of bacterial cells. The first name is the genus or family name (always capitalized) which represents a grouping of various bacteria into those that possess similar characteristics. The second name is the species name (always lowercase) which represents the specific characteristics of that particular bacteria. For example, *Staphylococcus aureus* and *Staphylococcus epidermis* are both members of the family of bacteria that share the *Staphylococcus* characteristics that we will shortly learn. However, these are two distinct species (*aureus* and *epidermis*) with unique characteristics that set them apart. As you may have noticed when writing the genus and species names, they should always be italicized.

Bacterial Structure and Morphology

As can be seen in Figure 28-1, a bacterial cell contains a cell membrane, a cell wall, and no nucleus. However, it does contain a nucleus-like (nucleoid) region where the DNA is stored. Some bacteria can form a protective covering around the cell wall known as a **capsule** which can increase their resistance to antibacterial agents. While many bacteria have no independent forms of locomotion or movement, others do possess short fine filaments called **flagella** that can provide motility.

Certain types of bacteria can even go into a state of suspension or inactivity for long periods of time. These bacteria produce **spores** which are highly resistant forms of the organism that develop in response to adverse environmental conditions. They can then regenerate and become active when the environmental conditions improve. Spores are extremely hard to kill and have been estimated to be able to remain in the dormant state for tens of thousands of years.

The morphology or shape of bacteria is an important diagnostic tool for identification. The three basic shapes are as follows:

- **cocci**: round or spherical shaped
- **bacilli**: rod shaped
- **spirilla**: spiral shaped

Cocci

In addition to the basic round shape of cocci bacteria, these bacteria will group together in distinct formations and can be named accordingly:

- *mono:* means spherical bacterial in single formation
- *diplo:* refers to bacteria occurring in pairs
- *strepto:* refers to a formation of bacteria in chain-like structures
- *staphylo:* literally means "bunch" and refers to bacteria that group together in clusters like a bunch of grapes

Diplococci have been associated with meningitis, pneumonia, and gonorrhea. Streptococci cause the familiar strep throat along with specific pneumonias, rheumatic fever, and some skin conditions like impetigo. *Staphylococcus epidermis* is the normal flora on your skin, mucous membranes of the nose, throat, and intestines where it does not normally present any problems. However, if you puncture your skin and allow this organism to enter the deeper tissue or bloodstream, a serious infection may result. Another species of the *Staphylococcus* family, *Staphylococcus aureus*, is pyogenic (pus producing) and can cause skin infections that result in abscesses, boils, and carbuncles.

See Figure 28-2 which illustrates bacterial morphology.

> **QUOTES & NOTES**
>
> **B**e careful to not confuse pyogenic (pus-producing bacteria) and pyrogenic (heat- or fever-producing bacteria).

Bacilli

The rod-shaped bacteria can possess flagella for motility and can also be found in pairs (diplobacillus) and chains (Streptobacillus) as shown in

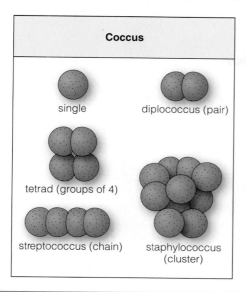
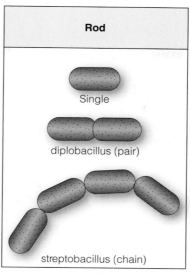
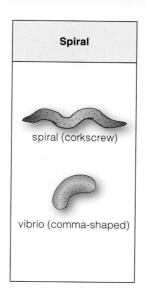

Figure 28-2 *Bacteria classification and morphology.*

Source: Ingraham, John L., & Ingraham, Catherine A., *Introduction to Microbiology: A Case-History Study Approach*, 3e, Brooks/Cole, Cengage Learning

Figure 28-2. Rod-shaped *Escherichia coli,* or *E. coli* for short, is the needed normal flora in your intestinal tract. However, if it migrates to the urinary tract due to poor hygiene, it can cause a urinary tract infection (UTI). If *E. coli* enters into the bloodstream, a very serious septicemia (infection in the blood) can result. Other bacillus type diseases include typhoid fever, diphtheria, tuberculosis, botulism, and tetanus. Bacilli can form spores and therefore live for a long time in harsh environmental conditions, within the soil, for example.

Spirilla

Most of the spiral-shaped bacteria are mobile due to their shape (think of the movement produced by a spring coiling and uncoiling) and are responsible for diseases such as syphilis and cholera.

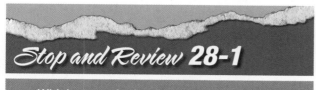

Stop and Review 28-1

a. Which area of microbiology focuses on the study of fungi, yeast, and molds?

b. List the three basic shapes of bacteria and how they relate to their names.

c. Describe the nomenclature system of naming bacteria.

Bacterial Staining

Using different dyes or stains to color the bacteria not only makes them easier to view under the microscope, but also gives important information about their classification and treatment. A *simple stain* would allow for contrast to better illustrate the structure and arrangement of bacterial cells. A *differential stain* would provide more information based on the composition of the bacterial wall.

A common differential stain developed more than 100 years ago, called the **Gram stain**, is still in use today. The Gram stain technique places the bacteria on a slide and stains them with a purple stain called crystal violet. All organisms will take up this stain and therefore turn purple. The slide is then covered with fixative agent (Gram's iodine) to help the stain adhere better. An acetone/alcohol decolorizing rinse is then applied that can wash away the stain depending on the type of bacteria. If the bacteria retain the purple color after the decolorizing rinse, they are called gram-positive or gram+ bacteria. The slide is then counterstained with a red dye (usually safranin) and those bacteria that decolorized with the acetone are now colored red or pink in color. These organisms that stain red or pink are called gram-negative (gram−) bacteria. The cell wall in gram-negative organisms has three layers, and since many antibacterial agents work by destroying cell wall function, the tougher cell wall of the gram-negative organisms make them harder to treat.

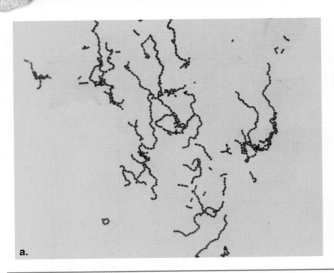
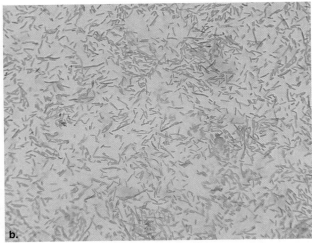

Figure 28-3 *(A) Gram-positive streptococci displaying purple stain. (B) Gram-negative rods displaying pink stain.*

Source: Delmar/Cengage Learning

Another type of differential stain used on bacteria in the genus *Mycobacterium,* the causative agent of tuberculosis (TB) and leprosy, is the **acid-fast (Zeil-Neelsen) stain**. Acid-fast organisms resist staining due to a waxy capsule that surrounds the cell wall. Acid-fast bacteria appear red against a blue background because they retain the carbolfushin (red) stain that is first applied to them and do not take on the second methylene blue stain.

See Figure 28-3 representing gram-positive and gram-negative organisms.

Clinical Relevancy

Specimen Collection

In order to assist in the diagnosis and treatment of the pathogen creating the disease, proper specimen collection procedures must be followed. The specimen collected can come from many body regions such as wounds; oral, nasal, or genital regions; or eyes or ears. In addition, specimen collection can come from body fluids such as urine, blood, sputum, or cerebral spinal fluid (CSF).

See Table 28-1 which lists specimen types or areas along with collection considerations and possible pathogens that may be found.

Regardless of the specimen type that is collected, the following general guidelines should be maintained to ensure accurate results:

- Ideally, collect specimens before antibiotics are begun.
- Use sterile supplies and collection containers. (See Figure 28-4 for examples of different transport media and specimen containers.)
- Collect the specimen from the site of infection and not surrounding areas.

- Collect and place the specimen in an appropriate container and/or transport media according to protocol.
- Collect a sufficient amount of specimen for testing.
- Appropriately label each specimen and transport to lab within an appropriate time.

Safe collection and handling of specimens is critical for accurate results, but also for prevention of the spread of the disease to other patients or health care workers. Always assume that all specimens potentially contain harmful pathogens and strictly follow the safety protocols of your institution.

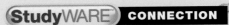

StudyWARE CONNECTION

To view a video on **Specimen Collection and Processing Procedures***, go to your StudyWARE™ DVD.*

(continues)

(continued)

TABLE 28-1
Specimen Samples, Collection Procedures, and Pathogens Related to Collection Sites

SPECIMEN SAMPLE	COLLECTION SITE/CRITERIA	SOME POSSIBLE PATHOGENS
Blood	Venipuncture or from an indwelling line using strict sterile technique	*Staphylococcus aureus* *Staphylococcus epidermis* *E. coli* *Pseudomonas* species
Urine	Clean catch midstream or from indwelling catheter	*E. coli* *Pseudomonas* species *Klebsiella-Enterobacter* species
Sputum	Morning collection preferred; collected from deep cough	*Streptococcus pneumoniae* *Staphylococcus aureus* *Haemophilus influenzae* *Legionella* species
Cerebral spinal fluid (CFS)	Lumbar puncture	*Haemophilus influenzae* *Neisseria meningitides*
Stool	While sterile container not required, several specimens may be needed and must be sure not to be contaminated with urine	*Salmonella* species *Shigella* species *Giardia* species
Wound	May be aspirated (drawn) from pus-filled area with needle or by placing a sterile swab deep within wound	*Staphylococcus aureus* *Streptococcus pyogenes* *E. coli* *Clostridium* species
Nasal	Sterile swab or thin wire in each nostril; use separate swab per nostril	*Bordatella pertussis* *Staphylococcus aureus*
Throat	Use sterile tongue depressor and swab back of throat and tonsils	*Streptococcus pyogenes* or group A strep
Eyes and ears	Sterile swabs are mainly used	*Staphylococcus aureus* *Streptococcus pyogenes* *Haemophilus influenzae*

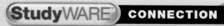

StudyWARE CONNECTION

To view videos on **Sputum Sampling and Throat Cultures**, *go to your StudyWARE™ DVD.*

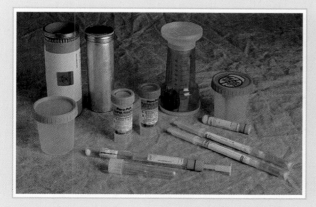

Figure 28-4 *An assortment of containers used to obtain and transport specimens.*
Source: Delmar/Cengage Learning

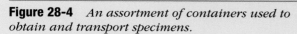

Growing and Testing Bacteria

Once a specimen has been obtained, it must be grown and tested to see what agents can harm or destroy it. The common test ordered is a **culture and sensitivity (C&S) test**. The culture contains nutrients allowing the organism to grow in sufficient quantities to identify the organism. The sensitivity portion determines what is the most effective antibiotic for treatment by subjecting the cultured organisms to various antibiotic agents to determine which will harm or kill it.

Culturing

The culture is a group of microbes (colonies) growing in a nutrient-rich environment. Once collected the specimen is place on a culture medium that varies in composition with the needs of specific bacteria. Cultures are usually grown on a Petri dish (see Figure 28-5) that is clear so that culture growth can be observed without removing the lid, which could introduce other organisms (contamination). In Figure 28-5, you can see bacterial colony growth on the nutrient-rich medium of the agar plate. Agar is a gelatin-like substance containing nutrients needed for microbial growth.

The first culture is called the *primary culture* and results after 24 to 48 hours of incubation (growth in a controlled environment). The colonies are observed for differing characteristics, and if more than one organism is identified, it is considered a *mixed culture*. The mixed culture must now be separated into subcultures until each culture yields a *pure culture* containing only one microorganism species.

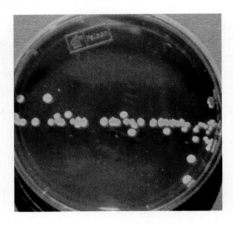

Figure 28-5 *Bacterial culture in an agar Petri dish.*
Source: Delmar/Cengage Learning

Most culture mediums contain simple nutrients such as water, carbon, hydrogen, nitrogen, oxygen, sulfur, calcium, potassium, and magnesium along with complex nutrients such as sugar, amino acids, and blood products. The media type can be a liquid broth, a semisolid, or a solid known as agar.

Inoculating the media refers to placing the microbes from the original sampling instrument, such as a swab, on the growth medium. The specimen is often spread or streaked on the Petri dish or plate in a specific pattern that divides the plate into four quadrants (see Figure 28-6). The culture plate is then placed in an incubator bottom up to prevent condensation from dripping onto the colonies. The incubator provides a stable temperature and humidity level for optimal growth.

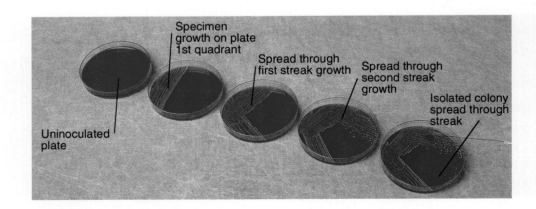

Figure 28-6 *Streaking and inoculating patterns on blood agar.*
Source: Delmar/Cengage Learning

Identification

Now that specific colonies of microorganisms have been isolated, initial examination and staining can be done to identify the unknown pathogen. Often microscopic examination and Gram staining are all that is needed to identify the pathogen. However, in some cases, further testing such as exposing the organism to biochemical reactants is required for accurate identification.

Sensitivity Testing

After an organism is identified, its sensitivity or susceptibility characteristics may be determined in order to guide antibiotic therapy. If a microorganism is susceptible to an antibiotic, the antibiotic has a better chance of fighting the infection. There are several methods by which microbial susceptibility may be determined. We will review **disk diffusion** and **broth dilution** methods.

Disk diffusion is a classic laboratory technique that provides qualitative information about susceptibility. The bacteria are cultured and grown on solid media (e.g., in a Petri dish). Different antibiotic-containing paper disks are then placed on the "lawn" of bacteria. The bacteria will not grow near the specific antibiotic disks that they are sensitive to, and therefore there will be a zone of no growth surrounding those disks. The areas without bacterial growth, known as the "zones of inhibition," are measured and compared with established standards to determine whether the bacteria are *sensitive* (the antibiotic will work), *intermediate* (the antibiotic may or may not work), or *resistant* (the antibiotic will not work). See Figure 28-7.

Broth dilution is a second, commonly used clinical method for determining bacterial sensitivity to an antimicrobial agent. This type of testing is more quantitative than the disk diffusion method; that is, it can more accurately identify the concentration or dosage of a drug needed to inhibit organism growth. The organism is placed in various test tubes containing defined concentrations of an antimicrobial agent (i.e., different drug doses) and a liquid growth medium. The test tubes are incubated for a designated amount of time and then visually inspected for organism growth. The test tube with the lowest concentration of antimicrobial agent that inhibits the growth of the organism is referred to as the *minimum inhibitory concentration,* or *MIC.* See Figure 28-8a.

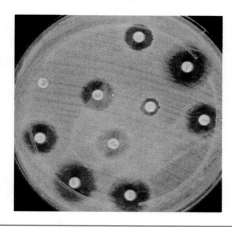

Figure 28-7 *A sensitivity testing indicating varying sizes of zones of inhibition for different antibiotics: (A) sensitive, and (B) resistant.*

Source: Delmar/Cengage Learning

Note that the MIC does not provide information about whether the organism is actually killed. The *minimum bactericidal concentration,* or *MBC,* determines this information. The MBC determines the killing activity associated with an antimicrobial agent. The MBC is determined by taking a sample from each clear MIC tube and culturing it on agar plates. The concentration in which no significant bacterial growth is observed is the MBC. See Figure 28-8b.

If the MIC is identified at a concentration that cannot be safely achieved in the patient, then the organism is considered resistant. If the MIC is identified at a clinically achievable level, the organism is considered sensitive. If the MIC is identified at a level that may or may not be clinically achievable, the organism is considered intermediate.

QUOTES & NOTES

Even though the term is a general term meaning "against life," antibiotics are used to treat bacterial infections only. You will shortly learn that there are other specific anti-infective agents to treat viruses (antiviral agents) and fungi (antifungal agents).

It's best to collect the sample of material from the infected area before an antibiotic is started, or you may not be able to grow and identify the pathogen. In patient care situations, antibiotics are often started before the results of laboratory tests are available. For serious infections, it's important to start an antibiotic as soon as possible and to adjust the drug or dose once a more precise diagnosis is available.

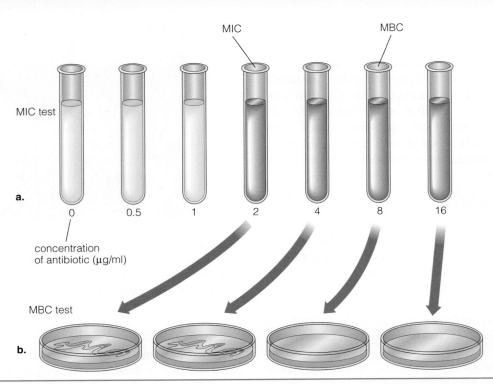

Figure 28-8   *MIC and MBC testing: (A) The minimum inhibitory concentration (MIC) is 2 micrograms/mL as shown in the middle tube. (B) The minimum bactericidal concentration (MBC) is at 8 micrograms/mL where you see no growth in the agar plate.*

Source: Ingraham, John L., & Ingraham, Catherine A., *Introduction to Microbiology: A Case-History Study Approach*, 3e, Brooks/Cole, Cengage Learning

Bacterial Disease

While bacteria can cause disease directly by destroying infected tissue, many bacteria cause disease due to the release of toxins into the host body. Toxins can cause many problems, including destruction of body tissues, destruction of blood cells, inhibition of ribosomes, fluid loss, high fever, decreased blood pressure, increased blood clotting, fluid in the lungs, and paralysis. Signs and symptoms of bacterial infection may include high fever; rapid pulse and breathing; abnormal, often foul-smelling discharge from the infected area; and pain and swelling at the site of infection. Other symptoms depend on the location of the infection.

Bacterial infections are treated with antibiotics, chemicals that can kill the prokaryotic bacteria without harming eukaryotic cells. See Table 28-2 for common bacteria and related diseases.

General Principles of Antibacterial Therapy

With the discovery of penicillin in the 1930s, the antibiotic era began. Antibiotic availability and widespread use have been both a tremendous

TABLE 28-2
Common Bacteria and Related Diseases

BACTERIA	DISEASE
Staphylococcus aureus (gram+)	Skin and wound infections, pneumonia, and food poisoning
Staphylococcus epidemis (gram+)	Wound and nosocomial infections
Streptococcus pyogenes (group A strep) (gram+)	Acute pharyngitis (sore throat)
Streptococcus pneumoniae (gram+)	Pneumonia
Enterococci (gram+)	Nosocomial infections
Escherichia coli or *E. coli* (gram−)	Urinary tract infections and sepsis
Neisseria species (gram−)	Meningitis and gonorrhea
Haemophilus influenzae (gram−)	Sinusitis, pneumonia, and otitis media
Salmonella species (gram−)	Typhoid fever and food poisoning
Shigella species (gram−)	Dysentery
Legionella (gram−)	Pneumonia (Legionnaire's disease)
Bacillus species (gram+)	Anthrax, endocarditis, food poisoning, and septicemia
Vibrio species (gram−)	Cholera

benefit and a burden to medical care. The beneficial effects are clear in the number of lives that have been spared. The burden has presented itself with a vengeance in the last several decades with the evolution of pathogens that are able to resist the effects of many antibiotic agents.

A chemotherapeutic substance derived from a living organism that kills microorganism growth is an **antibiotic**. *Antibiotic* is a general term derived from the Greek roots *anti-* (against) and *bios* (life). The term *antibiotic* was meant to distinguish between chemical therapeutic agents and those that come from living organisms (e.g., penicillin). Nowadays, drugs are made mainly in the lab, and the terms are used interchangeably. Traditionally, antibiotics refer to drugs for treating bacterial infections.

There are many ways to classify antibacterial drugs. Antibacterial drugs are classified as either bacteriostatic or bactericidal. **Bacteriostatic** agents inhibit the replication of microorganisms and prevent the growth of the organisms without destroying them. **Bactericidal** drugs actively kill bacteria. Most antibiotics are bacteriostatic at low concentrations, but at higher concentrations, bactericidal activity is more likely to be present.

Antibacterials can also be classified according to whether they are *broad-spectrum* or *narrow-spectrum*. Broad-spectrum antibiotics are effective against a wider range of bacteria than are narrow-spectrum antibiotics.

Another classification of bacteria is based on bacteria's need for oxygen. If a bacterium needs oxygen to survive, it is **aerobic**. If it does not, it is called **anaerobic**. Fewer antibiotic options are available to treat anaerobic infections, and those infections can be more serious. Remember that gram-negative infections, as a general rule, are harder to treat than gram-positive infections due to the bacterium's multilayered cell wall.

The development of so-called "super-bacteria" has been facilitated by the widespread misuse of antibacterial agents for infections of viral origin (e.g., common colds, influenza) and the continued use of broad-spectrum agents in the treatment of infections caused by single organisms, in which case a narrow-spectrum agent would do. Use of antibiotics effective against a wide range of microorganisms (**broad-spectrum** drug) can result in overkill if a drug effective against fewer microorganisms (**narrow-spectrum** drug) would be just as effective. Such use has resulted in the selective evolution of bacteria that have adapted to become **resistant** to certain antibiotics, leaving physicians with limited options for the management of some infections.

Resistance to antibiotics develops in many ways. One example is when the drug is destroyed by bacterial enzymes. Bacteria that produce the enzyme beta lactamase can make the penicillin group of antibiotic drugs inactive. Another method for resistance to occur is when some organisms develop enzymes that bind to the drug and prevent the drug from attaching to the binding site of the bacteria.

Resistance also develops when patients do not finish an anti-infective treatment. A rather common occurrence is patients who stop taking the drug once they begin to feel better. Think about this possible mechanism for resistance to occur. If you discontinue use of an antibiotic as soon as you feel better, the drug may have destroyed just enough of the weaker pathogens to give you symptomatic relief. However, there are still some minimal pathogenic bacteria remaining that haven't yet been killed and therefore represent a stronger strain. Once the anti-infective agent has been prematurely discontinued, these stronger pathogens can multiply, and when they reach a certain level, the symptoms reappear. Now, when the drug is restarted, it must contend with an overall stronger version of the pathogen.

Stop and Review 28-2

a. Contrast gram-negative and gram-positive bacteria.

b. State the purposes of a culture and sensitivity test.

c. Contrast bacteriostatic and bactericidal agents.

d. Why is it important to finish a complete regimen of antibiotics?

Virology

Viruses are the most common infectious agents in humans. Viruses (from a Latin term meaning "poison") are infectious particles that have a core containing genetic material (codes to replicate)

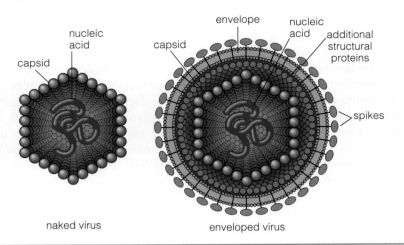

Figure 28-9 *Examples of viruses.*

Source: Ingraham, John L., & Ingraham, Catherine A., *Introduction to Microbiology: A Case-History Study Approach*, 3e, Brooks/Cole, Cengage Learning

surrounded by a protective protein coat called a **capsid**. A virus is an obligate parasite, which means it can only live and replicate in a living host cell. This makes it difficult to kill the virus without harming the host cell. Because this is a different situation than with bacteria, different drugs are needed to treat viruses than bacteria.

Viruses come in all shapes and sizes and are so small (.02–.03 microns) that they can only be seen under a powerful electron microscope. They contain no organelles and are basically a protein coat that covers a single strand of DNA or RNA. See Figure 28-9.

Viruses are classified by whether they contain RNA or DNA. RNA viruses cause diseases such as influenza, polio, human immunodeficiency virus (HIV), rabies, and encephalitis. DNA viruses cause adenovirus respiratory disease, papilloma warts, herpes simplex, and Epstein-Barr mononucleosis.

Viruses cause disease in two ways: directly, by shutting down a cell or destroying the cell outright (cell ruptures to release viruses), or indirectly, by making a favorable environment for the development of secondary bacterial or fungal infections. For example, influenza rarely kills people. The leading cause of death due to the flu is bacterial pneumonia which can easily infect lung tissue damaged by the flu virus.

Signs and symptoms of viral infection include low-grade fever (although it may also be high sometimes), muscle aches, and general fatigue, though some viral infections may cause no symptoms. Most viruses will be destroyed by the immune system within a few days of infection.

The treatment for most viral infections is rest, fluids, and treatment of symptoms to keep the patient comfortable.

Immunization has been the mainstay preventative treatment of many of the viral infections such as influenza, measles, mumps, polio, and rubella. Only recently have more antiviral drugs become available for diseases such as the common cold and flu. Viral infections are classified by their severity, length of time present, and body parts affected. Infections such as the common cold and influenza can be acute and quickly resolve in 7 to 14 days, or they can be slow and have a progressive course, as with HIV. Viral infections can be local and just affect the respiratory tract, for example, or generalized and spread throughout the bloodstream.

Some viruses can be dormant and then under certain conditions reproduce again. This is called *latency* and implies that a disease may surface years after transmission or after the initial breakout.

QUOTES & NOTES

Herpes and HIV can be in the cell, latent and undetectable, and surface long after the initial transmission.

Viral Identification

Several methods exist to isolate and identify viruses; these are often done at large medical laboratories. Identification can be accomplished by the following methods:

- *cell culture:* Viruses are grown in a layer or suspension of living tissues (since they require a host cell) and then are identified under electron microscopy.
- *direct detection:* The viral antigen is detected in the specimen showing that the patient was exposed to the virus.
- *seriodiagnosis:* Virus antibodies are detected in serum showing by special enzyme testing. Two examples are ELISA (enzyme-linked immunosorbent assay) and EIA (enzyme immunoassay).

Refer to Table 28-3 for a listing of common viruses and the pathogenic conditions they can cause. Also see Figure 28-10, which shows the relative sizes of viruses, bacteria, and human cells.

Parasitology

A parasite can be a one-celled (unicellular) or a multicellular organism that lives in or on another organism or host at the host's expense. Some parasites can cause illnesses that vary in severity from mild to life threatening. Parasites can exist in many areas of the human body, including blood, bone marrow, liver, spleen, urinary tract, intestines, skin, and hair.

Parasites are identified not only by their names but also according to their specific stages of development, as follows:

- *trophozite:* motile, multiplying form (feeding and growing stage)

TABLE 28-3
Common Viruses and the Pathogenic Conditions They Can Cause

VIRUS	DISEASE	IMMUNIZATION EXISTS
Rhinovirus or *coronavirus*	Common cold	No
Influenza A,B,C	Viral flu	Yes
Hepatitis B virus (HBV)	Hepatitis B	Yes
Hepatitis C virus (HCV)	Hepatitis C	No
Varicella zoster virus	Chicken pox and shingles	Yes
Epstein-Barr virus (EBV)	Infectious mononucleosis	No
Human immunodeficiency virus (HIV)	Acquired immunodeficiency disease syndrome (AIDS)	No
Human papilloma virus (HPV)	Genital warts	Yes
Herpes simplex type 1	Fever blisters	No
Herpes simplex type 2	Genital herpes	In progress
Respiratory syncytial virus (RSV)	Croup bronchitis	No

- *cyst:* dormant form
- *ova:* eggs of specific parasites
- *larvae:* immature form of the parasite
- *adult:* mature form of parasite

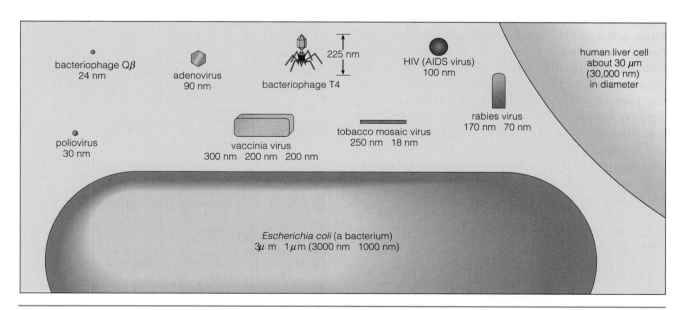

Figure 28-10 *Relative sizes of viruses, bacteria, and human cells.*

Source: Ingraham, John L., & Ingraham, Catherine A., *Introduction to Microbiology: A Case-History Study Approach*, 3e, Brooks/Cole, Cengage Learning

Clinical Relevancy

Antiviral Therapy

Antivirals do not typically cure the disease but, rather, lessen the severity of it. Herpes can be treated with antiviral medications. Herpes is a DNA virus that can cause the vesicular skin eruption most people know as fever blisters or cold sores. It can also cause genital herpes, which can be spread by sexual contact with an infected person. The main drugs to lessen the severity of herpes are acyclovir (Zovirax®), famciclovir (Famvir®), and valcyclovir (Valtrex®). These drugs interfere with viral DNA and inhibit viral replication.

Antiviral agents can also help in the treatment of influenza. The "flu" is a common viral infection due to different strains of the influenza virus. Certain patients are at higher risk for complications from influenza. These include the elderly, diabetics, and patients with cardiac,

renal, and respiratory problems. Influenza agents include amantadine (Symmetrel®), rimantadine (Flumadine®), zanamivir (Relenza®), and oseltamivir (Tamiflu®).

Respiratory syncytial virus (RSV) is a pathogen causing bronchiolitis and pneumonia; it is a major cause of acute respiratory disease in children. Ribavirin is an antiviral with inhibitory activity against RSV as well as influenzas A and B, and herpes simplex. Although its actual mechanism is not known, it inhibits essential nucleic acid formation in viral particles.

AIDS is a progressively fatal disease caused by the retrovirus human immunodeficiency virus (HIV). Treatment of HIV comprises several different drugs to suppress the virus. These drugs are termed *antiretrovirals*. In addition, several HIV vaccines are undergoing clinical testing.

Stool specimens are tested for ova and parasites, as are urine, vaginal secretions, blood, and areas of the skin.

Protozoa are unicelluar animals like microorganisms that can cause parasitic infections in humans. Most protozoan infections are caused by ingestion of contaminated water or from insect bites. Many of these protozoans are parasites, actually taking up residence in the human body and living off its cells. Most protozoans that infect humans cause disease. Symptoms of protozoan infections vary widely depending on the type of protozoan infection. Many are very serious diseases that cause long-term debilitating illness, such as malaria, which is transmitted by mosquitoes. Others are relatively mild illnesses, like "beaver fever" caused by *Giardia,* a protozoan that lives in streams and water supplies contaminated by fecal matter.

Table 28-4 shows some common parasites, mechanisms of transmission, and resulting diseases or conditions.

TABLE 28-4
Common Parasites and Their Mechanism of Transmission and Related Disease or Condition

PARASITE	ROUTE OF TRANSMISSION	SPECIMEN FOR TESTING	DISEASE OR CONDITION
Giardia lamblia	Drinking or eating contaminated feces	Feces	Severe diarrhea
Entamoeba histolytica	Drinking or eating contaminated food or water	Feces	Amoebic dysentery
Hookworm	Soil larvae can penetrate bare feet	Feces	Iron deficiency/anemia
Pinworm	Ingestion of infected food, or soiled bedding or clothing; common in children	Feces	Anal itching
Plasmodium	Bite of infected mosquito	Blood	Malaria

Mycology

Mycology is the study of fungi. A fungus is reproduced by spores, has a rigid cell wall, and has no chlorophyll. See Figure 28-11. Fungi include mushrooms, yeasts, and molds. Fungi have ergosterol instead of the cholesterol in human cells.

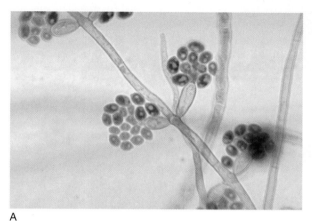

A

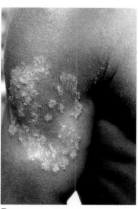

B

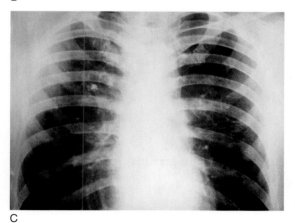

C

Figure 28-11   *(A) Shelf fungi growing on a tree trunk. (B) Grapes infected with mold. (C) Mycelium.*

Source: Ingraham, John L., & Ingraham, Catherine A., *Introduction to Microbiology: A Case-History Study Approach*, 3e, Brooks/Cole, Cengage Learning

Antifungals work by preventing the making of ergosterol, which is a building block for the cell membranes.

Fungal infections are most likely to develop in patients with an impaired immune system. In addition, antibiotics or steroids can destroy the body's natural flora, which can result in an opportunistic fungal infection. Fungal infections are identified by microscopic observation and biochemical reaction testing. Molds are identified by the spores they produce.

Most fungal infections are caused by the inhalation or ingestion of fungal spores, or the entrance of spores through open wounds. Spores are tiny bodies resistant to environmental changes, meaning they can stay dormant until conditions are just right. Most fungal spores do not cause disease in otherwise healthy individuals, though fungal infections of the skin, such as athlete's foot and jock itch, are common. Many fungal infections are opportunistic, causing disease in individuals with compromised immune systems or other underlying disease. Symptoms of fungal infection vary widely depending on the location of the infection.

Fungal infections are difficult to treat. Antifungal drugs are highly toxic, and many fungal infections are resistant to treatment. Fungal infections such as athlete's foot and jock itch can be treated with topical antifungal creams. More serious fungal infections include histoplasmosis within the lung and *Candida albicans* (thrush) of the oral cavity. These can progress to systemic infections.

Nystatin (Mycostatin®) is an antifungal agent available orally and as a topical cream; it is used to treat *Candida albicans* and skin fungal infections. Miconazole (Monistat®) is a topical cream used for vaginal yeast infections. Miconazole can also be administered by IV for systemic fungal infections.

See Table 28-5 which lists common fungal diseases and causative agents.

TABLE 28-5 **Common Fungal Diseases and Causative Agents**	
FUNGI	**DISEASE/CONDITION**
Tinea species	Dermatomycosis (ringworm)
Candida	Candidiasis, vaginal infections, thrush (white throat)
Histoplasma capsulatum	Histoplasmosis
Aspergillus	Systemic infections in immunocompromised patients

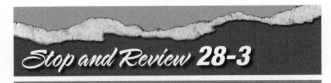

Stop and Review 28-3

a. List signs and symptoms that are typical of a viral infection.

b. Why is immunization important?

c. List four places parasites may exist in the human body.

■ CHAPTER REVIEW

Exercises

State whether the following diseases are caused by bacteria, fungi, parasites, or viruses.

1. _____ Ringworm

2. _____ Fever blisters

3. _____ Thrush

4. _____ *Giardia*

5. _____ Strep throat

6. _____ Influenza

7. _____ Shingles

8. _____ *Staphylcoccal* pneumonia

9. _____ Pinworm

10. _____ *E. coli* septicemia

11. _____ Athlete's foot

12. List the following organisms as gram+ or gram−.

   Bacillus species _____
   Escherichia coli or *E. coli* _____
   Staphylococcus aureus _____
   Haemophilus influenzae _____
   Staphylococcus epidemis _____

13. When viewing an agar plate for C&S, how do you know the bacteria are sensitive?

14. Why should you not use antibiotics on the common cold?

15. Describe the two ways that viruses can cause disease.

16. List and describe the stages of development of a parasite.

Real Life Issues and Applications

Drug-Resistant Tuberculosis (TB)

1. There has been a rise of drug-resistant tuberculosis (TB), which many feel is primarily caused by poor patient compliance in taking their full treatment of antibiotics. Debate whether, due to the risk to public health, forced compliance is an ethical and legal option.

2. Research the HIPPA regulations concerning patient confidentiality as it relates to infectious diseases.

Additional Activities

1. Invite a pathologist or laboratory technologist to discuss infectious disease identification and treatment.

2. Play "name that organism." Using the list of diseases and causative agents in this chapter, develop a game to identify organisms and their corresponding disease. Research more to add to the list.

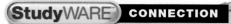

StudyWARE CONNECTION

Go to your StudyWARE™ DVD and have fun learning as you play interactive games, view animations and videos, and take practice tests to help reinforce key concepts you learned in this chapter.

Workbook Practice *Go to your Workbook for more practice questions and activities.*

CHAPTER 29

INFECTION CONTROL

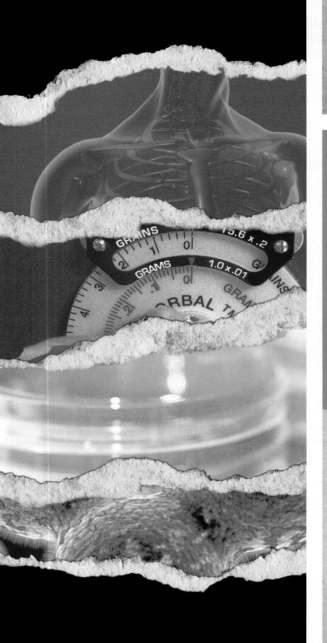

Objectives

Upon completion of this chapter, you should be able to

- Define the purpose of infection control

- Explain the key terms of infection control

- Describe various methods of cleaning, disinfecting, and sterilizing

- Define and describe the purposes of standard precautions

- List the specialized precautions and their indications

Key Terms

acetic acid
autoclave
bacteriostatic
chain of infection
chlorine
cleaning
contamination
decontamination
denatured
disinfection
ethanol (ethyl alcohol)
ethylene oxide (**ETO**)
gamma irradiation
germicidal
glutaraldehydes
hydrogen peroxide
infection
infection control

inflammation
isopropyl alcohol
nosocomial infections
pasteurization
personal protective equipment
    (**PPE**)
phenols
portals of entry
quaternary ammonium
    compounds
reservoir of
    infection
routes of transmission
sanitization
spores
standard precautions
sterilization
vegetative organisms

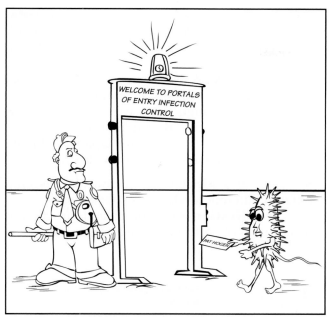

Source: Delmar/Cengage Learning

■ INTRODUCTION

To help protect the health of your patients, co-workers, and yourself, you need to have a basic understanding of **infection control**.

As a general term, infection control includes policies and procedures designed to monitor and control the transmission of communicable diseases. This also includes professionals who are involved with conducting infection control activities with other health care professionals, government agencies, and voluntary organizations. At the staff level, infection control includes education and performing basic procedures such as cleaning, sanitization, sterilizing, isolation procedures, and hand washing as well as performing various procedures in a manner that protects patients and staff from the spread of infection.

The **chain of infection**, a cycle or pathway of infection, begins with a creation of a source of infection, continues with the transportation of a given pathogen, and ends with the entry into the body. Our goal, then, is to prevent the spread of infection by breaking the chain of infection at some point along the way. See Figure 29-1.

Our patients may already be compromised due to the nature and severity of their disease(s) that have weakened their immunity. Possibly, their immune systems are impaired due to chemotherapy or anti-rejection drugs

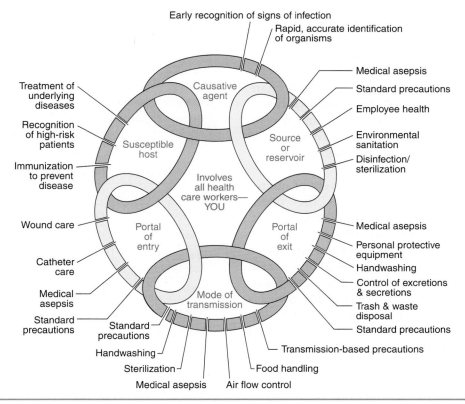

Figure 29-1 *Components of the chain of infection with ways it can be broken.*
Source: Delmar/Cengage Learning

used for organ transplants. They may be susceptible to organism exposure as a result of various procedures performed on them that breech their normal defenses such as the use of urinary catheters, bronchoscopies, or hip replacement surgery.

Basic Definitions

Before we go any further, it's important to learn a few basic terms. **Vegetative organisms** are organisms that are actively growing. **Spores** are a dormant, protective state of an organism. Spores are resistant to external environmental effects that would ordinarily damage or destroy that organism. In this form they are very hard to kill. **Denatured** means to structurally alter a substance or organism. **Contamination** is the presence of microorganisms without tissue reaction. **Infection** is the presence of microorganisms with a tissue reaction. **Inflammation** is a tissue's reaction to injury that may, or may not, be a result of infection. **Nosocomial infections** are infections acquired in health care settings such as hospitals or nursing homes.

There are several different levels of microorganism removal. **Cleaning** is the *physical* removal of all foreign matter such as dirt, blood, and sputum that may allow the growth of an organism. Cleaning exposes the surface to more intensive cleaners or chemicals by scrubbing with hot water and soaps or detergents. **Sanitization** is a general term for any process that reduces the total bacterial contamination to a level in which an object may be handled safely. **Decontamination** is the process used to remove contaminants by chemical or physical means. **Disinfection** is the process that eliminates vegetative, pathogenic microorganisms from an inanimate object. There are several levels of disinfectants.

- *Low-level disinfectants* are **germicidal** (*cide:* killing action) agents that can kill some but not all vegetative bacteria, fungi, and viruses.
- *Intermediate-level disinfectants* are germicidal agents that can kill all gram-negative bacteria and fungi, but have variable success against spores and certain viruses.
- *High-level disinfectants* are capable of killing all microorganisms except their spores.

See Table 29-1 which shows germicidal susceptibility to different levels of disinfectants.

Sterilization is the complete destruction or inactivation of all forms of microorganisms.

QUOTES & NOTES

In spite of all the best efforts to maintain sterility of the operating room and all the equipment, there is still an approximately 10% infection rate of patients undergoing surgery.

TABLE 29-1
Germicidal Susceptibility of Various Microorganisms

MICROORGANISM	GERMICIDAL SUSCEPTIBILITY		
	HIGH	INTERMEDIATE	LOW
Bateria			
Endospores	Killed	Not killed	Not killed
Vegetative cells[a]	Killed	Killed	Killed
Mycobacterium tuberculosis[b]	Killed	Killed	Not killed
Fungi	Killed	Killed	Some killed
Viruses			
Nonlipid and small	Killed	Some killed	Some killed
Lipid and medium-size	Killed	Killed	Killed

[a] Vegetative cells of most bacteria
[b] Owing to its resistance and special importance, *M. tuberculosis* is considerd separately.
Source: Ingraham, John L., & Ingraham, Catherine A. *Introduction to Microbiology: A Case-History Study Approach*, 3rd ed. Belmont, CA: Brooks/Cole, Cengage Learning.

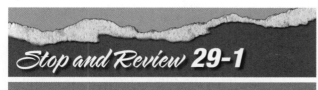

Issues to Consider When Killing an Organism

We need to kill microorganisms, or at the very least, keep them from reproducing. To accomplish this, there are several things that we need to consider. First, the initial number and type(s) of organisms we have to kill may dictate what methods and procedures we need to utilize. Some species can exist in protective spores and can't always be destroyed by means such as chemicals or dry heat. Some exist in different environments that require special techniques. Rough surfaces must be physically cleaned to expose all of the surfaces to disinfecting or sterilizing substances.

The time we have along with the intensity of the killing agent is another consideration in accomplishing our goal of sterilization. When disinfecting, the concentration of the agent used and the amount of exposure time are important factors to consider.

Temperature is another factor. Generally, killing action increases as the temperature increases. For example, in some situations at lower temperatures, a 10-degree temperature increase can double the killing rate.

Methods Used to Disinfect and Sterilize

A number of different methods can be used to disinfect and sterilize, including heat, dry heat, water below its boiling point, boiling water, steam and pressure, and various types of liquid, gas, and radiation.

Heat

The application of heat to disinfect and sterilize is very common. Generally, the higher the temperature of heat used, the less time is needed to disinfect or sterilize. Heat causes the denaturing of proteins and leads to cellular coagulation. While dry heat is fairly effective, the use of steam is more so due to its greater heat capacity since water molecules are involved. Steam can be even more effective if it is pressurized, as in an autoclave, as you will soon see.

Dry Heat

While not as effective as steam heat, dry heat is used on objects that moist heat could damage, such as oils, powders, or dressings. Glassware is normally sterilized by using dry heat. In the extreme form, incineration is used to destroy and thus "sterilize" disposable objects.

Water Below Its Boiling Point

Pasteurization is the use of water heated enough to kill vegetative cells, and most viruses such as HIV. Equipment is immersed in 70-degree Celsius water for 30 minutes. The object must then be dried and packaged in a sterile manner.

Boiling Water

Immersion in boiling water for at least 15 minutes will kill most bacteria and inactivate most viruses, but it is ineffectual against many bacterial and fungal spores. As a result, this method cannot be considered a true sterilizing process, but it does greatly reduce the number of pathogens when no other method is available. Altitude plays a factor in the effectiveness of using boiling water; for every 1,000-foot increase of altitude, increase your boiling time by 5 minutes.

Steam and Pressure

These two are effectively combined when using an **autoclave** (see Figure 29-2). This is the most efficient method of sterilizing. Items are usually packaged with a heat-sensitive indicator before being placed in an autoclave. This way you will know if the item has been heated sufficiently to be sterilized. This method can kill bacteria, fungi, viruses, and spores. The down side to this method

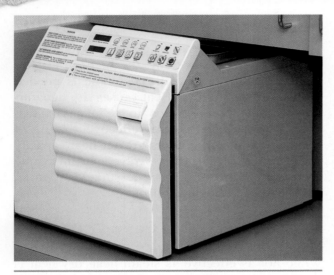

Figure 29-2 *Example of an autoclave that uses steam and pressure to sterilize items.*

Source: Delmar/Cengage Learning

is that it can melt some plastics and rubber, and corrode some metals. It also cannot be used on oils and waxes, as steam cannot penetrate those substances.

Liquids

Liquids used to disinfect and sterilize include alcohol, acetic acid, phenols, chlorine, hydrogen peroxide, quaternary ammonium compounds, and glutaraldehyde solutions.

Alcohol

If you have ever gotten an injection at the doctor's office, then you are familiar with the use of alcohol as a disinfectant. Your skin was rubbed with a small patch soaked in alcohol which cleaned your skin and removed any fats and lipids. Alcohol disorganizes the cell's lipid structures of the membrane and denatures the cellular proteins.

Alcohol is effective against gram-positive, gram-negative, and acid-fast bacteria. Although alcohol is effective against some viruses such as HIV, it is not sporicidal. Alcohol is also somewhat irritating to the skin and can damage some plastics and rubber materials.

There are two forms of alcohol that are commonly used. **Ethanol (ethyl alcohol)** is most effective when used at a 70% concentration. **Isopropyl alcohol** is most effective when used at a 90% concentration.

Acetic Acid

Acetic acid, commonly known as vinegar, has traditionally been used as a food preservative because it inhibits the growth of many bacteria **(bacteriostatic)** and fungi. Acetic acid's action is due to its acidity that denatures the cell's proteins. Normally, a 1.25% acetic acid solution is utilized for disinfecting by combining 1 part vinegar (5% strength acetic acid) with 3 parts water. White distilled vinegar is preferred over brown apple cider vinegar.

Phenols

Phenols are a result of coal tar distillation and are utilized because they cause cell leakage and inactivate enzymes in the cell membrane. This group has some virucidal properties but is not sporicidal. This class of liquids is commonly used for cleaning instruments and for general housekeeping activities.

Chlorine

If you have ever gone swimming in a public swimming pool, you are probably already familiar with this substance. **Chlorine** in both its gaseous and liquid forms is very effective against most bacteria, viruses, and fungi but is not sporicidal at room temperature. As a liquid, it is widely used in the dairy and food industry and is commonly used in hospitals and public buildings as a sanitizer. It is highly corrosive to some metals and cannot be used on rubber.

A common and very effective liquid form of chlorine is household bleach. In a 1:50 diluted bleach solution, it is effective against gram-negative bacteria, bacterial spores, and tuberculosis bacteria with a 10-minute exposure time. A 1:10 solution is recommended to clean up blood spills.

Hydrogen Peroxide

Hydrogen peroxide is a strong oxidizer that is as effective as chlorine against most bacteria. In a 3% solution, it is used as a mild antiseptic for wound cleaning. It is commonly used to clean tracheostomy tubes and incision sites as well as surgical devices and contact lenses. Caution should be exercised because a stronger solution can actually damage wound tissue. A 6% solution is bactericidal, virucidal, and fungicidal with a 10-minute exposure at room temperature. This same solution strength is sporicidal if given a 6-hour exposure.

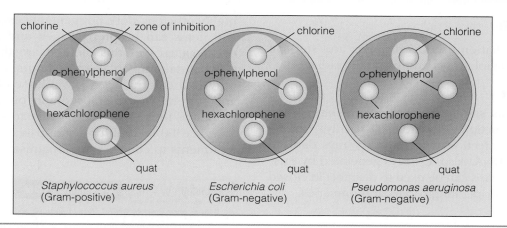

Figure 29-3 *Comparing the effectiveness of four germicides against pathogens.*

Source: Ingraham, John L., & Ingraham, Catherine A. *Introduction to Microbiology: A Case-History Study Approach,* 3rd ed. Belmont, CA: Brooks/Cole, Cengage Learning.

Quaternary Ammonium Compounds

The action of the group of agents known as **quaternary ammonium compounds** works by causing the cell's membrane's loss of semipermeability leading to lysis and denaturing of the cell's proteins. It is bactericidal to many organisms, especially gram-positive bacteria, but is ineffective against tuberculosis bacillus spores, bacterial spores, enteroviruses, hepatitis B, and some fungi.

See Figure 29-3 which shows the effects or noneffects of the liquid agents chlorine, hexachlorophene, O-phenylphenol, and quaternary ammonium on various pathogens.

Glutaraldehydes

Disinfecting and sterilizing agents in the glutaraldehyde group are widely used for cleaning surgical instruments and equipment parts. **Glutaraldehydes** are bactericidal, tuberculocidal, fungicidal, and virucidal with a 10- to 30-minute exposure and sporicidal in approximately 10 hours. Their action is through interrupting metabolism and reproduction. Caution must be taken when using agents in this group, as they can cause irritation to skin, mucous membranes, and eyes. They also can damage some rubbers and plastics and can corrode some metals. It is important to rinse, dry, and package cleaned objects in a sterile or clean manner after they have soaked in a glutaraldehyde solution.

Gas

A common gas used to disinfect and sterilize is ethylene oxide.

Ethylene oxide

Ethylene oxide (ETO) is extensively used in gas sterilization. ETO interrupts the normal metabolism and reproduction of organisms. Proper sterilization with gas is dependent on the following:

- Gas concentration
- Humidity
- Temperature
- Time

A typical setup for effective sterilization would be a gas concentration of 450 mg of ETO/L of air, 50 to 60 degrees Celsius, 30% relative humidity, at a pressure of 5 to 7 psi (pounds per square inch) for 1.5 to 6 hours of exposure.

The object to be sterilized with ETO is usually packaged with an indicator tape to ensure that there was exposure to the gas. This does not guarantee sterility so a biological indicator of a specific organism is utilized daily to ensure that sterilization is occurring (the biological indicator, a bacteria culture, dies).

Although the use of ETO is very effective, you need to be aware of some cautions. A mandatory airing time of at least 24 hours in a well-ventilated area is necessary to get rid of any residual gas. This gas can be toxic to humans. If objects made of PVC have been previously gamma irradiated, they may react with ETO to form thylene chlorhydrin which can be a skin irritant. Also, if an object to be sterilized contains water, it will react with ETO to form ethylene glycol (antifreeze) which is potentially poisonous.

Radiation

Types of radiation used to disinfect and sterilize include ultraviolet rays and gamma irradiation.

Ultraviolet

Something as simple as sunlight can have some bactericidal action. Ultraviolet (UV) rays can be used for disinfection where the UV rays damage a bacteria's DNA. Also, UV rays generated by mercury vapor lamps can be used to disinfect in closed areas such as operating rooms and nurseries.

Gamma

Gamma irradiation uses very short wavelengths of light that ionize water molecules, thus inactivating DNA molecules. This form of sterilizing is highly efficient, does not generate excessive heat, and items can be prepackaged and sealed. The disadvantages of this method are that sterilization can take up to 48 to 72 hours, it may cause polyvinyl chloride (PVC) to release chlorine gas, and currently it can be used only on a large-scale level, and thus is quite expensive to set up.

See Table 29-2 for a synopsis of the various treatments to control microorganisms.

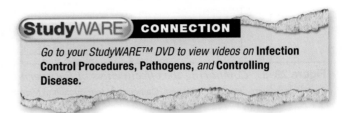

StudyWARE CONNECTION

Go to your StudyWARE™ DVD to view videos on **Infection Control Procedures, Pathogens,** *and* **Controlling Disease.**

TABLE 29-2
Examples of Methods of Sterilization and Disinfection, Modes of Actions, and Practical Uses

TREATMENT	EFFECT	MODE OF ACTION	USES
Physical Methods **Heat**			
Dry heat	Sterilizes	Denatures protein	In the laboratory, used to sterilize dry materials that can withstand high temperature and any materials damaged by moisture.
Moist heat	Sterilizes	Denatures protein	In the laboratory, used to sterilize liquids and material easily charred. Used in food canning.
Pasteurization	Kills certain microorganisms	Denatures protein	Eliminates pathogens and slows spoilage of milk and dairy products, wine, beer. (Canned evaporated or condensed milk is sterilized.)
Radiation			
UV light	Sterilizes	Damages DNA	In the laboratory, sterilizes surfaces.
X rays and gamma rays	Sterilizes	Strips electrons from atoms	Used to sterilize plastic equipment and surface of fresh fruits and vegetables.
Chemicals			
Phenols	Kills most microorganisms	Denatures protein	Germicides.
Phenolics	Kills most microorganisms	Denatures proteins and disrupts plasma membrane	Disinfectants, antiseptics.
Alcohols	Kills most microorganisms	Denatures proteins and disrupts plasma membrane	Disinfects surfaces, including skin and thermometers.
Hydrogen peroxide	Kills many microorganisms	Oxidizes vital biochemicals	Mild skin disinfectant.
Surfactants			
Soap detergent	Washes away microorganisms	Physically removes microbes	Disinfects surfaces, including skin, bench tops.
Quaternary ammonium salts	Kills microorganisms	Disrupts membranes	Widely used sterilizing agents.
Alkylating agents			
Formaldehyde and glutatraldehyde	Kills microorganisms	Inactivates enzymes by adding alkyl groups	Preserves tissues, prepares vaccine, sterilizes surgical instruments.
Ethylene oxide	Kills microorganisms	Inactivates enzymes by adding alkyl groups	Gas used to sterilize heat-sensitive materials and unwieldy objects in hospitals.

Source: Ingraham, John L., & Ingraham, Catherine A. *Introduction to Microbiology: A Case-History Study Approach*, 3rd ed. Belmont, CA: Brooks/Cole, Cengage Learning.

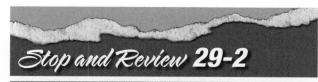

Stop and Review 29-2

1. Why is the use of an autoclave more effective than boiling water?

2. What are the four factors that determine the effectiveness of ETO sterilization?

3. Give the mode of disinfectant action for each of the following: alcohol, quaternary ammonium, glutaraldehydes, and phenols.

Protecting Our Patients and Ourselves

So far we have discussed ways of stopping the spread of infection through various methods of cleaning equipment and other inanimate objects. This section will deal with ways to protect your patients and yourself from the spread of pathogens.

It is important to always remember that many of our patients are immune-suppressed due to their disease state(s), chronic infections, and preexisting conditions. The medications they use, such as anti-rejection drugs for transplant procedures, chemotherapeutic agents, and corticosteroids, may lead to immune system suppression. As a result, common infective organisms that have little effect outside of the hospital may have a devastating effect once inside a health care facility.

Nosocomial infections, ones that are hospital-acquired, are a major cause of increased hospital stays and preventable deaths in a hospital, costing the health care system additional millions of dollars annually. It has been estimated that approximately 20,000 hospital deaths a year can be attributed to nosocomial infections.

Portals of Entry

Portals of entry are a limited number of openings by which infectious agents can gain access to the body. See Figure 29-4. These portals can include the respiratory tract, gastrointestinal tract, genitourinary tract, breeches in the skin, and wounds. Normally, pathogens entering one of these portals are stopped by the body's defense system, or at most, they create only a local

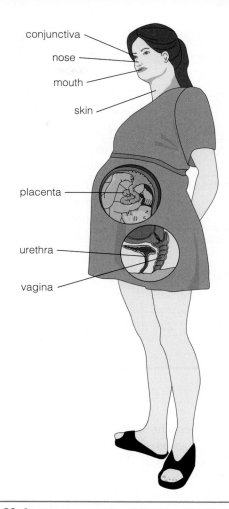

Figure 29-4 *Major portals of entry to the body.*

Source: Ingraham, John L., & Ingraham, Catherine A. *Introduction to Microbiology: A Case-History Study Approach,* 3rd ed. Belmont, CA: Brooks/Cole, Cengage Learning.

infection. However, depending on the type of organism and the patient's immune system, that invader may be able to spread systemically and establish infections in various parts of the body with potentially deadly results.

It is interesting to note that some individuals may be only *carriers* of a disease and possess no disease symptoms. Such individuals become what is known as a **reservoir of infection** and thus spread the disease to others. The classic example of this occurred in the early 1900s when Mary Mallon, a cook, spread typhoid fever from one community to another. She came to be known as "Typhoid Mary."

Quite often hospital procedures cause breeches in the natural defenses of the body. Surgical procedures that create deep wounds, such

TABLE 29-3
Portals of Entry with Examples of Related Microorganisms and Diseases

PORTAL OF ENTRY	MICROORGANISM	MICROORGANISM TYPE	DISEASE PRODUCED
Skin	*Staphylococcus aureus*	Bacterium	Impetigo
	Papilloma virus	Virus	Warts
	Trycophyton	Fungus	Ringworm
Wound	*Clostridium tetani*	Bacterium	Tetanus
	Rabies virus	Virus	Rabies
Respiratory tract	*Bordetella pertussis*	Bacterium	Whooping cough
	Influenza virus	Virus	Influenza
	Blastomyces dermatitidis	Fungus	Blastomycosis
Gastrointestinal tract	*Clostridum difficile*	Bacterium	Diarrheal illnesses (often accompanied by pseudomembranous colitis)
	Polio virus	Virus	Polio
	Giardia lambia (*G. duodenalis*)	Protozoan	Giardiasis
Gentourinary tract	*Treponema pallidum*	Bacteria	Syphilis
	Herpes simplex virus type II	Virus	Genital herpes
	Candida albicans	Fungus	Vaginitis

as hip replacement surgery, have the potential to deposit pathogens deep within the body. Once these are deposited, the wound is stitched up, sealing the pathogens inside where they can grow, colonize, and spread throughout the body via the circulatory and lymphatic systems. The insertion of an artificial airway to facilitate the use of a mechanical ventilator bypasses the natural defenses of coughing and the natural mucus removal by the cilia in the airways. This makes an individual more prone to respiratory infections. See Table 29-3 for the portals of entry and examples of related microorganisms and their diseases.

Routes of Transmission

So how do pathogens find their way inside of us and cause infections? The avenues used are known as the **routes of transmission**. These include contact, common vehicle, airborne, and vector routes.

Contact

Direct Contact

Direct contact is the spread of infective agents to an individual directly from a contaminated source. Shaking dirty hands and then rubbing your eyes, and kissing an individual with an open sore on the lip, are examples of direct contact spread of pathogens.

Indirect Contact

Indirect contact spread involves an infected individual and an improperly cleaned object that is then used on, or by, another individual. A clinical example would be performing a bronchoscopy on an individual to examine his or her lungs for tuberculosis. Tuberculosis is found and a sputum sample is taken to culture. The bronchoscope is then removed and improperly cleaned for use on the next patient, leaving tuberculosis bacilli in and on the bronchoscope. The next patient has the bronchoscope inserted into his or her lungs and the tuberculosis bacilli come off the bronchoscope, are deposited into that patient's lungs, and begin to grow there.

Common Vehicle

The common vehicle route occurs when there is a contamination of a specific substance, such as tainted blood supplies or *E. coli* in hamburger that is transported and consumed by a number of individuals. It is relatively easy to recognize this route as usually it occurs within a specific time frame, many individuals are affected at the same time, a patient history workup of each individual reveals the consumption of the same or very similar substance, and a specific pathogen is identified in all of the cases.

Airborne

Since we normally inhale between 10,000 and 20,000 liters of air a day with between 10,000 to 1,000,000 microorganisms riding those volumes, it shouldn't be a shocker that your respiratory tract is a main portal of entry for a of variety of pathogens. These pathogens are spread as a result of the aerosol generated from a sneeze or cough and can float around in the air for some time before being inhaled by another person. As you can see from Figure 29-5, an uncovered sneeze has the potential to spread a multitude of aerosol particles leading to the potential infection of others.

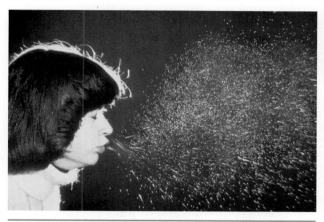

Figure 29-5 *A sneeze propels aerosols containing microorganisms. Can you now understand why it is important to cover your mouth?*

Source: Courtesy of Lester V. Bergman/Corbis.

Vector

Vectors are organisms that carry a disease agent to the host (the victim). See Figure 29-6. The vector doesn't need to develop the disease to be able to spread it to a human. It can merely serve as a reservoir of infection. Mosquitoes are frequently a vector for the spread of diseases such as malaria. Vector transmission can occur in two ways: biologically or mechanically.

Biological

A biological form of vector transmission occurs when the vector (a mosquito) ingests blood from an infected source, flies to a human, and bites that individual. Some of the tainted blood from the previous bite is injected into the fresh bite on that human. Now the pathogen can begin to grow in the new host.

Mechanical

The mechanical spread of infection by a vector occurs when the pathogen is located on the outside of the vector's body. A common example would be flies walking over fresh feces with pathogens attaching to their little "feet." They then fly to a nearby picnic table where there is a big bowl of uncovered potato salad and begin walking around on it. As they continue to walk around, the pathogens on their feet begin to slough off, contaminating the potato salad. If it is a nice warm day, the number of pathogens begins to grow, waiting for someone to consume them.

See Table 29-4 showing various routes of transmission and related diseases.

Alcohol-based, antiseptic hand sanitizers are useful when full hand washing cannot be performed. Just be sure to use the same hand cleaning

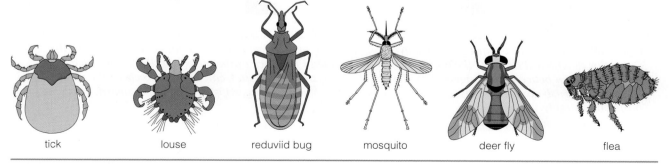

| tick | louse | reduviid bug | mosquito | deer fly | flea |

Figure 29-6 *Examples of arthropod vectors.*

Source: Ingraham, John L., & Ingraham, Catherine A. *Introduction to Microbiology: A Case-History Study Approach,* 3rd ed. Belmont, CA: Brooks/Cole, Cengage Learning.

Special Focus

Basics of Hand Washing

Arguably, the easiest, most cost-effective way to prevent the spread of infection is hand washing. However, there is a correct way to wash your hands:

■ Remove all jewelry from your hands.
■ Crank out enough paper towel to dry your hands, but don't tear it off.
■ Turn on the water as hot as tolerable.
■ Wet hands and apply soap.
■ Work the soapy water over your hands, between fingers and around nails.

■ Continue this action for at least 25 to 30 seconds (enough time to sing "Happy Birthday to You" or "Row, Row, Row Your Boat" twice).
■ Rinse with water, positioning your hands so the water flows from above the wrists, downward over the hands and then the fingers.
■ Tear off the paper towel, and dry hands.
■ Use the paper towel to turn off the water.
■ Discard the towel into the trash can.
■ See Figure 29-7 for the proper hand washing procedure.

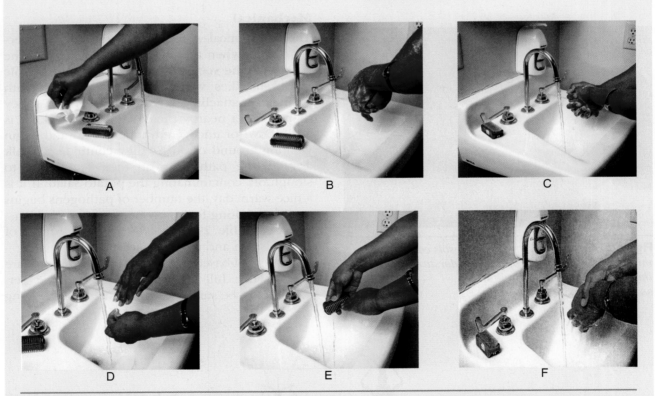

Figure 29-7 *Proper technique for hand washing. (A) Use a dry towel to turn the faucet on. (B) Point the fingertips downward and use the palm of one hand to clean the back of the other hand. (C) Interlace the fingers to clean between the fingers. (D) The blunt end of an orange stick can be used to clean the nails. (E) A hand brush can also be used to clean the nails. (F) With the fingertips pointing downward, rinse the hands thoroughly.*

Source: Delmar/Cengage Learning

TABLE 29-4
Routes of Transmission with Their Related Diseases

ROUTES OF TRANSMISSION	DISEASE EXAMPLES
Respiratory droplets	Pertussis, pneumonia, measles

Fomites
   Facial tissues, household surfaces
   Eating utensils
   Contaminated needles
	Common cold
	
	Typhoid
	HIV infection

Direct contact	Gonorrhea, herpes virus infections, syphilis, AIDS
Fecal-oral	Cholera, viral gastroenteritis, hepatitis A, giardiasis

Vectors
   Mechanical
   Biological
	Cholera, typhoid
	Malaria, yellow fever

Airborne	Tuberculosis, San Joaquin Valley fever
Parenteral By injection	Tetanus; gas gangrene *Hepatitis B, HIV infection*

Source: Ingraham, John L., & Ingraham, Catherine A. *Introduction to Microbiology: A Case-History Study Approach,* 3rd ed. Belmont, CA: Brooks/Cole, Cengage Learning.

action as described below. Continue that action until the sanitizer has evaporated and your hands are dry. See Figure 29-8.

Cover Your Mouth!

Another simple and effective way to prevent the spread of pathogens is to cover your mouth when coughing or sneezing. In the past it was suggested that you cover your mouth with your hand. This, however, is somewhat counterproductive, especially if you cover a sneeze with your hand and then shake someone else's hand, turn a door knob, or pick up a ketchup bottle to squeeze some on your fries. You've just spread the pathogens that your hand captured! It is better to use a tissue or cough/sneeze into the crook of your elbow if no tissue is available.

Personal Protective Devices and When to Use Them

Personal protective equipment (PPE) is a general term for clothing or equipment individuals use to protect their eyes, mucous membranes, skin, respiratory system, and clothing from exposure to hazardous/infectious agents. A type of PPE can be as simple as hospital gloves or as complex as a complete Hazmat suit. The Clinical Relevancy section will provide examples of which types of PPE to use in different situations.

QUOTES & NOTES

It is important to consider all blood and body fluid to be potentially infected. During the early stages of a disease, many people are unaware that they are even infected because signs and symptoms may not be present.

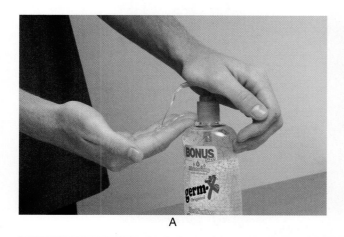

A

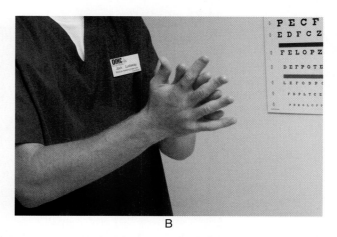

B

Figure 29-8 *Using alcohol-based, antiseptic hand sanitizers. (A) Apply the appropriate amount of alcohol-based hand rub. (B) Rub your hands together until all the hand rub is absorbed/evaporated. Be sure to rub between your fingers.*

Clinical Relevancy

Special Patient Precautions

Special precautions have been established to decrease the chances of contamination of yourself and the cross-contamination of patients under your care. The Centers for Disease Control have created several precaution guidelines that should be taken with all patient contact and in specific situations when certain infective agents are present.

Standard Precautions

Standard precautions are used to protect yourself and patients and should be utilized whenever there is a possible exposure to blood, body fluids, or any other excretions from any patient or equipment. These precautions include the following activities:

- Wash your hands before and after patient contact, after glove removal.
- Place used and unused sharps in a sharps container. Do NOT recap needles.
- Bag linens at the bedside if they are saturated with any body fluids.

- Discard all items that are saturated, dripping, or caked with human blood or infectious body fluids in an infectious waste bag (red in color).

In addition, you should use the following personal protective equipment (PPE):

- *Gloves* when touching blood, body fluids, mucous membranes, or contaminated medical equipment
- *Gowns* to protect your skin and clothing during any activity that may generate splashes or sprays of blood, body fluids, secretions, or excretions
- *Masks* and *eye protection* (or *face shields*) to protect your eyes, nose, and mouth during any activity that could cause a splash, of blood, body fluids, secretions, or excretions

See Figure 29-9 for some examples of PPE. Note that the types of PPE to be used will vary in different situations. Also review the standard precautions chart in Figure 29-10.

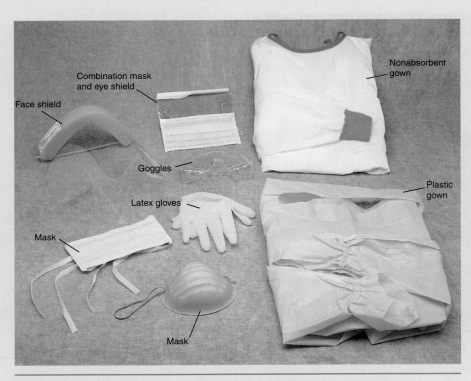

Figure 29-9 *Examples of personal protective equipment (PPE).*

(continues)

(continued)

STANDARD PRECAUTIONS

Assume that every person is potentially infected or colonized with an organism that could be transmitted in the healthcare setting.

Hand Hygiene

Avoid unnecessary touching of surfaces in close proximity to the patient.

When hands are visibly dirty, contaminated with proteinaceous material, or visibly soiled with blood or body fluids, wash hands with soap and water.

If hands are not visibly soiled, or after removing visible material with soap and water, decontaminate hands with an alcohol-based hand rub. Alternatively, hands may be washed with an antimicrobial soap and water.

Perform hand hygiene:
    Before having direct contact with patients.
    After contact with blood, body fluids or excretions, mucous membranes, nonintact skin, or wound dressings.
    After contact with a patient's intact skin (e.g., when taking a pulse or blood pressure or lifting a patient).
    If hands will be moving from a contaminated-body site to a clean-body site during patient care.
    After contact with inanimate objects (including medical equipment) in the immediate vicinity of the patient.
    After removing gloves.

Personal protective equipment (PPE)

Wear PPE when the nature of the anticipated patient interaction indicates that contact with blood or body fluids may occur.

Before leaving the patient's room or cubicle, remove and discard PPE.

Gloves

Wear gloves when contact with blood or other potentially infectious materials, mucous membranes, nonintact skin, or potentially contaminated intact skin (e.g., of a patient incontinent of stool or urine) could occur.

Remove gloves after contact with a patient and/or the surrounding environment using proper technique to prevent hand contamination. Do not wear the same pair of gloves for the care of more than one patient.

Change gloves during patient care if the hands will move from a contaminated body-site (e.g., perineal area) to a clean body-site (e.g., face).

Gowns

Wear a gown to protect skin and prevent soiling or contamination of clothing during procedures and patient-care activities when contact with blood, body fluids, secretions, or excretions is anticipated.

Wear a gown for direct patient contact if the patient has uncontained secretions or excretions.

Remove gown and perform hand hygiene before leaving the patient's environment.

Mouth, nose, eye protection

Use PPE to protect the mucous membranes of the eyes, nose and mouth during procedures and patient-care activities that are likely to generate splashes or sprays of blood, body fluids, secretions and excretions.

During aerosol-generating procedures wear one of the following: a face shield that fully covers the front and sides of the face, a mask with attached shield, or a mask and goggles.

Respiratory Hygiene/Cough Etiquette

Educate healthcare personnel to contain respiratory secretions to prevent droplet and fomite transmission of respiratory pathogens, especially during seasonal outbreaks of viral respiratory tract infections.

Offer masks to coughing patients and other symptomatic persons (e.g., persons who accompany ill patients) upon entry into the facility.

Patient-care equipment and instruments/devices

Wear PPE (e.g., gloves, gown), according to the level of anticipated contamination, when handling patient-care equipment and instruments/devices that are visibly soiled or may have been in contact with blood or body fluids.

Care of the environment

Include multi-use electronic equipment in policies and procedures for preventing contamination and for cleaning and disinfection, especially those items that are used by patients, those used during delivery of patient care, and mobile devices that are moved in and out of patient rooms frequently (e.g., daily).

Textiles and laundry

Handle used textiles and fabrics with minimum agitation to avoid contamination of air, surfaces and persons.

SPR

©2007 Brevis Corporation www.brevis.com

Figure 29-10 *Standard precautions for infection control.*

Source: Reprinted with permission from Brevis Corporation, www.brevis.com.

(continues)

(continued)

Contact Precautions

These precautions are instituted when there is a possibility of the transmission of pathogens by body-to-body contact. Utilize standard precautions plus the following additional precautions. Usually a private room should be used, although a multiple-patient room can be used if all patients have the same condition. Equipment should be dedicated to the individual patient during his or her length of stay. Any equipment removed from the room must be properly disinfected. Personal protective equipment used includes:

- *Gloves* when entering the room
- *Gowns* for any direct contact with the patient, environmental surfaces, or any equipment in the room

Airborne Precautions

When there is a concern about a possibility for pathogen transmission by droplet spread or by dust particles, initiate standard precautions plus the following procedures. Place the patient in a negative-pressure room and keep the door closed. That way no air will escape into the hall or other rooms. Your personal protective equipment will include:

- Mask, an N95 HEPA-filtered mask must be put on before entering the room. If the patient has chickenpox or measles and you are immune to those diseases, the mask is not necessary.

See figure 29-11 for an example for an N95 mask.

Droplet Precautions

Patients warranting this form of precaution are known to or are suspected of having a serious illness that is easily spread by large particle droplets (e.g., pneumonia, influenza, meningitis). Use standard precautions, plus use a private room

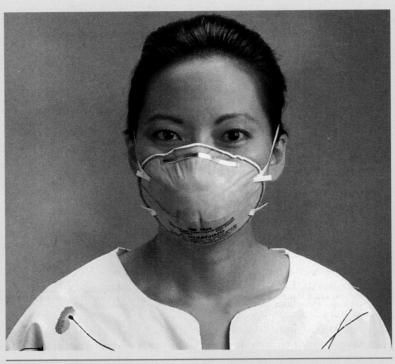

Figure 29-11   *Example of the N95 respirator mask.*
Source: Courtesy of 3M Company, St. Paul, MN.

(continues)

(continued)

or a multiple-patient room if all patients exhibit the same condition. The door to the room may be kept open. Utilize the following personal protective equipment:

■ Wear a surgical mask when entering a patient's room.

See Figure 29-12 for droplet precautions.

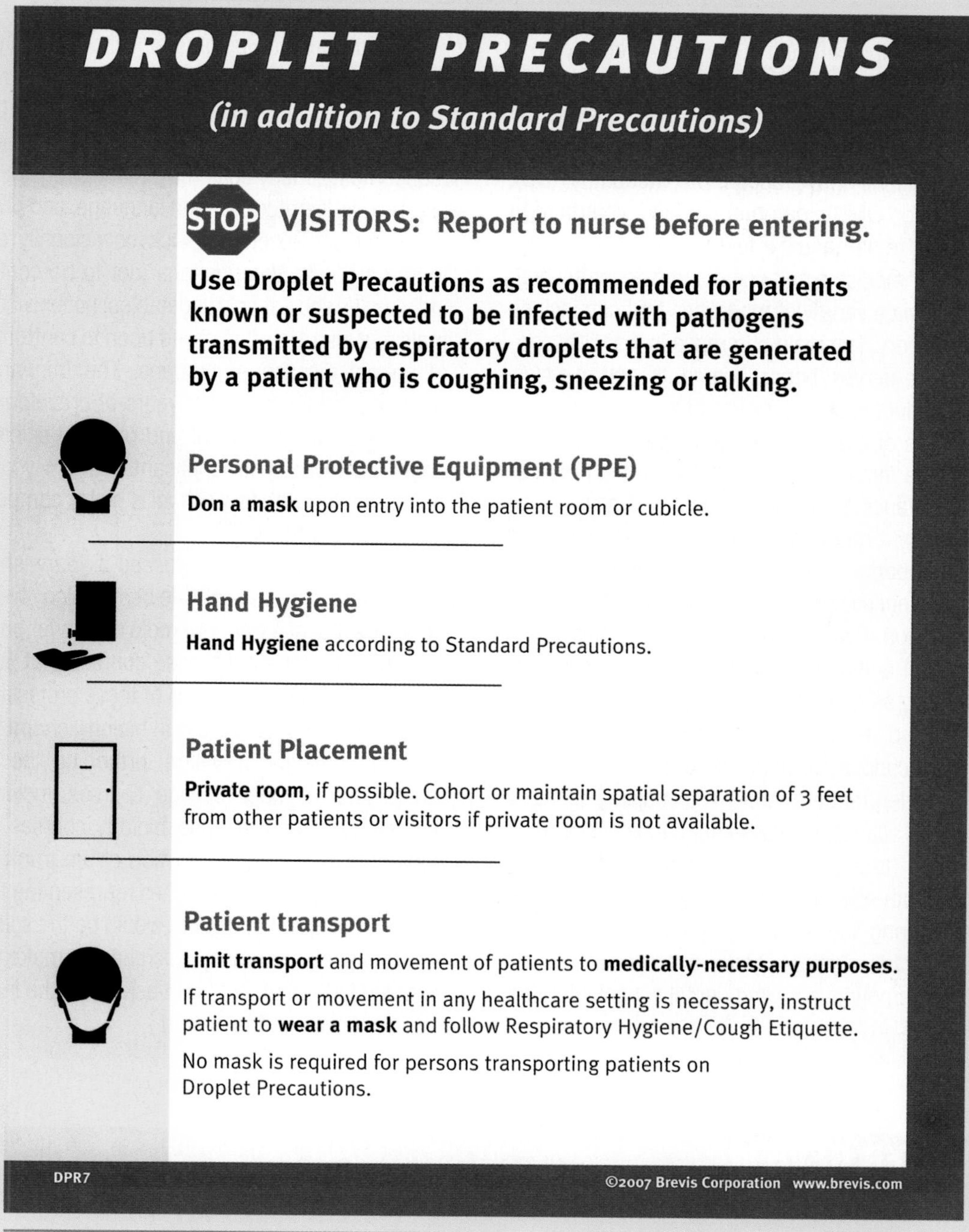

DROPLET PRECAUTIONS

(in addition to Standard Precautions)

STOP **VISITORS: Report to nurse before entering.**

Use Droplet Precautions as recommended for patients known or suspected to be infected with pathogens transmitted by respiratory droplets that are generated by a patient who is coughing, sneezing or talking.

Personal Protective Equipment (PPE)

Don a mask upon entry into the patient room or cubicle.

Hand Hygiene

Hand Hygiene according to Standard Precautions.

Patient Placement

Private room, if possible. Cohort or maintain spatial separation of 3 feet from other patients or visitors if private room is not available.

Patient transport

Limit transport and movement of patients to **medically-necessary purposes**.

If transport or movement in any healthcare setting is necessary, instruct patient to **wear a mask** and follow Respiratory Hygiene/Cough Etiquette.

No mask is required for persons transporting patients on Droplet Precautions.

DPR7

©2007 Brevis Corporation   www.brevis.com

Figure 29-12 *Droplet precautions.*

Source: Reprinted with permission from Brevis Corporation, www.brevis.com.

Professional Profile

Health Careers Requiring Postgraduate Degrees

While many health professions can be entered with a 2- or 4-year college degree, you may be interested in pursuing a career that requires a degree followed by advanced (postgraduate) study. These careers include doctor of medicine (MD), doctor of osteopathy (DO), dentist (DDS or DMD), optometrist, and veterinarian (DMV or VMD), to name just a few.

Doctors of medicine and doctors of osteopathy both treat patients via a variety of modalities that can include drugs and surgery. The main difference is that DOs concentrate on the nerves, bones, ligaments, and muscles. Both types of doctor can specialize in a variety of fields. Required areas of study when pursuing undergraduate work (usually a minimum of 3 years' worth) in preparation for acceptance to medical school typically include English, biology, organic and inorganic chemistry, and physics. It is important to note that courses in the humanities, social sciences, and mathematics are very important to make you a well-rounded student. Admission to medical school is highly competitive. Grade average is very important, as is your personality, including leadership abilities and, especially, self-motivation.

Dentistry candidates must perform a minimum of 3 years of undergraduate work. The majority of those entering dental school possess either bachelor's or master's degrees. Undergraduate courses should include those from both the sciences and humanities. Areas considered during the admission process can include your overall grade average, grade average for science courses, recommendations, and dental school interview results.

Candidates for optometry school usually need to complete at least 2 years of undergraduate work. Most optometry students have bachelor's degrees, however. It is interesting to note that in addition to the usual course requirements, many optometry schools require courses in psychology, literature, foreign language, and philosophy.

Even old Rover gets sick occasionally and needs to see a doctor. Veterinarians (not to be confused with individuals who eat only vegetables) not only care for animals, but also are often called upon to control the spread of animal disease to humans. The minimum undergraduate requirement is 2 years of preveterinary study focusing on the biological and physical sciences. Once again, however, most applicants have 4-year degrees. Admission to veterinary school is highly competitive—so keep your grades up!

So, how should you proceed if you wish to pursue one of these professions? The best analogy we can come up with is that of a tree. The roots and lower portion of the tree trunk represent the base courses that you need—those that are common to all of these professions. These include high school courses in biology, chemistry, health, and mathematics. Traveling further up the trunk, you would find the base college courses, including physics, various chemistry and biology courses, and math courses. The uppermost portion of the trunk before the tree branches out (the branches representing the courses in your profession of choice) would be the social science and humanities courses, which help to make you a well-rounded individual. But don't ask about the leaves—this analogy occurs in the winter!

■ CHAPTER REVIEW

Exercises

1. Match the following terms with their meanings:

_____ contamination

_____ infection

_____ inflammation

a. a generalized tissue reaction to injury

b. presence of microorganisms without tissue reaction

c. presence of microorganism with tissue reaction

2. Differentiate vegetative organisms and spores.

3. Contrast the following levels of disinfectants: low level, intermediate level, and high level.

4. List and describe the variables that determine the effectiveness of a disinfectant.

5. List three portals of entry and typical diseases that can be found in each region.

6. Give three examples of how to break the chain of infection.

7. List the steps in the proper hand washing technique.

8. Select three PPE devices and describe their usage.

9. Describe the before care, during care, and aftercare droplet precaution activities for a patient with infectious pneumonia.

Real Life Issues and Applications

Initiating Patient Precautions

A patient presents in the Emergency Department with the following signs/symptoms:

- Productive cough with occasional hemoptysis
- Recent weight loss
- Low grade fever with "night sweats"
- SOB
- Lethargy
- A recent Mantoux test that was positive. A second test was performed with the same results.

This patient states that she toured several Southeast Asian countries about 7 months ago. Sputum samples for culture and sensitivity are obtained from the patient, and she is admitted to the hospital. From the information you have been provided and any other research you may conduct, what patient precautions do you think should be initiated? Justify your answer.

Additional Activities

1. Invite the head of your local hospital's infection control department to your class to speak on his or her various responsibilities, methods for monitoring and controlling nosocomial infections, trends in patient infections, and the importance of his or her job in relationship to the patients and the hospital organization.

2. Invite the head of the local Health Department to your class to discuss preparedness for major influenza outbreaks, pandemic preparation, and the department's monitoring and reporting procedures.

StudyWARE CONNECTION

Go to your StudyWARE™ DVD and have fun learning as you play interactive games, view animations and videos, and take practice tests to help reinforce key concepts you learned in this chapter.

Workbook Practice *Go to your Workbook for more practice questions and activities.*

GLOSSARY

abdominal (ab-**DOM**-ih-nal).   Pertaining to (*al*) the stomach (*abdomen*).

abduction (ab-**DUCK**-shun).   Movement away (*ab*) from the body, such as in raising your arm away from your side.

absolute humidity.   The actual weight of the water present in a given amount of gas.

absolute temperature.   A measure of temperature based on the Kelvin temperature scale.

absolute zero.   The theoretical temperature at which there is a cessation of molecular movement.

acceleration.   The rate of change in speed.

accessory muscles.   Additional muscles utilized when the normal muscles of breathing are inadequate for the body's needs.

acetic acid.   The chemical name for vinegar.

acetylcholine (ACh) (as-eh-till-**KOH**-leen).   A substance vital to the transmission of nerve impulses at synaptic areas and at myoneural junctions.

acetylcholinesterase (AChE) (as-eh-till-**KOH**-lin-**ESS**-ter-ase).   An enzyme that stops the action caused by acetylcholine.

acid.   A substance that produces hydrogen ions in solution.

acid-base indicators.   Materials that are used to identify the pH of a substance.

acidosis.   A blood condition characterized by lower-than-normal pH.

acid-fast (Zeil-Neelsen) stain.   Staining technique to diagnose tuberculosis and leprosy.

acrocyanosis (ak-roh-**sigh**-ah-**NO**-sis).   A condition (*osis*) when the extremities (*acro*) of the body turn blue (*cyan/o*).

acromegaly (ack-roh-**MEG**-ah-lee).   A disease condition wherein the extremities (*acro*) become enlarged (*mega*) as a result of increased function of the pituitary gland after puberty.

action potential.   The term used to describe the change in electrical potential of nerves or muscle fibers when they are stimulated.

activation energy.   The amount of energy required to start a reaction.

activator.   A metal ion cofactor.

active site.   The region on the enzyme where catalytic reaction takes place.

acute disease.   A disease that is usually severe but short in duration.

acute kidney failure.   A condition wherein the kidneys are unable to properly excrete urine; also known as *renal failure*.

adaptation.   The adjustment an organism makes as a result of a change in its environment.

Addison's disease.   A condition of either partial or complete failure of adrenocortical function; can be fatal.

adduction (add-**DUCK**-shun).   Movement toward (*ad*) the body, such as in lowering a raised arm to your side.

adenoids (**AD**-eh-noids).   Lymphatic structures located in the upper portions of the nose and throat; also known as *nasopharyngeal tonsils*.

adhesive forces.   Forces of attraction between unlike particles.

adrenal cortex (ah-**DREE**-nal).   The outer portion of the adrenal gland; secretes the steroid hormones mineralcorticoids, glucocorticoids, and androgens.

adrenal glands (ah-**DREE**-nal).   The structures that secrete a variety of substances that control body system functions.

adrenocorticotropic hormone (ACTH) (ad-**REE**-no-**kor**-te-koh-**trawp**-ick).   A pituitary hormone that stimulates the adrenal cortex to secrete adrenal cortical hormones.

aerobic (er-**OH**-bick).   Taking place in the presence of oxygen.

aerobic bacteria.   A form of bacteria that requires oxygen to survive.

aldosterone (al-**DOS**-ter-own).   A hormone needed to regulate the amounts of sodium, chloride, and potassium in the body.

alimentary canal (al-ih-**MEN**-tair-ee).   A general term for the digestive system (and no relation to the Erie Canal!).

alkalosis.   A blood condition characterized by higher-than-normal pH.

alkane. Straight or branched-chain hydrocarbon compound wherein the carbon atoms are joined by single covalent bonds.

alkene. Straight or branched-chain hydrocarbon compound wherein at least two carbon atoms are joined by a double covalent bond.

alkyne. Straight or branched-chain hydrocarbon compound wherein at least two of the carbon atoms are joined by a triple covalent bond.

alpha cells. Cells that are located in the islands of Langerhans (the authors' favorite vacation spot) and that produce glucagon, which aids in maintaining normal glucose levels in the body.

alpha radiation. The radiation produced by helium nuclei.

alveoli (al-**VEE**-oh-lye). Air sacs located in the lungs and surrounded by a capillary network; where the act of respiration occurs.

amblyopia (am-blee-**OH**-pee-ah). Reduced or dimmed (*ambly/o*) vision not caused by an organic lesion of the eye.

amino acid (ah-**ME**-no). An organic compound used to make protein.

amplitude. The highest displacement from zero achieved by a wave.

amylopectin. A type of starch having a branched structure.

amylase (**AM**-eh-lace). Enzymes that break down starches.

amylose. A type of starch having a linear structure.

anabolic steroids. A class of steroids that stimulate body growth but that can lead to dangerous side effects.

anaerobic (an-er-**OH**-bick). Relating to a non-oxygen environment.

anaerobic bacteria. A form of bacteria that does not require oxygen to survive.

anatomy (ah-**NAT**-oh-me). The study of the form and structure of an organism.

anemia (uh-**NEE**-me-uh). Condition characterized by a deficiency in the number of red blood cells.

angina (an-**JIGH**-nah). A general term that usually refers to chest pain or discomfort resulting from a reduction in the amount of oxygen supplied to the heart muscle.

angina pectoris (an-**JIGH**-nah peck-**TORE**-is). The medical term for chest pain of cardiac origin.

angle of incidence. The angle between a ray of light and a line perpendicular to the surface struck by the ray of light.

angle of reflection. Angle between a reflected light ray and an imaginary line perpendicular to the surface from which the ray is reflected.

anion. A negatively charged ion.

anterior (an-**TEER**-ee-or). Pertaining to the front (*anter/o*).

anterior lobe. That portion of the pituitary gland also known as the *adenohypophysis*.

antibiotic. A chemotherapeutic substance that kills or prevents microorganism growth.

antibodies. Substances created by the body to combat harmful or potentially harmful substances (such as bacteria and viruses).

antidiuretic hormone (ADH). Substance that is produced by the pituitary gland and regulates the body's water balance by reducing urine output; also known as a *vasopressin*.

antipyretics. Chemicals that reduce fever.

antitussive. A medicine that prevents coughing.

anuria (an-**YOU**-ree-ah). A condition characterized by either no creation of urine or an inability to urinate; also known as *anuresis*.

anvil (**AN**-vil). A small bone found in the middle ear; also known as the *incus* (**IN**-kus).

aorta (ay-**OR**-tah). The largest artery in the body; originates at the left ventricle and eventually branches out to all parts of the body.

aortic valve (ay-**OR**-tick). A semilunar (that is, shaped like a half moon) valve positioned between the aorta and the left ventricle of the heart.

aphasia (ah-**FAY**-zee-ah). A condition resulting from brain damage and characterized by an inability to speak or write or to understand what is written or what is said (*a* meaning "not," *phasia* meaning "speak").

apoenzyme. The protein portion of an enzyme.

apoplexy (**AP**-oh-pleck-see). *See* **cerebrovascular accident.**

appendix (ah-**PEN**-dix). A structure located near the cecum.

aqueous humor. A watery substance that fills the eye (*aque/o* meaning "water," *humor* meaning "clear body liquid"); do not confuse this with "funny water."

arachnoid membrane (ah-**RACK**-noid). The second layer surrounding the brain and spinal cord.

arterial (ar-**TEER**-ree-al). Pertaining to the arteries (*arteri/o*), the vessels that carry oxygen-rich blood from the heart to all parts of the body.

arteries. Blood vessels that carry blood *away* from the heart (think *a*rteries and *a*way).

arterioles (ar-**TEER**-ee-ohlz). The smaller branches of the arteries; supply blood to the capillaries.

arteriosclerosis. Hardening of the arterial walls.

articular cartilage (ar-**TICK**-you-ler). Cartilage that covers bone surfaces where joints occur, such as at the knees.

articulation (ar-**TICK**-you-lay-shun). Another name for a joint (*arthr/o*).

asexual reproduction. Identical replication of the cell without the involvement of another cell.

associative neurons. Neurons that carry impulses from one neuron to another; also known as *connecting neurons*.

asthma (**AZ**-mah). A condition of the airways characterized by bronchospasm, increased mucous secretion, and blocked airways leading to gas trapping.

astringents. Chemicals having the ability to shrink organic tissue.

ataxia (ah-**TACK**-see-ah). A condition characterized by lack (*a* meaning "without") of muscle coordination (*tax/o*).

atelectasis (ah-tuh-**LEK**-tah-sis). A lung condition characterized by varying degrees of alveolar sac collapse.

atherosclerosis (ath-er-oh-skleh-**ROH**-sis). A condition characterized by decreased blood flow through the blood vessels as a result of plaque build-up; commonly referred to as hardening of the arteries.

atom. The smallest particle of an element.

atomic number. The number of protons in the nucleus of an atom.

ATPS. An environmental condition wherein there is *a*mbient *t*emperature (room temperature), *p*ressure (the current barometric pressure), and *s*aturation with water vapor (at that particular room temperature).

atria (**AY**-tree-ah). Singular, *atrium*; the upper chambers of the heart that act as blood-receiving chambers before the blood goes to the ventricles.

atrioventricular node (ay-tree-oh-ven-**TRICK**-you-lahr). The region of the heart that transmits electrical impulses to the bundle of HIS, thus allowing for the contraction of the ventricles; also known as the *AV node*.

atrium (**AY**-tree-um). Upper chamber of each side of the heart.

atrophy (**AH**-troh-fee). The wasting away of tissue or an organ often because of disuse (*a* meaning "without," *troph/o* meaning "growth").

auditory nerve. Nerve that transmits vibrations to the auditory center of the cerebral cortex (*audit/o* meaning "ear," "hearing," or "sense of hearing").

auricle (**AW**-reh-kul). The outer structure of the ear not located within the head (*aur/i* meaning "ear" or "hearing"); also known as the external ear, or *pinna* (*pinn/i* meaning "external ear").

autoclave. A device using steam and pressure to sterilize equipment.

autonomic nerves. Sometimes referred to as the *peripheral nervous system*; composed of two divisions, the sympathetic division and the parasympathetic division, that act to balance each other and maintain homeostasis in the body.

average. A method of referring to the center of a set of values.

Avogadro's law (av-oh-**GAH**-droe). Gas law stating that at any given temperature and pressure, equal volumes of all gases contain equal numbers of molecules (6.02×10^{23}).

Avogadro's number (av-oh-**GAH**-droe). The number of particles in one mole of a substance (that is, 6.02×10^{23}).

axon (**ACK**-son). Nerve cell structure that extends away from the cell body and conducts impulses away from that cell body (*ax/o* meaning "mainstem").

bacilli (bah-**SILL**-eye). A rod-shaped bacteria.

bactericidal. Agent that actively kills bacteria.

bacteriology (back-**TEER**-ih-**ol**-oh-jee). The study of (*ology*) bacteria.

bacteriostatic. Agent that inhibits the growth and replication of microorganisms but does not destroy them.

bar graph. A method of representing data using bars.

barometer. A device used to measure barometric pressure.

barometric pressure. The pressure or force exerted by the atmosphere.

Bartholin's glands. Mucus-secreting glands that are located on either side of the vaginal opening and provide lubrication.

base. Either a substance that produces hydroxide ions in solution or the number being multiplied in an exponential expression—or a foundation on which to build … or what you steal in baseball … or where military personnel work … or where you are safe in a children's game.

benign prostatic hypertrophy (BPH) (bee-**NINE PRO**-stat-ic high-**PER**-troh-fee). Abnormal enlargement of the prostrate gland.

beta cells. Cells that are found in the islands of Langerhans and produce insulin, which is needed for the utilization of glucose in the body.

beta radiation. The radiation produced by fast-moving electrons.

bile. A digestive juice manufactured by the liver.

binary fission. The normal reproductive process of bacteria.

body planes. Imaginary divisions of the body; used to describe locations of organs or conditions.

bolus. A mass of chewed food waiting to be swallowed.

Boyle's law. Gas law stating that if the temperature of a gas remains constant, the volume of the gas will vary inversely to the pressure of the gas. Thus, if the volume of a given gas increases, the pressure of the gas decreases.

brachial plexus (**BRAY**-kee-all **PLECK**-sus). One of the four main networks (*plex/o*; *plexi*, plural) of intersecting nerves. The other three networks are the *cervical plexus, lumbar plexus,* and *sacral plexus.*

bradycardia (**braid**-ee-**KAR**-dee-ah). A slow (*brady*) heart (*cardia*) rate (usually less than 60 beats per minute).

brain. Given that you have one, you probably do not need a definition; however, this is the organ that regulates and coordinates all activities in the body.

broad-spectrum drug. An antibiotic that is effective against a wide range of organisms.

bronchi (**BRON**-kye). Singular, *bronchus*; divisions of the main airways to the right and left lungs, which further branch out into smaller and smaller airways once in the lungs.

bronchiectasis (**bron**-kee-**ECK**-tah-sis). A condition characterized by irreversible dilation and injury to the bronchial wall (*ectasis* meaning "stretching" or "enlargement").

bronchioles (**BRON**-kee-ohlz). The smallest branches of the bronchi.

bronchitis (bron-**KYE**-tis). Inflammation of the bronchi.

bronchospasm (**BRON**-ko-spazm). Constriction and spasm of the smooth muscles of the airways.

broth dilution. A test used to determine bacterial sensitivity to an antibiotic and ideal dosing.

BTPS. An environmental condition wherein there is *b*ody *t*emperature (37°C), *p*ressure (barometric), and *s*aturation with water vapor at that given temperature.

buffer solution. A solution that will maintain a constant pH.

bulbourethral glands (**bol**-boh-you-**REE**-thral). Mucus-secreting glands that are located just below the prostate gland and provide lubrication; also known as *Cowper's glands.*

bundle of HIS (HISS). A group of nerves that carry impulses to the left and right ventricles of the heart, thus stimulating the ventricles to pump blood.

bursa (**BER**-sah). A sac found between certain tendons and bones; provides a cushion between bones; contains synovial fluid.

calcitonin. A hormone that is produced by the thyroid gland and aids in the regulation of calcium levels in the blood and tissues.

calculi (**KAL**-q-lye). Singular, *calculus*; a "stone" formed in the body from mineral salts.

capillaries. The microscopic blood vessels that allow for the exchange of oxygen, nutrients, and waste products between the tissues and the blood.

capillarity. A form of adhesive and capillary force that allows a fluid to rise up a tube having a small diameter.

capillary action. *See* **capillarity.**

capsid. A protective protein coat surrounding a virus.

capsule. The protective covering around a cell wall of certain bacteria.

carbohydrates. The class of nutrients that includes sugars, glycogen, and starches.

cardiac arrhythmias. Abnormal electrical patterns of the heart

cardiac cycle. The period of time beginning with the contraction of the atria and ending when the atria fill again with blood for the next contraction.

cardiac muscle. The special type of muscle that composes the heart walls and, through contraction, causes the heart to beat; also known as *myocardium* (*myo* meaning "muscle," *cardi/o* meaning "heart").

cardiac valve. The ring of muscle that surrounds the opening to the stomach and controls the flow of material between the esophagus and the stomach; often referred to as the *cardiac sphincter*.

cardiology (**kar**-dee-**OL**-oh-jee). The study of (*ology*) the heart (*cardi*).

cardiopulmonary. Pertaining to the respiratory and cardiac systems, and specifically, to gas exchange between the lungs and blood system.

cardiovascular (**kar**-dee-oh-**VAS**-kyou-lar). Pertaining to the heart and blood vessels.

cardiovascular system. The system that contains the heart (*cardi/o*) and all the blood vessels (*vascul/o*) that transports blood from the heart to the body and back again to the heart.

carina (kuh-**RINE**-uh). The area where the main airway bifurcates into the right and left mainstem bronchi.

cartilage (**KAR**-tih-lidj). Flexible and somewhat elastic connecting tissue. Some cartilage forms a protective cover for bone, while other cartilage provides form such as the tip of the nose.

catalyst. A substance that affects the rate of a reaction but is not itself consumed in the reaction.

cataract (**KAT**-a-rack). A pathological condition wherein the lens of the eye becomes opaque—not to be confused with a medieval feline torture device.

cation. A positively charged ion.

caudal (**KAWD**-al). Pertaining to, or towards the tail.

caustic. A strong alkali that is highly corrosive or burning in nature.

cavity. An opening or space.

cell body. Nerve cell portion that contains the nucleus.

cells (**SELLZ**). The individual building blocks of the body.

cellulose. The most abundant polysaccharide.

Celsius temperature scale. Temperature scale wherein 0 represents the freezing point of water and 1008 the boiling point.

centi. Prefix used in the metric system to mean times 10 to the power of 2 (10^2).

central chemoreceptors. Specialized brain cells that react to chemical stimuli.

central cyanosis. A condition (*osis*) wherein the central portion of the body (trunk and neck, for example) become blue (*cyan/o*).

central nervous system (CNS). The brain and spinal cord, and their nerves and end organs; controls voluntary and involuntary acts including mental activities.

central processing unit (CPU). That part of a computer that performs various operations when it receives data.

centriole (**SEN**-tree-ol). Organelles involved in cell division.

centrosome (**SEN**-tro-sohm). The area of a cell's cytoplasm that contains centrioles.

cerebellum (**ser**-eh-**BELL**-um). The second largest portion of the brain; responsible for coordinating voluntary activities as well as maintaining balance and correct muscle tone.

cerebral cortex (seh-**REE**-brawl). The outer portion of the cerebrum.

cerebrospinal fluid (CSF) (sir-**ee**-broh-**SPY**-nal). A clear, watery liquid that flows throughout the brain and spinal column, acting as a shock absorber and cushion to protect the brain and spinal cord from injury.

cerebrovascular accident (CVA) (**ser**-eh-bro-**VAS**-kyou-lar). Condition that occurs when blood flow is suddenly shut off from a portion of the brain; commonly known as a *stroke*, or *apoplexy*.

cerumen (see-**ROO**-men). Ear wax.

ceruminous glands (see-**ROO**-men-us). Modified sweat glands in the external auditory canal that produce cerumen (ear wax).

cervical plexus (**SER**-vih-kal). A network of intersecting nerves located in the neck (*cervic/o*) area.

chain of infection. Cycle or pathway of infection that can be broken at various points to stop the spread.

Charles' law. A gas law stating that if the mass and pressure of a gas remain constant, the volume and temperature of the gas will relate directly.

chlorine. A highly irritating poisonous gas that is a bleaching agent and germicidal.

cholesterol (koh-**LESS**-ter-ol). A sterol widely distributed in animal tissue important to body metabolism and a precursor to various steroid hormones in the body.

choroid (**KOH**-roid). The opaque middle layer of the eyeball; contains blood vessels; also known as the *choroid layer* or *choroid coat*.

choroid plexus (**KOH**-roid). That structure within the ventricles of the brain that manufactures cerebrospinal fluid.

chromatin (**KRO**-mah-tin). A substance found in chromosomes.

chromosome (**KROH**-moh-sohm). That part of a cell containing genetic information; also known as a *gene.*

chronic bronchitis. A long-term pulmonary disease characterized by productive cough, airway inflammation and airway obstruction.

chronic disease. A disease that occurs or reoccurs over a long period of time.

chronic renal failure. An ongoing or constantly occurring condition wherein the kidneys are unable to properly excrete urine.

chyme (**KYM**). Partly digested, semifluid food.

cicatrix (sih-**KAY**-tricks). The scarring normally found in a healing wound.

cilia (**SIL**-ee-ah). Microscopic hairs found in the airways; act as oars to move the mucous blanket toward the esophagus to be swallowed.

ciliary muscles (**SILL**-ee-air-ee). Muscles that adjust the thickness and shape of the eye lens.

circle graph. A method of representing data using a circle.

cleaning. The physical removal of all foreign matter such as dirt and blood.

clitoris (**KLIT**-oh-ris). A sensitive, erectile female organ located anterior to the vaginal opening.

cocci (**COCK**-sye). A round or spherical bacterial shape.

cochlea (**KOCK**-lee-ah). A spiral-shaped passage leading from the oval window of the ear (*cochle/o* meaning "snail" or "spiral").

coefficient. The leading factor in an algebraic expression.

coenzyme. A cofactor that is an organic compound.

cofactor. The nonprotein part of an enzyme.

cohesive forces. Forces of attraction between like particles.

combined gas law. A combination of Boyle's, Charles', and Gay-Lussac's gas laws wherein

$$\frac{P_1 V_1}{T_1} = \frac{P_2 V_2}{T_2}$$

combining form. A word root and a connecting vowel (for example, *path/o*).

comedo (blackhead) (**KOM**-ee-doh). Results from a buildup of sebum and keratin in the pores of the skin.

common denominator. A denominator that is the same in two or more fractions—or a denominator that is not of royal blood.

common fraction. An expression that represents the division of two quantities; usually used to indicate a part of a whole.

compact bone. Extremely hard, dense, and strong bone; forms the outer layer on the bones; also called *cortical bone.*

complete protein. A protein containing all the essential amino acids in the proper amounts.

compound. Two or more elements joined by a chemical bond.

compound words. Words made by combining more than one word root.

computerized tomography (CT). Radiologic imaging technique that takes pictures of extremely thin "slices" of the body, thus providing a three-dimensional picture as opposed to a flat, one-dimensional X-ray.

conchae (**KON**-kay). Nose structures that cause turbulence of inhaled air, and aid in moistening and warming air; also known as *turbinates.*

conductivity. The ability to transmit an electrical impulse.

cones. Specialized, cone-shaped cells located in the retina; receive color stimuli.

congenital (kon-**JEN**-ih-tal). Having occurred before or at birth (*con* meaning "with" or "together," *genic* meaning "generation" or "production").

congestive heart failure (CHF). Heart condition characterized by the heart's inability to maintain adequate circulation as a result of infarction of the ventricles, retained sodium and water, or a variety of other disorders.

conjunctiva (kon-junk-**TYE**-vah). A mucous membrane that lines the inner side of the eyelid and covers the exposed surface of the eyeball.

conjunctivitis (kon-**junk**-tih-**VYE**-tis). An in-flammation (*itis*) of the conjunctiva.

connecting neurons. *See* **associative neurons.**

connective tissue. Tissue that holds the organs in place and keeps all the body parts together.

constant. A value that does not change in a mathematical problem.

contamination. The presence of microorganisms without tissue reaction.

contusion (kon-**TOO**-zhun).   An injury to the body characterized by possible pain, swelling, and discoloration but not by broken skin.

core temperature.   The temperature inside the body where the vital organs are located.

corpus callosum (**KOR**-pus kah-**LOW**-sum). Located in the major division between the hemispheres of the brain, structure that aids in communication between the left side and right side of the brain.

cortical bone (**KOR**-tee-call).   *See* **compact bone.**

cortisol (**KOR**-tih-sol).   A steroid hormone that regulates the amount of fat, protein, and carbohydrates in the cells of the body and acts as an anti-inflammatory agent; also called a *hydrocortisone*.

counting numbers.   *See* **natural numbers.**

covalent bond.   A chemical bond formed by the sharing of two or more electrons.

Cowper's glands.   *See* **bulbourethral glands.**

cramp.   A painful muscular contraction or spasm.

cranial (**KRAY**-nee-al).   Pertaining to the skull region.

cranial nerves.   The twelve pairs of nerves that originate in the brain.

crenation (cree-**NAY**-shun).   The shrinking of cells.

cretinism (**CREE**-tin-izm).   A condition characterized by retarded physical and mental growth resulting from a congenital lack of thyroid gland secretion.

cross-multiplying.   The method of solving proportions whereby the numerator of one fraction is multiplied by the denominator of the other fraction, and vice versa.

culture and sensitivity (C&S) test.   A test in which bacteria is grown for identification and the organism is exposed to various antibiotics to determine which is most effective for its treatment.

cyanosis (**sigh**-ah-**NO**-sis).   A condition (*osis*) wherein the skin appears blue (*cyan/o*).

cytologist (sigh-**TOL**-oh-jist).   One who studies (*ologist*) cells (*cyt/o*).

cytology (sigh-**TOL**-oh-jee).   The study of (*ology*) cells (*cyt/o*).

cytoplasm (**SIGH**-toh-plaz-im).   The formative substance (*plasm*) of a cell (*cyt/o*).

Dalton's law.   Gas law stating that each type of gas in a gas mixture will exert a partial pressure equal to its fractional concentration of the whole gas mixture.

data.   Facts—or the android on *Star Trek: The Next Generation*.

deca (da).   Prefix used in the metric system to mean times 10 to the power of 1 (10^1).

deci (d).   Prefix used in the metric system to mean times 10 to the power of negative 1 (10^{-1}).

decimal.   A means of representing a fraction having a denominator that is a power of ten (for example .10 for 1/10).

decontamination.   The process of the removal of contaminants by chemical or physical means.

denaturation.   The disorganization of a protein structure in such a manner as to render the protein incapable of performing its function.

dendrite.   Cell structure that resembles a root and receives impulses that it conducts to the cell body.

denominator.   The bottom part of a fraction; indicates the number of equal parts into which a whole is divided.

density.   The "compactness" of a material as determined by the masses of the particles that compose the material and the space between those particles.

deoxygenated (dee-**ok**-see-jen-**AY**-ted).   The act of removing part or all of the oxygen present.

deoxyribonucleic acid (DNA) (dee-**ok**-see-**RI**-bo-nu-**klee**-ik).   Chemical found in cells; determines hereditary characteristics.

dermatitis (**der**-mah-**TYE**-tis).   An inflammation (*itis*) of the skin (*dermat/o*).

dermatologist (**der**-mah-**TOL**-oh-jist).   One who studies (*ologist*) the skin (*dermat/o*).

dermis (**DER**-mis).   A term for skin (*derm/o*).

diabetes insipidus (dye-ah-**BEE**-teez).   A disease found most often in young patients and characterized by either a deficiency in the production of antidiuretic hormone (ADH) or an inability of the kidneys to respond to ADH. Symptoms include extreme thirst (polydipsia) and extreme urination (polyuria).

diabetes mellitus (dye-ah-**BEE**-teez).   Term used to describe a number of disorders that result in inadequate amounts of insulin.

diagnosis (dye-ag-**NO**-sis).   A determination of the nature of an illness.

diaphragm (**DYE**-eh-fram).   The primary breathing muscle of the body; located below the lungs.

diaphysis (dye-**AF**-ih-sis).   The shaft of a long bone.

diastole (dye-**AH**-stol-ee). Portion of the cardiac cycle when the ventricles are resting and blood pressure is, thus, at its lowest.

diencephalon (**die**-in-**SEF**-ah-lawn). The region of the brain that includes the thalamus and hypothalamus.

diffusion. The movement of a gas from an area of high concentration of that gas to an area of low concentration of that gas so that there is an equal concentration of the gas in all involved areas.

disaccharide (dye-**SACK**-eh-ride). A carbohydrate consisting of two monosaccharides bonded together.

disinfection. The elimination of vegetative, pathogenic microorganisms from an inanimate object.

disk diffusion. A classic lab test to determine the susceptibility of bacteria to a variety of antibiotics.

dislocation. When a bone is forced out of its normal position.

distal (**DIS**-tal). Away from (*dist/o*) a point of reference.

distributive law. A mathematical law that states $a(b + c) = ab + ac$.

diuretic (**die**-you-**RET**-ick). A substance that increases urination.

dorsal (**DOOR**-sal). Pertaining to the back (*dors/o*).

dorsal root ganglia. The cerebrospinal ganglia that contain the cell bodies of primary sensory nerves.

duodenum (**dew**-oh-**DEE**-num). The upper portion of the small intestine, just below the stomach.

dura mater (**DOO**-rah **MAY**-ter). The tough membrane that covers the outside of the meninges.

dwarfism. A disease that can be caused by hyposecretions of the pituitary gland and that is characterized by small, underdeveloped bones and normal mental development.

dysrhythmias (dis-**RITH**-me-ahs). Abnormal heart rhythms.

eardrum. The structure located between the middle ear and outer ear; also known as the *tympanic membrane.*

ecchymosis (eck-eh-**MOH**-sis). The black-and-blue mark a person receives when bumping into a hard object.

ejaculation (ee-**JACK**-you-**lay**-shun). The expulsion or ejection of semen. A typical ejaculation contains approximately 2–5 milliliters (mL) of semen, with each milliliter of semen containing 60–150 million sperm.

ejaculatory duct (ee-**JACK**-you-lah-**tor**-ree). A pathway that allows semen to pass to the urethra.

electrolytes (ee-**LEC**-trow-lites). Ions dissolved within the bloodstream and important to physiologic functioning.

electromagnetic radiation. Radiation resulting from vibrations associated with atoms.

electromyography (ee-**leck**-tro-my-**OG**-rah-fee). A test that records (*graph/o*) the degree of muscle (*my/o*) contraction strength when a specific muscle is electrically (*electro*) stimulated.

electron. A subatomic particle that orbits the nucleus and has a mass number of zero and a negative charge.

electron dot structure. Schematic of an atom wherein dots are used to represent the electrons in the outermost energy level of the atom.

element. A pure substance that cannot be broken down by ordinary chemical means.

emboli (**EM**-boh-lie). Singular, *embolus*; in a blood vessel, a foreign object that partially or totally blocks blood flow.

embryo (**EM**-bree-oh). Name given to the unborn child up to the third month of the pregnancy.

emphysema (em-fih-**SEE**-mah). A chronic condition characterized by reversible destruction of the alveoli and corresponding capillary networks.

empirical formula. The simplest whole-number ratio of elements in an ionic compound.

empyema (em-pye-**EE**-mah). A condition characterized by accumulation of pus in the pleural cavity.

encephalitis (en-**sef**-ah-**LYE**-tis). An inflammation of the brain.

endocarditis (en-doh-kar-**DYE**-tis). Inflammation of the inner layer of the heart.

endocardium (en-doh-**KAR**-dee-um). The inner surface of the walls of the heart.

endocrine (**EN**-doh-krin). Pertaining to secretion (*crin/o*) directly into (*end/o*) the bloodstream.

endolymph (**IN**-dough-limf). The fluid found within the labyrinth of the ear (*endo* meaning "inner").

endometriosis (**en**-doh-**ME**-tree-oh-sis). An inflammatory disease in which endometrial tissue invades other tissues throughout the body.

endoplasmic reticulum (**en**-doe-**PLAZ**-mik ree-**TICK**-you-lim). The network of small canals or tubes that connect the nucleus of a cell to the cytoplasm.

endorphins (**en**-**DORF**-fins). The body's natural pain killers.

endosteum (en-**DOS**-tee-um). Tissue that lines the hollow areas of the bones.

endothelium (**en**-doh-**THEE**-lee-um). The tissue that lines the internal (*endo*) organs as well as the blood vessels.

endotoxins. A poison found within (*endo*) a bacterium's body that is released only upon the bacterium's death.

energy levels. The orbits of the electrons around the nucleus of an atom—or that with which young kids are blessed in abundance.

English system of measurement. The common household system of measurement that uses the units of miles, feet, ounces, pounds, etc.

enzymes. Complex chemical proteins that act as organic catalysts; cause the chemical changes necessary to break down food so it can be used by the body.

epidermis (**ep**-ih-**DER**-mis). The outermost (*epi*) layer of skin (*dermis*) found on the body.

epiglottis (ep-ih-**GLOT**-is). The lid-like structure that protects the airway during swallowing.

epiglottitis (**ep**-ih-glot-**TYE**-tis). Inflammation of the epiglottis; potentially life-threatening in infants.

epinephrine (**ep**-ih-**NEFF**-rin). Hormone that stimulates the sympathetic nervous system, thus increasing cardiac activity and blood pressure for the fight-or-flight response; also known as *adrenaline*.

epiphyses (eh-**PIF**-ih-sees). The wide ends of the long bones.

epithelium (**ep**-ih-**THEE**-lee-um). The outer (*epi* meaning "upon" or "upper") layer of skin.

equation. The setting of two expressions equal to one another.

erythrocytes (eh-**RITH**-roh-sites). Red(*eryth/o*) blood cells (*cyt/o*), abbreviated *RBCs*; responsible for carrying oxygen in the blood.

erythropoiesis (eh-**rith**-roh-poy-**EE**-sis). The process of forming red blood cells (RBCs).

esophagus (eh-**SOF**-ah-gus). The passageway from the mouth to the stomach; sometimes referred to as the *food tube* or the *gullet*.

essential amino acid. An amino acid that cannot be synthesized from the carbohydrates and lipids in the body.

estrogen (**ES**-troh-jin). Primary female sex hormone; secreted by the ovaries and responsible for the development of secondary sex characteristics and regulation of the menstrual cycle.

ethanol (ethyl alcohol). Alcohol derived from the distillation of grains used as a disinfectant.

ethylene oxide (ETO). A gas used to sterilize equipment and materials.

etiology (ee-tee-**ALL**-oh-jee). The study of (*ology*) the origin of a disease.

Eustachian tube (you-**STAY**-kee-an). A narrow, tube-like passageway extending from the middle ear to the pharynx; responsible for equalizing air pressure between the middle ear and the outside environment.

exocrine (**ECKS**-oh-krin). Pertaining to secretion (*crin/o*) out (*ex/o*) of the body or to other organs of the body.

exophthalmos (**ecks**-of-**THAL**-mohs). Abnormal protrusion of the eyeballs, a common symptom of the disease goiter.

expectorant. A medicine that facilitates the expulsion of mucus from the lungs.

exponent. The superscript number in an exponential expression; indicates the number of times the base is multiplied.

extension. Increasing the angle between two bones, as when straightening out a limb such as an arm or leg.

external auditory canal. The passageway from the auricle to the middle ear.

external ear. *See* **auricle.**

external respiration. *See* **respiration.**

extrasensory perception (ESP). Perception of external events via a sense or senses other than the five basic senses. (For example, we knew you would be reading this right now.)

factor-label method. A means of changing units through cancellation.

factors. Those parts of an algebraic expression that indicate multiplication.

Fahrenheit temperature scale. Temperature scale wherein 328 represents the freezing point of water and 2128° the boiling point.

fallopian tubes (fal-**LOH**-pee-on). The ducts that both transfer the ovum from the ovaries to the uterus and provide a pathway for sperm to travel from the vagina to the uterus.

fats. Lipids that are solids at room temperature.

fertilization. The uniting of the female's egg with the male's sperm; typically occurs in the fallopian tube.

fetus (**FEE**-tus). Name given to the unborn child from the third month of pregnancy to birth.

fibrous protein. A type of protein that is insoluble in water.

fight-or-flight response. Autonomic nervous system process wherein the nerves act without conscious control as a means of survival.

filtrate. A liquid that has been passed through a filter.

flaccid (**FLAS**-sid). Weak; characterized by greatly decreased or lack of muscle tone.

flagella (flah-**GELL**-eh). Short fine filaments that provide cell motility.

flexion (**FLECK**-shun). Decreasing the angle between two bones, as when bending an arm or leg.

flora. Microbial life that adapts to live in the body.

follicles (**FALL**-ih-kolz). Sacs or pouch-like structures.

force. The "push" or "pull" that causes a change in an object's state of motion.

formulas. Equations wherein the variables represent physical quantities.

fractional distillation of liquid air. The process whereby air is rapidly cooled to liquefy the gaseous constituents of that air and whereby gas is then boiled off at its own temperature and collected for further refining or use.

free fall. When an object falls to earth and is acted on by only the attraction of the earth.

frequency. The number of occurrences or events that happen in a given unit of time.

friction. A force that opposes motion when two objects are in contact with each other.

frontal lobe. That area of the cerebrum that controls motor functions.

frontal plane. An imaginary plane that divides the body into a front half and a back half.

fructose (**FROOK**-tohs). Sugar form that is derived from fruit.

gallbladder. An organ that stores and concentrates bile so that the bile can be used in the digestive process.

gamma radiation. The radiation produced by high-energy X-rays.

gamma rays. Electromagnetic waves having an extremely high frequency; form of radiation used to fight cancer.

ganglia (**GANG**-glee-ah). A group of nerve cell bodies located outside the central nervous system.

gastric juice. A general term for the substance that is found in the stomach and digests food; contains hydrochloric acid, and the enzymes *protease*, *lipase*, and *pepsin*.

gastrointestinal. Pertaining to the digestive system (*gastr/o* meaning "stomach," *intestin/o* meaning "intestine").

Gay-Lussac's law. A happy little gas law stating that if the volume and mass of a given gas remain constant, the temperature and pressure of the gas will relate directly.

gene (**JEEN**). *See* **chromosome.**

genitourinary (jin-eh-toh-**YUR**-ih-nair-ee). Pertaining to the kidneys, urinary bladder, and related parts, as well as to the reproductive organs (*urin/o* meaning "relating to urine," *genit/o* meaning "relating to birth").

germicidal. Pertaining to killing of germs.

giantism. A disease resulting from a pituitary gland that is overactive prior to puberty and characterized by abnormal overgrowth of the body.

giga (G). Prefix used in the metric system to mean times 10 to the power of 9 (10^9).

gland. An organ or structure in the body that manufactures and secretes a substance.

glaucoma (glaw-**KOH**-mah). A class of eye diseases characterized by an increase in intraocular pressure possibly resulting in damage to the optic disk.

glia cells (**GLEE**-uh). Nonnerve cells that provide support and act as connective cells for the nervous system (*gli/o* meaning "glue").

globular protein. A type of protein that is water soluble.

glucagon. A hormone that is produced by the pancreas and increases the level of glucose in the blood.

glucocorticoids. A steroid hormone that is secreted by the adrenal cortex and aids the body in battling stress and metabolizing proteins and carbohydrates.

glucose (GLOO-kohs**).** A sugar; the most important carbohydrate involved in body metabolism.

glucosuria (gloo-koh-**SEW**-ree-uh**).** Presence of sugar in the urine.

glutaraldehydes. Class of sterilizing agents that are effective on all microorganisms including viruses and spores.

glycerol (GLISS-er-all**).** Another term for *glycerin*, which is found in all fats.

glycogen. The storage form of glucose in animals.

glycosuria (glye-koh-**SOO**-ree-ah**).** A condition characterized by glucose (*glyc/o*) in the urine (*ur/o*).

goiter (GOI-ter**).** A condition characterized by an enlarged thyroid gland; also known as *thyromegaly*.

Golgi apparatus (GOAL-je**).** The organelle responsible for packaging the waste from a cell.

gonadocorticoids (gon-ah-do-**KORT**-ih-**KOYDZ**)**.** Any hormones that stimulate the ovaries in the female or the testes in the male; also known as *sex hormones*.

gonads. Generic term for male (testes) and female (ovaries) sex glands.

graafian follicles (GRAF-ee-an **FOL**-lick-kulz**).** Located in the ovaries, each one of these thousands of follicles contains a single ovum.

gram (g). The basic unit of mass in the metric system.

gram molecular weight. The weight in grams of a substance equal to its molecular weight.

Gram stain. Technique used to identify gram-positive (stains purple) and gram-negative (stains pink) bacteria.

graph. A visual representation of information.

Graves' disease. A condition caused by excessive thyroxine secretion; also known as *toxic goiter*, *hyperthyroidism*, and *exothalmic goiter*.

gravity. The pull of the earth.

growth hormone (GH). Hormone that is produced by the pituitary gland and accelerates growth of the body; also known as *somatotropic hormone*.

gullet. *See* **esophagus.**

gyri (JIGH-rye**).** Singular, *gyrus*; the elevated parts of the cerebral cortex surface (*gyro/o* meaning "turning, folding").

hammer. One of the three small bones found in the middle ear; also known as the *malleus*.

heart failure (HF). The inability of the heart to circulate blood effectively to meet the body's needs.

heat. The amount of thermal energy that transfers from one substance to another because of a difference in temperature between the two substances.

hecto (h). Prefix used in the metric system to mean times 10 to the power of 2 (10^2).

Heimlich maneuver (HIME-lick**).** A method of dislodging a foreign body lodged in the airway by applying pressure below the region of the diaphragm and, thus, propelling the foreign body from the airway.

hemiplegia (hem-ee-**PLEE**-jee-ah**).** A condition characterized by paralysis of half (*hemi*) of the body.

hemoglobin (hee-ma-**GLOW**-bin**).** The substance that carries oxygen in a red blood cell.

hemothorax (he-moh-**THOH**-racks**).** Abnormal leakage of blood (*hemo*) into the thoracic cavity, usually in the pleural space.

Henry's law. Gas law stating that the amount of gas that enters a physical solution in a liquid is directly related to the partial pressure of that gas above the surface of the liquid.

hernia (HER-nee-ah**).** An abnormal protrusion of an organ resulting from a tear in a muscle.

hilum (HIGH-lim**).** The root of the lungs usually located at the fourth and fifth thoracic vertebrae

histologist (hiss-**TOL**-oh-jist**).** One who studies (*ologist*) tissues (*hist/o*).

histology (hiss-**TOL**-oh-jee**).** The study of (*ology*) tissues (*hist/o*).

homeostasis (hoh-me-oh-**STAY**-sis**).** The state of balance maintained by the body despite internal and external forces that attempt to alter this state of balance. Regulation of a constant body temperature regardless of the climatic conditions is one example.

horizontal. Lying flat and going from right to left or left to right.

hormone. A substance that is produced by an organ or gland and that travels to another part of the body, causing chemical action leading to either increased function or the release of another hormone.

hydrocarbons. Compounds that consist of only carbon atoms and hydrogen atoms.

hydrogen peroxide. An antiseptic, germicide and cleansing agent.

hydronium ion ($H3O^+$). Also known as the hydrogen ion and its concentration determines pH.

hydrothorax (**high**-dro-**THOH**-racks). Abnormal amounts of blood serum in the thoracic cavity, usually in the pleural space (*hydro* meaning "water").

hypercalcemia. A condition characterized by an excessive (*hyper*) amount of calcium (*calc/o*) in the blood (*emia*), possibly leading to bone decalcification and spontaneous bone fracture.

hyperglycemia. A condition characterized by an excess (*hyper*) of glucose (*gluc/o*) in the blood (*emia*).

hypermetabolism. An excessive rate of metabolism, possibly resulting from fever.

hyperopia (**high**-per-**OH**-pee-ah). Far-sightedness; occurs when light rays focus beyond the retina.

hyperpyrexia. Higher-than-normal body temperature.

hypertension (**high**-per-**TEN**-shun). Higher-than-normal (*hyper*) blood pressure (*tension*).

hyperthyroidism. A condition (*ism*) caused by excessive (*hyper*) secretion by the thyroid gland and characterized by increased metabolic rate, goiter, and autonomic nervous system abnormalities.

hypertonic solution. A solution having a higher concentration than a reference solution.

hypertrophy (hi-**PER**-tro-fee). An abnormal increase (*hyper* meaning "excessive," *troph/o* meaning "growth") in the volume or size of an organ or tissue.

hypocalcemia. A condition characterized by lower-than-normal (*hypo*) levels of calcium (*calc/o*) in the blood (*emia*).

hypoglycemia. A condition characterized by a lower-than-normal blood sugar level.

hypotension (**high**-poh-**TEN**-shun). Lower-than-normal (*hypo*) blood pressure (*tension*).

hypothalamus (**high**-poh-**THAL**-ah-mus). The brain structure located below the thalamus and responsible for regulating the autonomic system, the cardiovascular system, appetite, metabolism of sugar and fat, water balance, body temperature, sleep, the gastrointestinal system, and emotional state.

hypothermia. Lower-than-normal body temperature.

hypothyroidism. A condition caused by lower-than-normal secretion by the thyroid gland and characterized by lowered metabolic rate and lethargy.

hypotonic solution. A solution having a lower concentration than a reference solution.

idiopathic disease (**id**-ee-oh-**PATH**-ic). A disease that cannot be traced to a specific cause.

immunology (**im**-you-**NOL**-oh-jee). The study of (*ology*) the immune system.

improper fraction. A fraction having a numerator as large as or larger than the denominator—or a fraction that has not learned its table manners.

incisors (in-**SIGH**-zorz). Specialized teeth used to cut food when biting.

incomplete protein. A protein that is low in one or more of the essential amino acids.

incontinence. This is a condition characterized by loss of sphincter control so that urine, semen, or feces cannot be retained.

incus (**IN**-kus). *See* **anvil.**

inertia. The tendency of an object to not change its direction.

infection. The presence of microorganism with a tissue reaction.

infection control. Policies and procedures designed to monitor and control the transmission of communicable diseases.

inferior. Below or lowermost (*infer/o*).

inflammation. A tissue's reaction to injury that may or may not be a result of infection.

infrared radiation. Radiation not in the visible spectrum of light; often called *heat radiation*.

insulin. A hormone that regulates the amount of glucose entering the body cells.

insulin-dependent diabetes. *See* **type I diabetes.**

intake and output (I&O). A measurement comparing the amount of fluid taken in by a given patient (*I* for input) to the amount of fluid excreted by that patient (*O* for output).

integers. { .... , –2, –1, 0, 1, 2, ...}

integumentary system (in-**teg**-you-**MEN**-tair-ee). The body system comprising the skin, sweat glands, hair, breasts, and nails.

intercalated discs (in-**ter**-kah-**LAY**-ted). Cardiac muscle structures that allow for rapid communication between the fibers and, thus, smooth contraction for the pumping of blood.

internal ear. That region of the ear containing the sensory receptors for hearing and balance; also known as the *labyrinth* (*labyrinth/o* meaning "maze").

internal respiration. *See* **respiration.**

ion. A particle having a positive or negative charge—or what your parents may do on your first date: that is, keep an "ion" you.

ionic bond. An attraction between oppositely charged ions.

iris. The colored, muscular layer of the eye that surrounds the pupil and can change the size of the pupil to allow varying amounts of light into the eye.

irrational number. A number that, when written as a decimal, never ends or repeats.

irritability. Excitability; the response of a nerve to stimuli.

ischemia (iss-**KEE**-me-ah). Injury to tissue resulting from insufficient blood and, therefore, oxygen supply to the tissue.

islands of Langerhans (**LAHNG**-er-hahnz). Specialized cells that are found in the pancreas and secrete hormones that aid the body in metabolizing sugar and starch; also known as *islets of Langerhans.*

isomers. Compounds having the same molecular formula but different structural formulas.

isopropyl alcohol. Rubbing alcohol used to sterilize equipment. Not to be ingested.

isotonic solution. A solution having the same concentration as a reference solution.

isotopes. Chemical elements that have nearly identical chemical properties but different atomic weights and electric charges. They are often radioactive.

isthmus (**IS**-mus). A narrow connecting passageway.

joint. The area where two or more bones join together.

juvenile diabetes. *See* **type I diabetes.**

keloid (**KEE**-loid). Thick, raised scar formation resulting from an injury.

Kelvin temperature scale. Temperature scale developed by Lord Kelvin wherein 0 is the lowest temperature possible. This is equal to $-273°$Celsius.

keratin (**KER**-ah-tin). The fibrous protein that composes fingernails and hair.

ketones (**KEY**-tonz). Substances that are not normally found in the body and are produced when there is increased metabolism of fat.

kidneys. Two organs needed to maintain fluid balance in the body, excrete urine, regulate electrolytes, and maintain proper acid-base balance of the blood.

kilo (k). Prefix used in the metric system to mean times 10 to the power of 3 (10^3).

kinetic energy. The energy of an object as a result of the object's motion.

kinetic theory. Theory stating that all matter is composed of small particles that are in constant, random motion.

labia majora (**LAY**-be-ah). Singular, *labium*; two folds of skin on either side of the vaginal opening.

labia minora (**LAY**-be-ah). Singular, *labium*; two thin folds of skin found within the labia majora.

labyrinth (**LAB**-ih-rinth). *See* **internal ear.**

labyrinthitis (lab-ih-rin-**THIGH**-tis). An inflammation of the labyrinth.

laceration (lass-er-**AY**-shun). A torn or ragged wound to the skin.

lacrimal glands (**LACK**-rih-mal). The glands that are located above the outer corner of each eye and produce tears.

lacteals (**LACK**-tee-ahls). Specialized lymph vessels located in the small intestine; absorb fat from the small intestine and put the fat into the bloodstream.

large intestine. A structure that begins at the ileum of the small intestine and ends at the anus; includes five main portions: the *cecum*, the *colon*, the *sigmoid colon*, the *rectum*, and the *anus.*

laryngitis (lar-in-**JIGH**-tis). Inflammation of the larynx.

laryngopharynx (lah-**ring**-goh-**FAIR**-inks). The airway region composed of the pharynx (also known as the throat) and the larynx (also known as the voice box).

larynx (**LAIR**-inks). Airway structure containing the vocal cords and protected by cartilage, some of which forms the Adam's apple; also known as the voice box.

latent disease. A nonactive disease that has the potential to return.

lateral. Toward the sides.

least common denominator (LCD). The smallest common denominator; also known as the *lowest common denominator.*

lens. A curved structure found behind the iris and pupil.

lesion (**LEE**-zhun). A general term used to describe a pathological change in tissue as a result of injury or disease.

leukocytes (**LOO**-koh-sites). White (*leuko*) blood cells (*cyt/o*), abbreviated *WBCs*; responsible for fighting infection and disease.

leukocytopenia (**loo**-koh-sigh-to-**PEE**-nee-ah). A decrease (*penia*) in white (*leuk/o*) blood cells (*cyt/o*).

ligament. Tough, fibrous band of connective tissue that connects to the bones at an articulation.

line graph. A method of representing data using lines.

lingula (**LING**-gu-lah). That region of the left lung considered to be the "left middle lobe."

lipids. Plant or animal product that is soluble in nonpolar solvents.

liter (L). The basic unit of liquid measure in the metric system; remember, you can "liter" a horse to water, but you can't make him drink.

liver. An organ that serves several functions in the body including removing from the bloodstream and storing excess glucose, destroying all RBCs, filtering toxins out of the blood, and manufacturing bile.

local infection. An infection confined to a small area.

lower esophageal sphincter (LES). A ringed muscle that prevents backflow of stomach contents into the esophagus.

lumbar plexus. A network of nerves located in the region of the lower back.

lungs. The two organs responsible for bringing fresh air in and sending old air out of the body, thus providing the body with needed oxygen and removing the carbon dioxide that is a waste product of metabolization.

lunula (**LOO**-new-lah). The white, half-moon formation visible at the nail root.

lymph (**LIMPF**). A clear fluid found in tissue and in the spaces between cells; carries materials from the cells back to the blood system.

lymph nodes (**LIMPF**). Small kidney shaped organs of the lymph tissues that filter pathogens and produce lymphocytes to fight infection.

lymphocyte (**LIM**-foh-site). A type of leukocyte that aids the body in developing immunities.

lymph vessels. Canals or passageways that conduct lymph fluid throughout the body.

lysosome (**LIE**-so-sohm). The organelle responsible for digestion in a cell.

magnetic resonance imaging (MRI). A type of noninvasive nuclear imaging that allows a view of high-fat and high-water content tissues normally not seen on regular X-rays; provides excellent information regarding the chemical makeup of tissues and in some cases can indicate whether tissues are cancerous or noncancerous. The procedure takes 15–90 minutes.

malleus (**MAL**-ee-us). *See* **hammer.**

mass. The amount of inertia possessed by an object, or an object's resistance to a change in its motion.

mass number. The sum of the protons and neutrons in an atom.

maturity-onset diabetes. *See* **type II diabetes.**

mean. Arithmetic average.

measures of central tendency. The mean, median, or mode.

medial (**MEE**-dee-all). Toward the middle (*medi/o*).

median. The middle value of a given set of values, when the values are arranged in order.

median plane (**MEE**-dee-an). Imaginary plane that divides the body into a left side and a right side; also known as the *midsagittal plane.*

medulla (meh-**DULL**-ah). The inner layer or portion of an organ.

medulla oblongata (ob-long-**GAH**-tah). That portion of the brain stem responsible for breathing, heart rate, and blood pressure (*medull/o* meaning "inner section").

mega (M). Prefix used in the metric system to mean times 10 to the power of 6 (10^6).

melanocyte-stimulating hormone (MSH). Hormone responsible for pigmentation of the skin in humans.

melatonin hormone (mel-ah-**TOE**-nin). A hormone that is produced by the pineal gland and influences sexual maturation.

Ménière's disease (main-ee-**AYRZ**). A chronic inner-ear disease that can produce vertigo, unilateral deafness, and tinnitus.

meninges (meh-**NIN**-jeez). The three layers of membrane that are composed of connective tissue and encapsulate the brain and spinal cord.

meningitis (men-in-**JIGH**-tis). An inflammation of the meninges.

metabolic acidosis. An acid condition of the blood caused by a metabolic problem.

metabolism. The use of energy and food stores within the body for mechanical energy or heat generation.

metastasis. The movement of cancer cells to other organs in the body.

meter (m). The basic unit of length in the metric system.

metric system of measurement. A system of measurement based on powers of ten.

micro (mc). Prefix used in the metric system to mean times 10 to the power of negative 6 (10^{-6}).

microbiology. The study of microorganisms.

microorganism (mi-kro-**OR**-gan-ism). A small (*micro*), living thing that can be seen only with the aid of a microscope.

microwaves. Electromagnetic waves used in both communication systems and cooking.

midbrain. Area of the brain where the pons and cerebellum connect with the hemispheres of the cerebrum.

middle ear. The region of the ear that is surrounded by hollow air spaces and contains three small, bony structures known as the auditory ossicles; also known as the *tympanic cavity*.

midsagittal plane (mid-**SADJ**-ih-tal). *See* **median plane.**

milli (m). Prefix used in the metric system to mean times 10 to the power of negative 3 (10^{-3}).

mineralcorticoids. Steroids involved in the regulation of fluids and electrolytes in the body.

mitochondria (my-toe-**KON**-dree-ah). The powerhouse of a cell.

mitosis (my-**TOH**-sis). A form of asexual reproduction in which cells divide to form identical copies.

mitral valve (MY-tral). Valve located between the left atrium and left ventricle of the heart; also known as the *bicuspid valve*.

mixed number. A number containing both whole numbers and fractions.

mode. The most-often-observed value in a given set of values.

molars. Specialized teeth used to crush food.

mole. *See* **Avogadro's number.**

monosaccharide. A carbohydrate consisting of a single sugar molecule.

motility. The ability to move spontaneously.

motion. When an object moves from one point to another.

motor cortex. That portion of the frontal lobe that controls voluntary (skeletal) muscle movements.

motor neurons. Neurons that innervate the muscles and initiate muscle contraction.

mumps. A condition characterized by swollen glands and caused by a virus.

muscles. A general term for a group of long, slender cells that form fibers capable of contracting. Movement is possible as a result of this contraction.

myasthenia gravis (my-as-**THEE**-nee-ah **GRAH**-vis). A long-term muscular condition characterized by profound muscle (*my/o*) weakness coupled with progressive degeneration of muscle fibers (*a* meaning "without," *esthesia* meaning "feelings" or "sensation").

mycology. The study of fungi, yeasts, and molds.

myelin sheath (MY-eh-lin). White, fatty tissue surrounding the axons of certain nerve cells.

myocardial infarction. Medical term for heart attack in which cardiac tissue death results from disrupted blood flow to the tissue.

myocarditis (my-oh-kar-**DYE**-tis). Inflammation of the heart muscle (*myocardium*).

myocardium (my-oh-**KAR**-dee-um). *See* **cardiac muscle.**

myopia (my-**OH**-pee-ah). Nearsightedness; occurs when light rays focus in front of the retina.

myxedema (mick-seh-**DEE**-mah). A condition resulting from hypothyroidism and characterized by abnormal deposits of mucin in the skin; also known as *nonpitting edema*, it usually occurs in older children and adults.

nano (n). Prefix used in the metric system to mean times 10 to the power of negative 9 (10^{-9}).

narrow-spectrum drug. An antibiotic that is effective against a narrow range of organisms.

nasal septum (SEPT-tum). The cartilaginous wall that divides the nose into a right nostril and a left nostril.

nasopharynx (nay-zoh-**FAIR**-inks). *See* **pharynx.**

natural numbers. $\{1, 2, 3, 4, \dots\}$

negative feedback loop. The way the body regulates the activity of the pituitary gland by monitoring the level of glucocorticoids in the blood.

neonate (NEE-oh-nate). A newborn (*neo* meaning "new," *natus* meaning "born") child up to the age of six weeks.

nephrolithiasis (nef-row-lith-**EYE**-ah-sis). Kidney (*nephr/o*) stones (*lith/o*).

nephron (**NEF**-ron).   Kidney structure having a funnel shape and a long, curving tail.   There are approximately 1 million nephrons in each kidney.

nerve plexuses (**PLECK**-us-sus).   A network of intersecting nerves.

nerves.   One or more bundles of fibers that transmit impulses to and from the brain and spinal cord and also to and from the rest of the body.

neurilemma (**new**-rih-**LEM**-mah).   A membrane that encases the myelin sheath of peripheral nerve cells (*emm/o* meaning "husk" or "bark").

neuroglia (new-**ROG**-lee-ah).   *See* **glia cells.**

neuromuscular (**new**-roh-**MUS**-ku-lar).   Pertaining to both the muscle (*musc/o*) system and the nervous (*neur/o*) system.

neuron (**NEW**-ron).   The basic cell of the nervous system.

neurotransmitter substance.   A chemical substance that travels across the synapse to act on a target site.

neutralization.   The process whereby an acid and a base combine to produce water.

neutron.   A subatomic particle having a mass number of 1 and a charge of zero.

nevus (**NEH**-vus).   An area of concentrated blood vessels and skin pigment; also known as a mole or birthmark.

node.   A general term for a small, rounded structure or organ.

non-insulin-dependent diabetes.   *See* **type II diabetes.**

noninvasive.   Requiring no puncturing of the skin or body.

norepinephrine (nor-**ep**-ih-**NEFF**-rin).   A hormone secreted by the adrenal glands; stimulates the sympathetic nervous system and raises blood pressure; also known as *noradrenaline*.

normal flora.   Microorganisms normally found in the body that are beneficial.

nose.   The structure on the front of the face that allows air to enter the nasal cavity.

nosocomial infections (**no**-soh-**KOME**-ee-al). Hospital-acquired infections.

nuclear medicine.   The branch of medicine involving diagnostic, therapeutic, and investigative uses of radiation or radioactive materials.

nucleolus (**NEW**-klee-**ol**-lus).   The part of the nucleus where RNA is made.

nucleus (**NEW**-klee-us).   That structure within a cell that controls many of the cell's functions; also, the dense, central portion of an atom.

numerator.   The top part of a fraction; indicates the number of parts represented by the fraction.

occipital lobe (ox-**SIP**-ih-tahl).   Cerebrum section that is involved with eyesight.

occlusion (oh-**CLUE**-zhun).   A blockage or closure of a passageway.

oils.   Lipids that are liquids at room temperature.

olfactory (ol-**FAK**-toh-ree).   Pertaining to the sense of smell (*olfact/o* meaning "smell").

oliguria (**ol**-ig-**YOU**-ree-ah).   Less than expected urination (*olig/o* meaning "scanty" or "few," *ur/o* meaning "urine").

ophthalmometer (off-thal-**MOM**-et-er).   A device that measures the error of refraction or the anterior curvature of the eye.

opportunistic infections.   Infections caused by normally benign organisms when a patient's immune system or protective flora is compromised.

oral cavity.   The mouth.

orbit.   The bony cavity in the skull that houses and protects the eyeballs.

order of operations.   The rules used to determine the order in which operations are performed in an algebraic expression.

organ (**OR**-gan).   A somewhat independently functioning part of the body that has a specialized purpose.

organelle (**or**-gah-**NEL**).   An organized cytoplasmic structure having a specific function.

organ of Corti.   Portion of the ear that contains receptors for heaing.

oropharynx (oh-roh-**FAIR**-inks).   *See* **pharynx.**

osmosis.   The movement of water across a membrane from an area of lower concentration to an area of higher concentration.

ossicle (**AHS**-ih-kul).   One of the three small bones of the middle ear.

osteoblasts.   The bone cells responsible for building new bone.

osteoclasts.   The cells that continually tear down bones, thus enabling the renewal of osteoblasts.

osteoporosis (**oss**-tee-oh-por-**OH**-sis).   A condition (*osis*) wherein the bone (*oste/o*) loses its normal density and becomes porous (*per/o*); often found in the aging population.

otitis media (oh-**TYE**-tis **ME**-dee-ah). An inflammation of the middle ear; also known as *tympanitis*.

oval window. The thin membrane that separates the middle ear from the inner ear—not to be confused with the window in the president's office.

ovaries (**OH**-vah-reez). Two almond-shaped organs found in the female; produce hormones and house thousands of eggs known as *ova*.

oxytocin (**auk**-see-**TOE**-sin). A pituitary hormone that stimulates contractions of the uterus during childbirth and causes milk to secrete from the mammary glands.

palatine (**PAL**-ah-tine). Pertaining to the palate region of the mouth.

pancreas (**PAN**-kree-ass). A digestive system organ that secretes both juices containing digestive enzymes and hormones involved in the body's use of glucose and starch.

pancreatic juices (**pan**-kree-**AT**-tick). A fluid secreted by the pancreas and containing digestive enzymes.

papilla (pah-**PILL**-ah). Little bumps that cover the tongue and contain cells that act as taste receptors.

paralysis (pah-**RAL**-ih-sis). A condition characterized by loss of voluntary muscle movement.

paraplegia (par-ah-**PLEE**-jee-ah). Paralysis of both legs and the lower portion of the body.

parasite (par-ah-**SITE**). An organism that can only live off of another organism. (Anyone you know?)

parasitology. The study of parasites.

parasympathetic nervous system. That portion of the autonomic nervous system that regulates normal body functioning during unstressful times.

parathyroid glands. Four small glands (each approximately the size of a grain of rice) located on the posterior surface of the thyroid gland and important in regulating the amount of calcium in the blood.

parathyroid hormone (PTH). A hormone that in combination with calcitonin regulates the amount of calcium in the blood.

parietal lobe (pah-**RYE**-eh-tal). That portion of the brain that accepts and then interprets nerve impulses from the sensory receptors.

parotid glands (pah-**ROT**-id). Salivary glands found in the area forward of and slightly lower than the ears.

pasteurization. The use of water heated enough to kill vegetative cells and most viruses.

pathogen (**PATH**-o-jen). A microscopic organism capable of causing disease (*path/o*).

pathologist (pah-**THOL**-oh-jist). One who studies (*ologist*) disease (*path/o*).

pathology. The study of the nature and cause of disease.

pathophysiology. The study of (*ology*) why disease (*path/o*) occurs and how the body reacts to disease.

pelvic (**PEL**-vick). Pertaining to the area of the body containing the reproductive organs, the excretory system, and the pelvic bones.

pelvic inflammatory disease (PID). A general term for any inflammation of the female reproductive system, especially if the causative agent is bacterial in nature.

penis (**PEE**-nis). The male sex organ responsible for transporting sperm to the female's vagina.

pepsin. A digestive juice enzyme needed to help break down food into usable substances.

percentage. A means of representing quantities in hundredths (for example 50% = 50/100).

percent solution. The strength of a solution as determined by comparing the solute to 100 mL of the total solution.

perfusion (per-**FEW**-zhun). The flow of a liquid through or around an organ or tissues.

pericarditis (**per**-ih-kar-**DYE**-tis). Inflammation of the pericardium.

pericardium (**per**-ih-**KAR**-dee-um). The sac that surrounds the heart.

perilymph (**PAIR**-eh-limf). A pale-colored fluid found in the labyrinth of the ear.

periosteum (**per**-ee-**OSS**-tee-um). The tough, fibrous, outermost (*peri* meaning "surrounding") covering of the bones (*oste/o*).

peripheral (per-**IF**-er-al). Pertaining to surrounding areas.

peripheral chemoreceptors. Specialized cells that react to chemical stimuli.

peripheral nervous system (PNS). That portion of the nervous system that includes the cranial nerves, which extend from the brain, and the spinal nerves, which extend from the spinal cord.

peristalsis (**per**-ih-**STAL**-sis). The wave-like, smooth muscle action of the digestive system; moves food through the digestive system.

personal protective equipment (PPE). Clothing , masks, gloves, and various gear that protects an individual from exposure to dangerous chemicals or transmissible diseases.

petechiae (peh-**TEE**-kee-ee). Skin hemorrhage approximately the size of a pinpoint.

pH. A measurement of hydrogen ion concentration.

phagocytosis (**fag**-oh-sigh-**TOH**-sis). A way that the body fights infection whereby certain cells engulf and destroy germs via digestion.

pharyngitis (**far**-in-**JIGH**-tis). Inflammation of the pharynx; more commonly known as a sore throat.

pharynx (**FAIR**-inks). That portion of the airway commonly known as the throat; includes three sections: the *nasopharynx*, which is closest to the nose, the *oropharynx*, which is in the middle of the pharynx and can be seen when you open your mouth, and the *laryngopharynx*, which is located near the larynx.

phenols. Distillates of coal tar used to clean equipment.

photopigments. Substances that cause chemical changes when exposed to light—not to be confused with pictures of breath fresheners for swine.

phrenic nerve (**FREN**-ick). The nerve that stimulates the diaphragm and, thus, promotes breathing.

physiology (**fiz**-ee-**OL**-oh-gee). The study of (*ology*) the processes of an organism (*phys* meaning "relating to nature").

pia mater (**PEE**-ah **MAY**-ter). The third layer of the meninges, which is located nearest to the brain and spinal cord.

pico (p). Prefix used in the metric system to mean times 10 to the power of negative 12 (10^{-12}).

picture graph. A method of representing data using pictures.

piloerection (**pie**-low-ee-**RECK**-shun). When the hair "stands on end" (*pilo* meaning "hair").

pineal body (**PIN**-ee-al). A gland located in the central region of the brain.

pineal gland. Endocrine gland that synthesizes melatonin.

pinna (**PIN**-nah). *See* **external ear.**

pituitary gland (pih-**TOO**-ih-**tair**-ee). A gland located at the base of the brain; secretes hormones that regulate the functions of other glands in the endocrine system; also known as the *hypophysis*.

placenta (plah-**SEN**-tah). The structure that provides for the transfer of nutrients and oxygen from the mother to the child during pregnancy; also called *afterbirth*.

plaque (**PLAK**). An abnormal accumulation of lipids or calcium that lines blood vessel walls.

plasma (**PLAZ**-mah). The straw-colored blood fluid that transports nutrients, waste products, and hormones throughout the body.

pleural effusion (**PLOOR**-all eh-**FEW**-zhun). An increase in the amount of fluid found in the pleural cavity.

pneumoconiosis (**new**-moh-**koh**-nee-**OH**-sis). A lung condition caused by inhaling dust either at work or from the environment; usually occurs after years of exposure.

pneumonia. An inflammation of the lungs due to infection usually caused by bacteria or viruses.

pneumothorax (**new**-moh-**THOR**-racks). Abnormal accumulation of air (*pneumo*) or gas in the pleural space, possibly leading to collapse of a portion of the lung.

polar covalent bond. A covalent bond wherein the electrons are not equally shared and partial charges on the involved atoms therefore result.

polydipsia (**pol**-ee-**DIP**-see-ah). Abnormally excessive thirst.

polyphagia (**pol**-ee-**FAY**-jee-ah). Abnormally excessive food consumption.

polysaccharide. A carbohydrate consisting of a long chain of monosaccharides, such as glucose molecules, bonded together.

polyuria (**pol**-ee-**YOU**-ree-ah). Abnormally excessive urination.

portals of entry. A limited number of body openings by which infectious agents can gain access.

positron emission tomography (PET). An imaging device that gives a clearer and more in-depth image than X-rays.

posterior (pos-**TEER**-ee-or). Pertaining to the back (*poster/o*).

posterior lobe. In the pituitary gland, that portion called the *neurohypophysis*.

potential energy. The energy of an object as a result of the object's position.

power. The rate at which work is done.

prefix. A word part that precedes a word root and alters the word root's meaning.

premolars.   Teeth used in combination with the molars to chew and grind food; also known as *bicuspids*.

prenatal (pre-**NAY**-tal).   Before (*pre*) birth (*natal*).

pressure.   A force exerted per a unit of area.

primary structural feature.   The sequence of amino acids in a protein chain.

progesterone (pro-**JES**-ter-own).   A female hormone responsible for preparing the uterus for pregnancy.

prognosis (prog-**NO**-sis).   The outlook regarding a patient's recovery.

prolactin (PRL).   Hormone responsible for the stimulation of the production of breast milk.

prolapse.   Pertaining to the falling down or dropping down of a structure in the body.

proper fraction.   A fraction having a numerator smaller than the denominator—or a fraction that has learned its table manners.

proportion.   A statement that two ratios are equal.

prostate (**PRAWS**-tayt).   A gland that secretes a fluid that mixes with sperm, thus providing more motility to the sperm.

prostate gland (**PRAWS**-tate).   A muscular gland that secretes an alkaline fluid that forms part of the seminal fluid.

protein.   A substance composed of long chains of amino acids bonded together.

prothrombin (pro-**THROM**-bin).   A protein found in blood plasma and needed for proper blood clotting.

proton.   A subatomic particle having a mass number of 1 and a positive charge.

protoplasm (**PRO**-toe-plaz-im).   The material of which all living things are made.

proximal (**PROCK**-sih-mal).   Near a point of reference.

pruritus (proo-**RYE**-tus).   An itching sensation.

pulmonary valve.   A semilunar (that is, shaped like a half moon) valve located between the pulmonary artery and the right ventricle of the heart.

pupil.   The circular opening in front of the choroid. Its size can be varied by the muscular action of the iris.

pure covalent bond.   A covalent bond wherein the electrons are shared equally between the atoms.

pyloric sphincter (py-**LOR**-ick).   A ring of muscle that controls the flow of materials from the stomach to the duodenum.

pyrogens (**PYE**-roh-genz).   Substances that can produce (*gen*) fever (*pyr* meaning "fire").

quadriplegia (**KWAD**-rih-**PLEE**-jee-ah).   Paralysis of both arms and legs (*quad/o* meaning "four").

quantitative terms.   Terms used to represent numbers (such as *dozen* for 12).

quaternary ammonium compounds.   A family of compounds used to sterilize equipment.

radiation therapy.   The branch of medicine that uses radiation to treat malignant growths.

radiology.   The broad branch of medicine that uses radioactive substances, X-rays, and ionizing radiations to diagnose and/or treat disease.

radiopharmaceuticals.   Radioactive chemicals used to detect various problems in the body or to treat disease.

radio waves.   Electromagnetic waves found in the lower frequency ranges of the electromagnetic spectrum.

ratio.   A comparison or fraction (for example, 1:2 or 1/2).

rational number.   A number that can be written in the form p/q, where p and q are integers and $q \neq 0$.

real number line.   A line on which all real numbers can be represented by indicated points.

reciprocal.   The inverse of a given number (for example, 2 and 1/2).

rectal.   Pertaining to (*al*) the rectum.

refraction.   The bending of an otherwise straight beam of light as it travels through substances having varying densities.

relative humidity.   The relationship between the actual amount of water found in a given amount of gas and the amount of water the gas is capable of holding at a given temperature.

remission.   The partial or complete disappearance of signs and symptoms of a disease.

renal threshold.   The blood sugar level at which glucosuria will occur.

reservoir of infection.   An individual or object that contains a source of pathogens for distribution.

resistant.   The ability of certain organisms to be less affected by certain antibiotics.

respiration.   Either the exchange of gases between the lungs and the capillary network surrounding each alveolar sac, known as *external respiration*, or the exchange of gases between the blood and the other cells of the body, known as *internal respiration*.

respirometer (res-per-**OM**-et-er). A device that measures the amount of air inhaled or exhaled by the lungs.

retina (**RET**-ih-nah). Structure located in the chamber of the eye; contains specialized, light-sensitive cells that send impulses to the brain via the optic nerve.

retroperitoneal (**ret**-roh-**pair**-eh-toe-**NEE**-all). Pertaining to the area or region behind (*retr/o*) or outside of the peritoneal cavity.

ribonucleic acid (RNA) (rye-bo-new-**KLEE**-ik). The substance involved in protein synthesis within a cell.

ribosomes (**RYE**-boh-sohmz). Particles found within a cell; involved in protein synthesis.

rickets (**RICK**-ets). A bone disease caused by a lack of calcium and vitamin D; can lead to bone deformities.

rods. Specialized, light-sensitive eye cells needed for vision in dim light.

rotation. Movement around an axis, such as in turning the head.

routes of transmission. Avenues used by pathogens to cause infection.

sacral plexus (**SACK**-ral **PLEX**-us). Group (*plexus*) of sacral nerves where the sciatic nerve originates.

saliva (suh-**LIE**-vah). A liquid secreted by the salivary glands; moistens food, starts the process of digestion, and helps clean the mouth.

salivary glands (**SAL**-ih-vair-ee). Any of three pairs of glands that secrete saliva, including the *parotid glands*, the *sublingual glands*, and the *submandibular glands*.

salt. An ionic compound formed from the positive ion of a base and the negative ion of an acid.

sanitization. A general term for any process that reduces the total bacterial contamination to a level in which an object may be handled safely.

saturated fatty acid. A fatty acid containing an alkane hydrocarbon chain.

scientific notation. A means of representing very large or very small numbers based on the power of ten, or the scribblings of Albert Einstein.

sclera (**SKLAIR**-ah). The fibrous, white tissue of the eye that gives the eye its shape (*scler/o* meaning "hard").

scrotum (**SKROH**-tum). The externally located sac of skin that contains and gives support to the testes.

sebaceous glands (seh-**BAY**-shus). Skin glands that provide oil to keep the skin from drying out.

semen (**SEE**-men). The fluid that contains sperm and secretions from the Cowper's glands, prostate gland, and seminal vesicles.

semicircular canals. Canals that are found in the inner ear and contain hair-like cells and fluid; important in maintaining balance.

seminal vesicles (**SEM**-ih-nal **VES**-ih-kulz). Male glands located at the base of the urinary bladder; secrete a thick, yellow fluid that serves as nutrition for the sperm.

semipermeable (**sem**-ee-**PER**-mee-a-bill). Allowing only certain molecules to pass through (*semi* meaning "partial").

sensory neurons. Neurons that are located in the skin or sense organs and that send impulses to the spinal cord and brain; often called *afferent neurons*.

septum (**SEP**-tum). A structure or wall that divides two chambers or cavities.

sexually transmitted disease (STD). A general term for an affliction acquired or spread through either sexual intercourse or genital contact; also known as a *social disease* or *venereal disease*.

signed numbers. Numbers that carry the positive sign or negative sign.

similar terms. Terms having the same variable factors.

sinoatrialnode (**sign**-oh-**AY**-tree-ahl). Structure located in the upper right arterial wall and responsible for starting each wave of each heart contraction; commonly called the heart's *pacemaker*.

sinuses (**SIGN**-us-ez). Spaces that are found in the skull and produce mucus, reduce the weight of the skull, and affect the sound of the voice.

skeletal muscle. Special muscle that is attached to the bones and allows for movement.

slope. A measure of the steepness of a graph—or where you ski.

small intestine. Structure extending from the pyloric sphincter to the beginning of the large intestine; where nutrients are absorbed into the bloodstream; also known as the *small bowel*.

smooth muscle. *See* **visceral muscle.**

soft palate (**PAL**-at). The soft, flexible portion of the roof of the mouth; located posteriorly.

solute. Not to be confused with how a private greets a captain, a substance that is dissolved into a liquid.

solution. A uniform mixture of two or more substances in which there is a solute and a liquid solvent.

solution to an equation. The value that makes an equation true.

solvent. The liquid that dissolves the solute when forming a solution.

somatic muscles (so-**MAT**-ick). The muscles that allow body movement.

somatic nerves (so-**MAT**-ick). The nerves responsible for controlling the muscles that cause body movement.

somatotropic hormone (so-**MAT**-to-**troe**-pick). *See* **growth hormone (GH).**

sonography. A form of noninvasive diagnostic testing that uses sound waves to obtain an image of various structures in the body.

spasm. The sudden and involuntary contraction of a muscle or a group of muscles; can vary in severity. Spasms can also occur in blood vessels, thus constricting blood flow.

speed. The rate at which an object travels from one point to another; a comparison of distance over a period of time.

sperm. The male sex cell manufactured by the testes; also known as *spermatozoa.*

spermatozoa (**sper**-mah-toh-**ZOH**-ah). *See* **sperm.**

spinal. Pertaining to the backbone or spinal column.

spinal cord (**SPY**-nal). The structure that carries impulses to and from the brain for the limbs and lower part of the body.

spinal nerves (**SPY**-nal). The thirty-one pairs of nerves that originate in the spinal cord.

spirilla (spur-**ILL**-ah). A spiral-shaped bacteria.

spleen. An organ that is actually a mass of lymphatic tissue; produces lymphocytes and monocytes, which are important to the body's immune system; filters the blood, stores red blood cells (RBCs), and destroys expired RBCs.

spore. A highly protective form of an organism that protects it in hostile environments.

sputum (**SPU**-tum). The technical, as well as being a more acceptable, word for phlegm.

squamous cells (**SKWAY**-mus). Flat, scaly epithelial cells that form the outermost body layer called the skin.

standard precautions. A group of guidelines to prevent the spread of disease among patients and health care workers.

stapes (**STAY**-peez). One of the three small bones found in the middle ear; also known as the *stirrup.*

statistics. The branch of mathematics concerned with the collection, organization, and display of information.

stenosis (steh-**NO**-sis). Constriction or narrowing of a passageway or opening.

sterilization. The complete destruction or inactivation of all forms of microorganisms.

stimulus. Anything that acts as a stimulant, thus causing a nervous impulse.

stirrup. *See* **stapes.**

stomach. An organ of the alimentary canal; churns food to mix it with gastric juices, thus converting the food to chyme.

stool. A solid waste product of digestion; also known as *feces.*

story problems. Mathematical problems written in words.

STPD. An environmental condition wherein there is standard pressure (760-mm Hg), temperature (0°C), and dryness (0 mm Hg water vapor pressure).

structural formula. A formula wherein lines are used to represent pairs of shared electrons.

subacute disease. A disease that falls somewhere between a chronic disease and an acute disease in terms of severity and duration. *See* **chronic disease** *and* **acute disease.**

subarachnoid space (sub-ah-**RACK**-noyd). Brain area located between the arachnoid membrane and the pia mater and filled with cerebrospinal fluid.

subcutaneous facia (sub-kyou-**TAY**-nee-us **FASH**-ee-ah). The layer (*fascia*) of tissue found below (*sub*) the skin (*cutaneous*) and above the bones.

sublingual. Pertaining to the area under the tongue (*sub* meaning "below," *lingu/o* meaning "tongue").

substrate. The substance acted on by an enzyme.

sudoriferous glands (su-dor-**IF**-er-us). A fancy name for the sweat glands.

suffix. A word that follows a word root and alters the word root's meaning.

sulci (**SUL**-kye). Singular, *sulcus*; the normal grooves found on the cerebral cortex.

superior. Above or upper (*super/o*).

sympathetic nervous system (SNS). That portion of the autonomic nervous system that controls body function during times of stress.

synapse (**SIN**-apps).   The gap between either two neurons or between a neuron and a receptor site (*synapt/o* meaning "point of contact").

synovial fluid (sih-**NO**-vee-al).   A fluid produced in the body to lubricate the joints; makes joint movement smoother.

system (**SIS**-tem).   A specialized organization of tissues and organs that performs specific functions of the body.

systemic infection.   An infection that travels throughout the body via the bloodstream.

systole (**SIS**-toll-lee).   Portion of the cardiac cycle when the ventricles contract and blood pressure is, thus, at its highest point.

tachycardia (**tack**-ee-**KAR**-dee-ah).   An above-normal (*tachy* meaning "fast") heart (*cardia*) rate (usually more than 100 beats per minute).

tachypnea (tah-**KIP**-nee-ah).   An above-normal (*tachy* meaning "fast") breathing (*pnea* meaning "breath") rate (usually more than 20 breaths per minute).

tactile corpuscles (**TACK**-tile).   Tiny, elongated bodies found in certain nerve endings that give us impulses of pressure and touch; also known as *Meissner's corpuscles*.

taste buds.   Sensory end organs located in the mouth (and not just on the tongue); provide the sensation of taste.

temperature.   A measure of the average kinetic energy of the molecules of a substance.

temporal lobe.   That portion of the brain that regulates the senses of hearing and smell.

tendinitis (**ten**-dih-**NIGH**-tis).   Inflammation of (*itis*) a tendon.

tendon (**TEN**-don).   A tough, fibrous band of tissue that connects muscles to bone.

terms.   Parts of an algebraic expression connected by addition and subtraction symbols.

testes (**TESS**-teez).   Two small, oval glands found in the male; manufacture sperm and produce the hormone testosterone; also known as the *testicles*.

testicles.   *See* **testes.**

testosterone.   Primary male sex hormone that is secreted by the testes and stimulates sexual characteristics.

tetany (**TET**-ah-nee).   A condition characterized by muscle twitching, cramps, and convulsions.

thalamus (**THAL**-ah-mus).   Brain area located below the cerebrum and capable of either magnifying or suppressing sensory input.

thermal energy.   The combination of potential and kinetic energy that results from the random motion of particles.   "Thermal" can also be the answer to the question "where is the mall?"

thermometer.   A device that measures temperature.

thoracic (tho-**RASS**-ick).   Pertaining to the rib cage and area of the body known as the thorax.

thrombocytes (**THROM**-boh-sites).   The smallest of the formed elements of the blood; needed for proper blood clotting; also known as *platelets*.

thymus gland (**THIGH**-mus).   Gland located behind the sternum; secretes thymosin, which stimulates the production of antibodies, and decreases in size as the body ages.

thyroid gland (**THIGH**-roid).   The butterfly-shaped gland located on either side of the larynx; secretes hormones that regulate metabolism, influences mental and physical development, and maintains proper calcium levels in the body.

thyroid-stimulating hormone (TSH).   A hormone secreted by the pituitary gland; stimulates the thyroid gland to grow and secrete.

thyroxine.   A hormone secreted by the thyroid gland; regulates the body's metabolism rate and influences mental and physical development.

tinnitus (tin-**EYE**-tus).   A ringing sound in the ears; causes are many.

tissue (**TISH**-you).   A group of similar, specialized cells that perform a special function or functions.

tonsils (**TON**-sillz).   Masses of lymphatic tissue located in the throat (*palatine tonsils*) and the back of the tongue (*lingual tonsils*).

tonus (**TOH**-nus).   The normal state of partial muscle contraction experienced in the awake state (*ton/o* meaning "tone" or "tension").

trachea (**TRAY**-kee-ah).   The structure that extends from the neck and into the chest, right in front of the esophagus; commonly called the *windpipe*.

transdermal.   Route of drug administration via patches on the skin.

transverse plane (trans-**VERSE**).   An imaginary plane that divides the body into a top section and a bottom section.

T-score.   A measure of bone density. A score of more than 2.5 indicates osteoporosis.

tuberculosis (too-**ber**-kew-**LOH**-sis).   A disease that is caused by a bacteria and affects areas of the body having high levels of oxygen; a newer strain is considered deadly.

turbinates. *See* **conchae.**

tympanic cavity (tim-**PAN**-ick). *See* **middle ear.**

tympanic membrane (tim-**PAN**-ick). *See* **eardrum.**

type I diabetes. An often difficult-to-manage disease that usually develops before the age of 25 and is caused by an absolute deficiency of insulin; also known as *juvenile diabetes* or *insulin-dependent diabetes.*

type II diabetes. A condition that normally occurs in adults, results from the body's inability to produce sufficient amounts of insulin, and is treated by way of dietary changes, oral medication, or supplemental insulin; also known as *non-insulin-dependent diabetes* or *maturity-onset diabetes.*

ultraviolet waves (UV). Electromagnetic waves found in the invisible portion of the light spectrum; responsible for suntans, premature aging of the skin, and cataracts. (Elvis Presley owned a pink Cataract— or was that a Cadillac? By the way, some people claim that Elvis is still in the visible light spectrum.)

units. The descriptive word, or words, attached to numbers to give further meaning.

unsaturated fatty acid. A fatty acid having one or more carbon-to-carbon double bonds.

upper respiratory infection (URI). General term used to describe any infectious condition involving the nasal passages, pharynx, or bronchi.

urea (you-**REE**-ah). The major by-product of the body's metabolism of protein; found in the urine, blood, and lymph.

ureter (you-**REE**-ter). Two narrow tubes that carry urine from the kidneys to the urinary bladder.

urethra (you-**REE**-thrah). A tube extending from the urinary bladder to the outside of the body.

urinary bladder. Structure that stores urine until urination occurs.

urine (**YOU**-rine). The opposite of "you're out," or the fluid excreted by the kidneys; contains water and waste products of the body.

urticaria (hives) (er-tih-**KAY**-ree-uh). Localized regions of swellings that itch.

uterus (**YOU**-ter-us). The female organ wherein the fetus is contained and nourished until born; also called the *womb.*

uvula (**YOU**-view-lah). The little, punching-bag-shaped structure that hangs from the soft palate; aids in sound production.

vagina (vah-**JYE**-nah). A muscular tube found in the female and extending from the cervix of the uterus outside the body.

variables. Letters used to represent numbers in an algebraic expression.

vascularization (vas-ku-lair-i-**ZAY**-shun). The formation of blood vessels (*vascul/o*) in the tissues of the body.

vas deferens (vas-**DEF**-er-enz). A duct, or passageway, found in the male; carries sperm from the testes, to the pelvic region, and down to the urethra.

vasoconstriction (vase-oh-**CON**-strict-shun). Constriction of (*constrictus* meaning "bound") the blood vessels (*vaso*).

vasodilation (vase-oh-dye-**LAY**-shun). An increase in (*dilation* meaning "enlargement") the caliber of the blood vessels (*vaso*).

vasodilator. A chemical that dilates arteries or veins.

vasopressin (**VAY**-zoh-press-in). *See* **antidiuretic hormone (ADH).**

vegetative organisms. Organisms that are actively growing.

veins. Blood vessels that carry blood to the heart; the venous system uses lower pressures than does the arterial system.

venous system (**VEE**-nus). The portion of the circulatory system (*ven/o* meaning "vein") that brings blood back to the heart; usually carries deoxygenated blood.

ventilation. The movement of air in and out of the lungs.

ventral (**VEN**-tral). Pertaining to the front (*ventr/o*).

ventral root. That portion of the spinal nerves that deals with the voluntary and involuntary muscles and glands.

ventricles (**VEN**-trih-kuhlz). The two large pumping chambers of the heart.

venules (**VEN**-youls). The small veins that collect blood from the capillaries and combine to form larger blood vessels called *veins.*

vertebral (**VER**-teh-brall). The bones of the spinal column.

vertigo (**VER**-tih-go). A sense of whirling, dizziness, and loss of balance resulting from a condition involving the inner ear. Also a good Alfred Hitchcock movie.

vestibule chamber (**VES**-tih-byule). Area of the inner ear, located behind the cochlea and in front of the semicircular canals.

villi (**VILL**-eye).   The tiny, hair-like or finger-like projections found in the lining of the small intestine (*vill/i* meaning "tuft of hair"); absorb nutrients into the bloodstream.

virology.   The study of viruses.

virulence.   The increased ability for an organism to produce infection.

visceral muscle (**VIS**-er-al).   Special muscle that composes the internal organs and blood vessels and allows for movement.   Movement of visceral muscle is relatively slow and not consciously controlled.

vital signs.   The traditional measurable indicators of life, including heart rate, body temperature, breathing rate, and blood pressure.

vitreous humor (**VIT**-ree-us).   A soft, jelly-like substance found in the area behind the lens of the eye (*vitre/o* meaning "glassy," *humor* meaning "clear body liquid").

voiding.   Urination; also known as *micturition*.

V/V solution.   A mixture wherein both the solute and the solvent are measured by volume to obtain the desired solution.

water vapor.   Substance composed of water molecules so small that they act like a gas and thus exert a pressure like a gas.

wavelength.   The distance between two corresponding points on two successive waves.

wave motion.   A disturbance that travels through a substance (as in "the wave" performed at sporting events, when done properly).

white matter.   The myelinated nerves, which have white-colored sheaths of myelin around their fibers.

whole numbers.   {0, 1, 2, 3, ...}

womb.   *See* **uterus.**

word root.   The stem or foundation of a medical term; usually derived from the Greek or Latin language.

work.   The end result of the combination of force and distance.

W/V solution.   A mixture wherein the solute is measured by weight and the solvent is measured by volume to obtain the desired solution.

X-ray.   A high-energy electromagnetic wave having a very short wavelength; able to penetrate the body and produce a one-dimensional image on film.

zygote (**ZYE**-goht).   The fertilized egg.

zymogen.   The inactive form of an enzyme.

INDEX

CD ROM WITH
BOOK

DISCARD

DATE DUE	RETURNED